Dictionary of
Nutraceuticals and Functional Foods

FUNCTIONAL FOODS AND NUTRACEUTICALS SERIES

Series Editor
G. Mazza, Ph.D.

Senior Research Scientist and Head
Food Research Program
Pacific Agri-Food Research Centre
Agriculture and Agri-Food Canada
Summerland, British Columbia

**Functional Foods: Biochemical and Processing Aspects
Volume 1**
Edited by G. Mazza, Ph.D.

Herbs, Botanicals, and Teas
Edited by G. Mazza, Ph.D. and B.D. Oomah, Ph.D.

**Functional Foods: Biochemical and Processing Aspects
Volume 2**
Edited by John Shi, Ph.D., G. Mazza, Ph.D., and Marc Le Maguer, Ph.D.

Methods of Analysis for Functional Foods and Nutraceuticals
Edited by W. Jeffrey Hurst, Ph.D.

Handbook of Functional Dairy Products
Edited by Collete Short and John O'Brien

Handbook of Fermented Functional Foods
Edited by Edward R. Farnworth, Ph.D.

Handbook of Functional Lipids
Edited by Casimir C. Akoh, Ph.D.

Dictionary of Nutraceuticals and Functional Foods
N. A. Michael Eskin, Ph.D. and Snait Tamir, Ph.D.

Dictionary of
Nutraceuticals and Functional Foods

N. A. Michael Eskin
Snait Tamir

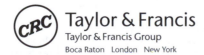

Taylor & Francis
Taylor & Francis Group
Boca Raton   London   New York

A CRC title, part of the Taylor & Francis imprint, a member of the
Taylor & Francis Group, the academic division of T&F Informa plc.

Published in 2006 by
CRC Press
Taylor & Francis Group
6000 Broken Sound Parkway NW, Suite 300
Boca Raton, FL 33487-2742

International Standard Book Number-10: 0-8493-1572-7 (Hardcover)
International Standard Book Number-13: 978-0-8493-1572-5 (Hardcover)
Library of Congress Card Number 2005050698

Library of Congress Cataloging-in-Publication Data

Eskin, N. A. M. (Neason Akivah Michael)
    Dictionary of nutraceuticals and functional foods / by N.A. Michael Eskin and Tamir Snait.
        p. cm. -- (Functional foods and nutraceuticals series ; no. 8)
    Includes bibliographical references.
    ISBN-13: 978-0-8493-1572-5 (acid-free paper)
    ISBN-10: 0-8493-1572-7 (acid-free paper)
    1. Functional foods--Dictionaries. 2. Dietary supplements--Dictionaries. I. Snait, Tamir. II. Title. III. Functional foods & nutraceuticals series ; no. 8.

QP144.F85E85 2005
613.2'03--dc22   2005050698

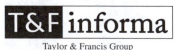

Taylor & Francis Group
is the Academic Division of T&F Informa plc.

Visit the Taylor & Francis Web site at
http://www.taylorandfrancis.com

and the CRC Press Web site at
http://www.crcpress.com

Dedication

This book is dedicated
to
a wonderful wife
Nella Eskin
and
a wonderful daughter
Orr Tamir

Preface

The current emphasis in preventative medicine encourages healthy lifestyles such as a balanced diet and exercise. In recent years a balanced diet has focused on ensuring functional foods are part of our diet. Functional foods are similar in appearance to conventional foods, but in addition to providing basic nutritional components, have physiological benefits that can reduce the risk of chronic diseases. The bioactive components responsible for the health benefits of functional foods are referred to as nutraceuticals. The past decade has witnessed a dramatic expansion in research activities worldwide to identify new functional foods and nutraceuticals. The latter will hopefully enhance the health and wellbeing of an aging population.

Research on functional foods and nutraceuticals is scattered throughout the scientific literature with only a very few journals devoted specifically to nutraceuticals. We have attempted to bring together, in a concise and informative manner, some of the literature published on 480 functional foods and nutraceuticals. This dictionary, which is more of a mini-encyclopedia, provides the reader with useful information on the nature of the bioactives in functional foods and their reported efficacy in cell cultures, animal studies, and, in some cases, human clinical trials. In addition to providing the structures of some of the bioactives or nutraceuticals, data showing their efficacy are also included. The information is presented alphabetically with some areas more extensively researched in the literature than others. We hope this book will prove a useful resource for researchers, teachers, as well as those working in the functional food and nutraceutical industry by providing reliable and accurate information based solely on peer-reviewed literature.

The authors acknowledge the professional help afforded by the staff of Taylor & Francis as well as the assistance of Marie Speare, reference librarian at the University of Manitoba. The authors are particularly appreciative of the support given by their respective families and academic institutions in preparing this unique volume.

N.A. Michael Eskin
S. Tamir

The Authors

Michael Eskin, PH.D., was born and educated in Birmingham, England. He completed his B.Sc. Hons. degree in biochemistry and Ph.D. in physiological chemistry at Birmingham University where he conducted research on toxicology focusing on mercapturic acid formation.

After teaching at the Borough Polytechnic (now Southbank University) in London, England for several years he joined the Department of Human Nutritional Sciences (formerly the Department of Foods and Nutrition) at the University of Manitoba in Winnipeg, Canada where he served a term as vice-chair and chair. He is currently an associate dean of the Faculty of Human Ecology

Professor Eskin holds several patents and has published 15 chapters and 100 scientific papers related to edible oils, methodology and mustard gum. He has authored and edited 8 books including *Biochemistry of Foods* which was translated into German, Japanese and Malay. He is currently working on a third edition of this book. Dr. Eskin also coedited *Methods to Assess the Stability of Oils and Fat-Containing Foods*, published by the American Oil Chemists' Society, and more recently *Food Shelf Life Stability*, published by CRC Press and translated into Portuguese.

Professor Eskin was the recipient of a number of awards including the 2001 W.J. Eva Award for outstanding contributions to research and service by the Canadian Institute of Food Science and Technology. He was recently honored by the Natural Sciences and Engineering Research Council of Canada (NSERC) for holding an NSERC grant for more than 25 years.

Dr. Eskin is a Fellow of the Canadian Institute of Food Science and Technology and the Institute of Food Science and Technology in the UK. In 2004, he was inducted a Fellow of the American Oil Chemists' Society at their Annual Meeting in Cincinnati for outstanding contributions to the society and to oilseed research. He is an associate editor of the *Journal of the American Oil Chemists' Society* as well as sits on the editorial boards of *Food Chemistry* (UK), *Journal of Food Lipids* (USA), *Indian Journal of Food Science and Technology* and served a term on the board of Food Hydrocolloids (USA). He also sits on the advisory board of *INFORM*, the technical publication of the American Oil Chemists' Society.

Snait Tamir, Ph.D., is professor of biochemistry and nutrition sciences, and head of the Department of Nutrition Sciences at Tel Hai Acadmeic College, Israel. In 1985 Dr. Tamir received her B.Sc. (cum laude), and in 1991 she received her Ph.D. (supervised by Prof. Yehudith Birk) in biochemistry and human nutrition from the Hebrew University of Jerusalem, Israel. In 1986 she completed her internship at Ichilov Medical Center in Tel Aviv, Israel and became a registered dietician. She conducted her postdoctoral study on "Nitric Oxide in DNA Damage and Repair" at the Division of Toxicology at the Massachusetts Institute of Technology, Cambridge, USA, with Professor Steven Tannenbaum, from 1992–1995.

In 1989, she studied, under the supervision of Professor T. Finlay, Medical Research Center, New York University, research techniques in breast cancer cells as part of a joint research project with Professor Yehudith Birk, the Hebrew University of Jerusalem.

In 1985 she was awarded The Dean's Scholarship at the Faculty of Agriculture Food and Environmental Sciences, The Hebrew University of Jerusalem. In 1987 she was awarded the Annual Distinction Award by the Women's Academic Association in Israel. She was also awarded the Rothschild Fellowship for the academic years 1992/3 by the Rothschild Foundation, Yad Hanadiv, Jerusalem, Israel, and the Guastella Fellowship for the academic years 1997/2000 by the Rashi Foundation, Jerusalem, Israel.

Dr. Tamir joined the academic staff at the Tel Hai Academic College in 1997 as a senior lecturer in the Department of Biotechnology and Environmental Sciences, in which she participated in the design, establishment, and management of the academic curriculum. Since 1999 she has served as head of the Nutrition Science Department and was head of the Biotechnology and Environmental Sciences Department in the years 2001–2002.

In 1999 Dr. Tamir joined the research group in the Laboratory of Natural Medicinal Compounds, Galilee Technological Center (MIGAL), which deals with the development of natural therapeutic compounds, mainly the isolation, characterization, and synthesis of new compounds, in collaboration with various leading academic institutes in Israel.

Dr. Tamir has published about 40 papers and book chapters. Her current research interest is the therapeutic actions of natural compounds such as phytoestrogens, antioxidants, whitening agents and psoriasis inhibitors. Based on the structure–activities relationship studies she aims to design the optimal anti-atherogenic compounds, hormone replacement agents, melanin biosynthesis inhibitors, and to develop new biological agents for psoriasis.

A

Acacia gum Acacia gums, or gum arabic, are Acacia-tree exudates that are highly branched galactan polymers with galactose or arabinose side chains terminated by rhamnose or glucuronic acid. It cannot be digested in the small intestine but behaves as a prebiotic by enhancing the growth of the probiotic bifidobacteria (Wyatt et al., 1986; Crociani et al., 1994). Michel and coworkers (1998) confirmed the similarity between two acacia gums and a prebiotic fructooligosaccharide with respect to their ability to decrease *Clostridium* sp. levels in human intestinal microbiota, as well as increase *Lactobacillus* sp. counts. However, the fructooligosaccharide preparation induced higher levels of *Lactobacillu* sp. The overall effect was attributed to increased production of short-chain fatty acids.

Hosobuchi et al. (1999) demonstrated the efficacy of supplementing diets with acacia gum, pectin, and guar gum for controlling hypercholesterolemia. A significant reduction was observed for both total and LDL cholesterol in 50 adults after four weeks on the supplemented diet.

Arabic gum was shown by Rehman et al. (2001) to scavenge nitric oxide. The decrease in the production of nitric oxide by arabic gum was later shown by Gamal el-adin et al. (2003) to protect against acetaminophen-induced hepatoxicity in mice. This reduction in oxidative stress (nitric-oxide production) was similar to the protection by arabic gum against gentamycin-induced nephrotoxicity reported previously by Al-Majed et al. (2002).

References

Al-Majed, A., Mostafa, A.M., Al-Rikabi, A.C., and Al-Shabanah, O.A., Protective effects of oral arabic gum administration in gentamycin-induced nephrotoxicity, *Pharmacol. Res.*, 47:4456–451, 2002.

Crociani, F., Alessandrini, A., Mucci, M.M., and Biavati, B., Degradation of complex carbohydrates by *Bifidobacterium* spp., *Int. J. Food Microbiol.*, 24:199–210, 1994.

Gamal el-adin, A.M., Mostafa, A.M., Al-Shabanah, O.A., Al-Bekairi, A.M., and Nagi, M.N., Protective effect of arabic gum against acetaminophen-induced hepatoxicity in mice, *Pharmacol. Res.*, 48:631–635, 2003.

Hosobuchi, C., Lapa Rutanassee, B.S., Bassin, S.L. and Wong, N.D., Efficacy of acacia, pectin, and guar gum-based fiber supplementation in the control of hypercholesterolemia, *Nutr. Res.* 19:643-649, 1999.

Michel, C., Kravtchenko, T.P., David, A., Gueneau, S., Kozlowski, F., and Cherbut, C., *In vitro* prebiotic effects of acacia gums onto the human intestinal microbiota depends on both botanical and environmental pH, *Anaerobe*, 4:257–266, 1998.

Rehman, K., Wingertzahn, M.A., Harper, R.G., and Wapnir, R.A., Proabsorptive action of gum arabic: Regulation of nitric oxide metabolism in basolateral potassium channel of the small intestine, *Gastroenterol. Nutr.*, 35:429–533, 2001.

Wyatt, G.M., Bayliss, C.E., and Holcroft, J.D., A change in human faecal flora in response to inclusion of gum arabic in the diet, *Br. J. Nutr.*, 55:261–266, 1986.

Acetyl-L-carnitine *see also* **Carnitine**
Acetyl-L-carnitine, an acetyl ester of carnitine, functions as a carrier of long-chain fatty acids into the mitochondria for β-oxidation. It also contributes to oxidative phosphorylation by the acetyl group forming acetyl-CoA, which enhances the supply of energy substrates to the Krebb's cycle (Dolezal and Tucek, 1981). During normal oxidative metabolism, the continuous production of reactive-oxygen metabolites (ROM) is extremely reactive, causing extensive mitochondrial DNA, cellular, and tissue damage over time. Such changes are associated with many chronic diseases, such as atherosclerosis, arthritis, autoimmune diseases, cancers, heart

disease, and cerebrovascular accidents, as well as aging. Seidman and coworkers (2000) examined the ability of two mitochondrial metabolites, including acetyl-L-carnitine, to enhance mitochondrial function and reverse age-related processes in experimental rats. Acetyl-L-carnitine was found to delay the decline in mito-

Acetyl-L-carnitine. (From Ilias et al., *Mitochondrion*. 4:163–168, 2004. With permission.)

chondrial function by reducing age-associated deterioration in auditory sensitivity and improving cochlear function. Kopke and colleagues (2002) also found that acetyl-L-carnitine reduced noise-induced hearing loss in animals due to cochlear injury from oxidative stress. Turpeinen et al. (2000) showed acetyl-L-carnitine prevented loss of myocardial sympathetic nervous function in patients with diabetes. Kaur and coworkers (2001) demonstrated new anti-aging effects of acetyl-L-carnitine by its ability to enhance glutathione *S*-transferase and multiple-unit activity and reduce lipid peroxidation and lipofuscin levels in the brain regions of aged rats. Biagiotti and Cavallini (2001) reported acetyl-L-carnitine was a far more effective and safer alternative to tamoxifen in the treatment of Peyronie's disease. A recent study by Mazzio et al. (2003) showed acetyl-L-carnitine prevented neurological damage in mouse brain neuroblastoma cells by 1-methyl-4-phenyl-1,2,3,6-tetrahydropyridine (MPTP+), a cogent Parkinson-causing agent. This beneficial effect may be due to its ability to sustain neuronal energy supplies in the absence of oxygen or when there is a malfunction of mitochondrial oxygen utilization, typical of Parkinson's disease. Recent studies by Loots et al. (2004) suggested acetyl-L-carnitine may prevent MPTP+ toxicity by denying cation access to the inner mitochondrial membrane, thereby attenuating its ability to produce radical-oxygen species via the electron-transport chain. These results suggest acetyl-L-carnitine may have

potential in the therapeutic treatment of Parkinson's disease.

Tomassini et al. (2003) found that acetyl-L-carnitine was well-tolerated as an alternative to the drug amantadine for the treatment of fatigue in multiple-sclerosis patients. A recent review by Ilias et al. (2004) pointed to the potential of acetyl-L-carnitine for treating complications associated with HIV infection and antiretroviral therapy. However, the data obtained so far were based on small, uncontrolled clinical trials and require further investigation.

References

Biagiotti, G. and Cavallini, G., Acetyl-L-carnitine vs tamoxifen in the oral treatment of Peyronie's disease: a preliminary report, *B.J.U. Int.*, 88(1):63–67, 2001.

Dolezal, V. and Tucek, S., Utilization of citrate, acetylcarnitine and carnitine palmityltransferase in the transport of fatty acyl groups across mitochondrial membranes, *J. Neurochem.*, 36:1323–1330, 1981.

Ilias, I., Manoli, I., Blackman, M.R., Gold, P.W., and Alesci, S., L-Carnitine and acetyl-L-carnitine in the treatment of complications associated with HIV infection and antiretroviral therapy, *Mitochondrion*. 4:163–168, 2004.

Kaur, J., Sharma, D., and Singh, R., Acetyl-L-carnitine enhances Na(+), K(+)-ATP-ase glutathione-*S*-transferase and multiple unit activity and reduces lipid peroxidation and lipofuscin concentration in aged rat brain regions, *Neurosci. Lett.*, 301:1–4, 2001.

Kopke, R.D., Coleman, J.K., Liu, J., Campbell, K.C., and Riffenburgh, R.H., Candidate's thesis: Enhancing intrinsic cochlear stress defenses to reduce noise-induced hearing loss, *Laryngoscope*, 112(9):1515–1532, 2002.

Loots, D.T., Mienie, L.J., Bergh, J.J., and Van der-Schyf, C.J., Acetyl-L-carnitine prevents total body hydroxyl free radical and uric acid production induced by 1-methyl-4-phenyl-1,2,3,6-tetrahydropyridine (MPTP) in the rat, *Life Sci.*, 75:1243–1253, 2004.

Mazzio, E., Yoon, K.J., and Soliman, K.F.A., Acetyl-L-carnitine protection against 1-methyl-4-phenylpyridinium toxicity in neuroblastoma cells, *Biochem. Pharmacol.*, 66:297–306, 2003.

Seidman, M.D., Khan, M.J., Bai, U., Shirwany, N., and Quirk, W.S., Biologic activity of mitochondrial metabolites on aging and age-related hearing loss, *Am. J. Otol.*, 21(2):161–167, 2000.

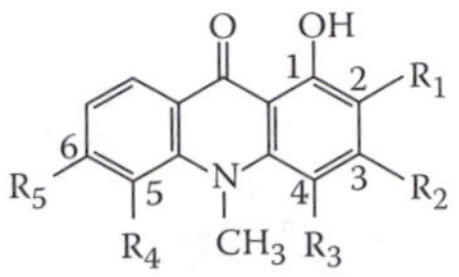

	R$_1$	R$_2$	R$_3$	R$_4$	R$_5$
1	H	OH	H	H	H
2	OCH$_3$	OCH$_3$	H	OH	H
3	H	OCH$_3$	H	OH	OCH$_3$
4	H	OCH$_3$	OCH$_3$	OH	H
5	H	OCH$_3$	OCH$_3$	OCH$_3$	OH
6	H	OH	prenyl	H	H
7	H	OCH$_3$	prenyl	H	H
8	geranyl	OH	H	OH	H
18	prenyl	OH	prenyl	H	H

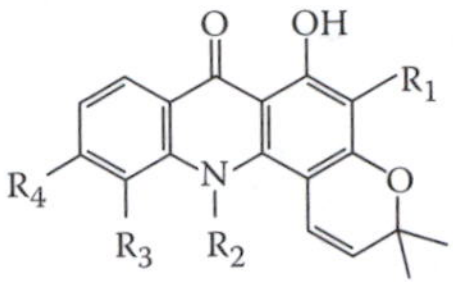

	R$_1$	R$_2$	R$_3$	R$_4$
9	H	H	H	H
10	H	CH$_3$	H	H
11	H	H	OCH$_3$	OH
12	prenyl	H	H	H
13	prenyl	H	OH	H
14	prenyl	CH$_3$	H	H
15	prenyl	CH$_3$	OH	H

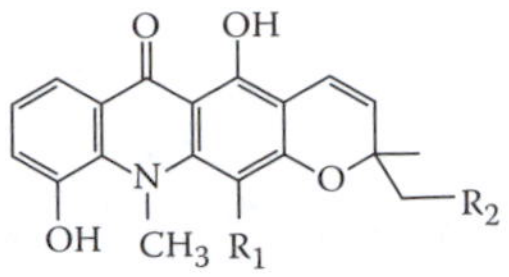

	R$_1$	R$_2$
16	OCH$_3$	H
17	H	prenyl

prenyl = ⟩⤻   geranyl = ⟩⤻⤻

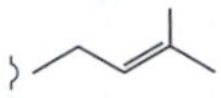

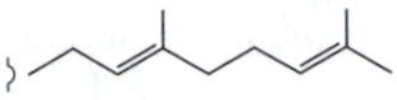

SCHEME A.1 Structures of acridone alkaloids tested for inhibition of TPA-induced EBV-EA activation. (From Itoigawa et al., *Cancer Lett.,* 193:133–138, 2003. With permission.)

Tomassini, V., Pozzilli, C., Onesti, E., Pasqualetti, P., Marinelli, F., Pisani, A., and Fieschi, C., Comparison of the effects of acetyl-L-carnitine and amantadine for the treatment of fatigue in multiple sclerosis: Results of a pilot, randomised, double-blind, crossover study, *J. Neurol. Sci.,* 218:103–108, 2004.

Turpeinen, A.K., Kuikka, J.T., Vanninen, E., Yang, J., and Uusitupa, M.I., Long-term effect of acetyl-L-carnitine on myocardial 1231-MIBG uptake in patients with diabetes, *Clin. Auton. Res.,* 10(1):13–16, 2000.

Acridone alkaloids Acridone alkaloids have been isolated from a number of plant sources, including citrus plants (family *Rutacea*). Some of them have been shown to exhibit cytotoxic, antiviral, and antimalarial properties (Kawaii et al., 1999; Yamamoto et al., 1989; Queener et al., 1991). A screening test showed that acridone alkaloids from citrus plants exhibited the most potent inhibition of 12-*O*-tetradecanoylphorbol-13-acetate (TPA)-induced Epstein–Barr virus early antigen (EBV-EA) activation (Takemura et al., 1995). Further studies by Itoigawa and coworkers (2003) isolated 17 acridone alkaloids from Rutaceous plants. Their structures are shown in Scheme A.1. Of these, the prenylated acridones were found to be the most potent cancer protective agents

when tested in a short-term, *in vitro* assay of 12-*O*-tetradecanoylphorbol-13-acetate (TPA)-induced Epstein–Barr virus early antigen (EBV-EA) activation in Raji cells. The prenylated acridone alkaloids included glycocitrin-II (6), *O*-methylglycocirine-II (7), severifoline (12), and ataphyllinine (13). The importance of the prenyl group was confirmed with the synthetic diprenylated acridone, 1,3-dihydroxy-10-methyl-2,4-diprenylacridone (18). Using an *in vivo*, two-stage mouse skin carcinogenesis model, it reduced the percentage of tumor-bearing mice to 73 percent after 10 weeks (Figure A.1), and the number of papillomas by approximately 48 percent after 20 weeks (Figure A.1B), compared to the nonprenylated acridones, 1,3-dihydroxy-10-methylacridone (1) and glycofilinine (5).

References

Itoigawa, M., Ito, C., Wu, T-S., Enjo, F., Tokuda, H., Nishino, H., and Furukawa, H., Cancer chemopreventive activity of acridone alkaloids on Epstein–Barr virus activation and two-stage mouse skin carcinogenesis, *Cancer Lett.,* 193:133–138, 2003.

Kawaii, S., Tomono, Y., Katase, E., Ogawa, K., Yano, M., Takemura, Y., Ju-ichi, M., Ito, C., and Furukawa H., The antiproliferative effect of acridone alkaloids on several cancer cell lines, *J. Nat. Prod.,* 62:587–589, 1999.

A

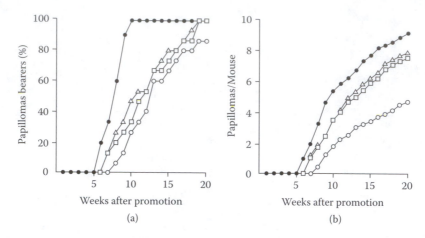

FIGURE A.1 Inhibitory effects of acridone alkaloids on DMBA-TPA mouse skin carcinogenesis. Tumor formation in all mice was initiated with DMBA (dimethylbenz[α]anthracene) (390 nmol) and promoted with TPA (1.7 nmol) twice weekly, starting one week after initiation. (a) Percentage of mice with papillomas. (b) Average number of papillomas per mouse: ●, control TPA alone; o, TPA + 85 nmol of 1,3-dihydroxy-10-methyl-2.4-diprenylacridone (18); Δ, TPA + 85 nmol of 1,3-dihydroxy-10-methylacridone (1); □, TPA + 85 nmol of glycofolinine (5). After 20 weeks of promotion, a difference in the number of papillomas per mouse between the groups treated with acridones and the control was evident ($p < 0.05$). (From Itoigawa et al., *Cancer Lett.*, 193:133–138, 2003. With permission.)

Queener, S.F., Fujioka, H., Nishiyama, Y., Furikawa, H., Bartlett, M.S., and Smith, J.W., *In vitro* activities of acridone alkaloids against *Pneumocystis carnii*, *Antimicrob. Agents. Chemother.*, 33:6–9, 1991.

Takemura, Y., Ju-Ichi, J., Ito, C., Furukawa, H., and Tokuda, H., Studies on the inhibitory effects of some acridone alkaloids on Epstein–Barr virus activation, *Planta Med.*, 61:366–368, 1995.

Yamamoto, N., Furukawa, H., Ito, Y., Yoshida, S., Maeno, K., and Nishiyama, Y., Anti-herpesvirus activity of citrusinine-1, a new acridone alkaloid, and related compounds, *Antiviral Res.*, 12:21–36, 1989.

Adlay   Adlay (*Coix lachryma-jobi* L.), a grass crop grown in China, is used as an herbal medicine and a food. A number of bioactive substances isolated from different parts of adlay were shown to exhibit anti-inflammatory, antitumor, and hypoglycemic activities. Early studies by Ukita and Tanimura (1961) and Tanimura (1961) showed the active component in adlay that inhibited the growth of Ehrlich ascites sarcoma was coixenolide. A number of benzoxazines isolated from adlay seeds were later found to have anti-inflammatory activity (Nagao et al., 1985). Chiang et al. (2000a)

showed dehulled adlay had a significant effect on the growth of intestinal bacteria in rats. Animals fed adlay had normal, healthy walls with no pathogenic signs. In addition, there were higher concentrations of short-chain fatty acids in the GI tracts. One of these, butyric acid, was shown to inhibit the growth of colonic tumors (Smith and German, 1995). Kuo and coworkers (2001) found that methanolic extracts of adlay hulls exhibited multiple antioxidant properties and induced apoptosis in human histolytic lymphoma monocytic cells. The antitumor properties of adlay were further demonstrated by Chiang et al. (2000b) by its inhibition of sarcoma-180 tumors in mice. A methanolic extract of adlay was subsequently shown by Chang et al. (2003) to be antiproliferative on A549 lung cancer cells in mice by inducing cell cycle arrest and apoptosis. Shih et al. (2004) recently found that a diet containing 20 percent dehulled adlay suppressed the early events in the development of cancer and not the formation of tumors in azoxymethane-induced colon carcinogenesis in rats.

Kuo and coworkers (2002) identified the antioxidants in a 1-butanol extract of adlay hulls exhibiting strong, radical-scavenging activity as coniferyl alcohol, syringic acid, ferulic acid,

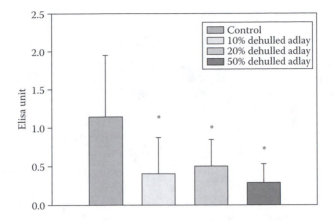

FIGURE A.2 Effects of different dosages of dehulled adlay on OVA-specific IgE levels in serum of mice consuming the test diets for six weeks and then intraperitoneally immunized with OVA plus alum. (From Hsu et al., *J. Agric. Food Chem.*, 51:3763–3769, 2003. With permission.)

syringaresinol, 4-ketopinoresinol, and a new lignan, mayuenolids. Hsu et al. (2003) showed that oral administration of several fractions obtained from dehulled adlay modulated Th1/Th2 cytokine production in cultured splenocytes obtained from ovalbumin (OVA)-immunized male BALB/c mice. This caused suppression of IgE biosynthesis (Figure A.2), which suggested it could be used to alleviate allergic symptoms.

A crude adlay-seed extract was shown by Kim and coworkers (2004) to exert hypolipidemic effects in obese rats maintained on a high-fat diet. The adlay extract modulated expression of both leptin and TNF-α, reducing body weight, food intake, fat size, adipose tissue mass, and serum hyperlipidemia. Adlay appears to have therapeutic potential for treating obesity.

References

Chang, H.-C., Huang, Y.-C., and Hung, W.-C., Antiproliferative and chemopreventive effects of adlay seed on lung cancer *in vitro* and *in vivo*, *J. Agric. Food Chem.*, 51:3656–3660, 2003.

Chiang, W., Cheng, C., Chiang, M., and Chung, K.-T., Effects of dehulled adlay on the culture count of some microbiota and their metabolism in the gastrointestinal tract of rats, *J. Agric. Food Chem.*, 48:829–832, 2000a.

Chiang, W., Shyu, M.-L., Su, J.-P., and Pangm V.F., Evaluation of the accessory anti-tumor effect of adlay processing food, *J. Health Sci.*, 2:113–122, 2000b.

Hsu, H.-Y., Lin, B.-F., Lin, J.-Y., Kuo, C.C., and Chiang, W., Suppression of allergic reactions by dehulled adlay in association with the balance of Th1/Th2 cell responses, *J. Agric. Food Chem.*, 51:3763–3769, 2003.

Kim, S.O., Yun, S.-J., Jung, B., Lee, E.H., Hahm, D.-Y., Shim, I., and Lee, H.-J. Hypolipidemic effects of crude extract of adlay seed (*Coix lachrymajobi* var: mayuen) in obesity rat fed high fat diet: Relation of TNF-α and leptin mRNA expressions and serum lipid levels, *Life Sci.*, 75:1391–1404, 2004.

Kuo, C.-C., Shih, M.-C., Kuo, Y.-H., and Chiang, W., Antagonism of free-radical-induced damage of adlay seed and its antiproliferative effect in human histolytic lymphoma U937 monocytic cells, *J. Agric. Food Chem.*, 49:1564–1570, 2001.

Kuo, C.-C., Chiang, W., Liu, G.-P., Chien, Y.-L., Chang, J.-Y., Lee, C.K., Lo, J.M., Huang, S.L., Shih, M.C., and Kuo, Y.H., 2,2′-Diphenyl-1-picrylhydrazyl radical-scavenging active components from Adlay (*Coix lachryma-jobi* L. var. *ma-yuen Stapf*) hulls, *J. Agric. Food Chem.*, 50:5850–5855, 2002.

Nagao, T., Otsuka, H., Kohda, H., Sato, T., and Yamasaki, K., Benzoxazinone from *Coix lachryma-jobi* var. *ma-yuen*, *Phytochemistry*, 24:2959–2962, 1985.

Shih, C.-K., Chiang, W., and Kua, M.-L., Effects of adlay on azoxymethane-induced colon carcinogenesis in rats, *Food Chem. Toxicol.*, 42:1339–1347, 2004.

Smith, M.L. and German, J.B., Molecular and genetic effects of dietary derived butyric acid, *Food Technol.*, 49:87–90, 1995.

Tanimura, A., Studies on the antitumor components in the seeds of *Coix lachryma-jobi* L. var. *ma-yuen*. Stapf. II. The structure of coixenolide, *Chem. Pharm. Bull.,* 9:47–53, 1961.

Ukita, T. and Tanimura, A., Studies on the antitumor components in the seeds of *Coix lachryma-jobi* L. var. *ma-yuen* (Roman.) Stapf. I. Isolation and antitumor activity of coixenolide, *Chem. Pharm. Bull.,* 9:43–46, 1961.

Adzuki beans   Adzuki beans (*Vigna angularis*), an important pulse crop in Asia, are particularly popular in Japan, China, and Korea. As a legume, its protein content and quality are high. A novel, antifungal peptide was recently isolated from adzuki beans by affinity chromatography and ion-exchange chromatography (Ye and Ng, 2002). The peptide, referred to as angularin, had a molecular weight of 8 kDa and was effective against fungal species, such as *Mycospharella arachidiocola* and *Botyris cinerea.*

Three triterpenoid saponins were isolated from the hypocotyls of adzuki beans by Iida et al. (1999). Related compounds are known to scavenge superoxide radicals, as well as exhibit antioxidant and chelating activities (Yoshiki et al., 1995, 1996, 1997).

References

Iida, T., Yoshiki, Y., Okubo, K., Ohrui, H., Kinjo, J., and Nohara, T., Triterpenoid saponins from *Vigna angularis, Phytochemistry,* 51:1055–1058, 1999.

Ye, X.Y. and Ng, T.B., Purification of angularin, a novel antifungal peptide from adzuki beans, *J. Peptide Sci.,* 8:101–106, 2002.

Yoshiki, Y., Kim, J.H., Okubo, K., Nagoya, L., Sakabe, T., and Tamura, N., A saponin in conjugated with 2,3-dihydro-2,5-dihydroxy-6-methyl-4H-pyran-2-ene from *Dolichos lablab, Phytochemistry,* 38:229–231, 1995.

Yoshiki,Y., Kinumi, M., Kahara, T., and Okubo, K., Chemiluminescence of soybean saponins in the presence of active oxygen species, *Plant Sci.,* 116:125–129, 1996.

Yoshiki, Y., Okuba, K., and Igarashi, K., In *Food Factors for Cancer Prevention,* H. Ogihashi, T. Osawa, J. Terao, S. Watanabe, and T. Yoshikawa, Eds., Tokyo, Spinger, Tokyo, 1997, p. 313.

Agrimony   Agrimony (*Agrimonia eupatoria*) is a valuable medicinal herb used mainly as a gastrointestinal tonic. It is characterized by long leaves with small, yellow flowers, one above the other in long spikes on a hairy, brown stalk, 2 to 3 feet high. A recent study by Gallagher and coworkers (2003) showed that compared to eight other plant sources, agrimony and avocado were the most effective in inhibiting the movement of glucose across a dialysis membrane. Previous research incorporating an aqueous extract of agrimony into the diet or drinking water of STZ-treated diabetic mice decreased weight loss, polydipsia, hyperphagia, and hyperglycemia (Swanston-Flatt et al., 1989; Gray and Flatt, 1998). This was accompanied by increased secretion of pancreatic insulin and insulin glucose uptake and metabolism *in vitro.* These studies suggest that the addition of agrimony as a dietary supplement could help to improve glycemic control in type 2 diabetic individuals.

References

Gallagher, A.M., Flatt, P.R., Duffy, G., and Abdel-Wahab, Y.H.A., The effects of traditional antidiabetic plants on *in vitro* glucose diffusion, *Nutr. Res.,* 23:413–424, 2003.

Gray, A.M. and Flatt, M., Actions of the traditional antidiabetic plant, *Agrimony eupatoria* (agrimony): effects on hyperglycaemia, cellular glucose metabolism and insulin secretion, *Br. J. Nutr.,* 80:109–114, 1998.

Swanston-Flatt, S.K., Day, C., Bailey, C.J., and Flatt, P.R., Evaluation of traditional plant treatments for diabetes: Studies in streptozocotin diabetic mice, *Acta Diabetol. Lat.,* 26:51–55, 1989.

Ajoene   Ajoene (*E,Z*)-4,5,9-trithiadodeca-1,6,11-triene 9 oxide), an organic trisulphur compound originally isolated from garlic, is formed from the spontaneous degradation of allicin.

$$CH_2{=}CHCH_2SSCH{=}CHCH_2S(O)CH_2CH{=}CH_2$$

Ajoene. (From MacDonald and Langler, *Biochem. Biophys. Res. Comm.,* 273:421–424, 2000. With permission.)

The possible pharmacological role of garlic in the prevention and treatment of cancers was attributed to the presence of ajoene. Rendu and coworkers (1989) reported ajoene was the antiplatelet compound in garlic responsible for inhibiting platelet aggregation. Later work by Apitz et al. (1992) showed the antiplatelet activity of ajoene prevented thrombus formation induced by vascular damage. Urbina and coworkers (1993) also found ajoene to be a potent antiplatelet compound capable of inhibiting both epimastogotes and amastigotes of *Trypanoso-ma cruiz*, the causative agent for Chaga's disease. Dirsch et al. (1998) reported ajoene-induced apoptosis in human promylelo-leukemic cells but not in periphereal mononuclear cells of healthy donors. The mechanism proposed was that ajoene stimulated peroxide formation in the leukemic cells and activated NF-κB. The antitumor properties of ajoene were demonstrated *in vivo* by Li et al. (2002ab, 2003), who showed it inhibited proliferation and induced apoptosis in several cancer-cell lines by activation of NF-κB and caspase-8. Hassan (2004) suggested that inhibition of proliferation and induction of apoptosis by ajoene was associated with blocking the G2/M phase of the cell cycle and activation of caspase-3 by ajoene, making it a new antileukemia agent for acute myeloid leukemia therapy (AML). Ajoene could be effective in elderly AML patients with poor tolerance to conventional chemotherapies. For example, Table A.1 shows the effect of ajoene with traditional drugs, cytarabine and fludarabine, on bcl-2 expression and caspase-3 activation in human-resistant myeloid leukemia cells. The most significant effect was activation of caspase-3, a prerequisite for apoptosis. A recent study by Ledezma et al. (2004) showed the cytotoxic effect of ajoene on murine melanoma B16F10 cells was also associated with activation of caspase-3 and subsequent apoptosis.

Using the water-maze test, Yamada et al. (2004) recently found that only Z-ajoene, and not alliin or diallyl disulfide, reduced acetylcholinesterase (AChE) activity in the brain of scopolamine-induced, memory-impaired mice. Excessive production of AChE leads to a deficiency of acetyl choline, resulting in a loss of memory and cognitive-impairment characteristic of Alzheimer's disease. Improvements observed following treatments with Z-ajoene suggest it could be used to treat this disease.

Gallwitz and coworkers (1999) also showed that the antiparasitic and cytostatic properties of ajoene were due to its effect on key enzymes involved in antioxidant thiol metabolism. Ajoene was previously found to inhibit HMG-CoA reductase, a key enzyme in cholesterol biosynthesis, as well as in the later steps of the mevalonate pathway in rat hepatocytes and HepG2 cells (Gebhardt et al., 1994). In addition to being a precursor of cholesterol, mevalonate is also a precursor of other nonsteroid isoprenoids (e.g., farnesyl and geranylgeranyl) that attach themselves to proteins and are crucial for cell proliferation (Grunler et al., 1994). Ferri and coworkers (2003) reported, for the first time, inhibition of protein prenylation and cell proliferation by ajoene in the smooth-muscle cells cultured from the aorta of Sprague–Dawley rats.

TABLE A.1
Bcl-2 Expression and Caspase-3 Activation in CD34 + CD7 + Human Resistant Myeloid Leukemia Cells Following Treatment with Cytarabine or Fludarabine in Presence or Absence of Ajoene

	Bcl-2 (U/million cells)			Activated caspase-3 (pg/million cells)		
	No ajoene	With ajoene	P	No ajoene	With ajoene	P
Control	227.7 ± 15.0	212.9 ± 14.	NS	51.4 ± 5.0	97.8 ± 9.0	NS
Cytarabine	24.8 ± 3.0	4.1 ± 0.3	< 0.001	210.5 ± 13.0	657.9 ± 11.0	< 0.001
Fludarabine	104.5 ± 12.0	70.3 ± 8.0	NS	183.7 ± 10.0	265.9 ± 16.0	NS

Source: From Hassan, *Leukemia Res.*, 28:667–671, 2004. With permission.

A

References

Apitz, C.R., Badimon, J.J., and Badimon, L., Effect of ajoene, the major antiplatelet compound from garlic, on platelet thrombus formation, *Thromb. Res.*, 68:142–145, 1992.

Dirsch, V.M., Gerbes, A.L., and Vollmar, A.M., Ajoene, a compound in garlic, induces apoptosis in human promyeloleukemic cells, accompanied by generation of reactive oxygen species and activation of nuclear factor κB, *Mol. Pharmacol.*, 53:402–407, 1998.

Ferri, N., Yokoyama, K., Sadilek, M., Paoletti, R., Apitz-Castro, R., Gelb, M.H., and Corsini, A., Ajoene, a garlic compound, inhibits protein prenylation and arterial smooth muscle cell proliferation, *Br. J. Pharmacol.*, 138:811–818, 2003.

Gallwitz, H., Bonse, S., Martinez-Cruz, A., Schlichting, I., Schumacher, K., and Krauth-Sigel, R.L., Ajoene is an inhibitor and subversive substrate of human glutathione reductase and *Trypanosoma cruzi* Trypanothione reductase: Crystallographic, kinetic, and spectroscopic studies, *J. Med. Chem.*, 42:364–372, 1999.

Gebhardt, R., Beck, H., and Wagner, K.G., Inhibition of cholesterol biosynthesis by allicin and ajoene in rat hepatocytes and HepG2 cells, *Biochem. Biophys. Acta*, 1213:57–62, 1994.

Grunler, J., Ericsson, J., and Dallner, G., Branch-point reactions in the biosythesis of cholesterol, dolichol, ubiquinone and prenylated proteins, *Biochem. Biophys. Acta*, 1212:259–277, 1994.

Hassan, H.T., Ajoene (natural garlic) compound: A new anti-leukemia agent for AML therapy, *Leukemia Res.*, 28:667–671, 2004.

Ledezma, E., Apitz-Castro, R., and Cardier, J., Apoptotic and anti-adhesion effect of ajoene, a garlic derived compound, on the murine melanoma B16F10 cells: possible role of caspase-3 and the $\alpha_4\beta_1$ integrin, *Cancer Lett.*, 206:35–41, 2004.

Li, M., Min, J.M., Cui, J.R., Zhang, L.H., Wang, K., and Valettle, A., Z-ajoene induces apoptosis in HL-60 cells: Involvement of bcl-2 cleavage, *Nutr. Cancer*, 42:241–247, 2002a

Li, M., Cui, J.R., Ye, Y., Min, J.M., Zhang, L.H., and Wang, K., Anti-tumor activity of z-ajoene, a natural compound purified from garlic: Antimitotic and microtubule-interaction properties, *Carcinogen*, 23:573–579, 2002b.

McDonald, J.A. and Langler, R.F., Structure-activity relationships for selected sulfur-rich antithrombotic compounds, *Biochem. Biophys. Res. Commun.*, 273:421–424, 2000.

Rendu, F., Daveloose, D., Debouzy, J.C., Bourdeau, N., Levy-Toledano, S., Jain, M.K., and Apitz-Castro, R., Ajoene, the antiplatelet compound derived from garlic, specifically inhibits platelet release reaction by affecting the plasma membrane internal microviscosity, *Biochem. Pharmacol.*, 38:1321–1328, 1989.

Urbina, J.A., Marchan, E., Lazardi, K., Visbal, G., Apitz, C.R., Gill, F., Aguirre, T., Piras, M.M., and Piras, R., Inhibition of phosphatidylcholine biosynthesis and cell proliferation in Trypanosoma cruzi by ajoene, an antiplatelet compound isolated from garlic, *Biochem. Pharmacol.*, 45:2381–2387, 1993.

Yamada, N., Hattori, A., Hayashi, T., Nishikawa, T., Fukuda, H., and Fujino, T., Improvement of scopolamine-induced memory impairment by Z-ajoene in the water maze in mice, *Pharmacol. Biochem. Behav.*, 78:787–791, 2004.

Alcohol *see also* **Ethanol** A considerable body of evidence associates moderate alcohol intake with a lower incidence of, and mortality from, coronary heart disease. Kannel and Ellison (1996) reviewed evidence of a protective effect due to alcohol raising HDL subfractions. A further discussion on the cardioprotective effects of alcohol by Gorinstein et al. (2002) suggested that, in addition to polyphenols, the antioxidant properties of ethanol can also prevent oxidation of LDL-cholesterol. This research further illustrates the importance of moderate alcohol consumption, as chronic alcohol consumption was shown to induce hepatic oxidation, leading to increased malondialdehyde levels in Wistar rats. Figure A.3 summarizes a study of 115 premenopausal, nonsmoking women conducted in four different regions in Europe. Bianchini et al. (2001) found an inverse correlation between alcohol consumption and 8-hydroxy-2′-deoxyguanosine (8-oxodGuo) lymphocyte levels (Figure A.3). The formation of 8-oxodGuo is a measure of oxidative damage to lymphocyte DNA. This unexpected finding pointed to the beneficial effects of moderate alcohol consumption. In a 12-year study of 38,077 males, Mukamal and coworkers (2003) confirmed the inverse relationship between alcohol consumption, at least three to

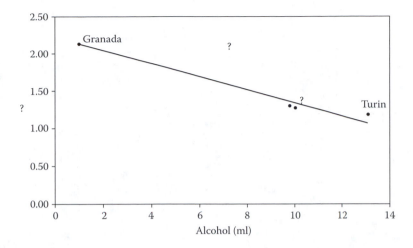

FIGURE A.3 Association between geometric mean 8-oxodGuo $\times 10^4$ levels and mean alcohol consumption among nonsmoking, premenopausal women between the four centers. (From Bianchi et al., *Carcinogenesis,* 22:885–890, 2001. With permission.)

four days a week, and the risk of coronary heart disease.

References

Bianchini, F., Jaeckel, A., Vineis, P., Martinez-Garcia, C., Elmstahl, S., van Kappel, A.-L., Boeing, H., Ohshima, H., Riboli, E., and Kaaks, R., Inverse correlation between alcohol and lymphocyte levels of 8-hydroxyguanosine in humans, *Carcinogenesis,* 22: 885–890, 2001.

Gorinstein, S., Caspi, A., Libman, I., and Trakhtenberg, S., Cardioprotective effect of alcohol consumption: Contemporary concepts, *Nutr. Res.,* 22:659–666, 2002.

Kannel, W.B. and Ellison, R.C., Alcohol and coronary heart disease: The evidence for a protective effect, *Clin. Chim. Acta,* 246:59–76, 1996.

Mukamal, K.J., Conigrave, K.M., Mittleman, M.A., Camargo, C.A., Jr., Stampfer, M.J., Willett, W.C., and Rimm, E.B., Roles of drinking pattern and type of alcohol consumed in coronary heart disease in men, *N. Eng. J. Med.,* 348:109–118, 2003.

Roig, R., Cascon, E., Arola, L., Blade, C., and Salvado, M.J., Effects of chronic wine and alcohol intake on glutathione and malondialdehyde levels in rats, *Nutr. Res.,* 20:1547–1555, 2000.

Alfalfa   Alfalfa (*Medicago satiova* L.) has been grown extensively as a livestock feed, while alfalfa sprouts are consumed as a garnish. It contains a large number of compounds, including saponins, flavonoids, tannins, coumestrol, carotenoids, and tocols. Flavonoids are known to have important health properties and include glycosides of apigenin, luteolin, and tricin (Packer et al., 1999). In addition to five known apigenin and luteolin glycosides and adenosine, Stochmal and coworkers (2001a) identified four new apigenin glycosides and a luteolin glycoside in alfalfa not reported previously. Further work by Stochmal et al. (2001b) characterized 10 flavone glycosides, including six tricin, one 3′-*O*-methyltricetin, and three chrysoeriol glycosides in the areial parts of alfalfa. Hwang et al. (2001) showed that pretreatment of soy and alfalfa extracts with acerola cherry extracts, a rich source of vitamin C, enhanced the antioxidant activity of soy and alfalfa extracts to inhibit LDL-oxidation (LDL⁻) (Figure A.4). The protective effect, only evident between alfalfa or soybean extracts and acerola cherry extracts, was attributed to synergistic interaction between its flavonoids and phytoestrogens with ascorbic acid in the cherry extract. In the case of alfalfa and acerola cherry extracts, this corresponded to 0.5 µM genistein and daidzein, 0.1 µM coumestrol and apigenin, and 102 µM ascorbic acid.

A

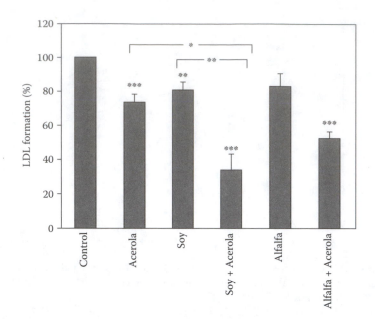

FIGURE A.4 LDL⁻ formation mediated by cells after addition of 100 µg/mL LDL protein. Cells were incubated under standard conditions (control) and preincubated with acerola, soy, soy and acerola, alfalfa, and alfalfa and acerola, extracts for five days, with male rabbit aortic endothelial cells. (From Hwang et al., *J. Agric. Food Chem.,* 49:308–314, 2001. With permission.)

References

Hwang, J., Hodis, H.N., and Sevanian, A., Soy and alfalfa phytoestrogen extracts become potent low-density lipoprotein antioxidants in the presence of acerola cherry extract, *J. Agric. Food Chem.,* 49:308–314, 2001.

Packer, L., Hiramatsu, M., and Yoshikawa, T., *Antioxidant Food Supplements in Human Health,* Academic Press, San Diego, 1999.

Stochmal, A., Piacente, S., Pizza, C., De Riccardis, F., Leitz, R., and Oleszek, W., Alfalfa (*Medicago sativa* L.) flavonoids. 1. Apigenin and luteolin glycosides from aerial parts, *J. Agric. Food Chem.,* 49:753–758, 2001a.

Stochmal, A., Simonet, S., Francisco, S., Macias, A., and Oleszek, W., Alfalfa (*Medicago sativa* L.) flavonoids. 2. Tricin and chrysoeriol glycosides from aerial parts, *J. Agric. Food Chem.,* 49:5310–5314, 2001b.

Allicin   Allicin (dially sulfonate) is one of the bioactive components of garlic (Rabinkov et al., 1994). It is formed in garlic by the action of the enzyme alliinase (alliin lyase, EC 4.4.1.4) on alliin [(+)*S*-2-propenyl L-cysteine *S*-oxide]

(Scheme A.2). Eilat and coworkers (1995) showed allicin altered the serum lipids in hyperlipidemic rabbits. Elkayam et al. (2001) found a synthetic preparation of allicin reduced blood pressure in fructose-induced hyperinsulenemic, hyperlipidemic, hypertensive rats from a maximum of 153.4 mm Hg to 139.7 mm after 2 weeks. Allicin acted similarly to enalapril with respect to blood pressure, insulin, and triglycerides, suggesting it as a potential alternative treatment of blood pressure. Kang et al. (2001) showed allicin had immunomodulating activity, especially on macrophages. Inflammatory murine peritoneal macrophages treated with increasing levels of allicin induced tumoricidal activity in a dose-dependent manner (Figure A.5). This was accompanied by corresponding increases in the production of the tumor necrosis factor (TNF-α) and nitric oxide.

Further research was recommended to establish the mode of this modulation and to what degree it occurs *in vivo.*

References

Eilat, S., Oestraqicher, Y., Rabinkov, A., Ohad, D., Mirelman, D., Battler, A., Eldar, M., and Vered, Z., Alteration of lipid profile in hyperlipidemic rabbits

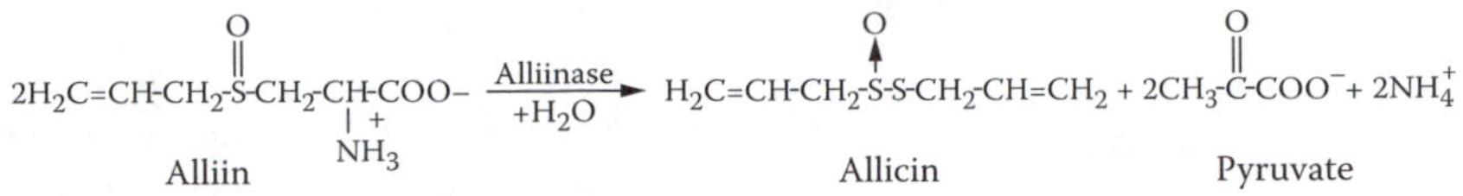

A

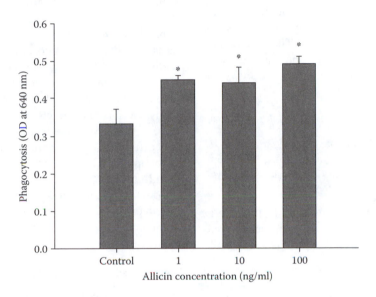

$$2H_2C=CH\text{-}CH_2\text{-}S\text{-}CH_2\text{-}CH\text{-}COO-\ \underset{+H_2O}{\xrightarrow{\text{Alliinase}}}\ H_2C=CH\text{-}CH_2\text{-}S\text{-}S\text{-}CH_2\text{-}CH=CH_2 + 2CH_3\text{-}C\text{-}COO^- + 2NH_4^+$$

Alliin   Allicin   Pyruvate

SCHEME A.2 Conversion of alliin to allicin by alliinase. (From Miron et al., *Anal. Biochem.,* 307:76–83, 2002. With permission.)

FIGURE A.5 Tumoricidal activities of allicin-treated murine peritoneal macrophages against a B16 melanoma-cell line. Results are the mean ± S.E.M. of quintuplicates. Differences were significantly different at $*p < 0.05$, and $**p < 0.01$ from the control (no treatment). (Kang et al., *Nutr. Res.,* 21:617–626, 2001. With permission.)

by allicin, an active constituent of garlic, *Coronary Artery Dis.,* 6:985–990, 1995.

Elkayam, E., Mirelman, D., Peleg, E., Wilchek, M., Miron, T., Rabinkov, A., Sadetzki, S., and Rosenthal, T., The effects of allicin and enalapril in fructose-induced hyperinsulinemic hyperlipidemic hypertensive rats, *Am. J. Hypertens.,* 14:377–381, 2001.

Kang, N.S., Moon, E.Y., Cho, C.G., and Pyo, S., Immunomodulating effect of garlic component, allicin, on murine peritoneal macrophages, *Nutr. Res.,* 21:617–626, 2001.

Miron, T., Shin, I., Feigenblat, G., Weiner, L., Mirelman, D., Wilchek, M., and Rabinkov, A., A spectrophotometric assay for allicin, alliin, and alliinase (alliin lyase) with a chromogenic thiol: reaction of 4-mercaptopyridine with thiosulfonates, *Anal. Biochem.,* 307:76–83, 2002.

Rabinkov, A., Xiao-zhu, Z., Graft, G., Galili, G., and Mirelman, D., Alliin lyase (alliinase) from garlic (*Allium sativum*): Biochemical characterization and cDNA cloning, *Appl. Biochem. Biotechnol.,* 48:149–171, 1994.

Allium fistulosum *Allium fistulosum* is a perennial herb grown around the world. However, most of the world's production is in China, Japan, and Korea. It is a member of the onion family and has been used in China to treat a wide range of diseases, including headache, abdominal pain, and diarrhea (Phay et al., 1999). Previous studies isolated a novel, antifungal compound in the roots of this herb, fistulosin.

Sang and coworkers (2002) isolated a new, unsaturated fatty-acid monoglyceride, glycerol mono-(E)-8,11,12-trihydroxy-9-octadecenoate, together with five compounds, tianshic acid, 4-(2-formyl-5-hydroxymethylpyrrol-1-yl) butyric

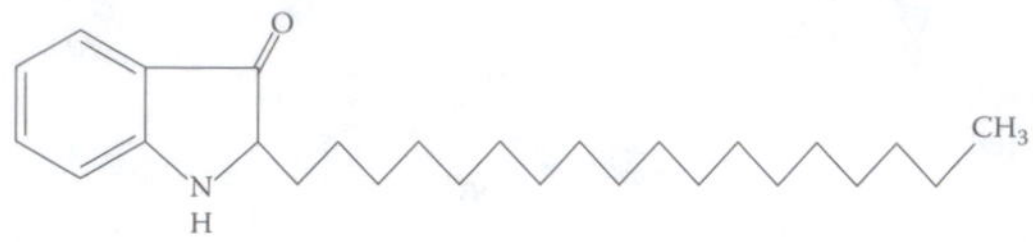

Fistulosin. (From Phay et al., *Phytochemistry*, 52:271– 274, 1999. With permission.)

acid, *p*-hydroxybenzoic acid, vanillic acid, and daucosterol. Some of these compounds are known to have bioactivity. The unsaturated fatty-acid monoglyceride and tianshic were both shown to inhibit the growth of *Phytophtohora capsici*.

References

Phay, N., Higashiyama, T., Tsuji, M., Matsuura, H., Fukushi, Y., Yokota, Y.A., and Tomita, F., An antifungal compound from roots of Welsh onion, *Phytochemistry*, 55:271–274, 1999.

Sang, S., Lao, A., Wang, L., Chin, C.-K., Rosen, R.T., and Ho, C.-T., Antifungal constituents from the seeds of *Allium fistulosum* L., *J. Agric. Food Chem.*, 50: 6318–6321, 2002.

Allium thiosulfinates *see also* **Methylmethane thiosulfinate**   The juice from onions and garlic both inhibited platelet aggregation in human blood *in vitro* (Bordia, 1978; Srivastava, 1984; Goldman et al., 1995). The compounds responsible were formed by alliinase action on *S*-alk(en)yl-L-cysteine sulfoxides producing sulfenic acid, ammonia, and pyruvate, with the sulfenic acid then forming thiosulfinates. For example, *S*-propenyl-L-cysteine sulfoxide, the main sulfoxide in garlic, is converted to 1-propylsulfenic acid (Scheme A.3), which oxidizes or cyclizes to form 1-propenyl-thiosulfinates (Block et al., 1992). Other sulfoxides in garlic and onion are also converted to thiosulfinates. Briggs and coworkers (2000) evaluated four

thiosulfinate inhibitors of platelet aggregation. These included methyl methane thiosulfinate, propyl propane-thiosulfinate, and 2-propenyl 2-propene-thiosulfinate (allicin), previously identified in freshly cut *Allium* vegetables, together with ethyl ethane-thiosulfinate, not previously identified. These researchers found propyl propane-thiosulfinate and alliicin, at 0.4 mM, strongly inhibited antiplatelet activity by 90 percent and 89 percent, respectively. In comparison, ethyl ethane thiosulfinate and methyl methane thiosulfinate at the same concentration were somewhat weaker, inhibiting antiplatelet activity by 79 percent and 24 percent, respectively. Because the effects of the thiosulfinates were not additive, these researchers pointed out the difficulty of predicting the antiplatelet potential of Allium extracts based on their quantitation. Nevertheless, the ethyl ethane thiosulfinate, methyl methane thiosulfinate, and allicin proved far more potent platelet inhibitors compared to an equivalent concentration of aspirins.

References

Block, E., Naganathan, S., Putman, D., and Zhao, S.H., *Allium* chemistry: HPLC analysis of thiosulfinates from onion, garlic, wild garlic (Ramsons), leek, scallion, shallot, elephant (great-headed) garlic, chive, and Chinese chive. Uniquely high allyl to methyl ratios in some garlic samples, *J. Agric. Food Chem.*, 40:2418–2430, 1992.

Bordia, A., Effect of garlic on human platelet aggregation *in vitro*, *Atherosclerosis*, 30:355–360, 1978.

Briggs, W.H., Xiao, H., Parkin, K.L., Shen, C., and Goldman, I.L., Differential inhibition of human platelet aggregation by selected *Allium* thiosulfinates, *J. Agric. Food Chem.*, 48:5731–5735, 2000.

Goldman, I.L., Schwartz, B.S., and Kopelberg, M., Variability in blood platelet activity of *Allium* (Alliaceae) species accessions, *Am. J. Bot.*, 82:827–832, 1995.

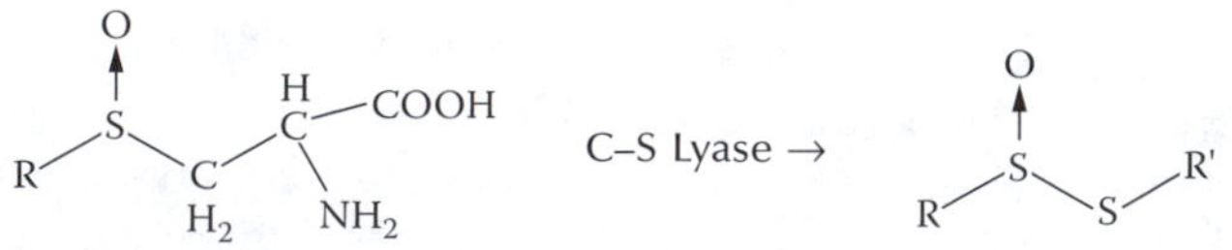

SCHEME A.3 Formation of thiosulfinate from *S*-propenyl-L-cysteine sulfoxide by cysteine sulfoxide lyase (C-S lyase) (where R and R′ = propenyl, CH_3-CH=CH-). (Adapted from Xiao and Parkin, *J. Agric. Food Chem.*, 50:2488–2493, 2002.)

Srivastava, K.C., Effects of aqueous extracts of onion, garlic, and ginger on platelet aggregation and metabolism of arachidonic acid in the blood vascular system: *in vitro* study. *Prostaglandins. Leukotrienes Med.*, 13:227–235, 1984.

Xiao, H. and Parkin, K.L., Antioxidant function of selected allium thiosulfinate and S-alky(en)yl-L-cysteine sulfoxides, *J. Agric. Food Chem.*, 50:2488–2493, 2002.

Allixin   Allixin (6-methyl-2-pentyl-4H-pyran-4-one) is one of the organosulfur compounds found in aged garlic extract. Kodera and coworkers (1989) identified this phenolic compound in garlic that had weak antimicrobial activity. Subsequent research by Nishino et al. (1990) showed allixin was an anticancer agent by inhibiting skin cancer in mice induced by 7,12-dimethylbenz[α]-anthracene (DMBA) and the promoter, 12-O-tetradecanoyl (TPA).

Allixin. (From Moriguchi et al., *Life Sci.*, 61:1413–1420, 1997. With permission.)

Allixin was also reported by Yamasaki et al. (1991) to inhibit aflatoxin B_1-induced mutagenesis in *Salmonella typhymurium,* as well as the formation of aflatoxin B10DNA adducts. Moriguchi and coworkers (1997) examined the effect of allixin and its analogues on the survival and morphology of primary cultured neurons from fetal-rat brain. Allixin (1–100 ng/mL) significantly promoted the survival of neurons, as well as increased the number of branching points per axon in the hippocampal region. At higher concentrations (> 1 microgram/mL), however, allixin was cytotoxic. Of the analogues examined, 2,6-dimethyl-3-hydroxy-4H-pyran-4-one (DHP) had potent neurotrophic activity at concentrations greater than 10 ng/mL without any cytotoxicity up to 10 microgram/mL. DHP was considered to be a useful prototype as a prophylactic drug for the treat-

ment of neurogenerative diseases. Allixin, a phytoalexin, is a stress compound produced by the plant when subjected to stress. Mahady and coworkers (2001) reported that allixin inhibited *Helicobacter pylori*. These researchers suggested reports that fresh garlic did not inhibit *H. pylori* growth were probably due to its absence of allixin, which is present only in stressed garlic.

References

Kodera, Y., Matsuura, H.m Susumu, Y., Toshihiko, S., Yoichi, I., Toru, F., and Hoyoku, N., Allixin, a stress compound from garlic, *Chem. Pharm. Bull.*, 37:1656–1658, 1989.

Mahady, G.B., Allixin, a phytoalexin from garlic, inhibits the growth of *Helicobacter pylori in vitro*, *Am. J. Gastroenterol.*, 96:3454–3455, 2001.

Moriguchi, T., Matsuura, H., Itakura, Y., Katsuki, H., Saito, H., and Nishiyama, N., Allixin, a phytoalexin produced by garlic, and its analogues as novel exogenous substances with neurotrophic activity, *Life Sci.*, 61:1413–1420, 1997.

Nishino, H., Nishino, A., Takayasu, J., Iwashima, A., Itakura, Y., Kodera, Y., Matsuura, H., and Fuwa, T., Antitumor-promoting activity of allixin, a stress compound produced by garlic, *Cancer J.*, 3:20–21, 1990.

Yamasaki, T., Teel, R.W., and Laum, B.H.S., Effect of allixin, a phytoalexin produced by garlic, on mutagenesid DNA-binding and metabolism of aflatoxin B_1, *Cancer Lett.*, 59:89–94, 1991.

S-Allyl-L-cysteine   S-Allyl-L-cysteine (SAC) is an organosulfur compound, which, together with allixin and its analogue, 2,6-dimethyl-3-hydroxy-4H-pyran-4-one (DHP), had antiaging,

S-Allyl-L-cysteine (SAC). (Adapted from Arnault et al., *J. Pharm. Biomed. Anal.*, 37:963–970, 2005.)

learning and memory improvement, neurotrophic effects, and antioxidant activity associated with aged garlic extract (Yamasaki et al.,

A

1994; Moriguchi et al., 1996, 1997; Nishiyama et al., 1997). Ito and coworkers (2003) showed SAC exerted a protective effect on amyloid β-protein-induced cell death in nerve growth, factor-differentiated PC 12 cells, a model of neuronal cells. Amyloid β-protein (Aβ), a 40-43 amino acid peptide, is involved with the formation of senile plaques in the brains of Alzheimer patients, as well as being cytotoxic to cultured neurons (Yao et al., 1999; Ekinci et al., 2000). SAC selectively protected neurons from Aβ-induced neurotoxicity. Kim and coworkers (2001) reported it was the antioxidant activity of garlic extract and SAC that differentially regulated nitric oxide in a murine macrophage by inhibiting iNOS expression and NF-κB activation while increasing nitric oxide in epithelial cells. This selectivity in regulation by garlic extract and SAC may contribute to their anti-inflammatory effect and ability to prevent atherosclerosis.

The ability of SAC to prevent gentamicin renal damage was attributed by Maldonado et al. (2003) to its antioxidant properties. SAC reduced oxidative stress through preservation of Mn-SOD, glutathione peroxidase, and glutathione reductase activities.

References

Arnault, I., Haffner, T., Siess, M.H., Vollmar, A., Kahane, R., and Auger, J., Analytical method for appreciation of garlic therapeutic potential for validation of a new formulation, *J. Pharm. Biomed. Anal.*, 37:963–970, 2005.

Ekinci, F.J., Linsley, M.D., and Shea, T.B., Beta-amyloid-induced calcium flux induces apoptosis in culture by oxidative stress rather than tau phosphorylation, *Brain Res. Mol. Brain Res.*, 76:389–395, 2000.

Ito, Y., Kosuge, Y., Sakikubo, T., Horie, K., Ishikawa, N., Obokata, N., Yokoyama, E., Yamashina, K., Yamamoto, M., Saito, H., Arakawa, M., and Ishige, K., Protective effect of *S*-ally-L-cysteine, a garlic compound, on amyloid β-protein-induced cell death in nerve growth factor-differentiated PC 12 cells, *Neurosci. Res.*, 46:119–125, 2003.

Kim, K.-K., Chun, S.-B., Koo, M.-S., Choi, W.-J., Kim, T.-W., Kwon, Y.-G., Chung, H.-T., Billiar, T.R., and Kim, Y.-M., Differential regulation of NO availability from macrophages and endothelial cells by the garlic component, S-ally cysteine, *Free Rad. Biol. Med.*, 30:747–756, 2001.

Maldonado, P.D., Barrera, D., Rivero, I., Mata, R., Medina-Campas, O.N., Hernandez-Pando, P., and Pedraza-Chaverri, J., Antioxidant S-allylcysteine prevents gentamicin-induced oxidative stress and renal damage, *Free Rad. Biol. Med.*, 35:317–324, 2003.

Moriguchi, T., Saito, H., and Nishiyama, N., Aged garlic extract prolongs longevity and improves spatial memory deficit in senescence accelerated mouse, *Biol. Pharm. Bull.*, 17:395–307, 1996.

Moriguchi, T., Saito, H., and Nishiyama, N., Trophic effects of aged garlic extract (AGE) and its fractions on primary cultured hippocampal neurons from fetal rat brain, *Phytother. Res.*, 10:472–486, 1997.

Nishiyama, N., Moriguchi, T., and Saito, H., Beneficial effects of aged garlic on learning and memory impairment in the senescence-accelerated mouse, *Exp. Gerontol.*, 32:149–160, 1997.

Yamasaki, T., Li, L., and Lau, B.H., Garlic compounds protect vascular endothelial cells from hydrogen peroxide-induced oxidative injury, *Phytother. Res.*, 8:408–412, 1994.

Yao, Z.X., Szweda, L.I., and Papadopoulus, V., Free radicals and lipid peroxidation do not mediate beta-amyloid-induced neuronal cell death, *Brain Res.*, 847:203–210, 1999.

Almonds (*Prunus amygdalus*)   Almonds, popular tree nuts worldwide, are used in snack foods and as ingredients in bakery and confectionery products. Fraser (1999) pointed out that substituting almonds or walnuts for traditional fats in the human diet reduced LDL cholesterol by 8–12 percent. Eating nuts is frequently associated with a substantial decrease in the risk of coronary heart disease of between 30–50 percent. In addition to their ability to reduce cholesterol, almonds have been reported to exhibit anticancer properties. Jenkins et al. (2002) compared whole almonds as a snack to low-saturated, whole-wheat muffins in a randomized, crossover study involving 27 men and women who consumed three isoenergetic supplements each for one month. The supplements contributed 22.2 percent of energy and were either full-dose almonds (73 ± 3 g/d), half-dose of

TABLE A.2
Effect of Almonds on Blood Lipids of Hyperlipidemic Subjects[1]

| | Control | | Almonds | | | |
| | | | Half-dose | | Full-dose | |
	Week 0	Treatment[2]	Week 0	Treatment[2]	Week 0	Treatment[2]
Cholesterol, mmol/L						
Total	6.45 ± 0.1	6.44 ± 0.15	6.47 ± 0.1	6.25 ± 0.15	6.60 ± 0.1	6.21 ± 0.15
LDL	4.34 ± 0.1	4.22 ± 0.13	4.30 ± 0.1	4.10 ± 0.12	4.45 ± 0.1	4.01 ± 0.12
HDL	1.43 ± 0.0	1.14 ± 0.08	1.38 ± 0.0	1.43 ± 0.08	1.40 ± 0.0	1.45 ± 0.09
Ratios						
Total:HDL Chol.	4.95 ± 0.2	4.89 ± 0.24	5.07 ± 0.2	4.68 ± 0.24	5.00 ± 0.2	4.58 ± 0.23
LDL:HDL Chol.	3.32 ± 0.0	3.23 ± 0.18	3.40 ± 0.2	3.11 ± 0.20	3.40 ± 0.18	2.99 ± 0.19
Cholesterol						
Oxidized LDL						
Conjugated dienes	64 ± 3	60 ± 2	65 ± 3	53 ± 3	62 ± 3	51 ± 2
Conjugated dienes/LDL	14.8 ± 0.6	14.3 ± 0.5	15.3 ± 0.8	13.4 ± 0.6	14.1 ± 0.6	12.9 ± 0.03

[1] Values are mean ± SEM. N = 27.

[2] Treatment values represent the mean of weeks 2 and 4.

Source: Adapted from Jenkins et al., *Circulation*, 106:1327–1332, 2002.

almonds plus half-dose muffin, or a full-dose muffin. Significant changes in serum lipids were observed for almonds, which are summarized in Table A.2. Both half- and full-dose almonds significantly reduced LDL cholesterol and LDL:HDL cholesterol, while only full-dose almonds significantly affected lipoprotein and oxidized LDL levels. A linear response to almonds was observed, which suggested that for each 7-g portion of almonds, there was a 1 percent reduction in LDL cholesterol. It was apparent from this study, together with epidemiological data, that the consumption of almonds may reduce the risk of coronary heart disease.

Davis and Iwahashi (2001) showed whole-almond consumption significantly reduced aberrant crypt foci compared to wheat bran and cellulose, suggesting a possible reduction in colon-cancer risk. Takeoka and coworkers (2000) identified three triterpenoids in the hulls of almonds, including betulinic, oleanolic, and ursolic acids. Sang and coworkers (2001) isolated a new, prenylated benzoic acid, together with catechin, protocatechuic, and ursolic acids, in almond hulls. Many of these triterpenoids have been shown previously to have anti-inflamma-

tory, anti-HIV, and anticancer activities, suggesting almond hulls are rich sources of these bioactive compounds. Pinelo et al. (2004) recently showed almond-hull extracts had almost 60 percent higher antioxidant capacity compared to pine sawdust, in spite of being much lower in phenolic compounds.

References

Davis, P.A. and Iwahashi, C.K., Whole almonds and almond fractions reduce aberrant crypt foci in a rat model of colon carcinogenesis, *Cancer Lett.,* 165: 27–33, 2001.

Fraser, G.E., Nut consumption, lipids, and risk of a coronary event, *Clin. Cardiol.,* 22(Suppl. 7):III, 11–5, 1999.

Jenkins, D.J.A., Kendall, C., Marchie, A., Parker, T., Connelly, P.W., Quian, W., Haight, J., Faulkner, D., Vidgen, E., Lapsley, K.G., and Spiller, G.A., Dose response of almonds on coronary heart disease risk factors: Blood lipids, oxidized low-density lipoproteins, lipoprotein (a), homocysteine, and pulmonary nitric oxide: A randomized, controlled, crossover trial, *Circulation*, 106:1327–1332, 2002.

Pinelo, M., Rubilar, M., Siniero, J., and Nunez, M.J., Extraction of antioxidant phenolics from almond hulls (*Prunus amygdalus*) and pine sawdust (*Pinus piaaster*), *Food Chem.,* 85:267–273, 2004.

A

Sang, S., Lapsley, K., Rosen, R.T., and Ho, C.-T., New prenylated benzoic acid and other constituents from almond hulls (*Prunus amygdalus* Batsch), *J. Agric. Food Chem.,* 50:607–609, 2001.

Takeoka, G., Dao, L., Teranishi, R., Wong, R., Flessa, S., Harden, L., and Edwards, R., Identification of three terpenoids in almond hulls, *J. Agric. Food Chem.,* 48:3437–3439, 2000.

Aloe vera   *Aloe vera*, a member of the *Liliaceae* family, is a tropical plant originating in the warm, dry climates of Africa. Of more than 360 *Aloe* species recognized, *Aloe barba-densis* Miller is the main commercial one used for its medicinal properties. Corsi and coworkers (1998) reported that *Aloe vera* had therapeutic potential by reducing the growth in pleural tumor-bearing rats. Shamaan et al. (1998) also found that vitamin C and *Aloe vera* both reduced the severity of chemical hepatocarcinogenesis in rats. An *Aloe vera* gel was found to contain small-molecular-weight immunomodulators, G1C2F1, capable of restoring ultraviolet B (UVB)-suppressed accessory-cell function of epidermal Langerhans cells (LC) *in vivo*. Lee and coworkers (1999) showed that topical application of G1C2F1 to the abdominal skin of mice reduced the suppression of contact sensitization exposed to UVB radiation. *Aloe vera* enhanced wound healing by increasing the levels of type III collagen in dermal wounds in rats (Chithra et al., 1998). Extracts of *Aloe vera* were found to exert anti-inflammatory activity by inhibiting cyclooxygenase (Vasquez et al., 1996). Avila and coworkers (1997), however, pointed out that *Aloe vera* gels contain cytotoxic, low-molecular-weight compounds, which must be removed or reduced in commercially prepared products. Pugh et al. (2001) identified a high-molecular-weight immunostimulatory polysaccharide from commercial *Aloe vera* juice, aloeride, containing glucose (37.2 percent), galactose (23.9 percent), mannose (19.5 percent), and arabinose (10.3 percent). While aloeride only accounted for 0.015 percent of the crude juice, it exhibited very potent immunostimulatory activity compared to the main carbohydrate component, acemannan. Aloeride as an immunostimulant could be beneficial for wound healing and immunotherapy.

A supercritical carbon dioxide extract from *Aloe vera* skin was shown by Hu et al. (2004) to be a superior antioxidant to BHT or α-tocopherol. A quality and safety (HACCP) management system was recently developed by He et al. (2005) for processing *Aloe vera* gel juice for the food industry.

References

Avila, H., Rivero, J., Herrera, F., and Fraile, G., Cytotoxicity of a low molecular weight fraction from Aloe vera (*Aloa barbadensis* Miller) gel, *Toxicon.,* 35: 1423–1430, 1997.

Chithra, P., Sajithial, G.B., and Chandrakasan, G., Influence of Aloe vera on collagen characteristics in healing dermal wounds made in rats, *Moll. Cell. Biochem.,* 181:71–76, 1998.

Corsi, M.M., Bertelli, A.A., Gaja, G., Fulgenzi, A., and Ferrero, M.E., The therapeutic potential of Aloe vera in tumor-bearing rats, *Int. J. Tissue React.,* 20: 115–118, 1998.

He, W., Changhong, L., Kojo, E., and Tian, Z., Quality and safety assurance in the processing of aloe vera gel juice, *Food Cont.,* 16:95–104, 2005.

Hu, Q., Hu, Y., and Xu, J., 2004. Free-radical scavenging activity of *Aloe vera* (*Aloe barbadensis* Miller) extracts by supercritical carbon dioxide extraction, *Food Chem.,* 2004 (in press).

Lee, C.K., Han, S.S., Kim, R.S., Chung, M.H., Park, Y.I., Lee, S.K., and Kim, Y.S., Prevention of ultraviolet radiation-induced suppression of sensory cell function of langerhans cells of *Aloe vera* gel components, *Immunopharmacology,* 37:153–162, 1997.

Pugh, N., Ross, S.A., ElSohly, M.A., and Pasco, D.S., Characterization of aloeride, a new high-molecular polysaccharide from *Aloe vera* with potent immunostimulatory activity, *J. Agric. Food Chem.,* 49:1030–1034, 2001.

Shamaan, A., Kader, K.A., Rahmat, A., and Ngah, W.Z.W., Vitamin C and aloe vera supplementation protects from chemical hepatocarcinogenesis in the rat, *Nutrition,* 14:846–852, 1998.

Vazquez, B., Avila, G., Segura, D., and Escalante, B., Anti-inflammatory activity of extracts from Aloe vera gel, *J. Ethnopharmacol.,* 55:69–75, 1996.

TABLE A.3
Total Cholesterol, LDL Cholesterol, HDL Cholesterol, and VLDL Cholesterol levels (mg/dL) of Hypercholesterolemic Rabbits

| | Diet | | | | | |
| Lipid parameters | Control | | Amaranth oil | | Extruded amaranth | |
	Day 1	Day 21	Day 1	Day 21	Day 1	Day 21
Total Cholesterol	201 ± 29.6	173 ± 38.8	219 ± 27.1	179 ± 27.6	196 ± 23.7	97.3 ± 20
LDL Cholesterol	159 ± 26.2	148 ± 36.6	183 ± 27.5	145 ± 26.7	162 ± 20.9	72.8 ± 20.8
HDL Cholesterol	34 ± 4.01	15.4 ± 1.75	28.3 ± 1.45	20.8 ± 4.10	31.3 ± 4.33	18.1 ± 1.37
VLDL Cholesterol	8.23 ± 1.06	9.63 ± 1.02	7.32 ± 1.27	4.08 ± 0.39	8.28 ± 1.94	4.52 ± 0.72

Source: Adapted from Plate and Areas, *Food Chem.,* 76:1–6, 2002.

Amaranth   Amaranth, a seed native to South America, has a protein content ranging from 14–18 percent and an excellent balance of amino acids. In addition, amaranth contains tocotrienols and squalene, both of which affect cholesterol biosynthesis. Chaturvedi and coworkers (1993) reported that amaranth seeds exerted a hypocholesterolemic effect in male Wistar albino rats compared to Bengal gram. Qureshi et al. (1996) found that serum total cholesterol and LDL cholesterol were 10–30 percent and 7–70 percent lower, respectively, in female chicks fed amaranth-containing diets. Grajeta et al. (1999) reported that the addition of sunflower oil augmented the hypolipidemic effect of amaranth. The hypocholesterolemic effect of extruded amaranth was reported by Plate and Areas (2002). A reduction in total cholesterol and LDL cholesterol occurred in hypercholesterolemic rabbits fed extruded amaranth for 21 days compared to the control and amaranth oil diets (Table A.3). VLDL levels were approximately 50 percent lower in rabbits fed either the extruded amaranth or amaranth oil diet compared to the control. Ethanolic extracts from two amaranth species were found by Klimczak and coworkers (2002) to exhibit strong antioxidant activity in a β-carotene-linoleic acid model system. Total phenolic content ranged from 39.17 to 56.22 mg/100 g for *Amaranthus cuadatus* and *Amaranthus paniculatus* seeds, respectively. Berger et al. (2003) showed a diet containing amaranth flakes (*Amaranthus cruentas*) decreased total cholesterol by 10 percent, but HDL and total cholesterol/HDL ratio remained unchanged. These researchers suggested that not all amaranth species have cholesterol-lowering properties, although they are still excellent sources of nutrients.

Tosi et al. (2001) obtained a high-fiber product from amaranth grain by differential milling. Using pneumatic classification, it was possible to obtain a high-fiber product that contained 63.9 percent insoluble fiber.

References

Berger, A., Monnard, I., Dionisi, F., Gumy, D., Hayes, K.C., and Lambelet, P., Cholesterol-lowering properties of amaranth flakes, crude and refined oils in hamsters, *Food Chem.,* 81:119–124, 2003.

Chaturvedi, A., Sarojini, G., and Devi, N.L., Hypocholesterolemic effect of amaranth seeds (*Amaranthus esculantus*), *Plant Foods Hum. Nutr.,* 44:63–70, 1993.

Grajeta, H., Effect of amaranth and oat bran on blood serum and liver lipids in rats depending on the kind of dietary fats, *Nahrung.,* 43:114–117, 1999.

Klimczak, I., Malecka, M., and Pacholek, B., Antioxidant activity of ethanolic extracts of amaranth seeds, *Nahrung,* 46:184–186, 2002.

Plate, Y.A.A. and Areas, J.A.G., Cholesterol-lowering effect of extruded amaranth (*Amaranthus caudatus* L.) in hypercholesterolemic rabbit, *Food Chem.,* 76:1–6, 2002.

Qureshi, A.A., Lehmann, J.W., and Peterson, D.M., Amaranth and its oil inhibit cholesterol biosynthesis in 6-week-old female chickens, *J. Nutr.,* 126:1972–1978, 1996.

Tosi, E.A., Lucero, E.R.H., and Masciarelli, R., Dietary fiber obtained from amaranth (*Amaranthus cruentus*) grain by differential milling, *Food Chem.*, 73:441–443, 2001.

Aminoethylcysteine ketimine Aminoethylcysteine ketimine is a natural, sulfur-containing, tricyclic member found in a variety of vegetables, including garlic, spinach, tomatoes, asparagus, aubergine, onion, pepper, and courgette (Macone et al., 2002). It is an antioxidant-protecting submitochondrial particle from lipid peroxidation (Pecci et al., 1995). The direct health benefits from aminoethylcysteine ketimine, however, remain to be determined.

Aminoethyl cysteine ketimine. (Adapted from Macone et al., *J. Agric. Food Chem.*, 50:2169–2172, 2002.)

References

Macone, A., Nardini, M., Antonucci, A., Maggio, A., and Matarese, R.M., Identification of aminoethylcysteine ketimine decarboxylated dimer, a natural antioxidant, in dietary vegetables, *J. Agric. Food Chem.*, 50:2169–2172, 2002.

Pecci, L., Fontana, M., Montefoschi, G., and Cavallini, D., Aminoethlcysteine ketimine decarboxylated dimer protects submitochondrial particles from lipid peroxidation at a concentration not inhibitory of electron transport, *Biochem. Biophys. Res. Commun.*, 205:264–268, 1994.

Angelica Angelica is a popular herb in North America, similar to the Chinese herb "Dong Quai." The most common use for angelica recommended by herbalists is as an "emmanagogic" agent to promote menstrual flow and regulate menstrual cycles. However, it contains compounds that are extremely carcinogenic to experimental animals. Fujioka et al. (1999) found a chloroform extract from the roots of *Angelica japonica* strongly inhibited human gastric adenocarcinoma. Several compounds, in addition to caffeic acid methyl ester, were identified, including a new furanocoumarin, named japoangelone, together with four furanocoumarin ethers and four polyacetylenic compounds. Furimi et al. (1998) found that a number of falcarindiol furanocoumarins exhibited antiproliferative activity using the MTT assay. Matsuda and coworkers (1998) previously showed that a methanolic extract from the roots of *Angelica furcijuga* protected the liver against injury induced by D-galactosamine (D-GaIN) and lipopolysaccharide (LPS). A comparison of the inhibitory activities of acetylated khellactones with coumarins found acyl groups were essential for potent activity. A polysaccharide, angelan, purified from the oriental herb *Angelica gigas* Nakai, was reported by Han et al. (1998) to stimulate immune function.

References

Fujioka, T., Furumi, K., Fujii, H., Okabe, H., Mihashi, K., Nakono, Y., Matsunaga, H., Katano, M., and Mori, M., Antproliferative constituents from umbelliferae plants. V. A new furanocoumarin and falcarindiol furanocoumarin ethers from the root of *Angelica japonica*, *Chem. Pharm. Bull. Tokyo*, 47: 96–100, 1999.

Furimi, K., Fujioka, T., Fujii, H., Okabe, H., Nakano, Y., Matsunaga, H., Katano, M., Mori, M., and Mihashi, K., Novel antiproliferative falcarindiol furanocoumarin ethers from the roots of *Angelica japonica*, *Bioorg. Med. Chem. Lett.*, 8:93–96, 1998.

Han, S.B., Kim, Y.H., Lee, C.W., Park, S.M., Lee, H.Y., Ahn, K.S.. Kim, I.H., and Kim, H.M., Characteristic immunostimulation by angelan isolated from *Angelica gigas* Nakai, *Immunopharmacology*, 40: 39–48, 1998.

Matsuda, H., Murakami, T., Kageura, T., Ninomiya, K., Toguchida, I., Nishida, N., and Yoshikawa, M., Hepatoprotective and nitric oxide production inhibitory activities of coumarin and polyacetylene constituents from the roots of *Angelina furcijuga*, *Bioorg. Med. Chem. Lett.*, 8:2191–2196, 1998.

Anise Anise (*Pimpinella anisum L.*), an annual herb with white flowers and small green-to-yellow seeds, is grown on a commercial scale in Southern Russia, Bulgaria, Malta, Spain,

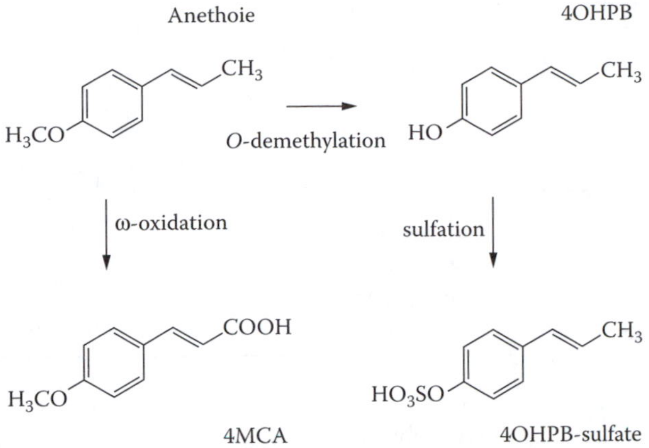

Anethoie 4OHPB

H_3CO — CH_3

O-demethylation HO — CH_3

ω-oxidation sulfation

H_3CO — COOH

4MCA

HO_3SO — CH_3

4OHPB-sulfate

SCHEME A.4 Proposed metabolism of anethole in rat hepatocytes. (From Nakagawa and Suzuki, *Biochem. Pharmacol.,* 66:63–73, 2003. With permission.)

Italy, North Africa, and Greece. It is grown for its fruits, commercially called seeds, which are used for flavoring. The fruit yields a syrupy, fragrant, volatile oil that accounts for 2.5–3.5 percent of the fruit. The major aromatic component in the oil is an alkylbenzene, anethole, which comprises around 90 percent of the oil. Anethole [1-methoxy-4-(1-propenyl) benzene] has been shown to exhibit both antimicrobial and antimutagenic activities (Rompelberg et al., 1993; Curtis et al., 1996). The *trans* isomer of anethole is the most abundant form, accounting for around 99 percent (Toth, 1967). Chainy et al. (2000) showed anethole suppressed TNF-induced lipid peroxidation and the generation of reactive oxygen (RO), which probably explains its ability to suppress inflammation and carcinogenesis. Elgayyar et al. (2001) found anise oil was highly inhibitory to molds. The total antioxidant activity of water and ethanol extracts obtained from anise seeds, using a linoleic-acid emulsion, was recently shown to be much stronger than α-tocopherol (Gulcin et al., 2003*)*. Nakagawa and Suzuki (2003) examined the metabolism of *trans*-anethole and its metabolites using freshly isolated rat hepatocytes and cultured MCF-7 human breast-cancer cells. Anethole was rapidly converted into at least three metabolites, 4-methoxycinnamic acid (4MCA), 4-hydroxy-1-propenylbenzene (4OHPB), and the monosulfate conjugate of 4OHPB, as shown in Scheme A.4.

The hydroxylated intermediate, 4OHPB, rather than the parent molecule appeared to be responsible for inducing cytotoxic effects in the liver and estrogenic-like effects in MCF-7 cells.

References

Chainy, G.B., Manna, S.K., Chaturvedi, M.M., and Aggarwal, B.B., Anethole blocks both early and late cellular responses transduced by tumor necrosis effect on NF-κB, AP-1, JNK, MAPK and apoptosis, *Oncogene*, 19:2943–2950, 2000.

Curtis, O.F., Shetty, K., Cassagnol, G., and Peleg, M., 1996. Comparison of the inhibitory and lethal effects of synthetic versions of plant metabolites (anethole, carvacrol, eugenol, and thymol) on a food spoilage yeast *(Debaromyces baromyces hansenii)*, *Food Biotechnol.,* 10:55–73, 1996.

Elgayyar, M., Draughton, F.A., Golden, D.A., and Mount, J.R., Antimicrobial activity of essential oils from plants against selected pathogenic and saprophytic microorganisms, *J. Food Prot.,* 64:1019–1024, 2001.

Gulcin, I., Oktay, M., Kirecci, E., and Kufrevioglu, O.I., Screening of antioxidant and antimicrobial activities of anise (*Pimpinella anisum* L.) seed extracts, *Food Chem.,* 83:371–382, 2003.

Nakagawa, Y. and Suzuki, T., Cytotoxic and xenoestrogenic effects via biotransformations of *trans*-anethole on isolated rat hepatocytes and cultured MCF-7 human breast cancer cells, *Biochem. Pharmacol.,* 66:63–73, 2003.

Rompelberg, C.J.M., Verhagen, H., and Van Bladeren, P.J., 1993. Effects of the naturally occurring alkylbenzenes eugenol and *trans*-anethole on drug metabolizing enzymes in the rat liver, *Food Chem.,* 31:637–645, 1993.

Toth, L., Untersuchungen uber das atherische Oil van *Foeniculum vulgare*, 1. Die Zusammensetzung des Frucht-und Wurselots, *Planta Med.*, 15:157–172, 1967.

Anka   Anka (or Red Mold Rice; Red rice), a fermented rice product with *Monascus* sp., is very popular in Asia. It has been used for more than 100 years in Chinese medicine to assist digestion and blood circulation. A number of secondary metabolites produced by *Monascus ruber* are mevilonin and lovastatin, monoacolins capable of inhibiting the rate-limiting enzyme in cholesterol synthesis, 3-hydroxy-3-methylglutaryl CoA reductase (Endo and Monoacotin, 1980). The hypocholesterolemic potential of these compounds was reported in mammalian species, including humans (Endo, 1985). Wang and coworkers (2000) fed a high-fructose (30 percent) diet containing dried Anka powder (2 percent) to experimental rats with hypertriglyceridemia. After six months, the levels of serum triacylglycerols, total cholesterol, VLDL-cholesterol, and LDL-cholesterol all decreased significantly, while HDL cholesterol increased significantly compared to the 30 percent fructose diet. This study showed Anka was capable of suppressing hypertriglyceridemia and hyperlipidemia in rats and has the potential to do the same for humans.

References

Endo, A. and Monoacolin, K., A new hypocholesterolemic agent that specifically inhibits 3-hydroxy-3-methylglutaryl coenzyme reductase A, *J. Antibiot.*, 33:334–336, 1980.

Endo, A., Compactin (MG236B) and related compounds as potential cholesterol lowering agents that inhibit HMG-CoA reductase, *J. Med. Chem.*, 28:401–405, 1985.

Wang, I.-K., Lin-Shiau, S.-Y., Chen, P.-C., and Lin, J.-K., Hypotriglyceridemic effect of Anka (a fermented rice product of *Monascus* sp.) in rats, *J. Agric. Food Chem.*, 48:3183–3189, 2000.

Anthocyanins   Anthocyanins are primarily responsible for the colors of fruits, fruit juices, wines, flowers, and vegetables. They are a subgroup within the flavonoids characterized by a

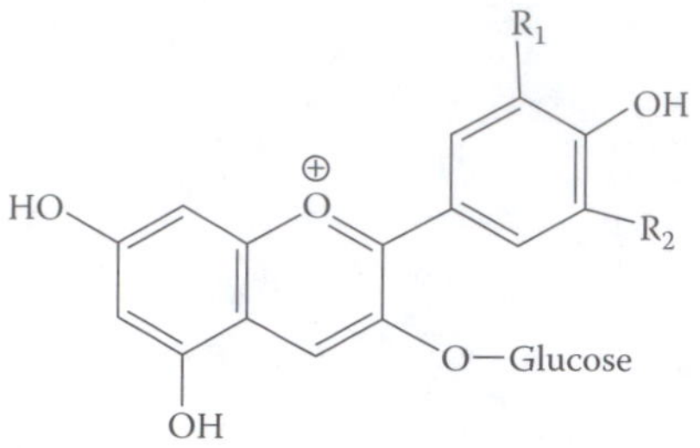

R_1	R_2	Anthocyanin
H	H	Pelargonidin-3-glucoside
OH	H	Cyanidin-3-glucoside
OH	OH	Delphinidin-3-glucoside
OCH_3	H	Peonidin-3-glucoside
OCH_3	OH	Petunidin-3-glucoside
OCH_3	OCH_3	Malvidin-3-glucoside

SCHEME A.5   Anthocyanin skeleton. (From Clifford, *J. Sci. Food Agric.*, 50:1063–1070, 2000. With permission.)

C-6-C-3-C-6 skeleton attached to a sugar (Scheme A.5). The six major anthocyanin aglycones or anthocyanidins are pelargonidin, cyanidin, delphinidin, peonidin, petunidin, and malvidin (Mazza and Miniati, 1993). These pigments have been reported to have a number of health benefits, particularly their antioxidant activity (Lapidot et al., 1999; Pratt, 1992; Wang et al., 1999). The low incidence of cardiovascular disease found in certain parts of France, known as the "French Paradox," was attributed to consumption of red wine, which contains substantial amounts of flavonoids, mostly anthocyanins, as high as 3200 mg/L (Lapidot et al., 1999). Seeram and Nair (2002) conducted the first study evaluating anthocyanidins, as well as several anthocyanins using a liposomal model system with antioxidant activities measured by their ability to inhibit the fluorescence intensity decay of an extrinsic probe, 3-[-(6-phenyl)-1,3,5-hexatrienyl]phenyl-proprionic acid, caused by free radicals generated during metal ion-induced peroxidation. Antioxidant activity increased with increasing number of hydroxyl groups on the B ring of the anthocyanidin, while methoxyl groups diminished the antioxidant activity. Anthocyanidins with a hydroxyl group at three position exhibited potent antioxidant activity. Substitution at position three

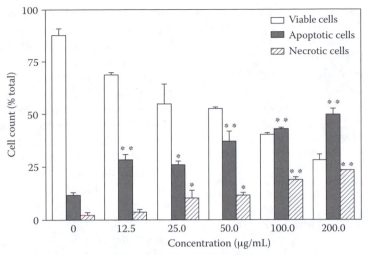

*p < 0.05, **p < 0.01 with respect to controls (Dunnet test)

FIGURE A.6 Fraction of viable, apoptotic, and necrotic cells, as detected in Jurkat cells treated with cyanidin-3-*O*-β-glucopyranoside at doses ranging from 12.5–200 μg/mL for 24 h. Cells were removed from treated and untreated cultures and stained with bannexin V flourecscein isothiocy-anate and propidium iodide. The presented is averaged from three independent experiments, with error bars denoting standard errors. (Fimognari et al., *Biochem. Pharmacol.,* 67:2047–2056, 2004. With permission.)

in the C ring also had a major effect on the antioxidant activity of anthocyanidins. Espin and coworkers (2000) found anthocyanin-based fruit extracts exhibited radical-scavenging capacity (RSC) using the 2,2-diphenyl-1-pic-ryl-hydrazyl radical (DPPH•). Of the fruits examined, black chokeberry and blackthorn were the most active, while strawberry and elderberry were the least active.

Lazze and coworkers (2004) examined the effects of two aglycone anthocyanins, delphini-din and cyanidin, on cell-cycle progression and induction of apoptosis in human uterine carci-noma and colon adenocarcinoma cells and in normal human fibroblasts. Over the concentra-tion range of 100–200 μM, cyanidin interfered with the cell cycle of normal cells, which con-trasted with delphinidin's inhibition of cell pro-liferation in both normal human fibroblasts and pro-apoptopic activity in cancer cells. The greater effect associated with delphinidin was attributed to the presence of three hydroxyl groups on the B ring, which may be important for biological activity.

Fimognari et al. (2004) showed that cyanidin-3-*O*-β-glucopyranoside, an anthocyanin found

in pigmented orange juice, induced apoptosis in two human leukemia cell lines, Jurkat T and HL-60 promyelocytic cells. For example, treat-ment of Jurkat cells with this anthocyanin, even at the lowest level tested (12.5 μg/mL), increased apoptotic cells (Figure A.6). The potential of cyanidin-3-*O*-β-glucopyranoside, as a chemo-preventive or chemotherapeutic agent, requires further study. To be effective, such compounds must be bioavailable; however, anthocyanins, like many other nutraceuticals, are very poorly absorbed. Netzel et al. (2001) reported that fol-lowing ingestion of 153 mg of anthocyanins by healthy volunteers, only 0.02 to 0.05 percent was detected in the urine. A review of the func-tional properties and health-related properties of anthocyanins was recently published by Stin-zing and Carle (2004).

References

Clifford, M.N., Anthocyanins — nature, occurrence and dietary burden, *J. Sci. Food Agric.,* 80:1063–1070, 2000.

Espin, J.C., Soler-Rivas, C., Wichers, H.J., and Garcia-Viguera, C., Anthocyanin-based natural colorants: A new source of antiradical activity in foodstuff, *J. Agric. Food Chem.,* 48:1588–1592, 2000.

A

Fimognari, C., Berti, F., Nusse, M., Cantelli-Forti, G., and Hrelia, P., Induction of apoptosis in two human leukemia cell lines as well as differentiation in human promyelocytic cells by cyanidin-3-O-β-glucopyranoside, *Biochem. Pharmacol.*, 67:2047–2056, 2004.

Lapidot, T., Harel, S., Granit, R., and Kanner, J., Bioavailability of red wine anthocyanins as detected in human urine, *J. Agric. Food Chem.*, 46:4297–4302, 1998.

Lazze, M.C., Savio, M., Pizzala, R., Cazzalini, O., Perucca, P., Scovassi, A.I., Stivala, L.A., and Bianchi, L., Anthocyanins induce cell cycle perturbations and apoptosis in different cell lines, *Carcinogenesis*, 25:1427–1433, 2004.

Mazza, G. and Miniati, E., *Anthocyanins in Fruits, Vegetables, and Grains*, CRC Press, Boca Raton, Florida, 1993.

Netzel, M., Strass, G., Janssen, M., Bitsch, I., and Bitsch, R., Bioactive anthocyanins detected in human urine after ingestion of blackcurrant juice, *J. Environ. Pathol. Toxicol. Oncol.*, 20:89–95, 2001.

Pratt, D.E., Natural antioxidants from plant materials, *ACS Symp. Ser.*, 507:54–71, 1992.

Seeram, N. and Nair, M.G., Inhibition of lipid peroxidation and structure-activity related studies of the dietary constituents anthocyanins, anthocyanidins, and catechins, *J. Agric. Food Chem.*, 50:5308–5312, 2002.

Stintzing, F.C. and Carle, R., Functional properties of anthocyanins and betalains in plants, food, and in human nutrition, *Trends Food Sci. Technol.*, 15:19–38, 2004.

Wang, H., Nair, H., Strasburg, G.M., Chang, Y.-C., Booren, A.M., Gray, J.I., and Dewitt, D.L., Antioxidant and anti-inflammatory activities of anthocyanins and their aglycone, cyanidin from tart cherries, *J. Nat. Prod.*, 62:294–296, 1999.

Antioxidants *see also* **Vitamins A, C, E, and K**   In addition to the natural antioxidant vitamins A, C, and E, there are a multitude of phenolic compounds that are responsible for the potent antioxidant properties of fruits, vegetables, and herbs. More than 200 epidemiological studies pointed to a strong association between the low consumption of fruits and vegetables and incidence of cancer (Willett and Trichopoulus, 1996). This association was attributed to the presence of antioxidants that protect cells from reactive-oxygen species that lead to DNA damage, mutation, and, ultimately, carcinogenesis (Boone et al., 1997). Thus, an increase in the consumption of some antioxidants can actually reduce oxidative damage and the development of some cancers. More recent data, however, suggests that reactive-oxygen species are used by cells in the signaling process that activates programmed cell death, or apoptosis, to eliminate cancer cells. Thus, inhibition of apoptosis by antioxidants may interfere with the elimination of precancerous or cancerous cells and actually promote cancers in individuals at risk for carcinogenic lesions. A review by Lopaczynski and Zeisel (2001) questioned whether cancer patients should be given dietary supplements containing much higher levels of antioxidants compared to a regular diet. This could explain why vitamin E and β-carotene enhanced lung cancer in heavy smokers, while protecting against prostate cancer (Heinonen et al., 1998). Further confirmation was provided by Wenzel et al. (2004) who showed that, while antioxidant vitamins, such as ascorbic acid, may play a role in cancer prevention, they could have different effects at different stages in the carcinogenic process. Using HT-29 human colon carcinoma cells, Wenzel and coworkers (2004) demonstrated the ability of ascorbic acid to interfere with apoptosis induced by the antitumor drug camptothecin or the flavonoid flavone. A significant increase in mitochondrial reactive-oxygen species (superoxide anion) by camptothecin and the flavone normally precedes down-regulation of bcl-X_L and apoptosis. This was prevented by the presence of 1 mM ascorbic acid, which reduced the amount of superoxide anion to that found in the control cells (Figure A.7). These results also raised concern regarding the high intake of antioxidant vitamins during chemotherapy.

References

Boone, C.W., Bacus, J.W., Bacus, J.V., Steele, V.E., and Kelloff, G.J., Properties of intraepithelial neoplasia relevant to the development of cancer chemopreventive agents, *J. Cell Biochem.*, 28–29:1–20, 1997.

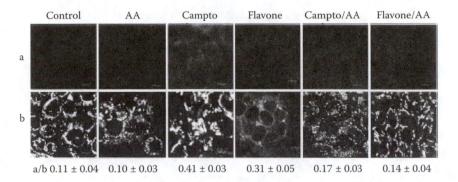

	Control	AA	Campto	Flavone	Campto/AA	Flavone/AA
a/b	0.11 ± 0.04	0.10 ± 0.03	0.41 ± 0.03	0.31 ± 0.05	0.17 ± 0.03	0.14 ± 0.04

FIGURE A.7 Ascorbic acid prevents the appearance of mitochondrial O_2. Cells were incubated with medium alone (control), or with 1 mM ascorbic acid (AA), or with 50 μM camptothecin (campto), or 150 μM flavone in the absence or presence of 1 mM ascorbic acid for 6 h. During the last period of incubation, cells were loaded with proxyfluorescamine for the detection of O_2 (a) in combination with MitoTracker for the visualization of mitochondria (b). The fluorescence ratios of a\over b were determined for the mitochondrial areas only. (Wenzel et al., *Carcinogenesis*, 25:703–712, 2004. With permission.)

Heinonen, O.P., Albanes, D., Virtano, J., Taylor, P.R., Huttunen, J.K., Harman, A.M., Hapakoski, J., Malila, N., Ratualahti, S., Maenpa, H., Teerenhovi, L., Koss, L., Virolainen, M., and Edwards, B.K., Prostate cancer and supplementation with alpha-tocopherol and beta-carotene: Incidence and mortality in a controlled trial, *J. Natl. Cancer Inst.,* 90:44–446, 1998.

Lopaczynski, W. and Zeisel, S.H., Antioxidants, programmed cell death, and cancer, *Nutr. Res.,* 21:295–307, 2001.

Wenzel, U., Nickel, A., Kuntz, S., and Daniel, H., Ascorbic acid suppresses drug-induced apoptosis in human colon cancer cells by scavenging mitochondrial superoxide anions, *Carcinogenesis,* 25:703–712, 2004.

Willett, W.C. and Trichopoulos, D., 1996. Nutrition and cancer: A summary of evidence, *Cancer Causes Control.,* 7:178–180, 1996.

Apigenin   Apigenin, a flavonoid compound, is the major constituent of the herb chamomile. It is a 4′,5,7-trihydroxyflavone, which appears to have a variety of medicinal uses, including the treatment of HIV, inflammatory-bowel disease, and skin conditions. It is also found in quite a number of other plant sources, including parsley, onions, tea, orange, wheat sprouts, and some seasonings (Birt et al., 1998; Duthie and Crozier, 2000). Chamomile flower is licensed in Germany as a medicinal tea, a rinse or gargle, cream, ointment, and vapor-inhalant bath additive. Apigenin

Apigenin. (From Zheng et al., *Life Sci.,* 76:1367–1379, 2005. With permission.)

was shown to inhibit tetradecanoyl-phorbol-13-acetate-(TBA)-mediated tumor promotion in mouse skin. Kavutcu and Melzig (1999) examined a number of flavonoids and found apigenin inhibited 5′-nucleotidase (5′-ribonucleotide phosphohydrolase, 5′-NT) activity, which could explain its pharmacological effects. Morton and Griffiths (1999) suggested a possible relationship between flavonoids, such as apigenin, and the prevention of prostate disease. Gupta et al. (2001) showed that apigenin caused selective cell-cycle arrest and apoptosis of several human prostate carcinoma cells but did not affect normal cells. An in-depth investigation by Gupta and coworkers (2002) showed apigenin inhibited serum- and androgen-stimulated, prostate-specific antigen (PSA) protein levels in human prostate carcinoma LNCaP cells concomitant with cell growth inhibition *via* G1-phase arrest and apoptosis. Based on this research, the following model was proposed (Scheme A.6), which confirms the potential of apigenin for the

A

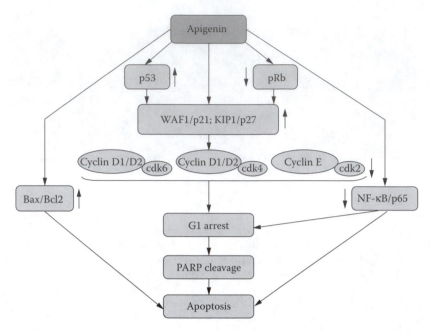

SCHEME A.6 Proposed model for apigenin-mediated cell dysregulation and apoptosis of human prostate carcinoma LNCaP cells. (From Gupta et al., *Oncogene*, 21:3727–3778, 2002.)

treatment of prostate cancer. A recent study by Zheng and coworkers (2005) also found apigenin had considerable potential for the treatment of cervical cancer by inducing p53 expression in human cervical carcinoma cells (HeLa), which resulted in cell-cycle arrest and apoptosis.

References

Birt, D.F., Shull, J.S., and Yaktrine, N.L., 1998. Chemoprevention of Cancer, In *Modern Health and Disease*; Shils, M.E., Olson, J.A., Shicke, M., and Ross, A.C., Eds., Williams and Wilkins, Ninth edition. Chapter 81, pp. 1263–1269, 1998.

Duthie, G. and Crozier, A., Plant-derived antioxidants, *Curr. Opin. Clin. Nutr. Metab. Care,* 3:447–451, 2000.

Gupta, S., Afaq, F., and Mukhtar, H., Selective growth-inhibitory, cell-cycle deregulatory and apoptic response of apigenin in normal versus human prostate carcinoma cells, *Biochem. Biophys. Res. Commun.,* 287:914–920, 2001.

Gupta, S., Afaq, F., and Mukhtar, H., Involvement of nuclear factor-κB, Bax and Bcl-2 in induction of cell cycle arrest and apoptosis by apigenin in human prostate carcinoma cells, *Oncogene,* 21: 3727–3778, 2002.

Kavatcu, M. and Melzig, M.F., *In vitro* effects of selected flavonoids on the 5′-nucleotidase activity, *Pharmazie,* 54:457–459, 1999.

Morton, D.L., and Griffiths, K., Diet and its preventive role in prostatic disease, *Eur. Urol.,* 35:377–387, 1999.

Zheng, P.-W., Chiang, L.-C., and Lin, C.-C., Apigenin induced apoptosis through p53-dependent pathway in human cervical carcinoma cells, *Life Sci.,* 76:1367–1379, 2005.

Apple Fruits, like vegetables, are known to have healthy properties. In fact it has been shown that the peels of fruit are among the major sources of antioxidants (Bocco et al., 1998; Gorinstein et al., 1998). An international study involving Israel, Spain, Poland, the Czech Republic, and Korea (Leontowicz and coworkers, 2002) examined the bioactive compounds in apples, peaches, and pears and their influence on lipids and antioxidant capacity in rats. The total polyphenols were almost three times higher in apple fruit and peels compared to the other fruit. Caffeic acid, *p*-coumaric, and ferulic acids, as well as the total radical-trapping antioxidative potential (TRAP), were also significantly higher in apple fruit and peels. No differences in dietary fiber were observed among the fruits examined. This study showed apples had the highest content of biologically active compounds, making them the preferred source for the dietary prevention of atherosclerosis. Knekt and coworkers (2000), in a large study involving 9,208 Finnish men and women 15 years and above, found a strong association between intake of apples and decreased risk of thrombotic stroke. A later study by Young and coworkers (2002) showed that a low-antioxidant diet supplemented with 10 percent apple/broccoli mixture fed to a chicken model stabilized erythrocytes, as well as reduced oxidation of muscle proteins and lipids in cooked liver. A number of *in vitro* studies attributed the ability of apple extracts to inhibit proliferation of tumor cells to the presence of phenolic/flavonoid antioxidants. Lapidot and coworkers (2002) cautioned that these results may be misleading, as the inhibition may be indirectly caused by hydrogen peroxide generated from interaction between the phenolics and the cell culture media. Consequently, the effects attributed to flavonoids and phenolics may be the result of the artifact production of oxidative stress. These researchers suggested that either catalase or metmyoglobin in the presence of a reducing agent be used to decompose any hydrogen peroxide formed so as to prevent such artifacts from occurring.

The high antioxidant capacity of apple polyphenols observed *in vitro* could not be found by Lotito and Frei (2004a) *in vivo*. No significant increase in resistance to oxidation was observed in the plasma of six healthy subjects up to four hours after eating five apples.

This suggested poor absorption and metabolic conversion of apple polyphenols, as previously observed for the consumption of black tea (Cherubini et al., 1999). A follow-up study by Lotito and Frei (2004b) showed that it was urate, not flavonoids, responsible for the increased plasma antioxidant activity following apple consumption. They suggested that the antioxidant health effects attributed to flavonoids in fruit may be confounded by the metabolic effect of fructose on urate. Increase in plasma urate had been reported previously in healthy individuals following consumption of tea (Natella et al., 2002) and red wine (Day and Stansbie, 1995).

Using a modified total-oxyradical scavenging (TOSC) assay, Wolfe et al. (2003) found the total antioxidant activity in the peels from four different apple varieties (Rome Beauty, Idared, Cortland, and Golden Delicious) were significantly ($p < 0.05$) higher compared to the flesh and flesh + peel. Based on the effective median dose (EC_{50}), they also showed, for the first time, that apple peels exhibited greater antiproliferative activity against $HepG_2$ human liver-cancer cells than did the corresponding flesh or flesh + peels (Table A.4). The low EC_{50} for Rome Beauty flesh and peel suggested synergism between the phytochemicals in the flesh and peel, as there was no measurable inhibition with the flesh alone. Antiproliferative activity on human liver-cancer cells had been reported previously by Liu and coworkers (2001) using extracts from Fuji, Gala, and Red Delicious apples.

TABLE A.4
[a]EC_{50} Values for Inhibition of $HepG_2$ Human Liver-Cancer Cell Proliferation by Phytochemical Extracts of Apples (Mean + SD, $n = 3$)

Apple	Flesh (mg/mL)	Flesh + Peel (mg/mL)	Peel (mg/mL)
Rome Beauty	a	26.5 + 0.3	12.4 + 0.4
Idared	a	125.1 + 58.8	16.6 + 0.2
Cortland	103.9 + 16.5	74.1 + 4.0	15.7 + 0.3
Golden Delicious	155.3 + 11.7	107.7 + 22.7	20.2 + 0.7

[a] The EC_{50} value could not be calculated from the dose–response curve.

Source: From Wolfe et al., *J. Agric. Food Chem.*, 50:5058–5062, 2003. With permission.

References

Boco, A., Cuvelier, M.E., Richard, H., and Berset, C., Antioxidant activity and phenolic composition of citrus and peel seed extracts, *J. Agric. Food Chem.*, 46:2123–2129, 1998.

Cherubini, A., Flint Beal, M., and Freir, B., Black tea increases the resistance of human plasma to lipid peroxidation *in vitro* but not *ex vivi*, *Free Rad. Biol. Med.*, 27:381–387, 1999.

Day, A. and Stansbie, D., 1995. Cardioprotective effect of red wine may be mediated by urate, *Clin. Chem.*, 41:1319–1320, 1995.

Gorinstein, S., Kulasek, G., Bartnikowska, E., Leontowicz, M., Zemser, M., Morawiec, M., and Trakhtenberg, S., The influence of persimmon peel and persimmon pulp on the lipid metabolism and antioxidant activity of rats fed cholesterol, *J. Nutr. Biochem.*, 4:223–227, 1998.

Knekt, P., Isotupa, S., Rissanen, H., Heliovaara, M., Jarvinen, R., Hakkinen, S., Aromaa, A., and Reunnanen, A., Quercetin intake and the incidence of cerebrovascular disease, *Eur. J. Clin. Nutr.*, 54:415–417, 2000.

Lapidot, T., Walker, M.D., and Kanner, J., Can apple antioxidants inhibit tumor cell proliferation? Generation of H_2O_2 during interaction of phenolic compounds with cell culture media, *J. Agric. Food Chem.*, 50:3156–3160, 2002.

Leontowicz, H., Gorinstein, S., Lojek, A., Leontowicz, M., Ciz, M., Soliva-Fortuny, R., Park, Y.-S., Jung, S.-T., Trakhtenberg, S., and Martin-Belloso, O., Comparative content of some bioactive compounds in apples, peaches and pears and their influence on lipids and antioxidant capacity in rats, *J. Nutr. Biochem.*, 13:603–610, 2002.

Liu, R.H., Eberhardt, M.V., and Lee, C.Y., Antioxidant and antiproliferative activities of selected New York apple cultivars, *N. Y. Fruit Q.*, 9:15–17, 2001.

Lotito, S.B. and Frei, B., Relevance of apple polyphenols as antioxidants in human plasma: Contrasting *in vitro* and *in vivo* effects, *Free Rad. Biol. Med.*, 36:201–211, 2004a.

Lotito, S.B. and Frei, B., The increase in human plasma antioxidant capacity after apple consumption is due to the metabolic effect of fructose on urate, not apple-derived antioxidant flavonoids, *Free Rad. Biol. Med.*, 36:251–258, 2004b.

Natella, F., Nardini, M., Giannetti, I., Dattilo, C., and Scaccini, C., Coffee drinking influences plasma antioxidant capacity in humans, *J. Agric. Food Chem.*, 50:6211–6216, 2002.

Wolfe, K., Wu, X., and Liu, R.H., Antioxidant activity of apple peels, *J. Agric. Food Chem.*, 51:609–614, 2003.

Young, J.F., Steffensen, C.L., Nielsen, J.H., Jensen, S.K., and Stagsted, J., Chicken model for studying dietary antioxidants reveals that apple (Cox's orange)/broccoli (*Brassica oleracea* L. var. *italica*) stabilizes erythrocytes and reduces oxidation of insoluble muscle proteins and lipids in cooked liver, *J. Agric. Food Chem.*, 50:5058–5062, 2003.

Apple juice *see also* **Phloridzin**   Pearson and coworkers (1999) examined the ability of six commercial apple juices to inhibit copper-catalyzed LDL-oxidation. Their results further support the inclusion of apple and apple products in a healthy diet. In addition, some apple phenolics also inhibited glucose transport *via* the Na-dependent glucose transporter (SGLT1). One such phenolic, phloridzin (phloretin 2′-O-β-D-glucoside), a flavonoid dihydrochalcone, is used in studies on glucose transport. Phloridzin and related dihydrochalcones are found in apple products, such as cider (Tomas-Barberan et al.,

Phloridzin. (From Lu and Foo, *Food Chem.*, 61:29–33, 1998. With permission.)

1993). Johnston and coworkers (2002) showed that apple-juice consumption modulated glucose uptake by delaying the intestinal absorption of glucose. Cloudy apple juice, containing higher levels of phloridzin and other phenols, suppressed glucose absorption in the proximal GI tract to a greater degree than clear apple juice. These researchers suggested that such plant phenols could play a role in determining the glycemic index of plant foods for the treatment of noninsulin-dependent diabetes mellitus

(NIDDM). In a recent paper by Andlauer et al. (2004), phloridzin amplified the absorption of the isoflavone genistin in isolated rat small intestine. Because of the cancer-protective effects associated with genistin, a functional food combining soy and apple may provide distinct health benefits.

References

Andlauer, W., Kolb, J., and Furst, P., Phloridzin improves absorption of genistin in isolated rat small intestine, *Clin. Nutr.*, 23:989–995, 2004.

Pearson, D.A., Tan, C.H., German, J.B., Davis, P.A., and Gershwin, M.E., Apple juice inhibits low density lipoprotein oxidation, *Life Sci.*, 64:1913–1920, 1999.

Johnston, K.L., Clifford, M.N., and Morgan, L.M., Possible role for apple juice phenolic compounds in the acute modification of glucose tolerance and gastrointestinal hormone secretions in humans, *J. Sci. Food. Agric.*, 82:1800–1805, 2002.

Lu, Y. and Foo, L.Y., Constitution of some chemical components of apple seed, *Food Chem.*, 61:29–33, 1998.

Tomas-Barberan, F.A., Garcia-Viguera, C., Nieto, J.L., Ferreres, F., and Tomas-Lorente, F., Dihydrochalcones from apple juices and jams, *Food Chem.*, 46: 33–36, 1993.

Apricot

Apricot   Apricots were shown to be rich sources of vitamins A and C, β-carotene, and selenium that met the RDAs of healthy individuals (Munzuroglu et al., 2003). In contrast, however, apricots were poor sources of vitamin E. Previous research also showed fresh apricots were significantly higher in selenium compared to other fruits and vegetables by a factor of up to fivefold (Kadrabova et al., 1997; Hussein and Bruggeman, 1999). The anticarcinogenic and antioxidant properties of vitamins A, C, β-carotene, and selenium makes apricots a potentially important functional food and source of nutraceuticals.

References

Hussein, L. and Bruggeman, J., Selenium analysis of selected Egyptian foods and estimated daily intakes among a population group, *Food Chem.*, 65: 527–532, 1999.

Kadrabova, J., Madaric, A., and Ginter, E., 1997. The selenium content of selected food from the Slovak republic, *Food Chem.*, 58:29–32, 1997.

Munzuroglu, O., Karatas, F., and Geckil, H., The vitamin and selenium contents of apricot fruit of different varieties cultivated in different geographical regions, *Food Chem.*, 83:205–212, 2003.

Arabinoxylan   Arabinoxylan, a major component of dietary fiber of cereals, is a hemicellulose composed of a xylose backbone and arabinose side chains (Amodo and Neukom, 1985). The outer layer of wheat bran and the inner layer of the endosperm are both rich sources of arabinoxylans. Lu and coworkers (2000) showed ingestion of arabinoxylan-rich fiber improved postprandial glucose and insulin responses in healthy patients. As a by-product of wheat processing, arabinoxylan-rich fiber could be beneficial for individuals with diabetes or impaired glucose tolerance.

Unlike *lactobacilli, enterococci, Eschrichia coli, Clostridium perfringens,* or *Clostrium difficile,* which are unable to ferment arabinoxylan, the probiotic *Bifidobacterium longum* strains grew well on it (Crittenden et al., 2002). As a consequence, arabinoxylan has potential to complement *Bifidobacterium longum* strains in synbiotic combinations.

References

Amodo, R. and Neukom, H., Arabinoxylan-rich fiber reduces blood glucose. Minor constituents of wheat flour: The pentosan, in *New Approaches to Research on Cereal Carbohydrates,* Hill, R.D. and Munch, L., Eds., Elsevier Science Publishers, Amsterdam, 1985, p. 241–251.

Crittenden, R., Karppinen, S., Ojanen, S., Tenkanen, M., Fagerstrom, R., Matto, J., Saarela, M., Mattila-Sandholm, T., and Poutanen, K., *In vitro* fermentation of cereal dietary fibre carbohydrates by probiotic and intestinal bacteria, *J. Sci. Food Agric.*, 82:781–789, 2002.

Lu, Z.X., Walker, K.Z., Muir, J.G., Mascara, T., and O'Dea, K., Arabinoxylan fiber, a byproduct of wheat flour processing, reduces the postprandial glucose response in normoglycemic subjects, *Am. J. Clin. Nutr.*, 71:1123–1128, 2000.

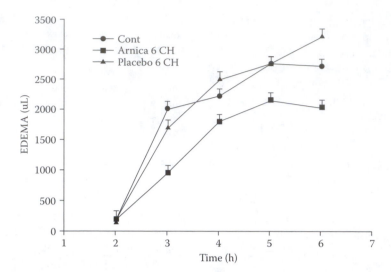

FIGURE A.8 Effect of oral treatment (0.1 mL) with *Arnica montana* 6cH and placebo, administered during three days (three times a day) prior to injection of carrageenan (1000 µg/paw). *$p < 0.05$. (Macedo et al., *Homeopathy*, 93:84–87, 2004. With permission.)

Arnica The flowering heads of the Arnica plant have been used in homeopathic medicine for many years. It is a perennial plant that is particularly popular in Germany. Puhlmann et al. (1991) isolated and characterized two homogeneous, immunologically active polysaccharides from *Arnica montana* cell cultures. One was a neutral fucogalactoxyloglucan, while the other was an acidic arabino-3,6-galactan-protein. Fucogalactoxyloglucan exhibited a marked enhancement of phagocytosis *in vivo*, while the acidic polymer showed a strong anti-complementary effect, stimulating macrophages to secrete the tumor necrosis factor (TNF-α). A more recent study by Koo et al. (2000) showed *Arnica montana* had only slight antibacterial activity against 15 oral pathogens *in vitro* compared to propolis. Using the acute carrageenan-induced rat-paw oedema-inflammation model, Macedo et al. (2004) observed a 30 percent inhibition when pretreated with *Arnica montana* 6cH (Figure A.8). Pretreatment of the chronic inflammation model with *Arnica montana* 6cH three days prior to application of nyastatin also significantly ($p < 0.05$) reduced inflammation. The mechanism of action appeared to involve blocking the action of histamine from increasing vascular permeability.

References

Koo, H., Gomes, B.P.F.A., Rosalen, P.L., Ambrosano, G.M.B., Park, Y.K., and Cury, J.A., *In vitro* antimicrobial activity of propolis and *Arnica montana* against oral pathogens, *Arch. Oral Biol.*, 45: 141–148, 2000.

Macedo, S.B., Ferreira, L.R., Perazzo, F.F., and Carvalho, J.C.T., Anti-inflammatory activity of Arnica montana 6cH: Preclinical study of animals, *Homeopathy*, 93:84–87, 2004.

Puhlmann, J., Zenk, M.H., and Wagner, H., Immunologically active polysaccharides of *Arnica montana* cell cultures, *Phytochemistry*, 30:1141–1145, 1991.

Artemisia Many spices belonging to the genus *Artemisia* are also known as aromatic plants. These spices, found in the Middle East, have been used in tonics, stomach, and as tinctures for the relief of rheumatic pains (Paris and Moise, 1971). A sesquiterpene lactone peroxide with antimalarial activity was isolated from selected chemotypes in the soil. One of these genera, *Artemisia judaica* L., has long been used in Egypt for medicinal purposes. Very strong antioxidant activity in *Artemisia judaica* L. oil was demonstrated by El-Massry and coworkers (2002), which was attributed to the

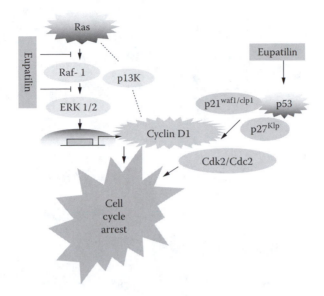

SCHEME A.7 Putative mechanism of eupatilin-induced cell-cycle arrest in MCF-1OA-*ras* cells. Eupatilin is proposed to inhibit expression of cyclin D1 via the Ras/Raf/MAPK signaling pathway, independently of the Akt pathway. In addition, eupatilin-induced cell-cycle arrest appears to be associated with upregulation of p53 and [p27kip1]. (From Kim et al., *Biochem. Pharmacol.,* 68:1081–1087, 2004. With permission.)

presence of 2,6-dimethyl phenol (1.39 percent) and camphor (0.38 percent).

Seo et al. (2001) identified eupatilin, a pharmacologically active flavone in extracts from *Aretemisia asiatica* Nakai. This flavone was

Eupatilin (5,7-dihydroxy-3′,4′,6′-trimmethoxy flavone). (From Kim et al., *Biochem. Pharmacol.,* 68: 1081–1087, 2004. With permission.)

found to induce apoptosis in human promyelocytic leukemia cells. Further studies by Kim and coworkers (2004) showed eupatilin inhibited the growth of H-*ras*-transformed human breast epithelial (MCF10A-*ras*) by modulating key cell-cycle growth regulators. The following scheme suggests eupatilin induces cycle arrest with down-regulation of cyclin D1 (Scheme A.7).

References

El-Massry, K.F., El-Ghorab, A.H., and Farouk, A., Antioxidant activity and volatile components of Egyptian *Artemisia judaica* L., *Food Chem.,* 79:331–336, 2002.

Kim, D.-H., Na, H.-K., Oh, T.Y., Kim, W.-B., and Surh, Y.-J., Eupatilin, a pharmacologically active flavone derived from *Artemisia* plants, induces cell cycle arrest in *ras*-transformed human mammary epithelial cells, *Biochem. Pharmacol.,* 68:1081–1087, 2004.

Paris, R.R. and Moise, H., *Matiere medicale, Vol. 3, Pharmacognice Speciale-Dicotyldones-Gamopetales,* Masson, Paris, 1971.

Seo, H.J. and Surh, Y.-J., Eupatilin, a pharmacologically active flavone derived from Artemisia plants, induces apoptosis in human promyelocytic leukemia cells, *Mutat. Res.,* 496:191–198, 2002.

Artichoke   Artichoke (*Cynara scolymus* L.) is an herbaceous perennial in which the head, an immature flower, is enjoyed as a vegetable throughout the world. Its leaves have been used as an herbal medicine for centuries. An artichoke dry extract was shown by Englisch et al. (2000) to substantially reduce total cholesterol

A

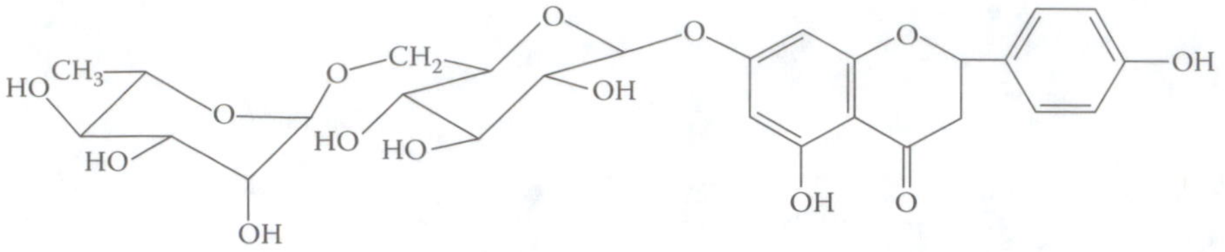

(Compound 1) (R&S)-narirutin

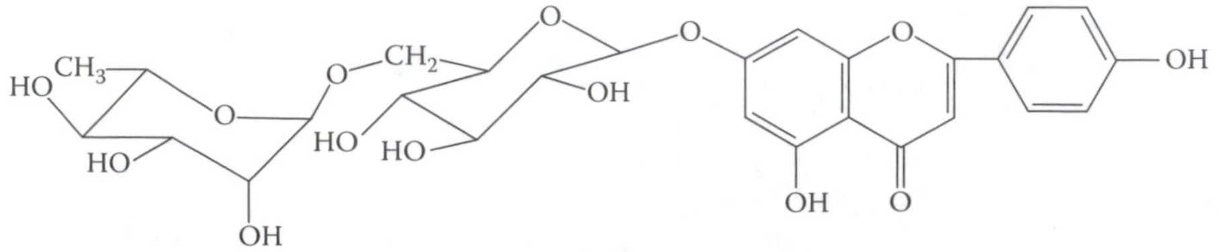

(Compound 2) apigenin-7-rutinoside

Apigenin-7-rutinoside and narirutin. (Adapted from Wang et al., *J. Agric. Food Chem.,* 51:601–608, 2003.)

and LDL-cholesterol levels in patients with hyperlipoproteinemia by 18.3 percent and 22.9 percent compared to 8.5 percent and 6.3 percent for the placebo, respectively. Perez-Garcia and coworkers (2000) found an artichoke-leaf extract reduced oxidative stress from reactive-oxygen species in human leukocytes. The antioxidant activity was concentration dependent and attributed to the presence of cynarin, caffeic acid, chlorogenic acid, and luteolin in the extract. Pittler and coworkers (2002) showed an artichoke-leaf extract significantly reduced blood cholesterol in patients suffering from hypercholesterolemia compared to the placebo. A growing body of evidence suggests that artichoke-leaf extract is beneficial for the treatment of irritable-bowel syndrome (IBS) and is supported from a surveillance study by Walker and coworkers (2001). The hepatoprotective effects of a water-soluble extract from artichoke (*Cynara scolymus* L.) leaves were shown by Gibhardt (2002) to prevent taurolithocholate-induced bile canalicular membrane transformations in cultured rat hepatocytes.

The previous studies all focused on artichoke leaves, a known rich source of polyphenols, while the components in the edible portion of the head remained unknown. A recent study by Wang et al. (2003), however, examined the leaves and heads of artichoke for total phenolic compounds, as well as the antioxidative active polyphenols, apigenin-7-rutinoside (compound 1) and narirutin (compound 2). The latter compounds were only found in the heads and increased in more mature vegetables; however, the level of total phenols was overall much higher in the leaves compared to the artichoke heads (Table A.5).

References

Englisch, W., Beckers, C., Unkauf, M., Ruepp, M., and Zinserling, V., Efficacy of artichoke dry extract in patients with hyperlipoproteinemia, *Arzneimittel-Forschung,* 50:260–265, 2000.

Gibhardt, R., Prevention of taurolithocholate-induced hepatic bile canicular distortions by HPLC characterized extracts of artichoke (*Cynara scolymus*) leaves, *Planta Med.,* 68:776–779, 2002.

Perez-Garcia, F., Adzet, T., and Canigueral, S., Activity of artichoke leaf extract on reactive oxygen species in human leukocytes, *Free Rad. Res.,* 33: 661–665, 2000.

Pittler, M.H., Thompson, C.O., and Ernst, E., Artichoke leaf extract for treating hypercholesterolaemia. *Cochrane Database Syst. Rev.,* Issue 3, Art No. 003335, 2002.

Walker, A.F., Middleton, R.W., and Petrowicz, O., Artichoke leaf extract reduces symptoms of irritable bowel syndrome in a post-marketing surveillance study, *Phytother. Res.,* 15:58–61, 2001.

Wang, M., Simon, J.E., Aviles, I.F., He, K., Zheng, Q.-Y., and Tadmor, Y., Analysis of antioxidative phenolic compounds in artichoke (*Cynara scolymus* L.), *J. Agric. Food Chem.,* 51:601–608, 2003.

TABLE A.5
Comparison of Purified Phenolic Compounds and Total Phenolic Content (Percent of Dry Weight) in Artichoke Variety (Green Globe) and Organs, Harvested on Two Dates and Oven- or Freeze-Dried, Based on HPLC Analysis of Methanolic Artichoke Extracts

Organ	1-Caffeoylquinic Acid	Chlorogenic Acid	Luteolin Rutinoside	Cyaroside	Narirutin	Apigenin 7-rutinoside	Cyarin	Total
Leaves[a,b]	0.149	4.158	0.213	0.314	0	0	1.619	6.455
Leaves[a,c]	0.064	4.654	0.275	0.114	0	0	0.924	6.031
Heads								
Young[a,b]	0.070	0.459	0.011	0.035	0.085	0.032	0.748	1.44
Young[b,d]	0.039	0.276	0.022	0.061	0.108	0.063	0.847	1.416
Mature[a,b]	0.020	0.186	0.025	0.024	0.182	0.050	0.309	0.795
Mature[b,d]	0.018	0.102	0.04	0.026	0.182	0.076	0.242	0.678

[a] Harvested Oct. 3, 2001.
[b] Oven-dried (70°C).
[c] Freeze-dried.
[d] Harvested Sept. 5, 2001.

Source: Adapted from Wang et al., *J. Agric. Food Chem.*, 51:601–608, 2003.

Ascorbic acid *see* Vitamin C

Asparagus *see also* Rutin

Asparagus (*Asparagus officinalis*) is readily available in grocery stores as canned or freshly packed. The major flavonoid in asparagus is rutin, which is a strong antioxidant (Makris and Rossiter, 2001). Earlier work by Vinson et al. (1998) showed asparagus ranked fourth out of 23 vegetables in the amount of total phenols, but first for antioxidant

Rutin. (Adapted from Deng et al., *Radiat. Phys. Chem.*, 53: 629–633, 1998.)

quality. Makris and Rossiter (2001) examined the effect of processing on the flavonol and antioxidant status of asparagus spears. The predominant flavonol was rutin, although a few minor peaks were also observed. The effect of processing is summarized in Table A.6. Boiling was a far more destructive process compared to chopping, with rutin losses being 18.5 percent and 43.9 percent for boiling and chopping, respectively.

Jang and coworkers (2004) recently isolated and characterized a number of natural chemopreventive agents from an ethyl acetate-soluble fraction of the methanol extract of the aerial parts of asparagus (*Asparagus officinalis*). Of 16 compounds identified, two were new natural products, asparagusic acid anti-*S*-oxide methyl ester and asparagusic acid syn-*S*-oxide methyl ester plus a new acetylenic compound, 2-hydroxyasaparenyn{3′,4′-*trans*-2-hydroxy-1-methoxy-4-[5-(4-methoxyphenoxy)-3-penten-1-ynyl]-benzene}. Of all the compounds identified, linoleic acid showed the most significant activity against COX-2 and moderate activity against COX-1 (Table A.7). Of the remainder, (±)-1-hexadececanoylglycerol (6) exhibited weak activity against COX-1 and moderate activity against COX-2, while ferulic acid (7),

A

TABLE A.6
Effect of Domestic Processes on Rutin Content of Asparagus[1]

Compound	Chopping			Boiling		
	Control	Chopped	Percent Change	Control	Chopped	Percent Change
Rutin	286.5 + 6.0	233.6 + 3.5	−18.50 percent	274.1 + 3.8	153.7 + 5.5	−43.90 percent

[1] Data expressed as $mgkg^{-1}$

Source: Adapted from Makris and Rossiter, *J. Agric. Food Chem.*, 49:3216–3222, 2001.

TABLE A.7
Inhibitory Activities of Compounds from *A. Officinalis* Against Cyclooxygenase-1 and -2[a]

Compound	COX-1		COX-2	
	% inhib at 100 µg/mL	IC_{50} (µg/mL)	% inhib at 100 µg/mL	IC_{50} (µg/mL)
6	50	ND[b]	67	45.4
7	55	33.7	1	ND
8	62	ND	30	ND
9	51	ND	0	ND
Linoleic acid	100	14.6	100	0.53
trans-resveratrol[b]	100	0.25	100	0.30

[a] ND Not determined.

[b] *trans*-Resveratrol was used as a positive control.

Source: From Jang et al., *J. Agric. Food Chem.*, 52:2218–2222, 2004. With permission

1,3-*O*-di-*p*-coumaroylglycerol (8) and 1-*O*-feruloyl-3-*O*-*p*-coumaroylglycerol (9) had only weak activity against COX-1. Inhibition of cyclooxygenase (COX) enzymes by nonsteroidal anti-inflammatory drugs (NSAIDs) are thought to hinder the development of colon cancer (Chan, 2002).

References

Chan, T.A., Nonsteroidal anti-inflammatory drugs, apoptosis, and colon-cancer chemoprevention, *Lancet Oncol.*, 3:166–174, 2002.

Deng, W., He, Y., Fang, X., and Wu, J., Radiolysis of rutin in aerated ethanolic solution, *Radiat. Phys. Chem.*, 53:629–633, 1998.

Jang, D.S., Cuendet, M., Fong, H.H.S., Pezzuto, J.M., and Kinghorn, A.D., Constituents of *Asparagus officinalis* evaluated for inhibitory activity against cyclooxygenase-2, *J. Agric. Food Chem.*, 52:2218–2222, 2004.

Makris, D.P. and Rossiter, J.T., Domestic processing of onion bulbs (*Allium cepa*) and asparagus spears (*Asparagus officinalis*): Effect on flavonol content and antioxidant status, *J. Agric. Food Chem.*, 49:3216–3222, 2001.

Vinson, J.A., Hao, Y., Su, X., and Zubik, L., Phenol antioxidant quantity and quality in foods, *J. Agric. Food Chem.*, 46:3630–3634, 2001.

Astaxanthin Astaxanthin, a carotenoid pigment, is responsible for the tinted red of crustaceans or the pink flesh of salmon. It is produced commercially worldwide from the microalga *Haemastoccus pluvialis* (Olaizola

Astaxanthin. (From Lai et al., *J. Chromatogr. B.*, 804:25–30, 2004. With permission.)

and Huntley, 2002). The structure of astaxanthin is very similar to β-carotene, but it has been shown to be a superior antioxidant (Lawlor and O'Brien, 1995; Palozza and Krinsky, 1992). Astaxanthin has also been shown to protect the skin and eyes from UV light (Papas, 1999). Other carotenoids, lutein and zeaxanthin, which are also structurally related to astaxanthin, do not have its strong antioxidant activity and UV-light-protective properties (O'Connor and O'Brien, 1998). When fed to humans at doses as low as 3.6 mg per day for two consecutive weeks, astaxanthin protected LDL cholesterol from induced *in vitro* oxidation (Miki et al., 1998). Jacobsson et al. (2004) found that LDL-oxidation time was significantly prolonged in Watanabe heritable hyperlipidemia (WHHL) rabbits in the presence of α-tocopherol but unaffected when treated with astaxanthin. However, the antioxidant treatment produced smaller lesions and intimal thickening. Further examination of atheroma by Li and coworkers (2004) showed astaxanthin had a protective role by reducing macrophage infiltration and modulated macrophage apoptosis and MMP3. A similar effect was evident for α-tocopherol, which suggested these antioxidants are both antiatherogenic, since lipid and macrophage infiltration is closely associated with early plaque development.

Astaxanthin has also been reported to significantly inhibit colon cancer in rats, as well as the enzyme 5-α-reductase involved in prostate growth (Anderson, 2001). The ability of astaxanthin to cross the blood–brain barrier in rats suggests it might be beneficial to neurological diseases, such as Alzheimer's (Tso and Lam, 1996). Evidence is also accruing regarding the immunomodulating activity of astaxanthin, including enhancement of immunoglobulin production in human blood cells in response to T-dependent stimuli (Jyonouchi et al., 1995). The bioavailability of astaxanthin was demonstrated in humans using a single, high dose of 100 mg and its transport by plasma lipoproteins (Osterlie et al., 2000).

The lipophilic nature of carotenoids, such as astaxanthin, renders it difficult to deliver it to target cells. One way to surmount this problem is to form water-soluble derivatives, such as the disodium salt disuccinate. Hix et al. (2004) showed this astaxanthin derivative was biologically active by upregulating expression of connexin protein (CX43), increasing the formation of CX43 immunoreactive plaques, as well as significantly upregulating intracellular communication. The enhanced delivery of these derivatives suggested greater potential for astaxanthin as an anticancer agent.

References

Anderson, M., Method of inhibiting 5-α reductase with astaxanthin to prevent and treat benign prostate hyperplasia (BPH) and prostrate cancer in human males, US Patent No. 6277417, 2001.

Hix, L.M., Lockwood, S.F., and Bertram, J.S., Upregulation of connexin 43 protein expression and increased gap functional communication by water soluble disodium discuccinate astaxanthin derivatives, *Cancer Lett.*, 211:25–37, 2004.

Jacobsson, L.S., Yuan, Y.-M., Zieden, B., and Olsson, A.G., Effects of α-tocopherol and astaxanthin on LDL oxidation and atherosclerosis in WHHL rabbits, *Atherosclerosis*, 173:231–237, 2004.

Jyonouchi, H., Sun, Y., and Gross, M.D., 1995a. Effect of carotenoids on *in vitro* immunoglobulin production by human peripheral blood mononuclear cells: Astaxanthin, a carotenoid without vitamin A activity, enhances *in vitro* immunoglobulin production in response to a T-dependent stimulant and antigen, *Nutr. Cancer*, 23:171–183, 1995a.

A

Jyonouchi, H., Sun, Y., Tomita, Y., and Gross, M.D., Astaxanthin, a carotenoid without vitamin A activity, *augments* antibody responses in cultures including T-helper cell clones and suboptimal doses of antigen, *J. Nutr.,* 124:2483–2493, 1995b.

Lai, J.-P., Jiang, Y., He, X.-W., Huang, J.-C., and Chen, F., Separation and determination of astaxanthin from microalgal and yeast samples by molecularly imprinted microspheres, *J. Chromatogr. B.,* 804:25–30, 2004.

Lawler, S.M. and O'Brien, N.M., Astaxanthin: Antioxidant effects in chicken embryo fibroblasts, *Nutr. Res.,* 15:1695–1704, 1995.

Li, W., Hellsten, A., Jacobsson, L.S., Blomqvist, H.A., Olsson, A.G., and Yuan, Y.-M., Alpha-tocopherol and astaxanthin decrease macrophage infiltration, apoptosis and vulnerability in atheroma in hyperlipidemia rabbits, *J. Mol. Cell. Cardiol.,* 37: 969–978, 2004.

Miki, W., Hosada, K., and Gross, M., Astaxanthin-containing drink, Japanese Patent No. 10155459, 1998.

O'Connor, I. and O'Brien, N., Modulation of UVA light-induced oxidative stress by beta-carotene, lutein and ataxanthin in cultured fibroblasts, *J. Dermatol. Sci.,* 16:226–230, 1998.

Olaizola, M. and Huntley, M.E., Recent advances in commercial production of astaxanthin from microalgae, in *Biomaterials and Bioprocessing,* Fingerman, M. and Nagabhushanam, R., Eds., Science Publishers, 9:143–164, 2002.

Osterlie, M., Bjerkeng, B., and Liaaen-Jenoen, S., Plasma appearance and distribution of astaxanthin E/Z isomers in plasma lipoproteins after a single dose administration of astaxanthin, *J. Nutr. Biochem.,* 11: 482–490, 2000.

Palozza, P. and Krinsky, N.I., Astaxanthin and canxanthin are potent antioxidants in a membrane model, *Arch. Biochem. Biophys.,* 297:291–295, 1992.

Papas, A., *Antioxidant Status, Diet, Nutrition and Health,* CRC Press, Boca Raton, Florida, 1999.

Tso, M.O.M. and Lam. T.T., Methods of retarding and ameliorating central nervous system and eye damage, U.S. Patent No. 1 5527533, 1996.

Astragalus Astragalus, a traditional Chinese herb derived from the root of *Astragalus membranaceus,* has been used to treat diabetes, heart disease, and high blood pressure. An extract from *Astragalus membranaceus* was shown by Zhao et al. (1990) to enhance the immune response in mice. Using a large-scale culture technique, Zheng and coworkers (1998) analyzed the hairy roots of *Astragalus membranaceus,* which contained 5.8 percent and 0.14 percent of crude saponins and astragaloside, respectively. They also demonstrated the ability of the hairy roots to increase immune function. Ma et al. (1998) demonstrated the therapeutic effects of *Astragalus membranaceus* on sodium and water retention in aortacaval fistula-induced heart failure. A clinical research trial by Zheng et al. (1995) showed astragalus improved the deformability of red blood cells and delayed aging in mice.

References

Ma, J., Peng, A., and Lin, S., Mechanisms of the therapeutic effect of *Astragalus membranaceus* on sodium and water retention in experimental heart failure, *Chin. Med. J.,* 111:17–23, 1998.

Zhao, K.S., Mancini, C., and Doria, G., Enhancement of the immune response in mice by *Astragalus membranaceus, Immunopharmacology,* 20:225–233, 1990.

Zheng, Z., Dai, J., and Zhu, M., Effect of injection of *Astragalus membranaceus* on the deformability of red blood cells, *Biorheology,* 32:322–, 1995.

Zheng, Z., Liu, D., Cheng, C., and Hu, Z., Studies on chemical constituents and immunological function activity of hairy roots of *Astragalus membranaceus, Chin. J. Biotechnol.,* 14:93–97, 1998.

Auraptene Auraptene (7-geranylcoumarin) is a natural component of citrus peel with chemoprotective properties against skin, tongue, esophagus, and colon carcinogenesis in rodents (Murakami et al., 1997; Tanaka et al., 1997, 1998a, b).

Auraptene. (From Tanaka et al., *Carcinogenesis,* 18:2155–2161, 1997.)

Tanaka et al. (1997) reported auraptene reduced the number of precancerous lesions in carcinogen-induced rat colons. A single oral dose of auraptene (200 mg/kg body weight) increased the activity of quinone reductase and glutathione S-transferase, two key Phase II detoxifying enzymes. *In vivo* studies showed auraptene suppressed the generation of superoxide anions ($\dot{O}_2$-) from inflammatory leukocytes. Murakami et al. (2004) found the inhibitory effects of auraptene were due to its selective blockage of the activation stage by attenuating the lipopolysaccharide-induced expression of inducible forms of both nitric-oxide synthase and cyclooxygenase in a murine macrophage line, RAW 264.7. It decreased the production of the nitrite anion and prostaglandin E_2, while suppressing the release of the tumor necrosis factor-α. The overall effect *in vivo* in ICR female rats was decreased levels of edema, H_2O_2 production, leukocyte infiltration, and PCNA-labeling index. *In vivo* data showed a marked suppression of iNOS/COX-2 expression and TNF-α release. Thus, auraptene could have application in preventing and medicating inflammation-related disorders, such as cancer.

References

Murakami, A., Kuli, W., Takahashi, Y., Yonei, H., Nakamura, Y., Ohto, Y., Ohigashi, H., and Koshimizu, K., Auraptene, a citrus coumarin, inhibits 12-*O*-tetradecanoylphorbol-13-acetate-induced tumor promotion in ICR mouse skin, possibly through suppression of superoxide generation in leukocytes, *Jpn. J. Cancer Res.,* 88:443–452, 1997.

Murakami, A., Nakamura, Y., Tanaka, T., Kawabata, K., Takahashi, D., Koshimizu, K., and Ohigashi, H., Suppression by citrus auraptene of phorbol ester- and endoxin-induced inflammatory responses, *Carcinogenesis,* 21:1843–1850, 2000.

Tanaka, T., Kawabata, K., Kakumoto, M., Hara, A., Mori, H., Satoh, K., Murakami, A., Kuki, W., Takahashi, Y., Yonei, H., Koshimizu, K., and Ohigashi, H., Citrus auraptene inhibits chemically induced colonic aberrant crypt foci in male F344 rats, *Carcinogenesis*, 18:2155–2161, 1997.

Tanaka, T., Kawabata, K., Kakumoto, M., Hara, A., Murakami, A., Kuki, W., Takahashi, Y., Yonei, H., Maeda, M., Otah, T., Odashima, S., Yamane, T., Koshimizu, K, and Ohigashi, H., Citrus auraptene exerts dose-dependent chemopreventive activity in rat large bowel tumorigenesis: The inhibition correlates with suppression of cell proliferation and lipid peroxidation and with induction of phase II drug-metabolizing enzymes, *Cancer Res.,* 58:2550–2556, 1998a.

Tanaka, T., Kawabata, K., Kakumoto, M., Matsunaga, K., Mori, H., Murakami, A., Kuki, W., Takahashi, Y., Yonei, H., Satoh, K., Hara, A., Maeda, M., Otah, T., Odashima, S., Koshimizu, K., and Ohigashi, H., Chemoprevention of 4-nitroquinoline 1-oxide-induced oral carcinogenesis by citrus auraptene in rats, *Carcinogenesis,* 19:425–431, 1998b.

Avocado Avocado is a type of pear (*Persea americana*) originating in Mexico that is processed for oil. Mexico (34 percent) is the largest producer of avocados, followed by the United States (8 percent), Israel (4 percent), South Africa (2 percent), and, recently, New Zealand (Eyres et al., 2001). Novel nitric-oxide and superoxide generation inhibitors, persenone A and B, were identified in avocado fruit by Kim and coworkers (2000a). These researchers showed persenone A suppressed expression of

Persenone A

Persenone B

Persenone (From Kim et al., *J. Agric. Food Chem.,* 48:1557–1563, 2000b. With permission.)

both inducible nitric-oxide synthase and COX-2 in mouse macrophages and inhibited H_2O_2 generation in mouse skin (Kim et al., 2000b). Their results suggest that persenone A may prevent inflammation-associated diseases, including cancer. Kawagishi and coworkers (2000) isolated five fatty-acid derivatives in avocado that showed extraordinary, potent liver-injury-suppressing activity against liver damage by D-galactosamine, a powerful liver toxin. The oil from avocado is highly valued by the cosmetic industry and in the food industry for the

A

TABLE A.8

β-Sitosterol of Eight of the Most Frequently Consumed Fruits in the U.S.A.

Fruit[1]	β-Sitosterol[2] (mg/100 g[2])
Apples	11
Avocado	76
Banana	11
Cantaloupe	8
Grapefruit	13
Strawberries	10
Sweet Cherries	12

[1] Raw, edible portion.

[2] β-Sitosterol values for all fruits, except avocado, Adapted from Moghadasian et al., 1999.

Source: Adapted from Duester, *Lipid Tec.,* 7:84–88, 2001.

beneficial effects of its monounsaturated fatty acid, oleic acid, which accounts for almost 80 percent of the total fatty acids. In addition, avocado oil also contains relatively high amounts of β-sitosterol (0.5–1.0 percent) reported to lower blood cholesterol levels (see Phytosterols). β-Sitosterol has also been attributed to alleviating the symptoms of benign prostatic hypertrophy in men over 50 years of age (Berges et al., 1995). Avocado appears to be one the richest sources of β-sitosterol compared to eight of the most popular fruits consumed in the United States, as seen in Table A.8. Lu and coworkers (2005) showed lipid-soluble bioactives in avocado extract inhibited the growth of prostate-cancer cells.

Avocado was also shown to have important antihyperglycemic properties in humans (Alvizouri-Munoz et al., 1994). Using an *in vitro* method for assessing glucose diffusion across the gastrointestinal tract, Gallagher and coworkers (2003) showed avocado decreased glucose movement by more than 50 percent. These researchers suggested that avocado could be used as a dietary supplement in the diet of type 2 diabetic subjects.

References

Alvizouri-Munoz, M., Carranza-Madrigal, J., Herrera-Abarca, J.E., Chavez, C.F., and Amezcua-Gastelum, J.L., Effects of avocado as a source of monounsaturated fatty acids on plasma lipid levels, *Arch. Med. Res.,* 23:163–167, 1992.

Berges, R.R., Winderler, J., Trampisch, H.J., Senge, T., and beta-sitosterol study group, Randomized, placebo-controlled, double-blind clinical trial of beta;-sitosterol in patients with benign prostatic hyperplasia, *Lancet,* 345:1529–1532, 1995.

Duester, K.C., Avocado fruit is the richest source of beta-sitosterol, *J. Am. Diet. Assoc.,* 101:404–405, 2001.

Eyres, L., Sherpa, S., and Hendriks, G., Avocado oil: A new edible oil from Australia, *Lipid Technol.,* 7:84–88, 2001.

Gallagher, A.M., Flatt, P.R., Duffy, G., and Abdel-Wahab, Y.H.A., The effects of traditional antidiabetic plants on *in vitro* glucose diffusion, *Nutr. Res.,* 23: 413–424, 2003.

Kawagishi, H., Fukumoto, Y., Hatakeyama, M., He, P.O., Arimoto, H., Matsuzawa, T., Arimoto, Y., Suganuma, H., Inakuma, T., and Sugiyama, K., *J. Agric. Food Chem.,* 49:2215–2221, 2001.

Kim, O.K., Murakami, A., Takahashi, D., Nakamura, Y., Torikai, K., Kim, H.W., and Ohigashi, H., An avocado constituent, persenone A, suppresses expression of inducible forms of nitric oxide synthase and cyclooxygenase in macrophages, and hydrogen peroxide generation in mouse skin, *Biosci. Biotechnol. Biochem.,* 64:2504–2507, 2000a.

Kim, O.K., Murakami, A., Nakamura, Y., Takeda, N., Yoshizumi, H., and Ohigashi, H., Novel nitric oxide and superoxide generation inhibitors, persenone A and B, from avocado fruit, *J. Agric. Food Chem.,* 48: 1557–1563, 2000b.

Lu, Q.-Y., Arteaga, J.R., Zhang, Q., Huerta, S., Go, V.L.W., and Heber, D., Inhibition of prostate cancer cell growth by an avocado extract: Role of lipid-soluble bioactive substances, *J. Nutr. Biochem.,* 16: 23–30, 2005.

Moghadisian, M.H. and Frolich, J.J., Effect of dietary phytosterols on cholesterol metabolism and atherosclerosis: Clinical and experimental evidence, *Am. J. Med.,* 107:588–594, 1999.

B

Baicalein and Baicalin   Baicalin, a flavonoid with a structure analogous to genistein, is found in *Scutellaria* species used widely in Chinese herbal medicine. It has a glucuronate group at the C-7 position, which is absent in its aglycone, baicalein. Baicalein and baicalin both appear to have antiviral (Kitamura et al. 1998), antioxidant (Shi et al., 1995), antitumor (Matsuzaki et al., 1996), and anti-inflammatory (Lin and Shieh, 1996) properties, as well as an ability to reduce blood pressure and relax arterial smooth-muscle cells (Chen et al., 1999). The antitumor effects of baicalin on human hepatoma cell lines was also reported by Motoo and Sabatu (1994). Po and coworkers (2002) showed baicalin, unlike genistein, suppressed 17β-estradiol-induced transactivation in MFC-7 cells expressing receptor α. Baicalin also proved to be a stronger apoptosis-inducing agent, making it a superior chemopreventive agent. Chan and coworkers (2000) reported baicalin induced apoptosis in several human prostate-cancer cell lines so that it had the potential to be a chemopreventive agent or an adjuvant for the treatment of prostate cancers.

Baicalin and baicalein were both found by Huang and coworkers (2004) to exhibit novel vascular effects by inhibiting endothelial aortic relaxation *via* inhibition of cyclic GMP accumulation in vascular smooth-muscle cells. If this occurred in small blood vessels, vascular permeability would be reduced, which may explain the anti-inflammatory action of these flavonoids against acute edema or by inhibiting lipoxygenase, a key enzyme involved in inflammatory response.

Shen and coworkers (2003) evaluated the mechanisms responsible for the anti-inflammatory properties of baicalin and baicalein in human leukocytes. They both reduced N-formyl-methionyl-leucyl-phenylalanine (fMLP)- and phorbol-12-myristate-13-acetate (PMA)-induced reactive-oxygen intermediates in neutrophils and monocytes. The anti-inflammatory activity of baicalin and baicalein was due to the combination of baicalin scavenging the reactive-oxygen intermediates and baicalein antagonizing ligand-initiated Ca^{2+} influx, both of which inhibit Mac 1-dependent leukocytes.

Li et al. (2000) reported that baicalin inhibited HIV-1 infection by interfering with the interaction of HIV-1 envelope proteins with chemokine coreceptors, blocking the entry of HIV into target cells. As a result, it is viewed as a possible natural chemotherapy for HIV infection (De Clerq et al., 2000). Recent studies by Wang and coworkers (2004) showed that coupling baicalein (BA) with zinc made it a far more effective inhibitor of recombinant reverse transcriptase (RT) and HIV-1 entry into the host cells. Figure B.9 shows that inhibition of recombinant RT was far greater in the presence of lower concentrations of BA-Zn with an EC50 25.09 μM which was threefold lower than the EC50 for BA of 83.48 μM.

Baicalein and Baicalin. (From Zhang et al., *J. Pharmaceut. Biomed. Anal.*, 36:637–641, 2004. With permission.)

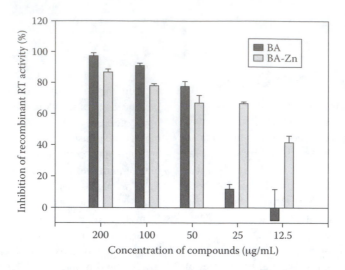

FIGURE B.9 Inhibition of recombinant HIV-1 RT activity by BA and BA-Zn. Inhibition rates were calculated according to the absorbance of the ELIZA Reader. Data expressed as means ±SEM of at least three independent measurements. (From Wang et al., *Biochem. Biophys. Res. Commun.,* 324:605–610, 2004. With permission.)

References

Chan, F.L., Choi, H.L., Chen, Z.Y., Chan, P.S.F., and Huang, C.Y., Induction of apoptosis in prostate cancer cell lines by a flavonoid, baicalin, *Cancer Lett.,* 160:219–228, 2000.

Chen, Z.Y., Su, Y.L., Lau, W.I., and Huang, Y., Endothelium-dependent contraction and direct relaxation induced by baicalin in rat mesenteric artery, *Eur. J. Pharmacol.,* 374:41-47, 1999.

De Clerq, E., Current lead natural products for the chemotherapy of human immunodeficiency virus (HIV) infection, *Med. Res. Rev.,* 20:323–349, 2000.

Huang, Y., Wong, C.M., Lau, C.-W., Yao, X., Tsang, S.Y., Su, Y.L., and Chen, Y., Inhibition of nitric oxide/cyclic GMP-mediated relaxation by purified flavonoids, baicalin and baicalein, in rat aortic rings, *Biochem. Pharmacol.,* 67:787–794, 2004.

Kitamura, K., Honda, M., Yoshizaki, H., Yamamoto, S., Nakane, H., Fukushima, M., Ono, K., and Tokunaga, T., Baicalin, an inhibitor of HIV-1 production *in vitro*, *Antiviral Res.,* 37:131–140, 1998.

Li, B.Q., Fu, T., Dongyan, Y. Mikovitz, J.A.n Ruscettim, F.W., and Wang, J.M., Flavonoid baicalin inhibits HIV-1 infection at the level of viral entry, *Biochem. Biophys. Res. Commun.,* 276:534–538, 2000.

Lin, C.C. and Shieh, D.E., The anti-inflammatory activity of *Scutellaria rivulas* extracts and its active components, baicalin, baicalein and wogonin, *Am. J. Clin. Chem.,* 24:31–36, 1996.

Matsuzaki, Y., Kurokawa, N., Terai, S., Matsumara, Y., Kobayashi, N., and Okita, K., Cell death induced by baicalein in human heptocellular carcinoma cell lines, *Jpn. J. Cancer Res.,* 87:170–177, 1996.

Motoo, Y. and Sawatu, N., Antitumor effects of saikosaponins, baicalin and baicalein on human heptoma cell lines, *Cancer Lett.,* 86:91–95, 1994.

Po, L.S., Chen, Z.Y,, Tsang, D.S.C., and Leung, L.K., Baicalein and genistein display differential actions on estrogen receptor (ER) transactivation and apoptosis in MCF-7 cells, *Cancer Lett.,* 187:33–40, 2002.

Shen, Y.-C., Chiou, W.-F., Chou, Y.-C., and Chen, C.-F., Mechanisms in mediating the anti-inflammatory effects of baicalin and baicalein in human leukocytes, *Eur. J. Pharmacol.,* 465:171–181, 2003.

Shi, H., Zhao, B., and Xin, W.J., Scavenging effects of baicalin on free radicals and its protection on erythrocyte membrane from free radical injury, *Mol. Bio. Int.,* 35:981–984, 1995.

Wang, Q., Wang, Y.-T., Pu, S.-P., and Zheng, Y.-T., Zinc coupling potentiates anti-HIV activity of baicalin, *Biochem. Biophys. Res. Commun.,* 324:605–610, 2004.

Zhang, L., Lin, G., and Zuo, Z. High-performance liquid chromatographic method for simultaneous determination of baicalein and baicalein 7-glucuronide in rat plasma, *J. Pharmaceut. Biomed. Anal.,* 36:637–641, 2004.

B

TABLE B.9
Effect of Various Fruit Extracts or Juices on NO Synthesis in Human Red-Cell Membrane

Addition to the Assay Mixture	nmol NO Produced/h/mg Residue
None	0.012 ± 0.005
Banana	8.45 ± 1.15
Cucumber	6.36 ± 0.057
Apple	6.07 ± 1.14
Lemon	6.05 ± 1.15
Pear	3.42 ± 0.14
Orange	2.57 ± 1.58
Grape (purple)	2.1 ± 0.054
Grape (green)	0.1 ± 0.011

Note: Results are the mean $\pm$ S.D. of six different experiments, each conducted in triplicate.

From Guha et al., *Nutr. Res.,* 23:1081–1088, 2003. With permission.

Banana   Bananas (*Musa Cavendish*), one of the most popular fruits worldwide, is a source of antioxidants, vitamin C, vitamin E, and β-carotene. Someya and coworkers (2002) found bananas were also high in flavonoids, with the peel being a richer source of total phenolics (907 mg/100 dry wt) compared to the pulp (232 mg/100g dry wt). This difference was reflected by the antioxidant activity of the peel extract being 2.2 times greater than the pulp. Several flavonoids were identified, including gallocatechin, catechin, and epicatechin. Of these, gallocatechin exhibited the greatest antioxidant activity and was much higher in banana peel (158 mg/100 g dry weight) compared to the pulp (29.6 mg/100 g dry weight). These researchers recommended that banana peels be considered a functional food source for combating chronic diseases and should not be discarded.

A study in India by Guha et al. (2003) showed ripe banana (*Musa paradisiacal sapientum*) extracts stimulated the production of nitric oxide (NO) in human erythrocyte membranes. Nitric oxide is tumoricidal, as well as induces apoptosis and differentiation in neoplastic cells (Farias-Eisner et al., 1994; Jun et al., 1996). Stimulation of nitric oxide is catalyzed by a family of isoenzymes, nitric synthase (NOS). Incubation of human red-cell membranes with different fruit extracts showed ripe banana was the most potent stimulator of NO, followed by cucumber, apple, and lemon, with pear lacking any activity (Table B.9). Inclusion of ripe bananas in the diets of mice administered Ehrlich's ascetic carcinoma cells showed that 70 percent of those animals receiving 2 g of ripe banana (wet weight/day) died within 35 days compared to the control group which died within 5–6 days. The ability of bananas to prevent or slow down the progression of ascetic carcinoma in mice could be extended to humans.

Vitamin A deficiency and chronic diseases are a particularly serious problem in Pacific Island countries. A recent paper by Englberger and coworkers (2003) pointed out the importance of bananas as significant sources of provitamin A and β- and α-carotenes, which could alleviate this problem in Micronesia.

References

Englberger, L., Schierle, J., Marks, G.C., and Fitzgerald, M.H., Micronesian banana, taro, and other foods: Newly recognized sources of provitamin A and other carotenoids, *J. Food Comp. Anal.,* 16:3–19, 2003.

Farias-Eisner, R., Sherman, M.P., Aeberhard, E., and Chaudhuri, G., Nitric oxide is an important mediator

B

for tumoricidal activity *in vivo, Proc. Natl. Acad. Sci. U.S.A.,* 91:9407–9411, 1994.

Guha, M., Basuray, S., and Sinha, A.K., Preventive effect of ripe banana in the diet on Ehrlich's ascetic carcinoma cell induced malignant ascites in mice, *Nutr. Res.,* 23:1081–1088, 2003.

Jun, C.-D., Lee, D.-K., and Cu, Y.-H., High-dose nitric oxide induces apoptosis in HL-60 human myeloid cells, *Korean J. Exp.. Mol. Med.,* 28:101– 108, 1996.

Someya, S., Yoshiki, Y., and Okubo, K., Antioxidant compounds from bananas (*Musa Cavendish*), *Food Chem.,* 79:351–354, 2002.

Barley Barley is one of the major cereals grown worldwide and is particularly important in China. The major uses for barley are in malting, as well as for the feed industry. Germinated barley foodstuff (GMF) obtained from the aleurone layer and scutellum fractions of malt consists mainly of dietary fiber and glutamine-rich protein. This material was found to have a preventive and therapeutic effect in an experimental colitis model (Kanauchi et al., 1997, 1998), as well as in patients with mild to moderate ulcerative colitis (Mitsuyama et al., 1998). Bamba and coworkers (2002) fed germinated barley to patients with mild to moderate active ulcerative colitis and found significant clinical and endoscopic improvements were associated with an increase in stool butyrate levels. These results suggested GMF was a new prebiotic for the treatment of ulcerative colitis. Deguchi and coworkers (2000) produced an anthocyanin-tannin type pigment from barley bran-fermented broth. The purple pigment, referred to as hordeumin, scavenged superoxide radicals in a dose-dependent manner, which was attributed to the bran polyphenols, such as proanthocyanidins.

Barley is also a good source of β-glucan, the mixed-linked $(1\rightarrow3)$, $(1\rightarrow4)$-β-D-glucan, which has been shown to have important health benefits. The β-glucan content of winter-barley cultivars grown in different locations in China were similar to those grown in Canada and Australia (Zhang et al., 2002). Because of the significant interaction between cultivars and

environment on β-glucan content, they emphasized the importance of planting appropriate barley cultivars in specific areas in order to maximize β-glucan levels.

References

Bamba, T., Kanauchi, O., Andoh, A., and Fujiyama, Y., A new prebiotic from germinated barley for nutraceutical treatment of ulcerative colitis, *J. Gastroeneterol. Hepatol.,* 17:818–824, 2002.

Deguchi, T., Ohba, R., and Ueda, S., Radical scavenging activity of a purple pigment, hordeumin, from uncooked barley bran-fermented broth, *J. Agric. Food Chem.,* 48:3198–3201, 2000.

Kanauchi, O., Nakamura, T., Agate, K., Mitsuyama, K., and Iwanaga, T., Effects of germinated barley foodstuff on dextran sulfate sodium-induced colitis in rats, *J. Gastroenterol.,* 33:179–188, 1998.

Kanauchi, O., Iwanaga, T., and Andoh, A., The dietary fibre fraction of germinated barley foodstuff (GMF) attenuated mucosal damage and diarrhea and accelerated repair of the colonic mucosa in a rate model of experimental colitis, *J. Gastroenterol. Hepatol.,* 16:160–168, 2001.

Mitsuyama, K., Saiki, T., and Kanauchi, O., Treatment of ulcerative colitis with germinated barley foodstuff: A pilot study, *Aliment. Pharmacol. Ther.,* 12:1225–1230, 1998.

Zhang, G., Junmei, W., and Jinxin, C., Analysis of β-glucan content in barley cultivars from different locations of China, *Food Chem.,* 79:251–254, 2002.

Basil (*Ocimum basilicum*) Basil (*Ocimum basilum* L. Laminiaceae) is a common herb used for culinary and medical purposes. The essential oil obtained from basil was reported to exhibit antimicrobial activity, as well as inhibit the fungus *Aspergillus ochraceus* and the production of ochratoxin A (Hili et al., 1997; Basilico and Basilico, 1999). A recent study by Opalchenova and Obreshkova (2003) identified the main components in basil by gas chromatography as linalool (59.5 percent), methylchavikol (12 percent), and methylcinnamate (7.2 percent). They also examined whether basil could inhibit multidrug-resistant clinical isolates of the genera *Staphyloccocus, Enterococcus,* and *Pseudomonas*. Basil proved

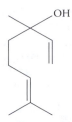

Linalool. (From Letizia et al., *Food Chem. Toxicol.*, 41:943–964, 2003. With permission.)

effective against these antibiotic-resistant tested bacteria with minimum inhibitory concentrations ranging from 0.0030–0.0007 percent.

Basil oil was also reported to exhibit anti-inflammatory properties against carrageenan, PGE_2, leukotriene, and arachidonic acid-induced paw edema in rats (Singh, 1998, 1999 a, b, c). Courreges and Benecia (2002) further explored possible immunomodulatory effects of basil oil on mouse macrophages. Exposure of macrophages to basil oil for a 24-hour period significantly inhibited phagocytosis, with complete inhibition with dilutions of 1:2000 and 1:1000 (Table B.10).

Javanmardi et al. (2003) screened 23 Iranian basils as sources of antioxidants and phenolics. They found them to be good sources of antioxidants because of their strong radical-scavenging activities. A positive linear relationship was observed between antioxidant activity and total phenolic acids for the basil samples examined.

References

Basilico, M.Z. and Basilico, J.C., Inhibitory effects of some spice essential oils on *Aspergillus ochraceus* NRRL 3174 growth and ochratoxin A production, *Lett. Appl. Micobiol.*, 29:135–141, 1999.

Courreges, M.C. and Benecia, F., *In vitro* antiphagocytic effect of basil oil on mouse macrophages, *Fitoterapia*, 73:369–374, 2002.

Hili, P., Evans, C.S., and Veness, R.G., Antimicrobial action of essential oils: The effect of dimethyl sulfoxide on the activity of cinnamon oil, *Lett. Appl. Microbiol.*, 24:269–275, 1997.

Javanmardi, J., Stushnoff, C., Locke, E., and Vivanco, J.M., Antioxidant activity and total phenol content of Iranian *Ocimum* accessions, *Food Chem.*, 83:547–550, 2003.

Letizia, C.S., Cocchiara, J., Lalko, J., and Api, A.M., Fragrance material review of linalool, *Food Chem. Toxicol.*, 41:943–964, 2003.

Opalchenova, G. and Obreshkova, D., Comparative studies on the activity of basil — an essential oil from *Ocimum basilicum* L., *J. Micobiol. Methods*, 54: 105–110, 2003.

Singh, S., Comparative evaluation of anti-inflammatory potential of fixed oil of different species of Ocimum and its possible mechanism of action, *Indian J. Exp. Biol.*, 36:1028–1031, 1998.

Singh, S., Mechanism of action of anti-inflammatory effect of fixed oil of *Ocimum basilicum* Linn, *Indian J. Exp. Biol.*, 37:248–252, 1999a.

TABLE B.10
Effect of Basil Oil and Phagocytic Activity and Respiratory Burst in Mouse Peritoneal Macrophages

Basil-oil Dilution	Percent of Phagocytosis	Percent Cells Including Precipitated Formazan
1:1000	0.6 ± 0.6^{1}	0.4 ± 0.6^{1}
1:2000	0.4 ± 1.3^{1}	3.4 ± 1.3^{1}
1:4000	45.2 ± 3.7^{1}	43.6 ± 5.2^{1}
1:8000	78.3 ± 6.6^{2}	82.2 ± 4.7^{2}
1:16000	89.4 ± 5.1^{ns}	92.7 ± 5.3^{ns}
Control	96.8 ± 5.8	98.3 ± 7.4

[1] $p < 0.005$; [2] $p < 0.05$; [ns] Not significant.

Source: From Courreges and Benecia, *Fitoterapia*, 73:369–374, 2002. With permission.

Singh, S., Evaluation of gastric antiulcer activity of fixed oil of *Ocumum basilicum* Linn and its possible mechanism of action, *Indian J. Exp. Biol.,* 37:253–257, 1999b.

Singh, S., Effect of *Ocimum sanctum* fixed oil on vascular permeability and leukocytes migration, *Indian J. Exp. Biol.,* 37:1136–1138, 1999c.

Beans   Beans are an important part of our diet and represent a good source of protein and nutrients. The consumption of beans, particularly in Mexico, has a long history and was estimated at 19.5 kg/annum per capita (Gonzalez de Mejia, 1990). The importance of phenolic compounds in plant foods, including beans, is related to their effect on nutritional and esthetic properties. In addition to their antioxidant and chelating properties, they are able to scavenge reactive-oxygen species and electrophiles, as well as modulate cellular-enzyme activities (Huang and Ferraro, 1992). The antimutagenic properties of the phenolic compounds from common beans (*Phaseolus vulgaris*) were reported by Gonzalez de Maija et al. (1999). The majority of polyphenols were located in the seed coat with negligible amounts in the cotyledons. The key antimutagenic compounds in beans, easily extracted with methanol, were phenols, while low-molecular-weight hydrolyzable phenols were present in the aqueous extract. The phenolic compounds specifically identified were catechin, tannic acid, and ellagic acid. These compounds were effective against the mutagenic activities of 1-nitropyrene (1-NP) and benzo[α]pyrene using the *Salmonella typhimurium* tester strain YG1024 in the plate-incorporation test. Dose-dependent inhibition was observed for all the samples tested. Doses of 500 µg equivalent catechin/plate resulted in 63%, 81%, and 83% inhibition for water, water/methanol, and methanol extracts, respectively. The greatest inhibition was evident for the methanol extract at lower doses of 50 µg equivalent catechin/plate. These results were consistent with earlier findings by Mandal and coworkers (1987) regarding the antimutagenic effects of ellagic acid.

References

Gonzalez de Mejia, E., Caracterizacion fiscoquimica e implicaciones nutricias de las lectinas de frijol tepari y sus hibridos, Ph.D dissertation, CIN-VESTAV-Unidad Irapuato, Irapuato, Gto, Mexico, 1990.

Gonzalez de Mejia, E., Castano-Tostado, E., and Loarca-Pina, G., Antimutagenic effects of natural phenolic compounds in beans, *Met. Res. Gen. Toxicol. Environ. Mutageneis.,* 441:1–9, 1999.

Huang, M. and Ferraro, T., Phenolic compounds in food and cancer prevention, in *Phenolic Compounds in Food and their Effects on Health. II. Analysis, Occurrence and Chemistry,* C. Ho, C., Lee, C.Y., and Huang, M., Eds., American Chemical Society, Washington, D.C., 1992, pp. 8–35.

Mandal, S., Ahuja, A., Shivapurkar, N.M., Sheng, S.J., Groopman, J.D., and Stoner, G.D., Inhibition of aflatoxin B in *Salmonella typhimurium* and DNA damage in cultured rat and human tracheobronchial tissues by ellagic acid, *Carcinogenesis,* 8:1651–1656, 1987.

Bearberry *see also* **Uva-ursi**   Bearberry (*Arctostaphylos uva-ursi* L.) is a small shrub that grows in the northern latitudes and high mountains of Europe, Asia, and America. Its astringent leaves have medicinal properties and are used as a disinfectant in the treatment of lower urinary-tract infections. One of the principal components of bearberry-leaf extracts is arbutin (hydroquinone-1-*O*-β-D-glucoside), which forms urinary metabolites that are conjugates with glucuronic and sulfuric acids (Paper et al., 1993; Siegers et al., 1997). These metabolites appear to be precursors of hydroquinone, which is released in the lower urinary tract where it kills or inhibits bacteria. Pegg and coworkers (2001) reported the presence of a natural antioxidant in the ethanol extracts of bearberry leaves, which proved to be very effective in nitrite-free processed meats. Bacterial surface hydrophobicity appears to be related to the ability of certain pathogens to cause infection. Thus, an increase in hydrophobicity is strongly correlated with enhanced pathogenic potential (Absolom, 1988; Andersson et al., 1998). Altering surface hydrophobicity could provide an effective way of decreasing the viability of pathogenic bacteria in food or in the

Arbutin (1, R = CH$_2$OH) and hydroquinone glucuronide (1, R = COOH) and hydroquinone sulfate potassium salt (2). (From Glockle et al., *J. Chromatogr. B*, 761:261–266, 2001. With permission.)

gastrointestinal tract. Annuk et al. (1999) compared aqueous extracts of four medicinal plants, including bearberry, on the cell surface hydrophobicity of the Gram-negative pathogen *Hylobacter pylori*. Bearberry extract proved to be the richest source of tannic acid and was attributed for the decrease in cell surface hydrophobicity and its antibacterial activity against *Hylobacter pylori*. Recent work by Dykes and coworkers (2003a) examined the effect of an antioxidant ethanolic extract from bearberry leaves on the surface hydrophobicity of 25 food-related bacteria. The bearberry extract significantly decreased the hydrophobicity of only four bacteria, while significantly increasing the hydrophobicity of 14. These researchers cautioned against marketing a particular extract, such as bearberry, based on a single claim, as there may be detrimental effects on food-related bacteria associated with such nutraceuticals. For example, increased antibiotic resistance in bacteria was recently associated with their exposure to certain neutraceutical extracts (Ward et al., 2002). However, Dykes et al. (2003b) also studied the effect of an ethanolic extract from bearberry, alone or in combination with nisin, on 25 food-related bacteria. Although bearberry did not exhibit any antimicrobial activity, it enhanced the antibacterial efficacy of nisin against Gram-positive bacteria, particularly *Brochothrix thermosphacta*.

References

Absolom, D.R., The role of bacterial hydrophobicity in infection: Bacterial adhesion and phagocyte ingestion, *Can. J. Microbiol.*, 34:287–298, 1988.

Andersson, A., Granum, P.E., and Ronner, U., The adhesion of *Bacillus cereus* spores to epithelial cells might be an additional virulence mechanism, *Internat. J. Food Microbiol.*, 39:93–99, 1998.

Annuk, H., Hirmo, S., Turi, E., Mikelsaar, M., Arak, E., and Wadstrom, T., Effect on cell surface hydrophobicity and susceptibility of *Helicobacter pylori*, *FEMS Microbiol. Lett.*, 172:41–45, 1999.

Dykes, G.A., Amarowicz, R., and Pegg, R.B., An antioxidant bearberry (*Arctostaphylos uva-ursi*) extract modulates surface hydrophobicity of a wide range of food-related bacteria: Implications for functional food safety, *Food Control*, 14:515–518, 2003a.

Dykes, G.A., Amarowicz, R., and Pegg, R.B., Enhancement of nisin antibacterial activity by a bearberry (*Arctostaphylos uva-ursi*) leaf extract, *Food Microbiol.*, 20:211–216, 2003b.

Glockl, I., Blaschke, G., and Veit, M., Validated methods for direct determination of hydroquinone glucuronide and sulfate in human urine after oral intake of bearberry leaf extract by capillary zone electrophoresis, *J. Chromatogr.*, B. 761:261–266, 2001.

Paper, D.H., Kohler, J., and Franz, G., 1993. Bioavailability of drug preparations containing a leaf extract of *Arctostaphylos uva-ursi* (L.), *Pharmaceut. Pharmacol. Lett.*, 3:63–66, 1993.

Pegg, R.B., Amarowicz, R., and Barl, B., Applications of plant phenolics in model and meat systems, in *Proceedings of the 47th International Congress of Meat Science. Technology*, Krakow, Poland, Vol. II, 234–235, 2001.

Siegers, C.P., Siegers, J.P., Pentz, C., Bodinet, C., and Freudenstein, J., Metabolism of arbutin from uva ursi-extracts in humans, *Pharm. Pharmacol. Lett.*, 7: 90–92, 1997.

Ward, P., Fasitsas, S., and Katz, S.E., Inhibition, resistance development, and increased antibiotic and antimicrobial resistance caused by nutraceuticals, *J. Food Prot.*, 65:528–533, 2002.

Beer   Epidemiological studies showed an inverse relationship between moderate ethanol consumption and risk of coronary heart disease

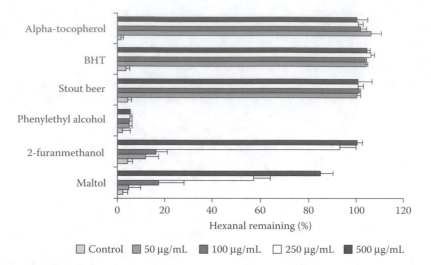

FIGURE B.10 Relative amounts of hexanal remaining in hexane samples containing volatiles, (a) phenylethyl alcohol; (b) 2-furanmethanol; (c) maltol. (From Wei et al., *J. Agric. Food Chem.,* 49:4097–4101, 2001. With permission.)

(Gronback et al. 1995; Kannel and Ellison, 1996). Reduced mortality was associated with the consumption of beer and wine but not with spirits. An increase in plasma antioxidant levels was reported by Ghiselli and coworkers (1999) in healthy, fasting nonsmokers consuming 500 mL beer in the morning. The antioxidants present in beer were phenolic acids, of which syringic and sinapic acids were the most significant. Wei et al. (2001) examined the antioxidant properties of volatiles extracted from stout beer, particularly phenylethyl alcohol, maltol, and 2-furanmethanol. Measuring antioxidant activity, as the reduction in the oxidation of hexanal to hexanoic acid, 2-furanmethanol and maltol were far more effective in preventing hexanal oxidation compared to phenylethyl alcohol (Figure B.10).

In addition to polyphenols, Gorinstein et al. (2002) reported the presence of protein and amino acids in beer. To assess whether these proteins were biologically active, these researchers examined the effect of lyophilized polyphenol-free beer and lyophilized polyphenol-free wine on rat-plasma lipids over four weeks. Only the group fed the diet supplemented with beer significantly lowered total cholesterol, LDL cholesterol, and triacylglycerols, pointing to the potential contribution by the proteins and essential amino acids present in beer. Thus, moderate consumption of beer

appears to be as beneficial as moderate consumption of wine.

Arimoto-Koyabashi and coworkers (1999) found native and freeze-dried Japanese-beer samples inhibited the genotoxicity of several heterocyclic amines and N-methyl-N'-nitro-N-nitrosoguani-dine (MNNG). Kimura et al. (1999) isolated an antimutagen in beer, glycine betaine, but it had no effect on MNNG. However, the first nucleoside with antimutagenic properties against MNNG was reported by Yoshikawa et al. (2002) who identified a pseudouridine compound in one of six antimutagenic fractions isolated from freeze-dried beer. Pseudouridine was present at around 0.4 mg/100 mL beer but only accounted for 3 percent of the beer's total antimutagenicity. The major compounds responsible for the bioactive properties of the beer still remained to be identified.

Nozawa et al. (2004) reported the inhibitory effects of four commercial beers, two pilsner-types, a black beer, and a stout beer, against five heterocyclic amine carcinogens. They all exhibited antimutagenic properties by inhibiting the genotoxic effects of these carcinogens, as well as significantly reducing the number of ACF in rats fed a diet containing these carcinogens.

Bamforth (2002), in reviewing the nutritional properties of beer, noted its contribution to certain B vitamins, minerals, antioxidants, and possibly fiber.

B

References

Arimoto-Kobayashi, S., Sugiyama, C., Harada, N., Takeuchi, M., Takemura, M., and Hayatsu, H., Inhibitory effects of beer and other alcoholic beverages on mutagenesis and DNA adduct formation induced by several carcinogens, *J. Agric. Food Chem.*, 47: 221–230, 1999.

Bamforth, C.W., Nutritional aspects of beer — a review, *Nutr. Res.*, 22:227–237, 2001.

Ghiselli, A., Natella, F., Guidi, A., Montanari, L., Fantozzi, P., and Scaccini, C., Beer increases plasma antioxidant capacity in humans, *J. Nutr. Biochem.*, 11:76–80, 2000.

Gorinstein, S., Leontowicz, H., Lojek, A., Leontowicz, M., Eiz, M., Stager, M.A.G., Montes. J.M.B., Toledo, F., Arancibia-Avila, P., and Trakhtenberg, S., Hypolipidemic effect of beer proteins in experiment on rats, *Lebensm. Wiss u-Technol.*, 35:265–271, 2002.

Gronback, A.M., Deis, A., Sorensen, T.I.A., Becker, U., Schnohr, P., and Jensen, G., Mortality associated with moderate intakes of wine, beer, or spirits, *BMJ*, 310:1165–1169, 1995.

Kannel, W.B. and Ellison, R.C., Alcohol and coronary disease: The evidence for a protective effect, *Clin. Chim. Acta*, 246:59–76, 1996.

Kimura, S., Hayatsu, H., and Arimoto-Kobayashi, S., Glycine betaine in beer as an antimutagenic substance against 2-chloro-4-methylthiobutanoic acid, the samma fish mutagen, *Mutat. Res.*, 439:267–276, 1999.

Nozawa, H., Tazumi, K., Sato, K., Yoshida, A., Takata, J., Arimoto-Kobayashi, S., and Kondo, K., Inhibitory effects of beer on heterocyclic amine-induced mutagenesis and PhIP-induced aberrant crypt foci in rat colon, *Mutat. Res.*, 559:177–187, 2004.

Wei, A., Mura, K., and Shibamoto, T., Antioxidative activity of volatile chemicals extracted from beer, *J. Agric. Food Chem.*, 49:4097–4101, 2001.

Yoshikawa, T., Kimura, S., Hatano, T., Okamoto, K., Hayatsu, H., and Arimoto-Kobayashi, S., Pseudouridine, an antimutagenic substance in beer towards N-methyl-N'-nitro-N-nitrosoguanidine (MNNG), *Food Chem. Toxicol.*, 40:1165–1170, 2002.

cells compared to capsanthin, cranberry, red onion skin, and short and long red bell peppers. The root extract also significantly inhibited tumors in mice skin and lungs. Bobek et al. (2000) fed diets supplemented with 15 percent fiber isolated from red beet to Wistar rats with hypercholesterolemia and chemically induced colon cancer. The red-beet diet significantly reduced serum cholesterol (–30 percent) and triacylglycerol (–40 percent) levels while significantly increasing HDL cholesterol. In addition, the number of animals bearing tumors was reduced by 30 percent, although it did not significantly affect the incidence of colon tumors.

Kanner and coworkers (2001) identified a new class of dietary cationized antioxidants in red beets, the betalains. The major one was betanin, a betanidin 5-O-β-glucoside. A relatively low concentration of betanin was found to inhibit lipid peroxidation of membranes or linoleate emulsion by the "free iron" redox cycle, H_2O_2-activated metmyoglobin, lipoxygenase. The bioavailability of betanin was demonstrated by the presence of betacyanin in the urine of four volunteers 2–4 h following the consumption of 300 mL of red beet juice containing 120 mg of the antioxidant.

References

Bobek, P., Galbavy, S., and Mariassyova, M., The effect of red beet (*Beta vulgaris* var. rubra) fiber on alimentary hypercholesterolemia and chemically induced colon carcinogenesis in rats, *Nahrung*, 44: 184–187, 2000.

Kanner, J., Harel, S., and Granit, R., Betalains — A new class of dietary cationized antioxidants, *J. Agric. Food Chem.*, 49:5178–5185, 2001.

Kapadia, G.J., Tokuda, H., Konoshima, T., and Nishino, H., Chemoprevention of lung and skin cancer by *Beta vulgaris* (beet) root extract, *Cancer Lett.*, 100:211–214, 1996.

Beets (*Beta vulgaris*) see also Betalains   Red beets are very popular vegetables used for the production of such ethnic foods as borscht. Kapadia and coworkers (1996) showed a root extract from red beet exhibited the strongest *in vitro* inhibitory effect on Epstein–Barr virus early antigen (ENV-EA) induction using Raji

---

Bell pepper (*Capsicum annuum*) see also Chili Peppers and Peppers   Bell pepper is used extensively in North Africa as a spice to enhance the flavor of food. Its juice was shown to inhibit N-methylnitrosourea-induced colon carcinogenesis in rats (Narisawa et al., 2000). Maoka and coworkers (2001) found that the

B

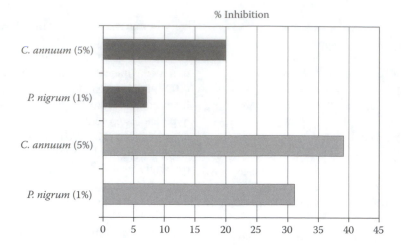

% Inhibition

FIGURE B.11 Pre-treatment effect with bell (*C. capsicum*) and black (*P. nigrum*) peppers on the mutagenicity of 10 mM EC (shaded) and 0.005 percent MMS (black). (Adapted from El Hamss et al., *Food Chem. Toxicol.,* 41:41–47, 2003. With permission.)

carotenoids obtained from the fruits of bell peppers exhibited potent antitumor properties both *in vivo* and *in vitro*. Carotenoids from bell pepper were previously shown to inhibit the mutagenicity of 1-nitropyrene, 1,6-dinitropyrene, and 1,8-dinitropyrene by 87 percent, 79 percent, and 73 percent, respectively (Gonzalez de Meija et al., 1998). Capsaicin, a major component in bell pepper, was shown to inhibit mutagens and carcinogens by modulating cytochrome P450 monooxygenases (Miller et al., 1993). El-Hamss et al. (2003) recently showed bell pepper had strong chemopreventive properties by its antimutagenic effect against promutagen ethyl carbamate (EC) and against the alkylating agent methyl methanesulfonate (MMS) in larvae of *Drosophila melanogaster,* using the wing Somatic Mutation and Recombination Test (SMART). The 2-day-old larvae were pretreated with bell and black peppers 24 h prior to treatment with EC and MMS. In the presence of 5 percent bell pepper, there was a significant reduction ($p < 0.05$) in mutational events by 39 percent from the original 1.02 spots/wing in the presence of EC (10 mM). This was somewhat greater than the 20 percent reduction of wing/spots in the presence of 5 percent bell pepper from the original 4.60 spots/wing in the presence of 0.005 percent MMS (Figure B.11). Black pepper was only effective in reducing mutations induced by EC. The inhibitory effect was attributed to such

compounds as β-carotene, together with small amounts of capsaicin.

References

El Hamss, R., Idaomar, M., and Alonoso-Moraga, A., and Munoz-Serrano, A., Antimutagenic properties of bell and black peppers, *Food Chem. Toxicol.,* 41:41–47, 2003.

Gonzalez de Mejia, E., Quintanar-Hernandez, A., Loarca-Pina, G., and Wurgler, F.A., Antimutagenic activity of carotenoids in green peppers against some nitroarenes, *Mutat. Res.,* 416:11–19, 1998.

Maoka, T., Mochida, K., Kozuka, M., Ito, Y., Fujiwara, Y., Hashimoto, K., Enjo, F., Ogata, M., Nabakuni, Y., Tokuda, H., and Nishino, H., Cancer chemopreventive activity of carotenoids in the fruit of red paprika *Capsicum anuum* L., *Cancer Lett.,* 172:103–109, 2001.

Miller, C.H., Zhang, Z., Hamilton, S.M., and Teele, R.W., Effects of capsaicin on liver microsomal metabolism of the tobacco-specific nitrosamine NNK, *Cancer Lett.,* 75:45–52, 1993.

Narisawa, T., Fukaura, Y., Hasebe, M., Nomura, S., Oshima, S., and Inakuma, Prevention of *N*-methylnitrosoreau-induced colon carinogenesis in rats by oxygenated carotenoid capsanthin and capsanthin-rich paprika juice, *Proc. Soc. Expt. Biol. Med.,* 224:116– 122, 2000.

Berries *see also* **Individual berries**   Berries are rich sources of phenolic pigments and anthocyanins. They are relatively high in phenolic antioxidants, which correlates with their

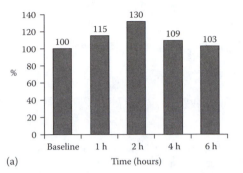

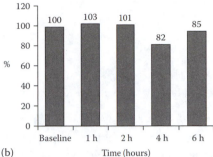

(a)   Time (hours)

(b)   Time (hours)

FIGURE B.12 (a) Relative changes in plasma antioxidant after juice consumption. (b) Relative changes in plasma MDA after juice consumption. (From Netzel et al., *Food Res. Intern.*, 35:213–216, 2002. With permission.)

anthocyanin and phenolic compounds (Heinonen et al., 1998; Prior et al., 1998). Berries, such as strawberries and black raspberries, have been shown to have chemopreventive properties against cancers. Ellagic acid, a major component in these fruits, was found to inhibit carcinogenesis in *in vitro* and *in vivo* studies. Xue et al. (2001) reported that in addition to ellagic acid, a methanolic extract of strawberries and

Ellagic acid. (Adapted from Mertens-Talcott and Percival, *Cancer Lett.*, 218:141–151, 2005.)

black raspberries also displayed chemopreventive properties. Miranda-Rottmann and coworkers (2002) showed Chilean berry [*Aristotelia chilensis* (*ach*)] was much higher in phenolics than blackberry, cranberry, and strawberry, with much higher scores for total radical-trapping potential (TRAP) and other *in vitro* antioxidant capacity tests. The anthocyanins present in *ach* juice prevented copper-induced LDL oxidation, indicating its possible antiantherogenic properties. Netzel et al. (2002) demonstrated the ability of a composite antioxidant-rich juice (30 percent grape, 25 percent black currant, 15 percent elderberry, 10 percent sour cherry, 10 percent blackberry, and 10 percent aronia) to significantly increase the plasma antioxidant

activity (30 percent after 2 h) and significantly reduce plasma MDA (18 percent after 4 h) in six healthy volunteers (Figure B.12 a, b).

References

Heinonen, I.M., Meyer, A.S., and Frankel, E.N., Antioxidant activity of berry phenolics on human low-density lipoprotein and liposome oxidation, *J. Agric. Food Chem.*, 46:4107–4112, 1998.

Mertens-Talcott, S.U. and Percival, S.S., Ellagic acid and quercetin interact synergistically with resveratrol in the induction of apoptosis and cause transient cell cycle arrest in human leukemia cells, *Cancer Lett.*, 218:141–151, 2005.

Miranda-Rottmann, S., Aspillaga, A.A., Pereez, D.D., Vasquez, L., Martinez, L., and Leighton, F., Juice and phenolic fractions of the berry *Aristotelia chilensis* inhibit LDL oxidation *in vitro* and protect human endothelial cells against oxidative stress, *J. Agric. Food Chem.*, 50:7542–7547, 2002.

Netzel, M., Strass, G., Kaul, C., Bitsch, I., Dietrich, H., and Bitsch, R., *In vivo* antioxidative capacity of a composite berry juice, *Food Res. Intern.*, 35:213–216, 2002.

Prior, R.L., Cao, G., Marton, A., Sofic, E., McEwen, J.J., O'Brien, C., Lischner, N.Y., Ehlenfeldt, M., Kalt, W., Krewer, G., and Mainland, C.M., Antioxidant capacity as influenced by total phenolic and anthocyanin content, maturity, and variety of *Vaccinium* species, *J. Agric. Food Chem.*, 46:2686–2693, 1998.

Xue, H., Aziz, R.M., Sun, N., Cassady, J.M., Kamendulis, L.M., Xu, Y., Stoner, G.D., and Klaunig, J.E., Inhibition of cellular transformation by berry extracts, *Carcinogenesis*, 22:831-833, 2001.

All *trans*-β-carotene. (Adapted from Keijer et al., *Biochem. Biophys. Acta,* 1740:139–146, 2005)

β-Carotene   β-Carotene is an important anti-oxidant present in fruits and vegetables. As a carotenoid it is a potent quencher of singlet oxygen and would be expected to exert a protective effect against sunlight-induced erythema in human skin (Gollnick et al. 1996; Biesalski and Obermiller-Jevic, 2001) and photoimmunosuppression (Fuller et al., 1992; Herraiz et al., 1992). Trekli and coworkers (2003) examined the effect of β-carotene on UVA-induced HO-1 gene expression in a cultured human fibroblast line FEK4. Activation of the HO-1 gene has become a sensitive marker for oxidative stress. These researchers showed β-carotene inhibited activation of the HO-1 gene, probably through scavenging singlet oxygen.

Considerable controversy surrounds β-carotene, as three randomized clinical trials showed that it alone, or in combination with vitamins A and E, increased lung-cancer incidence and mortality in heavy smokers and in asbestos workers (The Alpha-Tocopherol, Beta-Carotene Cancer Prevention Study Group, 1994; Stram et al., 2002; Omenn et al., 1996a, b). Paolini et al. (2003) reviewed the data on β-carotene and suggested it was harmful when given as the sole supplement to smokers or individuals exposed to environmental carcinogens. The high levels of cytochrome P450 isoforms induced by β-carotene under these conditions could predispose individuals to higher cancer risk as a result of bioctivation of procarcinogens or by increased production of reactive-oxygen species. Thus, β-carotene may act as a cocarcinogen, particularly in individuals exposed to tobacco smoke or industrial settings. However, under normal circumstances, β-carotene exhibits both antioxidant and anticancer properties.

References

The Alpha-Tocopherol, Beta-Carotene Cancer Prevention Study Group, The effect of vitamin E and β-carotene on the incidence of lung cancer and other cancers in male smokers, *N. Engl. J. Med.,* 330: 1029–1035, 1994.

Biesalski, H.K. and Obermueller-Jevic, U.C., UV light, β-carotene, and human skin: Beneficial and potentially harmful effects, *Arch. Biochem. Biophys.,* 389: 1–6, 2001.

Fuller, C.J., Faulkner, H., Bendich, A., Parker, R.S., and Roe, D.A., Effect of β-carotene supplementation on photosuppression of delayed-type hypersensitivity in normal young men, *Am. J. Clin. Nutr.,* 56:684–690, 1992.

Gollnick, H.P.M., Hopfenmueller, W., Hemmes, C., Chun, S.C., Schmid, C., Sundameier, K., and Biesalski, H.K., Systemic β-carotene plus topical UV sunscreen are an optimal protection against harmful effects of natural UV sunlight, *Eur. J. Dermatol.,* 6: 200–295, 1996.

Herraiz, L.A., Hsieh, W.C., Bendich, A., Parker, R.S., and Swanson, J.E., Effect of UV exposure and β-carotene supplementation on delayed-type sensitivity response in healthy older males, *J. Am. Coll. Nutr.,* 176:617–624, 1998.

Keijer, J., Bunschoten, A., Palou, A., and Franssen-van Hal, N.L.W., Beta-carotene and the application of transcriptomics in risk-benefit evaluation of natural dietary components, *Biochem. Biophys. Acta,* 1740:139–146, 2005.

Omenn, G.S., Goodman, G.E., Thornquist, M.D., Balmes, J., Cullen, M.R., Glass, A., Keogh, J.P., Meyskens, F.L., Jr., Valanis, B., Williams, J.H., Jr., Barnhartm S., Cherniack, M.G., Brodkin, C.A., and Hammer, S., Risk factors for lung cancer and for intervention effects in CARET, the beta-carotene and efficacy trial. *J. Ntl. Cancer Inst.,* 88:1550–1559, 1996a.

Omenn, G.S., Goodman, G.E., Thornquist, M.D., Balmes, J., Cullen, M.R., Glass, A., Keogh, J.P., Meyskens, F.L., Jr., Valanis, B., Williams, J.H., Jr., Barnhart, S., and Hammar, S., Effects of a combination of β-carotene and vitamin A on lung cancer and cardiovascular disease, *N. Engl. J. Med.,* 334:1150–1155, 1996b.

Paolini, M., Abdel-Rahman, S.Z., Sapone, A., Pedulli, G.F., Perocco, P., Cantelli-Forti, G., and Legator, M.S., β–Carotene: A cancer chemopreventive agent or a co-carcinogen, *Mut. Res.,* 543:195–200, 2003.

Stram, D.O., Huberman, M., and Wu, A., Is residual confounding a reasonable explanation for the apparent protective effects of β-carotene found in epidemiologic studies of lung cancers and smokers? *Am. J. Epidemiol.,* 155:622–628, 2002.

Trekli, M.C., Riss, G., Goralczyk, R., and Tyrrell, R.M., Beta-carotene suppresses UVA-induced HO-1 gene expression in cultured FEK4, *Free Rad. Biol. Med.,* 34:456–464, 2003.

Betalains   Betalains are water-soluble pigments containing nitrogen and include red-violet betacyanins and yellow betaxanthins. Betacyanins are a group of compounds exhibiting antioxidant and radical-scavenging activities (Escribano et al., 1998; Pedrano and Escribano, 2000). Betalains are a class of cationic antioxidants found in red beets. One of the major ones, betanin or betanidin 5-*O*-β-glucoside, was shown by Kanner and coworkers (2001) to inhibit linoleate peroxidation with an IC_{50} value of 0.4 µM compared to 1.2 and 5.0 for catechin and α-tocopherol, respectively. Betanin (IC_{50} < 2.5 µM) inhibited lipid peroxidation of membranes or linoleate emulsions catalyzed by the

"free iron" redox cycle, H_2O_2-activated met-myoglobin or lipoxygenase and was more effective than catechin. The bioavailability of betanin was demonstrated in four volunteers with 0.5–0.9 percent detected in the urine. An excellent review of betalain was published by Strack and coworkers (2002).

References

Escribano, J., Pedreno, M.A., Garcia-Carmona, F., and Munoz, R., Characterization of the antiradical activity of betalains from *Beta vulgaris* roots, *Phytochem. Anal.,* 9:124–127, 1998.

Kanner, J., Harel, S., and Granit, R., Betalains — A new class of dietary cationized antioxidants, *J. Agric. Food Chem.,* 49:5178–5185, 2001.

Pedreno, M.A. and Escribano, J., Studying the oxidation and antiradical activity of betalain from beetroot, *J. Biol.,* 35:49–59, 2000.

Strack, D., Vogt, T., and Schliemann, W., Recent advances in betalain research, *Phytochemistry,* 62: 247–269, 2002.

Bilberry   Bilberry, a low-growing shrub, grows mainly in the U.K., northern Europe, and Asia. Its dark-blue berries are used mainly for tarts and preserves. The main phenolic constituents in bilberry (*Vaccinium myrtillus* L.) are anthocyanins. Madhavi et al. (1998) identified

Betanin ($R^1 = R^2 = H$). (From Strack et al., *Phytochemistry,* 62:247–269, 2002. With permission.)

TABLE B.11
DPPH Radical-Scavenging Activity, Total Phenolic, and Anthocyanin Contents in Berry Extracts

	Total Phenolics (mg/g)	Anthocyanin (mg/g)	DPPH Radical-Scavenging Activity (µmol of Trolox/g)
Bilberry	55.1 ± 1.0	26.3 ± 1.5	287.9 ± 10.3
Blackberry	42.5 ± 0.3	10.0 ± 0.6	238.5 ± 5.9
Black Currant	40.9 ± 0.7	15.3 ± 0.7	200.3 ± 3.3
Raspberry	39.0 ± 0.6	4.4 ± 0.2	208.0 ± 8.5
Lowbush Blueberry	35.9 ± 0.4	12.1 ± 0.5	178.1 ± 5.4
Cowberry	35.4 ± 0.1	6.1 ± 0.4	196.9 ± 6.4
Highbush Blueberry	26.4 ± 0.4	6.3 ± 0.4	128.4 ± 8.2
Strawberry	22.5 ± 0.2	2.4 ± 0.2	121.6 ± 4.5
Cranberry	20.1 ± 0.4	3.1 ± 0.2	92.9 ± 2.3
Red Currant	13.0 ± 0.1	2.3 ± 0.1	71.3 ± 3.4

Source: From Katsube et al., *J. Agric. Food Chem.*, 51:68–75, 2003. With permission.

a major flavonoid fraction containing proanthocyanidins and anthocyanin pigments together with a hexane extract containing chlorophylls, carotenoids, sterols, and lipids in tissues extracted from bilberry fruits and callus cultures. Many of these constituents not only protected against initiation of carcinogenesis but prevented proliferation of the cancer cell lines. This was evident by the ability of the hexane extract to induce the phase II xenobiotic detoxification enzyme, quinone reductase (QR), in murine hepatoma cells.

A study by Logan and Wong (2001) showed bilberry may be beneficial in the treatment of chronic-fatigue syndrome through its control of oxidative stress. Head (2001) suggested a number of botanicals, including bilberries, could also prevent cataracts, particularly by inhibition of aldolase reductase activity. Katsube et al. (2003) recently reported that the phenolic and anthocyanin content, as well as DPPH radical-scavenging activity, was highest in the bilberry extract (Table B.11). Those anthocyanins eluted with 20–40 percent and 40 percent metanol were the more potent inhibitors of the growth of human promelocytic leukemia HL60 and HCT116 cancer cells, inducing apoptosis in the HL60 cells. The anticancer effects exhibited by bilberries make them a potential functional food.

References

Head, K.A., Natural therapies for ocular disorders, part two: Cataracts and glaucoma, *Altern. Med. Rev.*, 6:141–166, 2001.

Katsube, N., Iwashita, K., Tsushida, T., Yamaki, K., and Kobori, M., Induction of apoptosis in cancer cells by bilberry (*Vaccinium myrtillus*) and the anthocyanins, *J. Agric. Food Chem.*, 51:68–75, 2003.

Logan, A.C. and Wong, C., Chronic fatigue syndrome: Oxidative stress and dietary modifications, *Altern. Med. Rev.*, 6:450–459, 2001.

Madhavi, D.L., Bomser, J., Smith, M.A.L., and Singletary, K., Isolation of bioactive constituents from *Vaccinium myrtillus* (bilberry) fruits and cell cultures, *Plant Sci.*, 131:95–103, 1998.

Bitter tea (*Ligustrum pedunculare*) Bitter tea is a popular beverage in China. In contrast to green and oolong teas, which are prepared from the leaves of *Camellia sinensis*, bitter tea is brewed from the leaves of 10 species in five different families (He et al., 1992). Wong and coworkers (2001) characterized the antioxidants present in one of these species, *Ligustrum purpuracens,* as two phenylethanoid glycosides, acteoside and ligpurposide A. Both

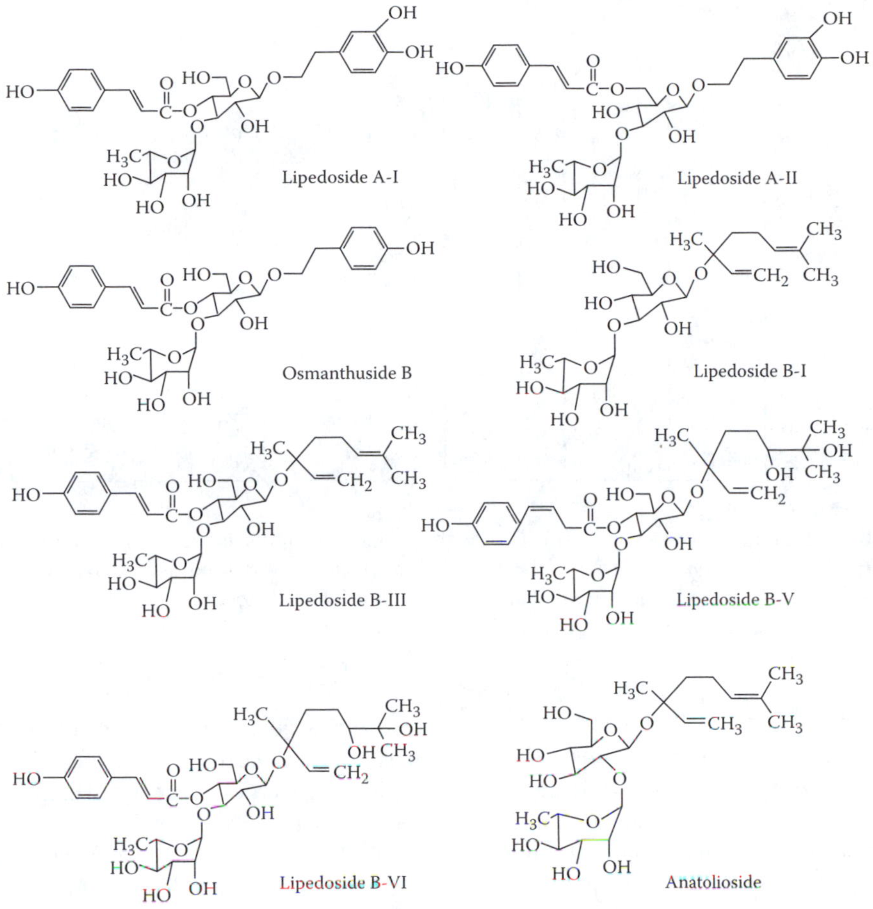

SCHEME B.8 Structures of phenylethanoid and monoterpene glycosides in bitter-tea beverage derived from the plant *L. pedunculare*. (From Chen et al., *J. Agric. Food Chem.,* 50:7530–7535, 2002. With permission.)

proved to be effective antioxidants comparable to green tea catechins. Further work by Chen and coworkers (2002) characterized the antioxidants in *Ligustrum pedunculare,* another species used for brewing bitter tea in Suchuan Province of China. He et al. (1994) previously isolated eight phenylethanoid or monoterpene glycosides in this species. Chen and coworkers (2002) showed the crude glycoside fraction prevented the oxidation of human low-density lipoprotein (Scheme B.8). Four out of the eight monoterpene glycosides (lipedosides B-V, B-VI, A-I and A-II) protected LDL from Cu^{2+}-mediated oxidation, as well as exhibited free-radical scavenging activity on DPPH equivalent to that of α-tocopherol (Figure B.13).

References

Chen, Z.Y., Wong, I.Y., Leung, M.W., He, Z.D., and Huang, Y., Characterization of antioxidants present in bitter tea (*Ligustrum pedunculare*), *J. Agric. Food Chem.,* 50:7530–7535, 2002.

He, Z.D., Liu, Y.Q., and Yang, C.R., Glycosides from *Ligustrum purpurascen, Acta Bot. Yunnanica.,* 14:328–336, 1992.

He, Z.D., Ueda, S., Akaji, M., Fujita, T., Inoue, K., and Yang, C., Monoterpenoid and phenylethanoid glycosides from *Ligustrum pedunculare, Phytochemistry,* 36:709–716, 1994.

Wong, I.Y., He, Z.D., Huang, Y., and Chen, Z.Y., Antioxidative activities of phenylethanoid glycosides from *Ligustrum purpurascens, J. Agric. Food Chem.,* 49:3113–3119, 2001.

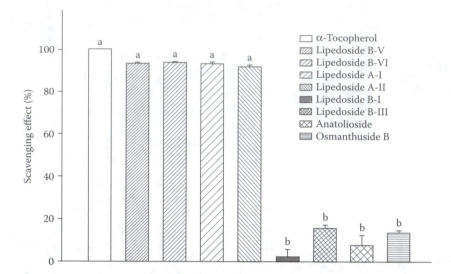

FIGURE B.13 Free-radical-scavenging effects of eight phenylethanoid or monoterpene glycosides (10 μM) isolated from *L. pedunculare*. 2,2-Diphenyl-1-picrylhydrazyl DPPH was used as a stable free radical. α-Tocopherol was used as a reference antioxidant. Means with different letters (a, b) differ significantly at $p < 0.05$. (From Chen et al., *J. Agric. Food Chem.*, 50:7530–7535, 2002. With permission.)

Black beans   Carmona et al. (1996) showed that condensed tannins isolated from black beans strongly inhibited α-amylase, maltase, sucrase, and lactase enzyme activities *in vitro*. The tannins also affected *in vitro* glucose uptake by rat-everted intestinal sleeves, which could explain the reduction in carbohydrate bioavailability found in animals fed high tannin diets. Chao and coworkers (1998) showed that water and organic-solvent extracts of black bean exhibited much higher antioxidant capacity compared to equivalent extracts from soybeans. The ability to inhibit LDL oxidation in plasma of patients suffering from cardiovascular disease was positively correlated with GSH, genistein, anthocyanin, and TAS in the water extract, and vitamin E, genistein, and anthocyanin in the organic extracts for all treatments.

The ability of black beans to bind bile acids *in vitro* was examined by Kahlon and Woodruff (2002). The cholesterol-lowering properties of food components can be predicted from their ability to bind bile acids, which in turn lowers the risk of cardiovascular disease. These researchers found that both black beans and pinto beans had much higher bile-acid-binding properties compared to soybean protein, suggesting black beans have important health-promoting properties. Recent research by Bawadi et al. (2004) showed that the water-soluble condensed tannins isolated from black beans inhibited the growth of Caco-2 colon, MCF-7 and Hs578T breast, and DV145 prostatic cancer cells without affecting normal human fibroblast lung cells.

References

Bawadi, H.A., Bansode, R.R., Trappey, A., Truax, R.E., and Losso, J.N., Inhibition of Caco-2 colon, MCF-7 and Hs578T breast, and DU145 prostatic cancer cell proliferation by water-soluble black bean condensed tannins, *Cancer Lett.*, 218:153–162, 2005.

Carmona. A., Borgudd, L., Borges, G., and Levy-Benshimol, A., Effect of black bean tannins on *in vitro* carbohydrate digestion and absorption, *J. Nutr. Biochem.*, 7:445–450, 1996.

Chao, P.-Y., Tai, W.-C., Wang, S.-P., and Hu, S.-P., The antioxidative capacity of black bean extract, *Atherosclerosis,* 136(1), P, S37–S61, 1998.

Kahlon, T.S. and Woodruff, C.L., *In vitro* binding of bile acids by soy protein, pinto beans, black beans and wheat gluten, *Food Chem.*, 79:425–429, 2002.

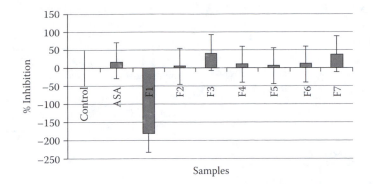

FIGURE B.14 Histogram of inhibition of hyaluronidase by crude extract (F1) and fractions (F2–F7) from chromatographic separation of blackberry fruit. (From Marquina et al., *Fitoterapia*, 73:727–729, 2002. With permission.)

Blackberry (*Rubus fructicosus* B.)   Blackberry is a small tree with red-blackish berries rich in polyphenols (Otaiza, 1997). It was reported that blackberry fruit exhibited anti-inflammatory activity (Thinquino, 1993). Marquina et al. (2002) assessed the anti-inflammatory activity of a number of different aqueous extract fractions from blackberry based on their ability to inhibit hyaluronidase activity. Several of these fractions were stronger inhibitors than aspirin (Figure B.14).

References

Marquina, M.A., Corao, C.M., Araujo, L., Buitrago, D., and Sosa, M., Hyaluronidase inhibitory activity from polyphenols in the fruit of blackberry (*Rubus fructicosus* B.), *Fitoterapia*, 73:727–729, 2002.

Otaiza, R., Plantas usuales en la medicina popular de Merida, Etidad por el consejo de desarrollo cientific, y tecnologia (C.D.C.H.T.) ULA, *Medria*, P, 177, 1997.

Thinquino, B., Terapias naturales. Publicaciones Latinoamericana Rayos de Luiz, Colombia, P, 330, 1993.

Black cohosh   Black cohosh (*Actea racemosa* and *Cimicifuga racemosa*) is related to the buttercup family, a perennial plant native to North America. Its botanical name was recently changed from *Cimicifuga racemosa* (L.) Nutt. to *Actea racemosa* (Ranunculaceae) (Compton et al., 1998a, b). Extracts prepared from its roots and rhizomes are standardized to 26-deoxy-actein content, a member of a group of compounds known as saponins (Chen et al., 2001). It is used as an alternative to hormone-replacement therapy to treat hot flashes and other menopausal symptoms (Lieberman, 1998; Hardy, 2000). A randomized, double-blind, placebo-controlled study of 80 menopausal women treated with a black-cohosh extract was compared to a control of conjugated estrogens over a 12-week period (Stoll, 1987). A marked decrease in hot flashes was observed for women on black-cohosh extract (4.9 to 0.7 hot flashes/day) compared to either the control (5.1 to 3.1 hot flashes/day) or estrogen group (5.2 to 3.2 hot flashes/day). A later study also found a similar decrease in hot flashes was experienced by breast-cancer survivors treated with black cohosh or an antiestrogen (Jacobson et al., 2002). The American College of Obstetricians and Gynecologists (ACOG) suggest black cohosh may be helpful in the short term for women with vasomotor symptoms of menopause (ACOG, 2001). Burdette and coworkers (2002) showed methyl caffeate, ferulic acid, and caffeic acid were the primary antioxidants present in methanol extracts of black cohosh that scavenged oxygen radicals and prevented menadione-induced DNA damage.

Li and coworkers (2003) attempted to analyze caffeic-acid derivatives in black cohosh using liquid chromatography/tandem mass spectrometry. A number of derivatives were detected, with six identified as caffeic acid, ferulic acid, isoferulic acid, fukinolic acid, cimicifugic acid A, and cimicifugic acid. Novel compounds with dehydrofukiic acid groups were also reported for the first time in black cohosh. The bioactive properties of these compounds require extensive investigations.

References

American College of Obstetricians and Gynecologists, Use of botanicals for management of menopausal symptoms, ACOG Practice Bulletin, 28:1–11, 2001.

Burdette, J.E., Chen, S.-N., Lu, Z.-Z., Xu, H., White, B.E., Fabricant, D.S., Liu, J., Fong, H.H., Farnsworth, N.R., Constantinou, A.I., van Breeman, R.B., Pezzuto, J.M., and Bolton, J.L., Black cohosh (*Cimicifua racemosa* L.) protects against menadione-induced DNA damage through scavenging reactive oxygen species: Bioassay-directed isolation and characterization of active principles, *J. Agric. Food Chem.*, 50:7022–7028, 2002.

Chen, S.-N., Li, W., Fabricant, D.S., and Santasiero, B.D., Isolation, structure and elucidation and absolute configuration of 26-deoxyactein from *Cimicifuga racemosa* and clarification of nomenclature associated with 27-deoxyactein, *J. Natural Prod.*, 65:601– 605, 2001.

Compton, J.A., Culham, A., Gibbings, J.G., and Jury, S.L., Phylogeny of *Actaea* including *Cimicifuga* (Ranunculaceae) inferred from nrDNA ITS sequence variation, *Biochem. System. Ecol.*, 26:185–197, 1998a.

Compton, J.A., Culham, A., and Jury, S.L., Reclassification of *Actaea* to include *Cimicifuga* and *Souliea* (Ranunculaceae); phylogeny inferred from morphology, nrDNA ITS, and cpDNA trnL-F sequence variation, *Taxon*, 47:593–634, 1998b.

Hardy, M.L., Herbs of special interest to women, *J. Am. Pharm. Assoc.*, 40:234–242, 2000.

Jacobson, J.S., Troxel, A.B., and Evans, J., Klaus, L., Vahdat, L., Kinne, D., Lo, M.S., Moore, A., Rosenmann, P.J., Kaufman, E.L., Neuget, A.I., and Grann, V.R., Randomized trial of black cohosh for the treatment of hot flashes among women with a history of breast disease, *J. Clin. Oncol.*, 19:2739–2745, 2001.

Li, W.L., Sun, Y., Liang, W., Fitzloff, J.F., and van Breeman, R.B., Identification of caffeic acid derivatives in *Actea racemosa* (*Cimicifuga racemosa*, black cohosh) by liquid chromatography/tandem mass spectrometry, *Rapid Commun. Mass Spectrom.*, 17: 978–982, 2003.

Lieberman, S., A review of effectiveness of *Cimicifuga racemosa* (black cohosh) for the symptoms of menopause, *J. Women's Health*, 7:525–529, 1998.

Stoll, W., Phytotherapy influences atrophic vaginal epithelium: Double-blind study of *Cimicifuga* vs estrogenic substances, *Therapeutikon*, 1:23–37, 1987.

Black currant (*Ribes nigrum*) see also Gamma Linolenic Acid (GLA)

Black currant berries have a very dark coloration due to their content of anthocyanin pigments. They also contain large amounts of flavonoids, phenolic acids and proanthocyanidins. The seeds are also recognized for their content of γ-linolenic acid (GLA), an important polyunsaturated fatty acid, which has important health-related properties. GLA remains stable in the seed due to the presence of large amounts of antioxidants. The berries are used in beverages due to their high content of these antioxidants (Constantino et al., 1993). Lu and Foo (2002) confirmed the presence of four major anthocyanins based on rutinosides and glucosides of delphinidin and cyanidin. They also identified for the first time aureisidin and 1-cinnamyl-β-D-glucoside in black currant. The importance of these anthocyanins is related to their antioxidant and pharmaceutical properties (Andersen et al., 1998; Constantino et al., 1992, 1993).

References

Andersen, O.M., Helland, D.E., and Andersen, K.J., Anthocyanidin and nthocyanidin derivatives, and their isolation, for treatment of cancer, diseases caused by lesions in connective tissues, and diseases caused by viruses, *PCT Int. Appl.*, WO 97 41,137 (Cl. C07H17/065), 6 November 1997, NO appl. 96/5,418 17 December 1996 (Chemical Abstracts 128, 10325k), 1997.

Constantino, L., Albasini, A., Rastelli, G., and Benvenuti, S., Activity of crude polyphenolic extracts as scavengers of superoxide radicals and inhibitors of xanthine oxidase, *Planta Med.*, 58:342–344, 1992.

Constantino, L., Rastelli, G., Rossi, T., Bertoldi, M., and Albasini, A., Antilipoperoxidant activity of polyphenolic extracts of *Ribes nigrum* L. *Plant Medicinales et Phytotherapie.*, 26:207–214, 1993.

Lu, Y. and Foo, L.Y., Polyphenolic constituents of blackcurrant seed residue, *Food Chem.*, 80:71–76, 2003.

Black pepper (*Piper nigrum*) *see also* Piperine   Black pepper is a common spice used in foods. It is rich in the alkaloid piperine, which is a member of a group of compounds based on the structure of vanillin, referred to as "vanilloids." It has been shown previously to enhance the serum levels of drugs and nutrients in animals and humans (Bano et al., 1991; Majeed et al., 1996). Badmaev and coworkers (2000) showed that piperine significantly increased the plasma levels of coenzyme Q10 by almost a third compared to the placebo. This effect could be attributed to an earlier study on its thermonutrient activity (Badmaev et al., 1999).

References

Badmaev, V., Majeed, M., and Norkus, E., Piperine, an alkaloid derived from black pepper increases serum response of beta-carotene during 14-days of oral beta-carotene supplementation, *Nutr. Res.*, 19: 381–388, 1999.

Badmaev, V., Majeed, M., and Prakash, L., Piperine derived from black pepper increases the plasma levels of coenzyme Q10 following oral supplementation, *J. Nutr. Biochem.*, 11:109–113, 2000.

Bano, G., Raina, R.K., Zutshi, U., Johri, R.K., and Atal, K., The effect of piperine on pharmacokinetics of phenytoin in healthy volunteers, *Planta Med.*, 53: 568–569, 1987.

Majeed, M., Badmaev, V., and Rajendran, R., Use of piperine to increase the bioavailability of nutritional compounds, US Patent No. 5,536,506 and No. 5,744,161, 1998.

Black tea   Black tea is the fermented tea, which contains a group of yellow- to dark-brown-colored polyphenolic compounds formed during fermentation (Xiao et al., 1998). Theaflavins (TF) and thearubigins (TR) are the two major classes of polyphenols responsible for its color and taste. During fermentation, these pigments form a mixture of catechin dimers, trimers, or multipolymers, referred to as tea pigments (Nursten, 1997). Animal and clinical studies have demonstrated the ability of tea pigments to treat hypertension, decrease blood sugar, and prevent atherosclerosis and cancer (Morse et al., 1997: Ye, 1997). Tea pigments were also shown to increase superoxide dismutase (SOD) activity and decrease lipid-peroxidation levels in experimental animals (Li et al., 1998; Ren et al., 1998). Cadneri et al. (2000) showed that polyphenolic extracts from black tea was similar to wine extracts in their ability to protect rats against AOM-induced colon carcinogenesis (Table B.12). Black-tea

---

TABLE B.12

Number of Adenomas or Cancers in the Colon/Rectum of AOM-Induced Rats Treated with Different Polyphenol Extracts

Group (n)	Tumors in the Colon-Rectum/ Rats Adenomas	Cancers
Controls (22)	1.72 ± 1.31	0.82 ± 1.00
Black tea (22)	$1.00 \pm 1.15^{*}$	0.54 ± 0.80
Green tea (22)	2.55 ± 1.50	0.70 ± 1.03
Wine extract (22)	1.09 ± 1.30	0.54 ± 0.74

Note: [*] Significantly different ($p < 0.05$) from control.

Source: From Caderni et al., *Carcinogenesis*, 21:1965–1969, 2000. With permission.

extracts were far more effective than green-tea extracts in increasing apoptosis of the tumors. The anticarcinogenic properties of black-tea extracts were demonstrated by Shukla and Taneja (2002), who reported significant decreases in the number of diethylnitrosamine (DEN)-induced pulmonary tumors in Swiss albino mice fed 2 percent and 4 percent black-tea extracts. Yaping and coworkers (2003) recently showed that tea pigments had similar free-radical-scavenging abilities to tea polyphenols, which further supports their role in disease prevention.

A melanin-like pigment was isolated by Sava et al. (2001) from black tea leaves by alkaline extraction, acid hydrolysis, and precipitation. The isolated pigment had immunostimulating activity, suggesting possible health benefits. Significant antimutagenic effects were also reported by Gupta et al. (2002) for black tea and its polyphenols using the Ames Salmonella assays. Recent work by Besra et al. (2003) also demonstrated the antidiarrheal properties of a hot-water extract of black tea.

References

Besra, S.E., Gomes, A., Ganguly, D.K., and Vedasiromoni, J.R., Antidiarrhoeal activity of hot water extract of black tea (*Camellia* sinensis), *Phytother. Res.,* 17:380–384, 2003.

Caderni, G., De Filippo, C., Luceri, C., Salvadori, M., Giannini, A., Biggeri, A., Remy, S., Cheynier, V., and Dolara, P., Effects of black tea, green tea and wine extracts on intestinal carcinogenesis induced by azoxymethane in F344 rats, *Carcinogenesis,* 21: 1965–1969, 2000.

Gupta, S., Chaudhuri, T., Seth, P., Ganguly, D.K., and Giri, A.K., Antimutagenic effects of black tea (World Blend) and its two active polyphenols theaflavins and thearubigins in *Salmonella* assays, *Phytother. Res.,* 16:655–661, 2002.

Li, N., Han, H., and Wang, Z., Protective effect of tea pigments on oxidative damage by free radical in guinea pig, *Zhong Guo Zhong Yi Yao Technology,* 29:23–24, 1998 (in Chinese).

Morse, M.A., Kresty, L.A., Steele, V.E., Kelloff, G.J., Boone, C.W., Balentine, D.A., Harbowy, M.E., and Stoner, G.D, Effects of theaflavins on N-nitrosomethylbenzylamine-induced esophageal tumorigenesis, *Nutr. Cancer Int. J.,* 29:7–12, 1997.

Nursten, H.E., 1997. Chemistry of tea infusions, in *Chemical and Biological Properties of Tea Infusions,* Schubert, R. and Spiro, M., Eds., German Medical Information Services, Frankfurt, 1997, pp. 10–83.

Ren, M., Zheng, Y., and Xu, S., 1998. The inhibitory effect of tea pigments on lipid peroxidation in mice, *Jiang Xi Med. Acta,* 38:49–51, 1998 (in Chinese).

Sava, V.M., Galkin, B.N., Hong, M.Y., Yang, P.C., and Huang, G.S., A novel melanin-like pigment derived from black tea leaves with immuno-stimulating activity, *Food Res. Inter.,* 34:337–343, 2001.

Shukla, Y. and Taneja, P., Anticarcinogenic effect of black tea on pulmonary tumors in Swiss albino mice, *Cancer Lett.,* 176:137–141, 2002.

Yaping, Z., Wenli, Y., Dapu, W., Xiaofeng, L., and Tianxi, H., Chemiluminescence determination of free radical scavenging abilities of "tea pigments" and comparison with "tea polyphenols," *Food Chem.,* 80:115–118, 2003.

Ye, W., The study and application of tea pigment, *China Food Add.,* 4:23–24, 1997 (in Chinese).

Xiao, W., Zhong, J., Xiao, H, and Li, D., The mechanism of formation of tea pigments during the industrial processing of tea known as "fermentation," *Fujian Tea,* 3:8–12, 1998.

Blueberries   Blueberries are rich sources of procyanidins and anthocyanins. Catechin and epicatechin were reported as monomers with (epi)catechin oligomer units exclusively singly linked (B-type) (Prior et al., 2001). Blueberries were among those fruit that strongly reduced the genotoxicity of 2-amino-1-methyl-6-phenylimidazo [4,5-b]pyridine (PhIP) in a dose-dependent manner in metabolically competent Chinese hamster-lung fibroblast V9 cells (Edenharder et al., 2002). Mazza and coworkers (2002) reported that 19 out of 25 anthocyanins, both intact glycosylated and possibly acylated forms, were absorbed by human subjects who consumed a high-fat diet together with a freeze-dried blueberry powder. The increase in serum anthocyanin levels correlated with an increase in serum antioxidant activity (ORAC) (Figure B.15).

Kay and Holub (2002) reported that consumption by healthy human subjects of a freeze-dried powder from wild blueberries

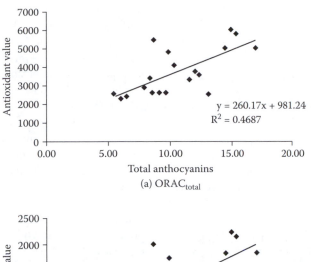

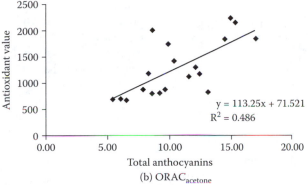

FIGURE B.15 Correlation between serum antioxidant capacity and concentration of serum total anthocyanins. Antioxidant value expressed as micromoles of Trolox equivalents per liter, and anthocyanins expressed (nanograms per milliliter of serum) as cyanidin 3-glucoside chloride. (From Mazza et al., *J. Agric. Food Chem.*, 50:7731–7737, 2002. With permission.)

(*Vaccinium angustifolium*), together with a high-fat meal, significantly increased serum-antioxidant status (determined by ORAC and TAS assays) compared to control diets. This increase in blood-antioxidant status has been associated with decreased risk in atherosclerosis (Durak et al., 2001) and cancer (Ching et al., 2002).

A number of proanthocyanidin fractions were recently separated from wild-blueberry extracts by Schmidt et al. (2004). Of these, only the high-molecular-weight proanthocyanidin oligomers exhibited antiproliferation and anti-adhesion properties. For example, two fractions composed predominantly of four to eight linked oligomeric proanthocyanidins with average degrees of polymerization of 3.25 and 5.65 prevented adhesion of the organism responsible for urinary infections, *Escherichia coli*. However, only the latter fraction exhibited significant antiproliferation activity against human prostate and mouse liver-cancer cells.

References

Ching, S., Ingram, D., Hahnel, R., Beilby, J., and Rossi, E., Serum levels of micronutrients, antioxidants and total antioxidant status predict risk of breast cancer in a case control study, *J. Nutr.*, 132: 303–306, 2002.

Durak, I.I., Kacmaz, M., Cimen, M.Y.B., Buyukkocak, U., and Ozturk, H.S., Blood oxidant/antioxidant status of atherosclerotic patients, *Int. J. Cardiol.*, 77:293– 297, 2001.

Edenharder, R., Sager, J.W., Glatt, H., Muckel, E., and Platt, K.L., Protection by beverages, fruits, vegetables, herbs, and flavonoids against genotoxicity of 2-acetylaminofluorene and 2-amino-1-methyl-6-phenylimidazo[4,5-b]pyridine (PhIP) in metabolically competent V9 cells, *Mutat. Res.*, 521:57–62, 2002.

Kay, C.D. and Holub, B.J., The effect of wild blueberry (*Vaccinium angustifolium*) consumption on postprandial serum antioxidant status in human subjects, *Br. J. Nutr.*, 88:389–397, 2002.

Mazza, G., Kay, C.D., Cottrell, T., and Holub, B.J., Absorption of anthocyanins from blueberries and serum antioxidant status in human subjects, *J. Agric. Food Chem.*, 50:7731–7737, 2002.

Prior, R.L., Lazarus, S.A., Cao, G., Muccitelli, H., and Hammerstone, J.F., Identification of procyanidins and anthocyanins in blueberries and cranberries (*Vaccinium* spp.) using high-performance liquid chromatography/mass spectrometry, *J. Agric. Food Chem.*, 49:1270–1276, 2001.

Schmidt, B.M., Howell, A.B., McEniry, B., Knight, C.T., Seigler, D., Erdman J.W., Jr., and Lila, M.A., Effective separation of potent antiproliferation and antiadhesion components from wild blueberry (Vaccinium angustifolium Ait.) fruits, *J. Agric. Food Chem.*, 52:6433–6442, 2004.

Borage oil   Borage oil is a high gamma-linolenic acid (GLA; C18:3n-6) oil extracted from borage seeds (*Borago officinalis* L.). The composition of the oil is shown in Table B.13. GLA accounts for almost 25 percent of the total fatty acids in borage oil. Mounting evidence points to GLA as a potent blood-pressure-lowering nutrient, making it a potential dietary intervention for hypertension (Das, 1995; Narce and Poisson, 1995; Engler et al., 1992). Engler and Engler (1998) found GLA-rich oils, such as borage oil, increased the composition of GLA and dihomogamma-linolenic acid in the plasma, hepatic, and vascular tissue of spontaneously hypertensive rats. The changes in fatty-acid profiles brought about by GLA-enriched oils were attributed to its favorable blood-pressure-lowering effect.

Another role for GLA is its ability to attenuate body-fat accumulation in rats. Obese Zucker rats fed black currant oil containing 70 percent GLA were found to have lower body-fat content compared with those animals fed soybean oil (Phinney et al., 1993). Takahashi and coworkers (2000) showed that GLA-rich borage oil reduced white adipose tissue weight compared to safflower oil by increasing gene expressions of the uncoupling protein 1 in brown adipose tissue.

Consumption of borage oil was also shown by Brosche and Platt (2000) to significantly and statistically improve skin function in the elderly. They reported a 34 percent reduction in itching, as well as in dry skin from 42 to 14 percent. Another benefit of borage oil is in the treatment of rheumatoid arthritis, due to its ability to decrease the tumor necrosis factor (TNF-α), a central tissue destructive mediator in rheumatoid arthritis (Belch and Hill, 2000). Kast (2001) reviewed double-blind studies suggesting borage oil was beneficial for treating rheumatoid arthritis. He proposed a mechanism whereby GLA in borage oil raised protaglandin E levels, which in turn increased cAMP levels that suppressed TNF-α. He further cautioned against the use of nonsteroidal anti-inflammatory drugs, which would undermine the effects of borage oil.

Gadek and coworkers (1999) showed that enteral nutrition with special diets containing either EPA or GLA reduced the number of neutrophils in brochoalveolar lavage fluid, as well as reducing pulmonary inflammation. This resulted in improved clinical outcomes in patients suffering from acute respiratory distress syndrome (ARDS). To explain the anti-inflammatory effects of EPA and GLA, Gillis and coworkers (2002) hypothesized this was due to induction of neutrophil apoptosis. Their studies showed that EPA and GLA, alone or in combination, triggered the induction of apoptosis and secondary necrosis in human promy-

TABLE B.13
Typical Fatty-Acid Composition of Borage Oil

Fatty Acid	Percent of Total Fatty Acids
C16:0	12.1
C18:0	3
C18:1	18.1
C18:2n-6	37.7
C18:3n-6	24.6
C18:3n-3	4.5
Total PUFA	66.7

Source: Adapted from Takahashi et al., *Comp. Biochem. Physiol.*, Part B, 127:213–222, 2000.

elocytic HL-60 cells. Thus, inclusion of GLA and EPA could improve clinical outcomes in ARDS.

Using a double-blind, monocentric trial with parallel groups of healthy male volunteers between the ages of 18 and 30, Duriez et al. (1997) showed it was possible to provide oral supplements of borage oil (3 g/day) over six weeks without having any adverse effects on platelet aggregation.

References

Belch, J.J. and Hill, A., Evening primrose oil and borage oil in rheumatic conditions, *Am. J. Clin. Nutr.,* 71:352–356S, 2000.

Brosche, T. and Platt, D., Effect of borage oil consumption on fatty acid metabolism, transdermal water loss and skin parameters in elderly people, *Arch. Gerontol. Geratr.,* 30:139–150, 2000.

Das, U.N., Essential fatty acid metabolism in patients with essential hypertension, diabetes mellitus and coronary heart disease, *Prostaglandins Leukotr. Essen. Fatty Acids,* 52:387–391, 1995.

Duriez, P., Luc, G., Jude, B., Bordet, J.C., Lacroix, B., Bonte, J.P., Parra, H.J., and Bard, J.M., A therapeutic dosage (3 g/day) of borage oil supplementation has no effect on platelet aggregation in healthy volunteers, *Atherosclerosis,* 134:189, 1997.

Engler, M.M. and Engler, M.B., The effects of dietary evening primrose, blackcurrant, borage and fungal oils on plasma, hepatic and vascular tissue fatty acid composition in the spontaneously hypertensive rats, *Nutr. Res.,* 18:1533–1544, 1998.

Gadek, J.E., DeMichele, S.J., Karlstad, M.D., Pacht, E.R., Donahoe, M., Alberston, T.E., Van Hoozen, C., Wennberg, A.K., Nelson, J.L., and Noursalehi, M., Effect of enteral feeding with eicosapentaenoic acid, gamma-linolenic acid, and antioxidants in patients with acute respiratory distress syndrome, *Crit. Care Med.,* 27:1409–1420, 1999.

Gillis, R.C., Daley, B.J., Enderson, B.L., and Karlstad, M.D., Eicosapentanoic acid and γ-linolenic acid induce apoptosis in HL-60 cells, *J. Surgical Res.,* 107:145–153, 2002.

Kast, R.E., Borage oil reduction of rheumatoid arthritis activity may be mediated by increased cAMP that suppresses tumor necrosis factor-alpha, *Int. Immunopharmacol.,* 1:2197–2199, 2001.

Narce, M. and Poisson, J-P., Age-related depletion of linoleic acid desaturation in liver microsomes from young spontaneously hypertensive rats, *Prostaglandins Leukotr. Essen. Fatty Acids,* 53:59–63, 1995.

Phinney, S.D., Tang, A.B., Thurmond, A.C., Nakamura, M.T., and Stern, J.S., Abnormal polyunsaturated-lipid metabolism in the obese Zucker rat with partial metabolic correction by γ-linolenic acid administration, *Metabolism,* 42:1127–1140, 1993.

Takahashi, Y., Ide, T., and Fujita, H., Dietary gamma-linolenic acid in the form of borage oil causes less body fat accumulation accompanying an increase in uncoupling protein 1 mRNA level in brown adipose tissue, *Comp. Biochem. Physiol., Part B,* 127:213–222, 2000.

Bovine lactoferrin *see also* **Lactoferrin**

Lactoferrin, an iron-binding protein found in milk, also possesses bacteriocidal activity. A 25-residue peptide released from the amino-terminal region of bovine lactoferrin catalyzed at acidic pH by pepsin was shown to have potent bacteriocidal activity (Bellamy et al., 1992). Such a reaction can occur in the stomach, in which a stable lactoferricin B is released into the intestine (Kuwata et al., 1998a, b). The intact peptide is extremely basic, with five arginine and three lysine residues. Lactoferrin appears to regulate immune and inflammatory responses by regulating the production of some cytokines, including interleukins and tumor necrosis factor-α (TNF-α) (Brock et al., 2000; Choe and Lee, 1999). Strom and coworkers (2001) examined the effects of charge and lipophilicity on the antibacterial activity of an undacapeptide (FKCRRWQWRMK) derived from bovine lactoferricin. All undecapeptides had Tryp residues in positions 6 and 8 and Arg in positions 5 and 9 and were more effective against Gram-positive bacteria, such as *Staphyloccus aureus,* with a higher bacteriocidal effect against *Escherichia coli* than *Pseudomonas aeruginosa.*

References

Bellamy, W., Takase, M., Yamauchi, K., Wakabayashi, H., Kawasa, T., and Tomita, M., Antibacterial spectrum of lactoferricin B, a potent bacteriocidal peptide derived from the N-terminal region of bovine lactoferrin, *J. Appl. Bacteriol.,* 73:472–479, 1992.

B

Brock, J.H., Guillen, G., and Thompson, C., Anti-inflammatory and immuno-regulatory properties of lactoferrin, in *Lactoferrin, Structure, Function and Applications,* Shimazaka, K., Ed., Elsevier Science, New York, 2000, pp. 119–128.

Choe, Y.H. and Lee, S.W., Effect of lactoferrin on the production of tumor necrosis factor-α and nitric oxide, *J. Cell Biochem.,* 76:30–36, 1999.

Kuwata, H., Yip, T.T., Tomita, M., and Hutchens, T.W., Direct evidence of the generation in human stomach of an antimicrobial peptide domain (Lactoferrin) from ingested lactoferrin, *Biochem. Biophys. Acta,* 1429:129–141, 1998a.

Kuwata, H., Yip, T.T., Yamauchi, K., Teraguchi, S., Hayasawa, H., Tomita, M., and Hutchens, T.W., The survival of ingested lactoferrin in the gastrointestinal tract of adult mice, *Biochem. J.,* 334:321–323, 1998b.

Strom, M.B., Rekdal, O., and Svendsen, J.S., The effects of charge and lipophilicity on the antibacterial activity of undecapeptides derived from bovine lactoferricin, *J. Peptide Sci.,* 8:36–43, 2001.

Bovine plasma   Only a small portion of blood taken from an animal after slaughter is used as emulsifiers, stabilizers, clarifiers, and as nutrients for foods. Interest in identification of bioactive peptides led to isolation of bovine blood plasma hydrolysates, including opioid peptides (Zhao et al., 1997), bradykinin-potentiating peptides (Piot et al., 1992), and several angiotensin 1-converting enzymes (ACE) (Hyun and Shin, 2000; Suetsuna, 1995). Janitha et al. (2002) reported the production of a number of bioactive peptides, following hydrolysis of defribinated plasma (DBP), a by-product of meat-processing plants, with a microbial protease. Examination of the different protein hydrolysates, following various degrees of hydrolysis (DH), showed an increase in ACE inhibition accompanied an increase in DH. The highest inhibitory activity was found for the 42 percent DH hydrolysate. Peptides were separated by size-exclusion chromatography, and the fraction with the greatest inhibitory activity contained peptides with GYP, HL(1), HPY, HPGH, L(1)F, SPY, and YPH sequences. Park and Hyun (2002) reported the production of bioactive peptides with antigenotoxic activity following enzymatic hydrolysis of bovine plasma proteins with several different proteases.

References

Hyun, C-K. and Shin, H-K., Utilization of bovine blood plasma proteins for the production of angiotensin 1 converting inhibitory peptides, *Process Biochem.,* 36:65–71, 2000.

Janitha, P.K., Wanasundara, P.D., Ross, A.R.S., Amarowicz, R., Ambrose, S.J., Pegg, R.B., and Shand, P.J., Peptides with angiotensin 1-converting enzyme (ACE) inhibitory activity from defibrinated, hydrolyzed bovine plasma, *J. Agric. Food Chem.,* 50: 6981–6988, 2002.

Park, K-J. and Hyun, C-K., Angenotoxin effects of the peptides derived from bovine blood plasma proteins, *Enz. Microb. Technol.,* 30:633–638, 2002.

Piot, J.M., Zhao, Q., Guillochon, D., Ricart, G., and Thomas, D., Isolation and characterization of a bradykinin-potentiating peotide from a bovine peptic hemoglobin hydrolysate, *FEBS Lett.,* 299:75–79, 1992.

Suetsuna, Y., Novel tripeptides and angiotensin converting enzyme inhibitors, Japanese Patent 07-188183, 1995.

Zhao, Q., Coeur, C.L., and Piot, J.M., Analysis of peptides from bovine hemoglobin and tuna myoglobin enzymatic hydrolysate: Use of HPLC with on-line second order derivative spectroscopy for the characterization of biologically active peptides, *Anal. Chim. Acta,* 352:201–220, 1997.

Bowman-Birk protease inhibitor The Bowman-Birk protease inhibitor (BBI), is a family of different forms and isoforms of natural polypeptide serine protease inhibitors of trypsin and chymotrypsin found in legume seeds, such as soybeans, chickpeas, and peanuts, and, to a lesser extent, in cereals, such as barley. Preclinical studies showed BBIs were effective suppressors of carcinogenesis both *in vivo* and *in vitro* (Kennedy, 1998). While the specific target(s) affected by BBIs have yet to be identified, indirect targets appear to be a modulation of superoxide anion radical production, oncongene levels, DNA repair, immune effects, and arachidonic-acid metabolism (Lippmann and Matrisian, 2000).

TABLE B.14
Clinical Response to BBI Concentrate with Respect to Dose Administered

Dose[1]	Prog[2]	NR[3]	PR[4]	CR[5]	N	Response
200	0	7	1	0	8	12.5
533	0	7	3	1	11	36.36
800	2	5	2	0	9	22.22
1066	0	1	2	1	4	75
Total	2	20	8	2	32	31.25

[1] CIU (chymotrypsin inhibitor units).
[2] Prog (progression), appearance of new lesions, or > 50 percent increase in total lesion area.
[3] NR (no response), < 50 percent reduction in total area of all lesions.
[4] PR (partial response), at least 50 percent reduction in total area of all lesions.
[5] CR, complete resolution of all lesions at completion of one month of BBI concentrate.

Source: From Armstrong et al., *Clin. Cancer. Res.,* 6:4684–4691, 2000b. With permission.

Early work by von Hofe et al. (1991) noted soybean BBI effectively inhibited esophageal carcinogenesis induced by *N*-nitrosomethylbenzylamine (NMBzA) in male Sprague–Dawley rats. A reduction of 45 percent in the frequency of papillomas and carcinomas was observed in rats receiving BBI in three tablets a week. The ability of BBI to prevent the development of malignancies has been demonstrated in a number of animal models (Kennedy, 1993). A phase I clinical trial conducted by Armstrong et al. (2000a) showed an oral dose of a BBI concentrate given to 24 patients suffering from oral leukoplakia was nontoxic. This was followed by a phase IIa clinical trial by Armstrong et al. (2000b) in which the same BBI concentrate was administered to 32 patients with oral leukoplakia. A 31 percent clinical response was observed, including two complete and eight partial, determined by pretreatment and post-treatment for individual and total lesion areas and analysis (Table B.14). The mean total lesion area decreased significantly ($p < 0.004$) from 614 to 435 mm² following treatment with BBI concentrate with a linear dose–response relationship observed. The absence of toxicity combined with a dose-dependent decrease in oral leukoplakia area will require further randomized clinical trials to determine the efficacy of BBI concentrate in treating this condition.

References

Armstrong, W.B., Kennedy, A.R., Wan, X.S., Atiba, J., McLaren, C.E., and Meyskens, F.L., Jr., Single-dose administration of Bowman-Birk inhibitor concentrate in patients with oral leukoplakia, *Cancer Epidemiol. Biomark. Prev.,* 9:43–47, 2000a.

Armstrong, W.B., Kennedy, A.R., Wan, X.S., Taylor, T.H., Nguyen, Q.A., Jensen, J., Thompson, W., Lagerberg, W., and Meyskens, F.L., Jr., Clinical modulation of oral leukoplakia and protease activity by Bowman-Birk inhibitor concentrate in a phase IIa chemoprevention trial, *Clin. Cancer. Res.,* 6:4684–4691, 2000b.

Kennedy, A.R., Overview: Anticarcinogenic activity of protease inhibitors, in *Protease Inhibitors as Cancer Chemopreventive Agents,* Troll, W. and Kennedy, A.R., Eds., Plenum Press, New York, 1993, pp. 9–64.

Kennedy, A.R., Chemopreventative agents: Protease inhibitor, *Pharmacol. Ther.,* 78:167–209, 1998.

Lippmann, S.M. and Matrisian, L.M., Protease inhibitors in oral carcinogenesis and chemoprevention, *Clin. Cancer Res.,* 6:4599–4603, 2000.

Von Hofe, E., Newberne, P.M., and Kennedy, A.R., Inhibition of *N*-nitrosomethylbenzylamine-induced esophageal neoplasms by the Bowman Birk protease inhibitor, *Carcinogenesis,* 12:2147–2150, 1991.

Boxwood   (*Buxus sempervirens*)   Boxwood is a popular woody, ornamental plant grown throughout Europe and North America. In folk

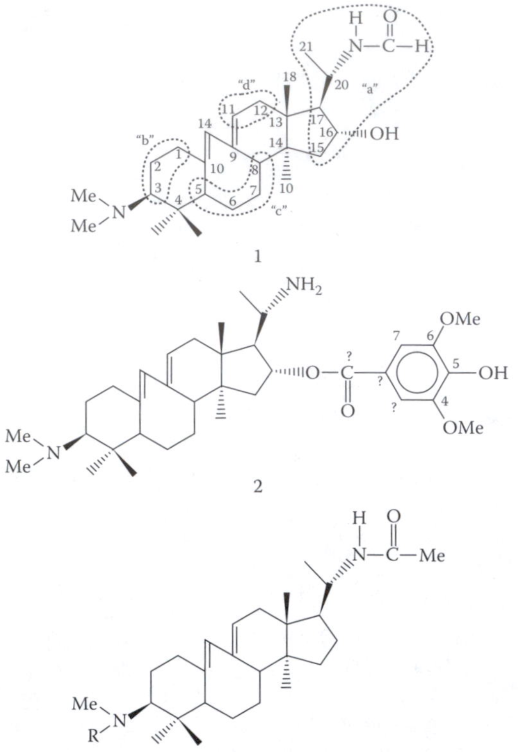

B

SCHEME B.9 Structure of four new alkaloids isolated from *Buxus sempervirens*. (From Loru et al., *Phytochemistry*, 54:951–957, 2000. With permission).

medicine, extracts from *Buxus* are used to cure different diseases, including the treatment of HIV infections (Valmet, 1983; Durrant et al., 1996, 1998). It is a rich source of steroidal alkaloids, with four new alkaloids extracted from its leaves by Loru and coworkers (2000). Some of these alkaloids may be responsible for some of the health-related properties attributed to boxwood (Scheme B.9).

References

Durant, J., Chantre, P., Gonzalez, G., Vandermander, J., Halfon, P., and Rousse, B., Efficacy and safety of *Buxus sempervirens* L. preparations (SPV30) in HIV-infected asymptomatic patients: A multicentre, randomized, double-blind, placebo-controlled trial, *Phytochemistry*, 5:1–10, 1998.

Durant, J., Vandermander, J., Chanre, P., and Dellamonica, P., in *Communication at conference on AIDS*, Vancouver, Canada (Abstr. LB6040), 1996.

Loru, F., Duval, D., Aumelas, A., Akeb, F., Guedon, D., and Guedj, R., Four steroidal alkaloids from the leaves of *Buxus sempervirens*, *Phytochemistry*, 54:951–957, 2000.

Valmet, J., *Phytotherapie traitement des maladies par les plantes*, Maloine, Paris, 1983.

Brassica vegetables   *see also* Crucifera

Brassica vegetables are among the most frequently consumed vegetables around the world (Lange et al., 1992a, b). They include white cabbage, red cabbage, broccoli, cauliflower, Brussels sprouts, and Savoy cabbage, as well as rape and mustard. They all contain glucosinolates, which undergo degradation to isothiocyanates, indoles, and nitriles (Scheme B.10). The chemopreventive properties of these vegetables are related to the ability of their bioactive components to inhibit phase I enzymes and to activate phase II enzymes, such as glutathione *S*-transferase (GST).

Brassica vegetables, such as broccoli, cauliflower, Brussels sprouts, and kale, have been reported to exhibit strong anticancer properties. A diet rich in Brussels sprouts decreased urinary excretion of 8-oxidG, indicative of DNA damage (Verhagen et al., 1997), while a low risk of lung cancer in Chinese men was associated with a high urinary excretion of isothiocyanates (London et al., 2000). One explanation for the decreased cancer risk associated with vegetable intake is related to induction or inhibition of biotransformation enzymes. Lampe and coworkers (2000) found Brassica vegetables increased while apiceous vegetables decreased cytochrome P450 1A2 in human subjects. Steinkellner et al. (2001) showed that it was the degradation compounds of glucosinolates in Brassica vegetables that were responsible for the protective effect against carcinogens. For example, indoles and isothiocyanates attenuated the carcinogenic effects of polycyclic aromatic hydrocarbons (PAHs), as well as against heterocyclic amines.

References

Lampe, J.W., King, I.B., Li, S., Grate, M.T., Barale, K.V., Chen, C., Feng, Z., and Potter, J.D., Brassica vegetables increase apiceous vegetables decrease

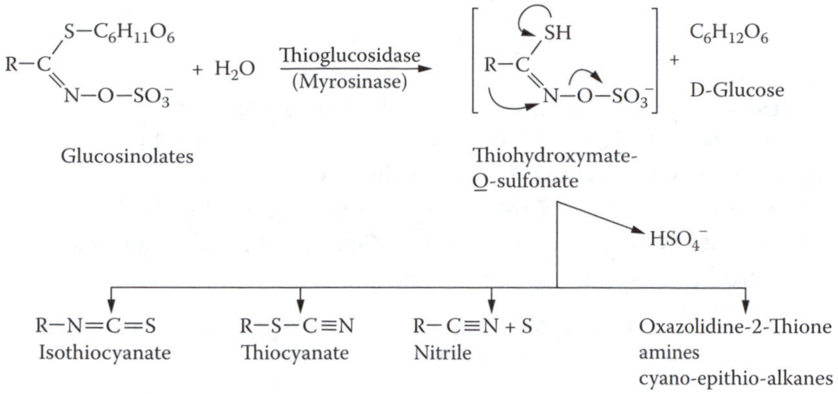

SCHEME B.10 Chemical structures of glucosinolates and their breakdown products following enzymatic hydrolysis by myrosinase. (Adapted from Pessina et al. (1990) by Steinkellner et al., *Mutat. Res.*, 480–481:285–297, 2001. With permission.)

cytochrome P450 1A2 activity in humans: Changes in caffeine metabolite ratios in response to controlled vegetable diets, *Carcinogenesis,* 21:1157–1162, 2000.

Lange, R., Baumgrass, R., Diedrich, M., Henschel, K.-P., and Kujawa, M., Glucosinolate in der Ernahrung-Pro und Contra einer Naturstoffklasse. Teil I: Ausgangssituation, Problem stellung, Analytik, Verzehr, Ernahr, *Umsch,* 39:252–257, 1992a.

Lange, L., Baumgrass, R., Diedrich, M., Henschel, K.-P., and Kujawa, M., Glucosinolate in der Ernahrung-Pro und Contra einer Naturastoff. Teil II: Abbau und Stoffwechsel Ernahr, *Umsch,* 39:252–257, 1992b.

London, S.J., Yuan, J.M., Chung, F.L., Gao, Y.T., Coetzee, G.A., Ross, R.K., and Yu, M.C., Isothiocyanates, glutathione C-transferase M1 and T1 polymorphisms, and lung-cancer risk: A prospective study of men in Shangai, China, *Lancet,* 356:724–729, 2000.

Pessina, A., Thomas, R.M., Palmieri, S., and Lussi, P.L., An improved method for the purification of myrosinase and its physicochemical characterization, *Arch. Biochem. Biophys.,* 280:383–389, 1990.

Steinkellner, H., Rabot, S., Fretwald, C., Nobis, E., Scharf, G., Chabicovsky, M., Knasmuller, S., and Kassie, F., Effects of cruciferous vegetables and their constituents on drug metabolizing enzymes involved in the bioactivation of DNA-reactive dietary carcinogens, *Mutat. Res.,* 480–481:285–297, 2001.

Verhagen, H., de Vries, A., Nijhoff, N.A., Schouten, A., van Poppel, G., Peters, W.H., and van den Berg, H., Effects of Brussels sprouts on oxidative DNA-damage in man, *Cancer Lett.,* 114:127–130, 1997.

Broccoli Consumption of Brassica vegetables, such as broccoli, leads to excretion of isothiocyanates (ITCs) in the urine. These compounds are produced by enzymic hydrolysis of intact thioglucoside conjugates or glucosinolates and may have a role as cancer chemopreventative agents (Conaway et al., 2002). The major glucosinolate in broccoli, glucoraphanin, is hydrolyzed by myrosinase to sulforaphane or sulforaphane nitrile (Scheme B.11). Matusheski and Jeffery (2001) compared the biactivity of these metabolites in mouse hepatoma cells.

Sulforaphane proved to be the most potent in inducing phase II detoxification enzymes and had

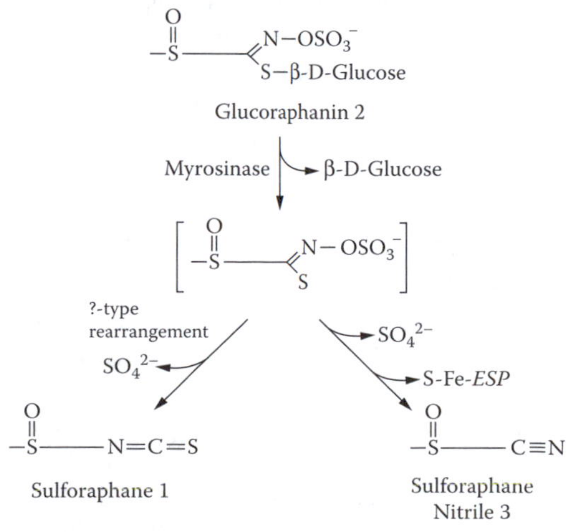

SCHEME B.11 Hydrolysis of glucoraphanin to sulforaphanes. (From Matusheski and Jeffery, *J. Agric. Food Chem.,* 49:5743–5749, 2001. With permission.)

B

TABLE B.15

Effect of Diets Containing 20 Percent Prehydrolyzed Broccoli (Broccoli-HP), 20 Percent Unhydrolyzed Broccoli with Intact Glucosinolates (Broccoli-GS), or Purified Sulforaphane (5.0 mmol of SFG/kg of Diet) Compared to a Control-Modified, AIN-76 B-40 Diet (C) on Hepatic and Colonic Mucosal Quinone Reductase (QR) of Rats Fed These Diets for Five Days[2]

Diet	Colonic QR Activity[2] (mmol of DPIP/min/mg of Protein)	Hepatic QR Activity[2] (mmol of DPIP/min/mg of Protein)
C	122.1 ± 17.4a	68.3 ± 6.1a
Broccoli-HP	396.6 ± 29.6b	77.3 ± 7.4ab
Broccoli-GS	543.7 ± 33.9c	94.4 ± 8.7b
SF	559.0 ± 43.2c	97.3 ± 6.5b

[1] Values shown are means ± SE, n = 5. Different letters within a column indicate values that differ significantly ($p \le 0.05$).

[2] QR activity measured using 2,6-dichlorophenolindophenol (DPIP) as the substrate.

Source: Adapted from Keck et al., *J. Agric. Food Chem.,* 51:3320–3327, 2003.

much greater potential as a chemoprotective agent than the corresponding nitrile. Keck et al. (2003) showed intact broccoli glucosinolates (Broccoli-GS) enhanced quinone reductase (QR) in the liver and colon of Fischer 344 rats far more than when fed hydrolyzed broccoli (Broccoli-HP) (Table B.15). There were no significant differences in the colonic or hepatic QR activity of rats fed a purified sulforaphane (SF) diet or the intact Broccoli-GS diet. They suggested that urinary sulforaphane conjugate of mercapturic acid was a useful biomarker for assessing the effects of dietary broccoli on QR induction in the liver and colon and could be extrapolated to measure the relative cancer prevention effects of broccoli. Based on the oxygen-radical absorbance capacity (ORAC) assay, broccoli was shown to be seventh in antioxidant capacity after kale, Brussels sprouts, alfalfa sprout, beets, and spinach broccoli (Cao et al., 1996). However, using linoleic-acid emulsions and phospholipid bilayers, Azuma and coworkers (1999) found broccoli (*Brassica oleraceae* var *italica*) exhibited the greatest antioxidant activity compared to 25 vegetable extracts (Wallig et al., 1999). The many antioxidants present in broccoli include carotenoids, tocopherols, acorbic acid, and flavonoids (Kurilich et al., 1999; Plumb et al., 1997). Using the ORAC assay, Kurilich et al. (2002) showed considerable variability in the antioxidant capacity of eight broccoli genotypes. They were unable to explain the variability based on ascorbic acid and flavonoid content of the hydrophyllic extracts suggesting the presence of other antioxidants or synergism. The carotenoids in the lipophylic extracts correlated with antioxidant capacity and accounted for the majority of the variability in this fraction.

References

Azuma, K., Ippoushi, K., Ito, H., Higashio, H., and Terao, J., Evaluation of the antioxidant activity of vegetable extracts in linoleic emulsion and phospholipid bilayers, *J. Sci. Food Agric.,* 79:2010–2016, 1999.

Cao, G., Sofic, E., and Prior, R., Antioxidant activity of tea and common vegetables. *J. Agric. Food Chem.,* 44:3426–3431, 1996.

Conaway, C.C., Yang, Y., and Chung, F.-L., Isothiocyantes as cancer chemopreventive agents: Their biological activities and metabolism in rodents and humans, *Curr. Drug Metab.,* 3:233–255, 2002.

Keck, A.-S., Qiao, Q., and Jeffery, E.H., Food matrix effects on bioactivity of broccoli-derived sulforaphane in liver and colon of F344 rats, *J. Agric. Food Chem.,* 51:3320–3327, 2003.

Kurilich, A.C., Tsau, G.J., Brown, A., Howard, L., Klein, B.P., Jeffery, E.H., Kushad, M., Wallig, M.A., and Juvik, J.A., Carotene, tocopherol, and ascorbate contents in subspecies of *Brassica oleracea, J. Agric. Food Chem.,* 47:1576–1581, 1999.

Kurilich, A.C., Jeffery, E.H., Juvik, J.A., Wallig, M.A., and Klein, B.P., Antioxidant capacity of different broccoli (*Brassica oleracea*) genotypes using the oxygen radical absorbance capacity (ORAC) assay, *J. Agric. Food Chem.*, 50:5053–5057, 2002.

Matusheski, N.V. and Jeffery, E.H., Comparison of the bioactivity of two glucoraphanin hydrolysis products found in broccoli, sulforaphane and sulforaphane nitrile, *J. Agric. Food Chem.*, 49:5743–5749, 2001.

Plumb, G.W., Price, K.R., Rhodes, M.J.C., and Williamson, G., Antioxidant properties of the major polyphenolic compounds in broccoli, *Free Radical Res.*, 27:429–435, 1997.

Wallig, M.A., Azuma, K., Ippoushi, K., Ito, H., Higashio, H., and Terao, J., Evaluation of the antioxidant activity of vegetable extracts in linoleic emulsion and phospholipid bilayers, *J. Sci. Food Agric.*, 79:2010–2016, 1999.

Broccoli sprouts   Research conducted at Johns Hopkins University School of Medicine showed that broccoli sprouts contain from 20 to 50 times higher levels of sulforaphane glucosinolates than adult cooked broccoli and

Sulforaphane. (From Konwinski et al., *Toxicol. Lett.*, 153:343–355, 2004. With permission.)

could provide better anticancer protection (Nestle, 1998). Previous studies by Fahey et al. (1997) showed that broccoli sprouts were rich in enzyme inducers that protect against carcinogenesis. For example, broccoli contains large amounts of isothiocyanates, sulforaphane, or 4-methyl-sulfinyl-butyl isothiocyanate, that are potent inducers of phase II enzymes. Isothiocyanates occur naturally as thioglucoside conjugates and appear to inhibit the development of cancerous tumors. Chung et al. (2000) confirmed the ability of sulforaphane and phenylethyl isothiocyanate to inhibit the development of colonic aberrant crypt foci during the initiation period in experimental male rats treated with azoxymethane (AOM), an initiator of colon cancer. Based on their observations,

Fahey and Talalay (2001) patented their discovery for the development of cancer chemoprotective food products based on broccoli sprouts.

References

Chung, F.L., Conaway, C.C., Rao, C.V., and Reddy, B.S., Chemoprevention of colonic aberrant crypt foci in Fischer rats by sulforaphane and phenylethyl isothiocyanate, *Carcinogenesis*, 21:2287–2291, 2000.

Fahey, J.W. and Talalay, P., Cancer Chemoprotective Food Products, U.S. Patent 6,177,122 B1, 2001.

Fahey, J.W., Zhang, Y., and Talalay, P., Broccoli sprouts; An exceptionally rich source of inducers of enzymes that protect against chemical carcinogens, *Proc. Natl. Acad. Sci.*, 94:10367–10367, 1997.

Konwinski, R.R., Haddad, R., Chun, J.A., Klenow, S., Larson, S.C., Haab, B.B., and Furge, L.L., Oltipraz, 3*H*-1, 2-thione and sulforaphane induce overlapping and protective antioxidant responses in murine microglial cells, *Toxicol. Lett.*, 153:343–355, 2004.

Nestle, M., Broccoli sprouts in cancer prevention, *Nutr. Rev.*, 56:127–130, 1998.

Brussels sprouts   Brussels sprouts (*Brassica oleracea* var. gemmifera) are particularly rich in the glucosinolate sinigrin. Sinigrin is hydrolyzed by myrosinase to allyl isothiocyanate (AITC), which was shown to induce glutathione

Sinigrin structure. (From Jen et al., *J. Chromatogr.*, A., 912:363–368, 2001. With permission.)

S-transferase activity in the liver and small intestine of rats (Bogaards et al., 1990). Musk and Johnson (1993) found that AITC selectively induced cell death in the undifferentiated phenotype of the HT29 human cell tumor cell line. Smith et al. (1998) reported that ingestion of sinigrin inhibited dimethylhydrazine-induced aberrant crypt foci, as well as induced apoptosis in the rat colon. The ability of AITC to act as a suppressor of colorectal carcinogenesis was further investigated by Smith and coworkers (2003). Freeze-dried raw and microwave-cooked Brussels sprouts containing high levels of glucosinolates significantly enhanced apoptosis and reduced mitosis in 1,2-dimethylhydrazine (DMH)-induced colonic mucosal crypts. The absence of any effect in blanched-sprout tissue was attributed to the inactivation of myrosinase and the presence of only intact glucosinolates. This study confirmed the importance of glucosinolate degradation products in affecting cell proliferation and apoptosis.

References

Bogaards, J.J., vav Ommen, B., Falke, H.E., Willems, M.I., and van Bladeren, P.J., Glutathione S-transferase subunit induction patterns of Brussels sprouts, allyl isothiocyanate and goitrin in rat liver and small intestinal mucosa: A new approach for the identification of inducing xenobiotics, *Food Chem. Toxicol.,* 28:81–88, 1990.

Jen, J.-F., Lin, T.-H., Huang, J.-W., and Chung, W.-C., Direct determination of sinigrin in mustard seed without desulatation by reversed phase ion-pair liquid chromatography, *J. Chromatogr.,* A., 912:363–368, 2001.

Musk, S.R. and Johnson, I.T., Allyl isothiocyanate is selectively toxic to transformed cells of the human colorectal tumor line HT29, *Carcinogenesis,* 14:2079–2083, 1993.

Smith, T.K., Lund, E.K., and Johnson, I.T., Inhibition of dimethylhydrazine-induced aberrant crypt foci and induction of apoptosis in rat colon following oral administration of the glucosinolate sinigrin, *Carcinogenesis,* 19:267–273, 1998.

Smith, T.K., Mithen, R., and Johnson, I.T., Effects of Brassica vegetable juice on the induction of apoptosis and aberrant crypt foci in rat colonic mucosal crypts, *Carcinogenesis,* 24:491–495, 2003.

Bryonolic acid

Bryonolic acid   Bryonolic acid is a multiflorane compound found in saffron as the p-aminobenzoate derivative. In his discussion of medicinal plants, Thatte et al. (2000) suggested compounds, such as bryonolic acid, induced programmed cell death arresting the proliferation of cancerous cell lines. Two novel multiflorane p-aminobenzoates were detected by Appendino and coworkers (2000) in zucchini seeds, while bryonolic acid was the sole multiforane constituent found in zucchini sprouts.

Bryonolic acid. (Adapted from from Appendino et al., *Fitoterapia,* 71:258–263, 2000.)

References

Appendino, G., Japukovic, J., Belloro, E., and Marchesini, A., Triterpenoid p-aminobenzoates from seeds of zucchini, *Fitoterapia,* 71:258–263, 2000.

Thatte, U., Bagadey, S., and Dahanukar, S., Modulation of programmed cell death by medicinal plants, *Cell. Mol. Biol.,* 46:199–214, 2000.

Bryostatins   Bryostatins, a group of marine macrocyclic lactones with a unique polyacetate backbone, have considerable potential as chemopreventive agents (Petite, 1996). Their low toxicity combined with their antineoplastic activity has made bryostatins ideal for treating cancer. Bryostatin 1, first isolated and characterized in 1982, is recognized for its immune stimulation, growth inhibition, induction of differentiation, and enhancement of cytotoxicity of other drugs directed at target cells (Watters and Parsons, 1999).

Bryostatin 1. (Baryza et al., *Chem. Biol.,* 11:1261–1267, 2004. With permission.)

Studies on bryostatins have focused on their interaction with enzymes and cell lines or on

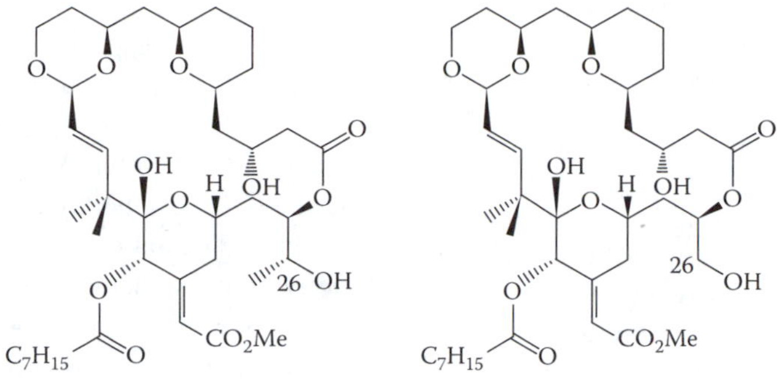

SCHEME B.12 Structures of analogs 1 and 2. (From Baryza et al., *Chem. Biol.*, 11:1261–1267, 2004. With permission.)

how these enzyme activities or cellular events affect apoptosis. For example, the effect of bryostatin 1 on protein kinase C isoenzymes has been studied extensively. This family of 12 isoenzymes plays a central role in cell signaling and other processes and is activated by bryostatin 1, phorbol esters (a group of tumor promoters), and diacylglycerol. Hennings et al. (1987) showed bryostatin 1 inhibited tumor promotion by phorbol esters in SENCAR mouse skin.

Preclinical trials to investigate bryostatin 1 as an anticancer drug showed it inhibited the growth of rabbit papillomas in a dose-dependent manner but did not provide a cure (Bodily et al., 1999). Other studies showed that bryostatin 1, in combination with anticancer drugs, proved more effective. For example, a cure was reported for WSU-CLL-bearing SCID mice (5/5) using a combination of auristatin PE followed by bryostatin every second day over a six-day period (Mohammed et al., 1998). A phase II trial by Nezhat et al. (2004) found a combination of bryostatin 1 and the drug cisplatin ineffective in patients with advanced-stage or recurrent cervical cancer. However, several analogs (analogs 1 and 2) of bryostatin 1 were later shown by Baryza and coworkers (2004) to be 50 times more potent than bryostatin at inducing translocation of PKCδ-GFF from the cytosol of rat basophilic leukemia (RBL) cells, suggesting great potential in cancer therapy (Scheme B.12). A review on bryostatins by Mutter and Wills (2000) is strongly recommended.

References

Baryza, J.L., Brenner, S.E., Craske, M.L., Meyer, T., and Wender, P.A., Simplified analogs of bryostatin with anticancer activity display greater potency for translocation of PKCδ-GFB, *Chem. Biol.*, 11:1261–1267, 2004.

Bodily, J.M., Hoopes, D.J., Roeder, B.L., Gilbert, S.G., Pettit, G.R., Herald, C.L., Rollins, D.N., and Robinson, R.A., The inhibitory effects of bryostatin 1 administration on the growth of rabbit papillomas, *Cancer Lett.*, 136:67–74, 1999.

Hennings, H., Blumberg, P.M., Pettit, G.R., Herald, C.L., Shores, R., and Yuspa, S.H., Bryostatin 1, an activator of protein kinase C, inhibits tumor promotion by phorbol esters in Sencar mouse skin, *Carcinogenesis*, 8:1343–1346, 1987.

Mohammed, R.M., Varterasian, M.L., Almatchy, V.P., Hannoudi, G.N., Pettit, G.R., and Al-Katib, A., Successful treatment of human chronic lymphatic leukemia xenografts with combination biological agents auristatin PE and bryostatin 1, *Clin. Cancer Res.*, 4:1337–1343, 1998.

Mutter, R. and Wills, M., Chemistry and clinical biology of the bryostatins, *Bioorg. Med. Chem.*, 8:1841–1860, 2000.

Nezhat, F., Wadler, S.W., Muggia, F., Mandeli, J., Goldberg, G., Rahaman, J., Runowicz, C., Murgo, A.J,. and Gardner, G.J., Phase II trial of the combination of bryostatin-1 and cisplatin in advanced or recurrent carcinoma of the cervix: A New York Gynecologic Oncology Group Study, *Gynecol. Oncol.*, 93: 144–148, 2004.

Petite, G.R., Progress in the discovery of biosynthetic anticancer drugs, *Nat. Prod.*, 59:812–821, 1996.

B

Watters, D.J. and Parsons, P.G., Critical targets of protein kinase C in differentiation of tumor cells, *Biochem. Pharmacol.*, 58:383–388, 1999.

Buckwheat Buckwheat is a pseudocereal grown in North America, including Western Canada. The protein in buckwheat was shown by Kayashita and coworkers (1997) to lower plasma cholesterol and raise fecal neutral sterols in cholesterol-fed rats because of its low digestibility. In addition, buckwheat protein was found to retard the ability of 7,12-dimethylbenzyl[α]anthracene-induced mammary carcinogenesis in rats by lowering serum estradiol. The ability of buckwheat protein to suppress plasma cholesterol in rats fed a cholesterol-free diet was shown by Tomotake et al. (2001) to be stronger than a soybean protein isolate. The effect was attributed to the enhanced excretion of fecal neutral and acidic steroids. Yokozawa et al. (2001) reported that an aqueous extract from buckwheat ameliorated renal injury in rats induced by ischemia-reperfusion. The buckwheat extract also protected cultured proximal tubule cells subjected to hypoxia-reoxygenation, which was attributed to preventing oxygen free radicals from attacking the cell membranes. Earlier work by Lee et al. (1998) reported antioxidant and free-radical-scavenging activities among buckwheat-seed components. Holasova et al. (2002) showed the antioxidant activity of buckwheat seeds was higher than those of oats, barley, and buckwheat straws and hulls. The antioxidant activity resided primarily with the methanol-soluble components.

The hypoglycemic effects of consuming buckwheat flour or biscuits containing buckwheat flour in patients with diabetes was first reported in 1992 by several researchers (Lu et al., 1992; Wang et al., 1992). Kawa and coworkers (2003) recently showed that a single, oral dose of buckwheat concentrate significantly lowered elevated serum-glucose concentrations in streptozotocin-diabetic rats by 12–19 percent at 90 and 120 minutes after administration (Figure B.16). The active component in buckwheat responsible for the glucose-lowering effect appeared to be d-*chiro*-inositol, which is present at 0.2 percent in the concentrate. Fonteles et al. (2000) reported that a singe dose of intragastric d-*chiro*-inositol (10 mg/kg) fed to streptozotocin-treated rats resulted in a 30–40 percent decrease in plasma-glucose concentrations. Buckwheat concentrate, a good source of

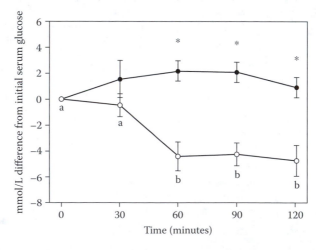

FIGURE B.16 Effect of low-dose buckwheat concentrate (10 mg of D-chiro-inositol/kg of body weight) or placebo given to STZ rats in the fed state on serum-glucose concentration. Data are expressed as the mmol/L difference from initial serum glucose concentrations (28.4 ± 0.95 mmol/L) for the placebo low-dose (, n = 9) and the low-dose buckwheat concentrate (, n = 8) groups. Asterisks (*) indicate differences (*p* < 0.001) between placebo-treated and buckwheat-treated rats. Data points with different letters indicate differences (*p* < 0.01) within a group, determined by Duncan's multiple range. (From Kawa et al., *J. Agric. Food Chem.*, 51:7287–7291, 2003. With permission.)

d-*chiro*-inositol, could be beneficial for the treatment of diabetes.

A statistically significant correlation was observed between total phenolics and rutin and antioxidant activity of buckwheat. Steadman et al. (2000, 2001a) reported buckwheat bran was a good source of protein, lipid and dietary fiber, fagopyritols, d-*chiro*-inositol, and other soluble carbohydrates. Steadman and coworkers (2001b) cautioned against the use of buckwheat bran for medicinal purposes because of the high levels of phytate and tannin present. Li and coworkers (2002) reported the production of peptides from buckwheat protein that inhibited angiotensin 1-converting enzymes, which lowered the systolic pressure in hypertensive rats. While the intact protein had some ACE inhibitory activity, it was enhanced substantially by hydrolysis with chymotrypsin and trypsin. This effect was not exhibited by rutin. A recent study by Prestamo et al. (2003) showed buckwheat acted as a prebiotic by increasing lactic-acid bacteria while decreasing mesophilic bacteria in the intestine of rats.

References

Fonteles, M.C., Almeida, M.Q., and Larner J., Antihyperglycemic effects of 3-*O*-methyl-D-*Chiro*-inositol and D-*chiro*-inositol associated with manganese in Sreptozotocin diabetic rats, *Horm. Metab. Res.,* 32:129–132, 2000.

Holasova, M., Fiedlerova, V., Smrinova, H., Orsak, M., Lachman, J., and Vavreinova, S., Buckwheat — the source of antioxidant activity in functional foods, *Food Res. Inter.,* 35:207–211, 2002.

Kawa, J., Przybylski, R., and Taylor, C., Buckwheat concentrate reduces serum glucose in streptozotocin-diabetic rats, *J. Agric. Food Chem.,* 51:7287–7291, 2003.

Kayashita, J., Shimoaka, I., Yamazaki, M., and Kato, N., Consumption of buckwheat protein lowers plasmas cholesterol and raises fecal neutral sterols in cholesterol-fed rats because of its low digestibility, *J. Nutr.,* 127:1395–1400, 1997.

Kayashita, J., Shimoaka, I., Nakajoh, M., Kishida, N., and Kato, N., Consumption of a buckwheat protein extract retards 7,12-dimethylbenz[alpha] anthracene-induced mammary carcinogenesis in rats, *Biosci. Biotechnol. Biochem.,* 63:1837–1839, 1999.

Lee, Y.C., Przbylski, R., and Eskin, N.A.M., Antioxidant and radical scavenging activities of buckwheat seed components, *J. Am. Oil Chem. Soc.,* 75:1595–1601, 1998.

Li, C.H., Matsui, T., Matsumoto, K., Yamasaki, R., and Kawasaki, T., Latent production of angiotensin 1-converting enzyme inhibitors from buckwheat protein, *J. Peptide Sci,.* 8:267–274, 2002.

Lu, C., Zu, J., Zho, P., Ma, H., Tong, H., Jin, Y., and Li, S., Clinical application and therapeutic effect of composite tartary buckwheat flour on hyperglycemia and hyperlipidemia, in *Proceedings of the 5th International Symposium on Buckwheat,* Lin, R., Zhou, M., Tao, Y., Li, J., and Zhang, Z., Eds., Agriculture Publishing House, Beijing, China, 1992, pp. 458–462.

Prestamo, G., Pedrazuela, A., Penas, E., Lasuncion, M.A., and Arroyo, G., Role of buckwheat diets on rats as prebiotic and healthy food, *Nutr. Res.,* 23:803–814, 2003.

Lee, Y.C., Przybylkski, R., and Eskin, N.A.M., Antioxidant and radical-scavenging activities of buckwheat seed components, *J. Am. Oil Chem. Soc.,* 75:1595–1601, 1998.

Steadman, K.J., Burgoon, M.S., Schuster, R.L., Lewis, B.A., Edwardson, S.E., and Obendorf, R.L., Fagopyritols, D-*chiro*-inositol, and other soluble carbohydrates in buckwheat seed milling fractions, *J. Agric. Food Chem.,* 48:2843–2847, 2000.

Steadman, K.J., Burgoon, M.S., Lewis, B.A., Edwardson, S.E., and Obendorf, R.L., Buckwheat seed milling fractions: Description, macronutrient composition, and dietary fiber, *J. Cereal Sci.,* 33:271–278, 2001a.

Steadman, K.J., Burgoon, M.S., Lewis, B.A., Edwardson, S.E., and Obendorf, R.L., Minerals, phytic acid, tannin and rutin in buckwheat seed, milling fractions, *J. Sci. Food Agric.,* 81:1094–1100, 2001b.

Tomotake, H., Shimaoka, I., Kayashita, J., Yokoyama, F., Nakajoh, M., and Kato, N., Stronger suppression of plasma cholesterol and enhancement of the fecal excretion of steroids by a buckwheat protein product than by a soy protein isolate in rats fed on a cholesterol-free diet, *Biosci. Biotechnol. Biochem.,* 65:1412–1414, 2001.

Wang, J., Liu, Z., Fu, X., and Run, M., A clinical observation on the hypoglycemic effect of Xinjiang buckwheat, in *Proceedings of the 5th International Symposium on Buckwheat,* Lin, R., Zhou, M., Tao,

Y., Li, J., and Zhang, Z., Eds., Agriculture Publishing House, Beijing, China, 1992, pp. 465–467.

Yokozawa, T., Fujii, H., Kosuna, K., and Nonaka, G., Effects of buckwheat in a renal ischemia-reperfusion model, *Biosci. Biotechnol. Biochem.*, 65:396–400, 2002.

Butyric acid   Butyric acid, a short-chain fatty acid, is a by-product of bacterial fermentation of dietary fiber. In addition to making the fecal pH more acid, short-chain fatty acids, such as butyric acid, decrease the activity of bacterial

$$CH_3–CH_2–CH_2–CH_2–COOH$$

7α-dehydroxylase, which converts bile acid from primary to secondary (Hill, 1975), a cancer promoter. Butyric acid appears to be responsible for the beneficial effect of fiber on bowel cancer (Riggs and coworkers, 1977). *In vivo* and *in vitro* studies with rats showed butyric acid acts as a potent anti-inflammatory agent (Andoh et al., 1999) while another study showed it induced apoptosis in myeloid leukemia (HL-60) cell lines (Celabresse et al., 1993). Abrahamse and coworkers (1999) found butyrate reduced DNA damage induced by hydrogen peroxide in rat colon cells, pointing to butyrate having anticarcinogenic effects *via* its antioxidant properties. Rosignoli et al. (2001) confirmed butyrate's ability to reduce H_2O_2-induced DNA damage in colon cells, although the mechanism of action still remains unknown. Sodium butyrate was also shown by Sasahara and coworkers (2002) to inhibit the growth of colon cancer by suppressing expression of inducible nitric-oxide synthase (iNOS) involving mechanisms independent from histone acetylation. An oral butyrate derivative, tributyrin, was reported by Clarke et al. (2001) to be a potent inhibitor of colorectal cancer by inducing apoptosis through activation of caspase-3 activity. Chethankumar and coworkers (2002) reported that butyric acid that supplemented high-fiber diets fed to streptozotocin-induced diabetic rats slowed down the diabetic process by inhibiting intestinal and renal disaccharidases, slowing down the release of glucose and its absorption.

References

Abrahamse, S.L., Pool-Zobel, B.L., and Rechkemmer, G., Potential of short chain fatty acids to modulate the induction of DNA damage and changes in the intracellular calcium concentration by oxidative stress in isolated rat distal colon cells, *Carcinogenesis*, 20:629–634, 1999.

Andoh, A., Kimura, T., Fukuda, M., Araki, Y., Fuyiyama, Y., and Bamba, T., Rapid intestinal ischemia reperfusion injury is suppressed in genetically mast cell deficient Ws/Ws rats, *Clin. Exp. Immunol.*, 116:90–93, 1999.

Celabresse, C., Venturini, L., Ronco, G., Villa, P., Chomienne, C., and Belpomme, D., Butyric acid and its monosaccharide ester induce apoptosis in the HL-60 cell line. *Biochem. Biophys. Res. Commun.*, 195:31–38, 1993.

Chethankumar, M., Salimath, P.V., and Sambiah, K., Butyric acid modulates activities of intestinal and renal disaccharidases in experimentally induced diabetic rats, *Nahrung*, 46:345–348, 2002.

Clarke, K.O., Feinman, R., and Harrison, E., Tributyrin, an oral butyrate analogue, induces apoptosis through activation of caspase-3, *Cancer Lett.*, 171:57–65, 2001.

Hill, M.J., The role of colon anaerobes in the metabolism of bile acids and steroids, and its relation to colon cancer, *Cancer*, 36(6):2387–2400, 1975.

Riggs, M.G., Whittaker, R.G., Neumann, J.R., and Ingram, V.M., Butyrate causes histone modification in HeLa and Friend erytholeukemia cells, *Nature*, 268:462–464, 1977.

Rosignoli, P., Fabiani, R., De Bartolomeo, A., Spinozzi, F., Agea, E., Pelli, M.A., and Morozzi, G., Protective activity of butyrate on hydrogen peroxide-induced DNA damage in isolated human colonocytes and HT29 tumor cells, *Carcinogenesis*, 22:1675–1680, 2001.

Sasahara, Y., Mutoh, M., Takahashi, M., Fukuda, K., Tanaka, N., Sugimura, T., and Wakabayashi, K., Suppression of promoter-dependent transcriptional activity of inducible nitric oxide synthase by sodium butyrate in colon cancer cells, *Cancer Lett.*, 177:155–161, 2002.

C

Cabbage *see also* Brassica and Crucifera

The antioxidant and antiproliferative activities of 10 common vegetables (broccoli, spinach, yellow onion, red pepper, carrot, cabbage, potato, lettuce, and celery) were recently studied by Chu and coworkers (2002). The phenolic content and antioxidant activity of cabbage fell in the middle, while antiproliferative activity, using HepG(2) human liver cells, was highest in spinach, followed by cabbage. Thus, cabbage had the second-highest bioactivity index (BI) suggested as an alternative biomarker for future dietary cancer-prevention studies.

Bresnick and coworkers (1990) reported that a diet containing cabbage significantly decreased the incidence of mammary cancer in female Sprague–Dawley rats injected with a carcinogen, *N*-methyl-*N*-nitrosourea (MNU). Later work by Mehta et al. (1995) reported that a synthetic brassinin [3-(*S*-methyldithiocarbamoyl)aminomethylindole], a phytoalexin first identified in cabbage, inhibited 7,12-dimethylbenz[α]anthracene (DMBA) induction of mouse skin tumors.

References

Bresnick, E., Birt, D.F., Wolterman, K., Wheeler, M., and Markin, R.S., Reduction in mammary tumorigenesis in the rat by cabbage and cabbage residue, *Carcinogenesis,* 11:1159–1163, 1990.

Chu, Y.F., Sun, J., Wu, X., and Liu, R.H., Antioxidant and antiproliferative activities of common vegetables, *J. Agric. Food Chem.,* 50:6910–6916, 2002.

Mehta, R.G., Liu, J., Constantinou, A., Thomas, C.F., Hawthorne, M., You, M., Gerhauser, C., Pezzuto, J.M., Moon, R.C., and Moriarty, R.M., Cancer chemopreventive activity of brassinin, a phytoalexin from cabbage, *Carcinogenesis,* 16:399–404, 1995.

Cacao *see* Cocoa

Caesalpinia ferrea

Caesalpinia ferrea The fruit of *Caesalpinia ferrea* or Juca*,* a leguminous tree in northern and northeastern regions of Brazil, was reported to have analgesic and anti-inflammatory properties (Carvalho et al., 1996). In addition, it was also used to treat diabetes (Balbach, 1972) and coughs and injuries (Hashimoto, 1996). The popular use of aqueous extracts of these fruit to treat cancer led to an investigation of its antitumor properties by Nakamura and coworkers (2002) using the *in vitro* Epstein–Barr virus early-antigen (EBV-EA) screening test. They identified the active constituents in *Caesalpinia ferrea* fruits responsible for antitumor effects as gallic acid and methylgallate. A total of 49 related compounds were also identified, of which three acetophenone derivatives, 2,6-dihydroxyacetophenone, 2,3,4-trihydroxyacetophenone, and 2,4,6-trihydroxyacetophenone, proved to be the most potent activity.

Acetophenone structure. (From Nakamura et al., *Cancer Lett.,* 177:119–124, 2002.)

References

Balbach, A., in *As Plantas que Curam*, Tree Press, Sao Paulo, 1972, pp. 302–303.

Carvalho, J.C.T., Teixeira, J.R.M., Souza, P.J.C., Bastos, J.K., Santos Filho, D., and Sarti, S.J., Preliminary studies of analgesic and anti-inflammatory properties of *Caesalpinia ferrea* crude extract, *J. Ethnopharm.,* 53:175–178, 1996.

Hashimoto, G., in *Illustrated Cyclopedia of Brazilian Medicinal Plants.* Japan, pp. 552–558, 1996.

Nakamura, E.S., Kurosaki, F., Arisawa, M., Mukainaka, T., Okuda, M., Tokuda, H., Nishino, H., and Pastore, F., Jr., Cancer chemoprotective effects of constituents of *Caesalpinia ferrea* and related compounds, *Cancer Lett.,* 177:119–124, 2002.

Caffeic acid Caffeic is one of the phenolic compounds in fruits and vegetables with strong antioxidant properties. Uz and coworkers (2002) showed that caffeic acid phenethyl ester (CAPE), a new antioxidant and anti-inflammatory agent, had a protective role on rat testicular tissue from reactive-oxygen species produced by testicular artery occlusion. In propolis (honeybee resin), caffeic acid is also present as

Caffeic acid phenethyl ester
(CAPE)

(From Celli et al., *J. Chromatogr. B.*, 810:129–136, 2004.)

the phenylethyl ester (Michaulart et al., 1999). Like caffeic acid, CAPE was shown in both *in vivo* and *in vitro* studies to be an anti-inflammatory compound (Huang et al., 1996; Michaulart et al., 1999; Orban et al., 2000). The anti-inflammatory properties of CAPE were attributed by Natarajan and coworkers (1996) to its inhibitory action on the transcription factor nuclear factor-B (NF-B). CAPE was also reported to induce apoptosis (Chiao et al., 1995; Chen et al., 2001). Fitzpatrick and coworkers (2001) showed CAPE inhibited NF-B and cytokine production in cell types for inflammatory-bowel disease (IBD). Lee and coworkers (2000) showed that synthetic caffeic phenylethyl ester-like compounds were cytotoxic on oral submucous fibroblasts, neck metastasis of Gigiva carcinoma, and tongue squamous-cell carcinoma cells. Further work was proposed to establish the efficacy of CAPE-like compounds as chemopreventive agents against oral cancer.

References

Celli, N., Mariani, B., Dragani, L.K., Murzulli, S., Rossi, C., and Rotilio, D., Development and validation of a liquid chromatographic-tandem mass spectrometric method for the determination of caffeic acid phenylether ester in rat plasma and urine, *J. Chromatogr. B.*, 810:129–136, 2004.

Chen, Y.J., Shiao, M.S., and Wang, S.Y., The antioxidant caffeic acid phenylethyl ester induces apoptosis associated with selective scavenging of hydrogen peroxide in human leukemic HL-cells, *Anticancer Drugs,* 12:143–149, 2001.

Chiao, C., Carothers, A.M., Grunberger, D., Solomon, G., Preston, G.A., and Barret, J.C., Apoptosis and altered redox state induced by caffeic acid phenylethyl ester (CAPE) in transformed rat fibroblast cells, *Cancer Res.,* 55:3576–3583, 1995.

Fitzpatrick, L.R., Wang, J., and Lee, T., Caffeic acid phenylethyl ester, an inhibitor of nuclear factor-B, attenuates bacterial peptidogylcan polysaccharide-induced colitis in rats, *J. Pharmacol. Therapeutics,* 299:915–920, 2001.

Huang, M.T., Ma, W., Yen, P., Xie, J.G., Han, J., Frenkel, K., Grunberger, D., and Conney, A.H., Inhibitory effects of caffeic acid phenylethyl ester (CAPE) on 12-*O*-tetradecanoylphorbol-13-acetate-induced tumor promotion in mouse skin and synthesis of DNA, RNA and protein in HeLa cells, *Carcinogenesis,* 17:761–765, 1996.

Lee, Y.-J., Liao, P.-H., Chen, W.-K., and Yang, C.-C., Preferential cytoxicity of caffeic acid phenylester analogues on oral cancer cells, *Cancer Lett.,* 153:51–56, 2000.

Michaulart, P., Masferer, J.L., Carothers, A.M., Subbaramaiah, K., Zweifel, B.S., Koboldt, C., Metre, J.R., Grunberger, D., Sacks, P.G., and Tanabe, T., Inhibitory effects of caffeic acid phenylethyl ester on the activity and expression of cyclooxygenase-2 in human oral epithelial cells and in a rat model of inflammation, *Cancer Res.,* 59:2347–2352, 1999.

Natarajan, K., Singh, Burke, T., Jr., Grunberger, D., and Aggarwal, B.B., Caffeic acid phenylethyl ester is a potent and specific inhibitor of activation of nuclear transcription factor NF-κB, *Proc. Natl. Acad. Sci.,* 93:9090–9095, 1996.

Orban, Z., Mitsiades, N., Burke, T.R., Grunberger, D., and Aggarwal, G.P., Caffeic acid phenylethyl ester induces leukocytes apoptosis, modulates nuclear factor-κB and suppresses acute inflammation, *Neuroimmunomodulation,* 7:99–105, 2000.

Uz, E., Sogut, S., Sahin, S., Var, A., Ozyyurt, H., Gulec, M. and Akyol, O., The protective role of caffeic acid phenyl ester (CAPE) on testicular tissue after testicular torsion and detorsion, *World J. Urol.,* 20:264–270, 2002.

Caffeine   Caffeine, 1,3,7-trimethylxanthine, consumed in such drinks as coffee and tea, is well-known for its biochemical and physiological activities. In recent years, evidence has accrued that caffeine can inhibit carcinogenesis

Structure of caffeine. (From Nafisi et al., *J. Mol. Struct.,* 705:35–39, 2004. With permission.)

in mice and rat lungs exposed to a nicotine-derived carcinogen (Chung, 1999; Chung et al., 1998), in mice skin exposed to ultraviolet light (Lu et al., 2001), and in rat stomachs exposed to a carcinogen and sodium chloride (Nishikawa et al., 1995). In contrast, however, no inhibition was observed when mammary glands were exposed to specific carcinogens in the presence of caffeine (VanderPloeg et al., 1991). Hagiwara and coworkers (1999) reported caffeine exerted a chemoprotective action against the carcinogen 2-amino-1-methyl-6-phenyl-imidazo [4,5-*b*]pyridine (PhIP) in female F344 rats for 54 weeks by significantly reducing mammary-gland tumor formation. Takeshita et al. (2003) were unable to explain how caffeine differentially modifies PhIP-induced colon and mammary carcinogenesis. The only parameter they found contributing to the elevation of colon carcinogenesis was elevation in PhIP-DNA adduct formation. Caffeine at a concentration of 2 mM enhanced the radiosensitivity of two rat yolk-sac cell lines with a mutant-type p53 by inducing apoptosis through a p53-independent pathway (Higuchi et al., 2000). Ito et al. (2003) also showed caffeine-induced G_2/M phase cell-cycle arrest in NB4 promyelocytic leukemia cells and apoptosis via activation of p53 by a novel pathway.

Kitamoto et al. (2003) reported that caffeine, combined with paclitaxel, a naturally occurring chemotherapeutic agent from the bark of the Western yew, suppressed cell proliferation in a dose-dependent manner. Examination of the

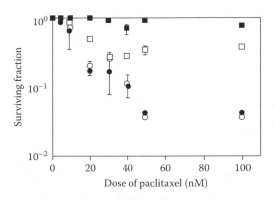

FIGURE C.17   Dose-response of A549 on paclitaxel alone, paclitaxel with 1, 5, and 20 mM of caffeine for 24 h, paclitaxel alone, (○), paclitaxel + caffeine 1.0 mM, (●), paclitaxel + caffeine 5.0 mM, (□), paclitaxel + caffeine 20 mM (■). Bar shows ± SE where these exceed the size of the symbol. (From Kitamoto et al., *Cancer Lett.,* 191:101–107, 2003. With permission.)

dose responses of paclitaxel alone and in combination with caffeine on the survival of a human lung adenocarcinoma cell line, A549, is shown in Figure C.17. The cell-killing effect of paclitaxel increased in a dose–response manner up to a maximum of 50 nM, with no further improvement at 100 nM. Combining with 5 mM caffeine, however, reduced the cytotoxicity of paclitaxel, which was further dramatically suppressed in the presence of 20 mM caffeine. These researchers showed that in the cell-cycle analysis, caffeine caused early G1 accumulation, while paclitaxel caused an early increase in G2-M and a decrease in G1. These effects suggested that while cell-modifying agents, like caffeine, can diminish the cytotoxic effects of paclitaxel, caution should be exercised in combining these substances.

References

Chung, F.L., The prevention of lung cancer induced by a tobacco-specific carcinogen in rodents by green and black tea, *Proc. Soc. Exp. Biol. Med.,* 220:244–248, 1999.

Chung, F.L., Wang, M., Rivenson, A., Iatropoulos, M.J., Reinhardt, J.C., Pittman, B., Ho, C.T., and Amin, S.G., Inhibition of lung carcinogenesis by black tea in Fischer rats treated with a tobacco-specific carcinogen: Caffeine as an important constituent, *Cancer Res.,* 58:4096–4101, 1998.

Hagiwara, A., Boonyaphiphat, H., Tanaka, H., Kawabe, M., Tamano, S., Kaneko, H., Matsui, M., Hirose, N., Ito, N., and Shirai, T., Organ-dependent modifying effects of caffeine, and two naturally occurring antioxidants -tocopherol and n-tritriacontane-16,18-dione, on 2-amino-1-methyl-6-phenylimidazo[4,5-b]pyridine(PhIP)-induced mammary and colonic carcinogenesis in female F344 rats, *Jpn. J. Cancer Res.,* 90:399–405, 1999.

Higuchi, K., Mitsuhashi, N., Saitoh, J., Maebayashi, K., Sakurai, H., Akimoto, T., and Niibe, H., Caffeine enhanced radiosensitivity of rat tumor cells with a mutant-type p53 by inducing apoptosis in a p53-independent manner, *Cancer Lett.,* 152:157–162, 2000.

Ito, K., Nakazato, T., Miyakawa, Y., Yamato, K., Ikeda, Y., and Masahiro, K., Caffeine induces $G_2.M$ arrest and apoptosis via a novel p53-dependent pathway in NB4 promyelocytic leukemia cells, *J. Cell. Physiol., 2003* (in press).

Kitamoto, Y., Sakurai, H., Mitsuhashi, N., Akimoto, T., and Nakano, T., Caffeine diminishes cytotoxic effects of paclitaxel on a human lung adenocarcinoma cell line, *Cancer Lett.,* 191:101–107, 2003.

Lu, Y.P., Lu, Y.R., Lin, Y., Shih, W.J., Huang, M.T., Yang, C.S., and Conney, A.H., Inhibitory effects of orally administered green tea, black tea and caffeine on skin carcinogenesis in mice previously treated with ultraviolet B light (high-risk mice): Relationship to decreased tissue fat, *Cancer Res.,* 61:5002–5009, 2001.

Nafisi, S., Manajemi, M., and Ebrahimi, S., The effects of mono- and divalent metal cations on the solution structure of caffeine and theophylline, *J. Mol. Struct.,* 705:35–39, 2004.

Nishikawa, A., Furukawa, F., Imizaka, T., Ikezaki, S., Hasegawa, T., and Takahasi, M., Effects of caffeine on glandular stomach carcinogenesis induced in rats by N-methyl-N-nitro-N-nitrosoguanidine and sodium chloride, *Food Chem. Toxicol.,* 33:21–26, 1995.

Takeshita, F., Ogawa, K., Asomoto, M., and Shirai, T., Mechanistic approach of contrasting modifying effects of caffeine on carcinogenesis in the rat colon and mammary gland induced with 2-amino-1-methyl-6-phenylimidazo [4,5-b]pyridine, *Cancer Lett.,* 194:25–35, 2003.

VanderPloeg, L.C., Wolfrom, D.M., and Welsch, C.W., Influence of caffeine on development of benign and carcinomatous mammary gland tumors in female rats treated with the carcinogens, 7,12-dimethylbenz(a)anthracene and N-methyl-N-nitrosourea, *Cancer Res.,* 51:3399–3404, 1991.

Calcium   Because of its importance in bone formation, particularly in relation to osteoporosis, calcium is now added to such beverages as orange juice. In addition, calcium also appears to exert cancer-preventive properties. Enhanced cell proliferation, an early biological event in the carcinogenesis process, combined with an abnormal distribution of proliferating cells in the colon, was evident in animals exposed to carcinogens and in humans with a high risk for colon cancer. Studies with human subjects have shown that calcium supplementation may reduce epithelial-cell proliferation, particularly in patients with a high risk for colon cancer (Wargovich et al., 1992; Bostick et al., 1993; O'Sullivan et al., 1993). Karkare et al. (1990) reported that supplemental calcium, relative to the standard concentration of 5.07 g/kg diet, decreased colon-tumor incidence in rats, although a lower concentration of 2.0 g/kg also reduced the incidence. However, Whitfield et al. (1995) cautioned that increasing calcium in the diet could actually promote colon cancer. Nevertheless, there is a large body of scientific evidence that increasing dietary calcium above normal levels may reduce colon cancer (Wargovitch et al., 1990; Bostick et al., 1993; O'Sullivan et al., 1993) and that this risk could also be reduced by decreasing calcium below this level (Karkare et al., 1990).

Li and coworkers (1998) showed that both low (0.5 and 1.0 g/kg) and high (10.0 and 15.0 g/kg) levels of calcium reduced the yield of azoxymethane (AOM)-induced aberrant crypt foci (ACF) in rat colons, relative to 5.0 g/kg of calcium (Figure C.18). A reduction in the yield of ACF with two or more crypts suggested that calcium levels above and below the standard level of 5.0 g/kg inhibited the promotion/progression of foci into tumors. A decrease in cell proliferation was also observed in the presence of low and high calcium levels by a reduction in both the PCNA-labeling index and the size of the PCNA-proliferative. Beaty and coworkers (1993) reported a nonstatistically significant reduction in tumor incidence of 1,2-dimethylhydrazine-induced colon carcinogenesis in rats fed high-fat diets containing vitamin D and calcium. Using diets containing 5000 and 15,000 ppm calcium with and without the presence of

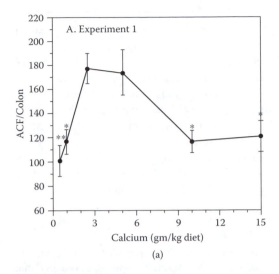

A. Experiment 1

ACF/Colon

Calcium (gm/kg diet)

(a)

FIGURE C.18 Effect of calcium on the yield of AOM/induced ACF. Results of means ± SE treatment group containing 12 rats. Statistically different results for the treatment group administered 5.0 g/kg as calcium are labeled, respectively, $*p < 0.05$ and $**p < 0.01$. (From Li et al., *Cancer Lett.*, 124:39–46, 1998. With permission.)

vitamin D and acetylsalicylic acid (ASA), Molck et al. (2002) found calcium levels affected ACF and tumor development differently. The number of ACF decreased with the higher calcium concentration, while the number of tumor-bearing animals increased with increasing calcium, either directly or indirectly, by adding vitamin D_3 together with ASA. This study showed calcium was a strong modulator of ACF and tumor development and masked the effect of vitamin D and ASA. Low calcium levels increased both the development of advanced ACF, as well as tended to increase tumor incidence. The latter can be avoided by adding vitamin D and ASA. These findings suggest that a high calcium intake may interact with other dietary or therapeutic components. These researchers cautioned against increasing calcium levels above recommended levels, as it could give initiated cells growth advantages compared to normal cells.

References

Beaty, M.M., Lee, E.Y., and Glauert, H.P., Influence of dietary calcium and vitamin D on colon epithelial cell proliferation and 1,2-dimethylhydrazine-induced colon carcinogenesis in rats fed high-fat diets, *J. Nutr.*, 123:144–152, 1993.

Bostick, R.M., Potter, J.D., Fosdick, L., Grambsh, P., Lampe, J.W., Lampe, J.R., Wood, T.A., Louis, T.A., Ganz, R., and Grandits, G., Calcium and colorectal epithelial cell proliferation: A preliminary randomized, double-blind, placebo-controlled clinical trial, *J. Natl. Cancer Inst.*, 85:132–141, 1993.

Karkare, M.R., Clark, T.D., and Glauert, H.P., Effect of dietary calcium on colon carcinogenesis induced by a single injection of 1,2-dimethylhydrazine in rats, *J. Nutr.*, 121:568–577, 1990.

Li, H., Kramer, P.M., Lubet, R.A., Steele, V.E., Kelloff, G.J., and Pereira, M.A., Effect of calcium on azoxymethane-induced aberrant crypt foci and cell proliferation in the colon of rats, *Cancer Lett.*, 124:39–46, 1998.

Molck, A.-M., Poulsen, M., and Meyer, O., The combination of $1\alpha,25(OH)_2$-vitamin D_3, calcium and acetylsalicylic acid affects azoxymethane-induced aberrant crypt foci and colorectal tumors in rats, *Cancer Lett.*, 186:19–28, 2002.

O'Sullivan, K.R., Mathias, P.M., Beattie, S., and O'Morain, C., Effect of oral calcium supplementation on colonic crypt cell proliferation in patients with adenomatrous polyps of the large bowel, *Eur. J. Gastroenterol. Hepatol.*, 5:85–89, 1993.

Wargovich, M.J., Allnut, D., Palmer, C., Anaya, P., and Stephens, L.C., Inhibition of the promotional phase of azoxymethane-induced colon carcinogenesis in theF344 rats by calcium lactate: Effect of stimulating two human nutrient density levels, *Cancer Lett.*, 53:17–25, 1990.

Whitfield, J.F., Bird, R.P., Chakravarhy, B.R., Isaacs, R.J., and Morley, P., Calcium-cell cycle regulator, differentiator, killer, chemopreventor, and maybe tumor promotor, *J. Cell Biochem.*, Issue 22 Suppl., 74–91, 1995.

***

***Calendula officinalis* L.** *Calendula officinalis* L. (Marigold), an annual herb found in the Mediterranean region, is grown for ornamental and medicinal purposes in Europe and North America. Many properties have been associated with tinctures and decoctions from its flowers, including anti-inflammatory, antitumoral, and analgesic (Duke, 1991). Cytotoxic effects were reported for extracts from its leaves, flowers, and whole plant against three cells lines from Ehrlich carcinoma. One of these extracts, rich

C

C

in saponins, exhibited antitumoral activity in an *in vivo* Ehrlich mouse carcinoma model (Boucaud-Maitre et al., 1988). Ramos and coworkers (1998) found a 60 percent aqueous-alcohol extract from *Calendula* flowers was not mutagenic in the Ames test but did report a genotoxic effect in the mitotic segregation assay of the heterozygous diploid D-30 of *Aspergillus nidulans*. This fraction was shown to contain a terpene lactone, tentatively identied as (–) oliolide (calendin), together with acyclic hydrocarbons. Two polar (aqueous and aqueous-alcohol) extracts from *C. officinalis* flowers were shown by Perez-Carreon et al. (2002) to be antigenotoxic at low concentrations by protecting rat-liver cell cultures from diethylnitrosamine (DEN) treatment. The opposite was observed at high concentrations, in which genotoxic effects were observed by the same extracts containing flavonols. These researchers pointed out that the concentration effect of these extracts must be clarified if these polyphenols are to be considered for therapeutic treatment.

Hamburger and coworkers (2003) developed a relatively simple, efficient preparative method for purifying the major anti-inflammatory triterpenoid esters from *Calendula* flower heads. The major compounds identified were faradiol esters, while the minor triterpenoid esters included maniladiol 3-*O*-laurate and myristate.

References

Boucaud-Maitre, Y., Algernon, O., and Raynaud, J., Cytotoxic and antitumoral activity of *Calendula officinalis* extracts, *Die Pharmazie,* 43:220–222, 1988.

Duke, J.A., in *Handbook of Medicinal Herbs,* CRC Press, Boca Raton, Florida, 1991, pp. 87–88.

Hamburger, M., Adler, S., Baumann, D., Forg, A., and Weinreich, B., Preparative purification of the major anti-inflammatory triterpenoid esters from Marigold (*Calendula officinalis*), *Fitoperia,* 74:328–338, 2003.

Perez-Carreon, J.I., Cruz-Jimenez, G., Licea-Vega, J.A., Popoca, E.A., Fazenda, S.F., and Villa-Trevino, S., Genotoxic and anti-genotoxic properties of *Calendula officinalis* extracts in rat liver cell cultures treated with diethytlnitrosamine, *Toxicol. In Vitro,* 16:253–258, 2002.

Ramos, A., Edeira, A., Vizoso, A., Betancourt, J., Lopez, M., and Decalo, M., Genotoxicity of an extract of *Calendula officinalis* L., *J. Ethnopharmacol.,* 61:49–55, 1998.

Cane sugar   The pressed juice from sugar cane (*Saccharum officinarum* L.) is used in Japan for the production of *Kokuto*. Previous studies isolated and characterized a number of phenolic compounds in *Kokuto* exhibiting antioxidant activity (Nakasone et al., 1996; Takara et al., 2000). Takara and coworkers (2002) recently isolated seven new phenolic glycosides, together with two known phenolic glycosides. Using the 2-deoxyribose oxidation method, all of these compounds exhibited antioxidant activity.

References

Nakasone, Y., Tanakara, K., Wada, K., Tanaka, J., and Yogi, S., Antioxidative compounds isolated from *Kokuto*, non-centrifuged cane sugar, *Biosci. Biotechnol. Biochem.,* 60:1714–1716, 1996.

Takara, K., Kinjo, A., Matsui, D., Wada, K., Nakasone, Y., and Yogi, S., Antioxidative compounds from the non-sugar fraction in *Kokuto*, non-centrifuged cane sugar, *Nippon Nogeikagaku Kaishi,* 74:885–890, 2000.

Takara, K., Matsui, D., Wada, K., Ichiba, T., and Nakasone, Y., New antioxidative phenolic glucosides isolated from *Kokuto* non-centrifuged cane sugar, *Biosci. Biotechnol. Biochem.,* 66:29–35, 2002.

Canola   Canola oil, the major edible in Canada, is recognized as a well-balanced oil, low in saturates, high in monounsaturates, and a good source of polyunsaturated acids (Table C.16). It is particularly low in saturated fatty acids (< 7.0 percent), accounting for half the level found in olive or soybean oil. In addition, the high level of monounsaturated fatty acids in canola oil provides possible protection against oxidation of LDL. This is important as uptake of LDL and formation of fatty streaks in the intima of blood vessels, an early lesion of atherosclerosis, is characterized by enhanced oxidation of LDL (Steinberg et al., 1989; Parathasarathy and Rankin, 1992). Canola oil is high in linoleic acid (> 20 percent), a member of the ω-6 family of essential fatty acids that are precursors of arachidonic acid and eicosanoids, hormone-like substances involved in many functions, such as blood clotting to immune responses. Canola oil is one of the few

TABLE C.16
Fatty-Acid Composition of Canola Oil

Fatty Acid	(%)
C14:0	0.1
C16:0	3.6
C18:0	1.5
C20:0	0.6
C22:0	0.3
C24:0	0.2
Saturated	**6.3**
C16:1	0.2
C18:1	61.6
C20:1	1.4
C22:1	0.2
Monounsaturated	**62.4**
C18:2n-6	21.7
C18:3n-3	9.6
Polyunsaturated	**31.3**

Source: Adapted from Przybylski et al., 2004. With permission.

oils high in α-linolenic acid (> 9 percent), an essential ω-3 fatty acid that is a precursor of docosahexaenoic acid (C22:6 ω-3), a major component of lipids in the brain and retina of the eye, and eicosapentaenoic acid (C22:5 ω-3), a precursor of another group of eicosanoids. There is a favorable balance in canola oil of 1:2 for the ratio of α-linolenic acid (10 percent) and linoleic acid (21.7 percent).

Animal studies have shown that diets high in polyunsaturated and monounsaturated fatty acids promote reduced fat accumulation compared to diets high in saturated fatty acids. Ellis and coworkers (2002) confirmed the ability of canola oil (high in monounsaturated fatty acids) to reduce fat deposition in growing female rats compared to corn oil (high in polyunsaturated fatty acids) and coconut oil (high in saturated fatty acids). In high-fat diets (40 percent calories), rats fed corn oil had a much larger fat-cell size compared to either canola or coconut oils, although the number of fat cells was much greater in coconut-oil-fed animals than the other oils. On the low-fat diet (6 percent calories), canola oil had a definite advantage over corn oil, as the animals had a lower body-weight gain. This study demonstrated the benefits of a diet

high in monounsaturated fatty acids because of its ability to reduce adiposity and plasma lipids.

Wakamatsu (2001) isolated a potent antioxidant in crude canola oil, which was subsequently identified as 4-vinyl-2,6-dimethoxylphenol, or canolol. Recent work by Kuwahara

Canolol. (From Kuwahara et al., *J. Agric. Food Chem.,* 52:4380–4387, 2004.)

et al. (2004) found canolol prevented apoptosis in mammalian cells induced by oxidative stress. Canolol proved toxic to cultured human colon cancer cells *in vitro* when present at 560 μM (Figure C.19A) as well as prevented apoptosis induced by oxidative stress by *tert-butyl hydroperoxide* (t-BuOOH) (Figure C.19B).

In addition, canolol also prevented DNA-strand breakage by peroxynitrite in a dose-dependent manner. The chemopreventive effects of canolol indicate its potential as a new nutraceutical.

References

Ellis,, J., Lake, A., and Hoover-Plow, J., Monounsaturated canola oil reduces fat deposition in growing female rats fed a high or low fat diet, *Nutr. Res.,* 22: 609–621, 2002.

Kuwahara, H., Kanazawa, A., Wakamatu, D., Morimura, S., Kida, K., Akaike, T., and Maeda, H., Antioxidative and antimutagenic activities of 4-vinyl-2,6-dimethoxyphenol (canolol) isolated from canola oil, *J. Agric. Food Chem.,* 52:4380–4387, 2004.

Mattson, R.S. and Grundy, S.M., Comparison of effects of dietary saturated, monounsaturated and polyunsaturated fatty acids on plasma lipids and lipoproteins in man, *J. Lipid Res.,* 26:194–202, 1985.

Parathasarathy, S. and Rankin, S.M., Role of oxidized low density lipoprotein in atherogenesis, *Prog. Lipid Res.,* 31:127–143, 1992.

Przybylski, R., Eskin, N.A.M., Mag, T., and McDonald, B.E., Canola/rapeseed oil, in *Bailey's Industrial Oil & Fat Products, Edible Oil & Fat Products: Oils and Oilseeds,* vol. 7, Hui, Y., Ed., John Wiley & Sons Inc., New York, 2003, chap. 1, pp. 1–95.

C

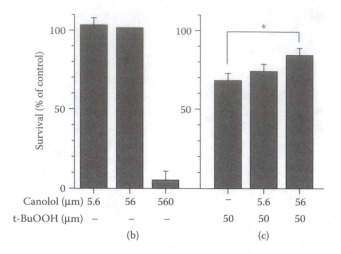

(b)　　　　　　　　(c)

FIGURE C.19 (a,b) Inhibition of t-BOOH-induced cytotoxicity in mammalian cells by canolol [values are means (n = 6 wells); bars indicate SE; *$p < 0.05$]. (From Kuwahara et al., *J. Agric. Food Chem.,* 52:4380–4387, 2004. With permission.)

Steinberg, D., Parthasarathy, S., Carew, T.E., Khoo, J.C., and Witztum, J.L., *N. Engl. J. Med.,* 320:915–, 1989.

Wakamutsa, D., Isolation and identification of radical scavenging compound, canolol, in canola oil, Master's thesis, Graduate School of Natural Science, Kumamoto University, Kumamoto City, Japan, 2001, pp. 1–48.

Capsaicin Capsaicin (*trans*-8-*N*-vanillyl-6-nonenamide) is an acrid, volatile alkaloid responsible for hotness in peppers. While it is used as an ingredient in pepper sprays, capsaicin and its dihydro derivatives all exhibit anti-inflammatory properties (Sancho et al., 2002). Kim et al. (2003) examined the anti-inflammatory mechanism of capsaicin on the production of inflammatory molecules in liposaccharides (LPS)-stimulated murine peritoneal macrophages. Capsaicin suppressed PGE2 production by inhibiting COX-2 enzyme and inducible nitric-oxide synthase (iNOS) expression in a

dose-dependent manner. The inflammatory action of capsaicin was independent of the vanilloid-receptor 1 (VR-1) but involved the following signaling pathway (Scheme C.13). Capsazepine, a known VR-1 antagonist, did not eliminate capsaicin action, but inhibited COX-2 and iNOS expression. Both compounds inactivated NF-κB via stabilization of IkB-a protein and may be useful in ameliorating inflammatory diseases and cancer.

Capsaicin is also used as a topical cream for treating various neuropathic conditions. Richeux and coworkers (1999) cautioned against the misuse of preparations containing 0.075 percent of capsaicin, which could lead to DNA-strand lesions, with detrimental effects to cellular functions, resulting in cell death or mutagenesis. The chemoprotective effects of topical application of capsaicin on the dorsal skin of female ICR mice was attributed by Han et al. (2001) to its suppression of phorbol ester-induced activation of NF-κB and activator protein-1 (AP-1) transcription factors. Lee et al.

Capsaicin. (Adapted from Zhou et al., *Life Sci.,* 74:935–968, 2004.)

C

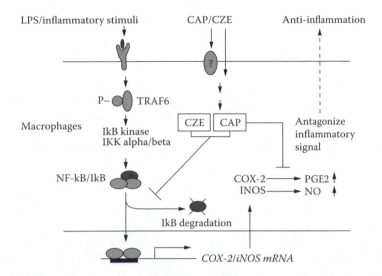

LPS/inflammatory stimuli   CAP/CZE   Anti-inflammation

SCHEME C.13 Proposed intracellular signaling pathways for the anti-inflammatory action of capsaicin or capsazepine in perotoneal macrophages, TRAP, tumor necrosis factor; CAP capsaicin; CZE Capsazepine. (From Kim et al., *Cell. Sig.,* 15:299–306, 2003. With permission.)

(2000) showed capsaicin induced apoptosis in A172 human glioblastoma cells in a time- and dose-dependent manner. The mechanism whereby capsaicin induced apoptosis may involve reduction of the basal generation of ROS. Capsaicin's ability to induce apoptosis in SK-Hep-1 heptacarcinoma cells was shown by Jung and coworkers (2001) to be due to its ability to reduce the ratio of antiapoptotic Bcl-2 to proapoptotic Bax and by activation of caspase-3.

While an early Italian case-control study showed chili consumption protected against stomach cancer (Buiatti et al., 1989), a subsequent epidemiologic study in Mexico City found a greater risk of developing stomach cancer (Lopez-Carrillo et al., 1994). Based on a number of studies, capsaicin appeared to both promote and inhibit chemically induced carcinogenesis. Further work is needed to confirm its chemopreventive properties.

References

Buiatti, E., Palli, D., Decarli, A., Amadori, D., Avellini, S., Biachi, S., Biserni, R., Cipriani, F., Cocco, P., and Giacosa, A., A case-control study of gastric cancer and diet in Italy, *Int. J. Cancer,* 44:611–616, 1989.

Han, S.S., Keum, Y.S., Seo, H.J., Chun, K.S., Lee, S.S., and Surh, Y.J., Capsaicin suppresses phorbol ester-induced activation of NF-κB/Rel and AP-1 transcription factors in mouse epidermis, *Cancer Lett.,* 164:119–126, 2001.

Jung, M.Y., Kang, H.J., and Moon, A., Capsaicin-induced apoptosis in SK-Hep-1 hepatocarcinoma cells involves Bcl-2 down-regulation and caspase-3 activation, *Cancer Lett.,* 165:139–145, 2001.

Kim, C.-S., Kawada, T., Kim, B.-S., Han, I.-S., Choe, S.-Y., Krata. T., and Yu, R., Capsaicin exhibits anti-inflammatory property by inhibiting IkB-a degradation in LPS-stimulated pertiotoneal macrophages, *Cell. Sig.,* 15:299–306, 2003.

Lee, Y.S., Nam, D.H., and Kim, J.A., Induction of apoptosis by capsaicin in A172 human glioblastoma cells, *Cancer Lett.,* 161:121–130, 2000.

Lopez-Carrillo, L., Hernandez, A.M., and Dubrow, R., Chili pepper consumption and gastric cancer in Mexico: A case control study, *Am. J. Epidemiol.,* 139: 263–271, 1994.

Richeux, F., Cascante, M., Ennamay, R., and Saboureau, D., Cytotoxicity and genotoxicity of capsaicin in human neuroblastoma cells SHSY-5Y, *Arch. Toxicol.,* 73:403–409, 1999.

Sancho, R., Lucena, C., Machio, A., Caldzado, M.A., Blanco-Molina, M., Minassi, A., Appendino, G., and Munoz, E., Immunosupresive activity of capsaicinoids: Capsiate derived from sweet peppers inhibits NF-κB activation and is a potent anti-inflammatory compound *in vivo, Eur. J. Immunol.,* 32:1753– 1763, 2002.

Zhou, S., Koh, H.-L., Gao, Y., Gong, Z.-Y., and Lee, E.J., Herbal bioactivation: The good, the bad and the ugly, *Life Sci.,* 74:935–968, 2004.

Capsicum *see* Paprika

L-Carnitine. (From Ilias et al., *Mitochondrion*, 4: 163–168, 2004. With permission.)

Caraway A reference-controlled double-blind equivalence study by Madisch et al. (1999) showed a mixture of caraway and peppermint oil was comparable to the prokinetic agent cisapride in the treatment of functional dyspepsia. Further research by Freise and Kohler (1999) on nonulcer dyspepsia confirmed that an enteric-coated capsule containing peppermint and caraway oil was comparable in efficacy to that of an enteric-soluble formulation composed of peppermint and caraway oil. Micklefield and coworkers (2000) subsequently demonstrated the safe application of enteric-coated and nonenteric-coated peppermint–caraway oil combinations for the treatment of gastroduodenal motility.

References

Freise, J. and Kohler, S., Peppermint oil–caraway oil fixed combination in non-ulcer dyspepsia-comparison of the effects of enteric preparations, *Pharmazie*, 54:210–215, 1999.

Madisch, A., Heydenreich, C.J., Wieland, V., Hufnagel, R., and Holtz, J., Treatment of functional dyspepsia with a fixed peppermint oil and caraway oil combination as preparation as compared to cisapride. A multicenter, reference-controlled double-blind equivalence study, *Arzneimittel-Forschung*, 49:925–932, 1999.

Micklefield, G.H., Greving, I., and May, B., Effects of peppermint oil-caraway oil on gastroduodenal motility, *Phytotherap. Res.,* 14:20–23, 2000.

L-Carnitine L-Carnitine (β-hydroxy-γ-trimethylammonium butyric acid), a small, water-soluble compound, is synthesized endogenously in humans, but most comes from the diet. The majority of L-carnitine on the market is produced by chemical synthesis. L-Carnitine plays an important role in mammalian fat metabolism as a fatty-acid carrier across the inner mitochondrial membrane, which undergoes β-oxidation for energy production. It has a number of important clinical applications, including the treatment of heart disease, hemodialysis, and Alzheimer's disease (Cederbaum et al., 1984; Breningstall, 1990; Seim et al., 2001). Dayanandan and coworkers (2001) showed L-carnitine protected atherosclerotic rats by significantly reducing lipid-peroxidation levels in their hearts, as well as restoring the levels of enzymatic oxidants, superoxide dismutase (SOD), catalase, glutathione peroxidase (GPx), and glucose 6 phosphate dehydrogenase (G6PD), and antioxidant vitamins C, E, and B_6 (Table C.17). A similar pattern was observed for the antioxidants and lipid peroxidation in the liver from the same atherosclerotic rats. By restoring the levels of these antioxidants, carnitine ensured that normal cell function was maintained.

Doxorubicin (DOX), an anthracycline antibiotic, is effective in reducing soft and solid tumors. However, its clinical application is somewhat limited by its severe cardiotoxicity due to the generation of cytotoxic aldehydes (Luo et al., 1999). These same researchers showed it was possible to attenuate the production of these peroxidation products by DOX by administering L-carnitine. The protective effect of L-carnitine was attributed to improving cardiac-energy metabolism and reduction in lipid peroxidation.

Male infertility is a serious problem in Western countries due, in part, to a decline in semen quality. The drugs used by practitioners and specialists for improving sperm quality have never really been tested. Lenzi et al. (1993) examined the effect of antioxidant therapies on sperm maturation. Both free and acetylated forms of L-carnitine are used by the spermatozoa for β-oxidation and for the transfer of acyl to mitochondrial CoA (Frenkel and McGarry, 1980; Peluso et al., 2000). Lenzi and coworkers (2003) treated 100 infertile patients (20–40 years) in a placebo-controlled, double-blind, crossover study with 2 g/day L-carnitine or the

TABLE C.17

Lipid Peroxidation and Antioxidant Levels in the Heart of Normal and Atherosclerotic Rats[1]

	Normal Rats Treated with Saline	Atherosclerotic Rats Treated with	
		Saline	Carinitine (14 days)
Lipid peroxidation (nmoles MDA released/mg protein)	1.8 + 0.12	2.3 + 0.21*	1.9 + 0.14**
SOD (units/min/mg/protein)	8.4 + 0.71	5.3 + 0.58*	6.7 + 0.63**
CATALASE (μmoles of GSH utilized/min/mg protein)	49.1 + 3.61	37.3 + 3.10*	45.7 + 3.70**
GPx (μmoles of GSH utilized/min/mg protein)	5.8 + 0.48	4.1 + 0.32*	5.4 + 0.45**
G6PD (μmg/mg protein)	1.8 + 0.18	1.5 + 0.14*	1.8 + 0.17**
Vitamin C (μmg/mg protein)	2.1 + 0.13	1.4 + 0.14*	1.9 + 0.18**
Vitamin E (μmg/mg protein)	1.3 + 0.16	1.0 + 0.09*	1.2 + 0.09**
Vitamin B$_6$ (μmg/mg protein)	133.6 + 12.0	93.7 + 11.0*	120.2 + 13.3**

[1] Values expressed as mean ± SD for six animals in each group.

[2] Amount of enzyme to inhibit autoxidation of pyrogallol by 50 percent in a standard 3 mL assay. For statistical evaluation, saline-treated atherosclerotic rats were compared with saline-treated normal *$p < 0.05$ and on comparing saline-treated atherosclerotic rats with carnitine treated atherosclerotic rats ** $p < 0.01$, *** $p < 0.001$.

Source: Adapted from Dayanandan et al., *J. Nutr. Biochem.,* 12:254–257, 2001.

placebo over two two-month periods. L-Carnitine therapy significantly improved semen quality, as measured by sperm concentration and total and forward motility. The potential of L-carnitine as a treatment for male infertility needs to be repeated using a much larger clinical trial and *in vitro* studies.

References

Breningstall, G.N., Carnitine deficiency syndromes, *Pediatr. Neurol.,* 6:75–81, 1990.

Cederbaum, S.D., Auestad, N., and Bernar, J., Four-year treatment systemic carnitine deficiency, *N. Engl. J. Med.,* 10:1395–1396, 1984.

Dayanandan, A., Kumar, P., and Panneerselvam, C., Protective role of L-carnitine on liver and heart lipid peroxidation in atherosclerotic rats, *J. Nutr. Biochem.,* 12:254–257, 2001.

Frenkel, R.A. and McGarry, J.D., *Carnitine Biosynthesis, Metabolism, and Function,* Italian ed., Academic Press, New York, pp. 321–340, 1980.

Ilias, I., Manoli, I., Blackman, M.R., Gold, P.W., and Alesci, S., L-Carnitine and acetyl-L-carnitine in the treatment of complications associated with HIV infection and antiretroviral therapy, *Mitochondrion,* 4:163–168, 2004.

Lenzi, A., Culasso, F., Gandini, L., Lombardo, L., and Dondero, F., Placebo-controlled, double-blind, cross-over trial of glutathione therapy in male infertility. *Hum. Reprod.,* 8:1657–1662, 1993.

Lenzi, A., Lombardo, F., Sgro, P., Salacone, P., Caponecchia, L., Dondero, F., and Gandini, L., Use of L-carnitine therapy in selected cases of male factor infertility: A double-blind crossover trial, *Fertil. Steril.,* 79:292–300, 2003.

Luo, X., Reichietzer, B., Trines, J., Benson, L.N., and Lehotay, D.C., L-Carnitine attenuates doxorubicin-induced lipid peroxidation in rats, *Free Rad. Biol. Med.,* 26:1158–1165, 1999.

Peluso, G., Nicolai, R., Reda, E., Benatti, P., Barbarisi, A., and Calvai, M., Cancer and anticancer therapy-induced modifications on metabolism mediated by carnitine, *J. Cell. Physiol.,* 182:339–350, 2000.

Seim, H., Eichler, K., and Kleber, H.-P., L(−)-Carnitine and its precursor, γ-butyrbetaine, in *Neutraceuticals in Health and Disease Prevention,* Kramer, K., Hoppe, P.-P., and Packer, L., Eds., Marcel Dekker, New York, 2001, pp. 217–256.

L-Carnosine   L-Carnosine (β-alanyl-L-histidine) and its related compounds, anserine and homocarnosine, are found in the skeletal muscle and brain of mammals (Kohen et al., 1988). In addition to their antioxidant properties, they are efficient, copper-chelating agents with a possible role in copper metabolism (Gercken et al., 1980). Choi and coworkers (1999) showed carnosine-related compounds protected Cu,

C

L-Carnosine. (From Hobart et al., *Life Sci.,* 75:1379–1389, 2004. With permisson.)

Zn-SOD (superoxide dismutase) from fragmentation by hydrogen peroxide. Carnosine and related compounds were shown by Ukeda and coworkers (2002) to protect human Cu, Zn-SOD from inactivation by glycoaldehyde, a Maillard-reaction intermediate, and from fructose. This protection was attributed to its hydroxyl radical-scavenging activity. Kang and coworkers (2002) showed L-carnosine's antioxidant properties protected rat liver epithelial cells from 12-*O*-tetradecanoyl-phorbol-13-acetate (TPA) or hydrogen peroxide-induced apoptosis via the mitochondria.

Carnosine, a histidine dipeptide in mammalian brain, has been shown to prevent neural-cell toxicity (Hipkiss et al., 1997), ischemic injury (Stvolinsky et al., 1999), thermal injury (Deev et al., 1997), and β-amyloid aggregation (Munch et al., 1997). The anticross-linking property of carnosine appeared to be responsible for its potential use in the treatment of Alzheimer's disease (Hobart et al., 2004). The imidazolium group of histidine in carnosine may stabilize adducts formed with the primary amino group.

References

Choi, S.Y., Kwon, H.Y., Kwon, O.B., and Kang, J.H., Hydrogen peroxide-mediated Cu, Zn-superoxide disutase fragmentation: Protection by carnosine, homocarnosine and anserine, *Biochem. Biophys. Acta,* 1472:651–657, 1999.

Deev, L.I., Goncharenko, E.N., Baizhumanov, A.A., Akhalaia, M.Ia., Antonova, S.V., and Shestokova, S.W., Protective effect of carnosine in hyperthermia, *Bull. Experiment. Biolog. Med.,* 124(7):50–52, 1997.

Gercken, G., Bischoff, H., and Trotz, M., Myocardial protection by a carnosine-buffered cardioplegic solution, *Arzneimmitelforschung,* 30:2140–2143, 1980.

Hipkiss, A.R., Michaelis, J., and Syms, P., Non-enzymatic glycosylation of the dipeptide L-carnosine, a potential anti-protein-cross-linking agent, *FEBS Lett.,* 371:81–85, 1995.

Hobart, L.J., Seibel, I., Yeargans, G.S., and Seidler, N.W., Anti-crosslinking properties of carnosine: Significance of histidine, *Life Sci.,* 75:1379–1389, 2004.

Kang, K.-S., Yun, J.-W., and Lee, Y.-S., Protective effect of L-carnosine against 12-*O*-tetradecanoylphorbol-13-acetate- or hydrogen peroxide-induced apoptosis on *v-myc* transformed rat liver epithelial cells, *Cancer Lett.,* 178:53–62, 2002.

Kohen, R., Yamamoto, Y., Cundr, K.C., and Ames, B.N., Antioxidant activity of carnosine, homocarnosine and anserine present in muscle and brain, *Proc. Natl. Acad. Sci. U.S.A.,* 85:3175–3179, 1988.

Munch, G., Mayer, S., Michaelis, J., Hipkiss, A.R., Riederer, P., Muller, R., Neumann, A., Schinzel, R., and Cunningham, A.M., Influence of advanced glycation end-products and AGE-inhibitors on nucleation-dependent polymerization of beta-amyloid peptide, *Biochem. Biophys. Acta,* 1360:17–19, 1997.

Stvolinsky, S.L., Kukley, M.L., Dobrata, D., Matejovicova, M., Tkac, I., and Boldyrev, A.A., Carnosine: An endogenous neuroprotector in the ischemic brain cell, *Mol. Neurobiol.,* 19:45–56, 1999.

Ukeda, H., Hasegawa, Y., Harada, Y., and Sawamura, M., Effect of carnosine and related compounds on the inactivation of human Cu, Zn-superoxide dismutase by modification of fructose and glycoaldehyde, *Biosci. Biotechnol. Biochem.,* 66:36–43, 2002.

Carnosol *see also* **Rosemary**   Carnosol is a phenolic dieterpene antioxidant obtained from the herb rosemary (*Rosemarinus officinalis Labiatae*). Its anticancer properties were demonstrated in animal models for breast and skin

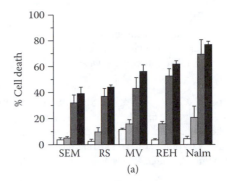

Carnosol. (From Huang et al., *Biochem. Pharmacol.*, 69:221–232, 2005. With permission.)

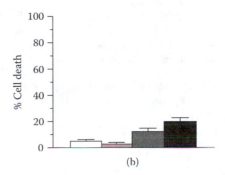

FIGURE C.20 Carnosol is cytotoxic to the leukemia cells (a). The leukemia cells lines; or (B), Peripheral blood mononuclear cells (PMBCs) from healthy volunteers were untreated, or treated with 3 (gray), 6 (hatched), and 9 μg/mL (black) carnosol, and the percentage cell death was measured after four days by propidium iodide staining of nuclei and a FACS-Calibur fluorescence-activated cell scorer (FACS). The data presented represent the mean of the percentage cell death ± SE of five separate experiments for (A) and three healthy donors for (b). The control is white. (From Dorrie et al., *Cancer Lett.*, 170:33–39, 2001. With permission.)

tumors (Huang et al., 1994; Singletary et al., 1996). Carnosol was shown to strongly inhibit the activity of phase I enzyme, CYP 450, while stimulating the activities of phase II enzymes, glutathione *S*-transferase (GST), and NAD (P)H-quinone reductase (QR) in the liver (Offord et al., 1998). Dorrie and coworkers (2001) showed carnosol was effective against several pro-B and pre-B acute lymphoblastic leukemia (ALL) lines, a disease prevalent among infants during early childhood. Carnosol induced apoptosis in B-lineage leukemias by down-regulating the antiapoptotic protein Bcl-2, suggesting it was a novel chemotherapeutic agent against other types of cancers. It proved cytotoxic against all five acute leukemia lines, with the percentage of dead cells ranging from 40 to 75 percent with the effect of 6 μg/mL of carnosol not statistically different from that of 9 μg/mL (Figure C.20). A recent study by Huang et al. (2005) showed the potential of carnosol for treating lung metastasis of B16/F10 mouse melanoma cells by inhibiting NF-6B and AP-1 binding activity. Following this, carnosol inhibited metalloproteinase (MMP)-9 gene expression which is associated with increased matastic potential for many types of cancers.

The antioxidant properties of carnosol were demonstrated by Lo and coworkers (2002) by its ability to scavenge DPPH free radicals and protect DNA from the Fenton reaction.

Carnosol markedly reduced lipopolysaccharide (LPS)-stimulated NO production in mouse macrophages in a concentration-dependent manner, with an IC_{50} of 9.4 μM, while only slight changes were observed for the other rosemary compounds (carnosic, rosmarinic, and ursolic acids). Multiple stages of carcinogenesis and inflammation are characterized by large amounts of NO produced by inducible NO synthase (iNOS). The mechanism for carnosol's anticancer and anti-inflammatory properties appears to be related to its suppression of NO production and iNOS gene expression through inhibition of nuclear factor-κB (NF-κB).

C

References

Dorrie, J., Sapala, K., and Zunino, S.J., Carnosol-induced apoptosis and down regulation of Bcl-2 in B-lineage leukemia cells, *Cancer Lett.*, 170:33–39, 2001.

Huang, S.-C., Ho, C.-T., Lin-Shiau, S.-Y., and Lin, J.-K., Carnosol inhibits the invasion of B16/F10 mouse melanoma cells by suppressing metalloproteinase-9 through down regulating nuclear factor-κB and c-Jun, *Biochem. Pharmacol.*, 69:221–232, 2005.

Huang, M.-T., Ho, C.T., Yuan Wang, Z., Ferraro, T., Lou, Y.-R., Stauber, K., Ma, W., Georgiadis, C., Laskin, J.D., and Conney, A.H., Inhibition of skin tumorigenesis by rosemary and its constituents carnosol and ursolic acid, *Cancer Res.*, 54:701–708, 1994.

Lo, A.-H., Liang, Y.-C., Lin-Shiau, S.-Y., Ho, C.-T., and Lin, J.-K., Carnosol, an antioxidant in rosemary, suppresses inducible nitric oxide synthase through down-regulating nuclear factor-κB in mouse macrophages, *Carcinogenesis*, 23:983–991, 2002.

Offord, E.A., Mace, K., Avanti, O., and Pfeifer, A.M., Mechanisms involved in the chemoprotective effects of rosemary extract in human liver and bronchial cells, *Cancer Lett.*, 114:275–281, 1997.

Singletary, K., MacDonald, C., and Wallig, M., Inhibition by rosemary and carnosol of 7,12-dimethylben[α]anthracene (DMBA)-induced rat mammary tumorigenesis and *in vivo* DMBA-DNA adduct formation, *Cancer Lett.*, 104:43–48, 1996.

Carotenoids   Consumption of diets high in fruits and vegetables has been associated with a decrease in cancer and cardiovascular diseases and possibly other degenerative diseases (Block et al., 1992; Willett, 1994; Ames et al., 1995). Of the 600 dietary carotenoids identified in fruits, vegetables, and fish, many of them are reported to protect against atherosclerosis, cancer, and macular degeneration, as well as act as photoprotectants against sun damage to the skin (Mares-Perlman et al., 1995; D'Odorico et al., 2000; Nishino et al., 2000; Ziegler and Vogt, 2002). As antioxidants, they scavenge free radicals or quench singlet oxygen. The association between oxygen radicals, such as superoxide ($\cdot O_2^-$) and nitric oxide (NO), and chronic diseases, such as cancer, makes carotenoids potentially important antioxidants in human health.

However, a recent ATBC Study suggested that β-carotene, under certain circumstances, may enhance carcinogenesis (Rautalahtu et al., 1997). In addition to β-carotene, Murakami and coworkers (2000) examined the ability of 18 natural carotenoids to inhibit tumor-promoting 12-*O*-tetradecanoylphorbol-13-acetate (TPA)-induced $\cdot O_2^-$ generation in differentiated human promyelocytic cell HL-60 cells (Scheme C.14). No cytotoxicity was observed for any of the carotenoids at 25 μM with inhibitory rates (IRs) ranging from –3.4 percent (for β-cryptoxanthin) to 52.6 percent (for halocynthiaxanthin). The 11 carotenoids all had superior or similar inhibitory rates (IRs = 25.1–52.6 percent) to β-carotene (21.3 percent) and the green tea polyphenol, (–) epigallocatechin gallate (IR = 15.6 percent). Murakami et al. (2000) proposed that carotenoids in fruits and vegetables suppressed leukocyte-induced oxidative stress by attenuating $\cdot O_2^-$ production systems, such as NADPH oxidase. From a structural point of view, the presence of a single, 3-hydroxy-κ-end group in carotenoids appeared important for this activity. For example, capsanthin 3,6-epoxide, with 3-hydroxy-κ-end group, had a significantly higher inhibitory rate of 40.9 percent compared to 28.4 percent for cucurbitaxanthin, with a 3-hydroxy-β-end group. The ability of these same carotenoids to inhibit lipopolysaccharide (LPS)- and interferon (IFN-γ)-induced NO generation by mouse macrophage RAW 264.7 cells ranged from –45.2 percent to + 94.7 percent with no cytoxicity reported for any of carotenoids at 50 μM. Halocynthiaxanthin from the Sastumas mandarin (*Citrus unshui*) exhibited the greatest inhibitory activity of 94.7 percent, indicating the importance of the 3-hydroxy-κ-end group for inhibiting NO production.

Kozuki and coworkers (2000) suggested the antioxidant properties of carotenoids, α-carotene, β-carotene, lycopene, β-cryptoxanthin, zeaxanthin, lutein, canthaxanthin, and astaxanthin, were responsible for inhibiting invasion of rat ascites hepatoma AH109A cells in a dose-dependent manner up to 5 μM. Using a model membrane environment composed of unilamellar dipalmitoyl phosphatidylcholine, Cantrell and coworkers (2003) found singlet oxygen quenching varied with the particular carotenoid incorporated. Lycopene and β-carotene had the

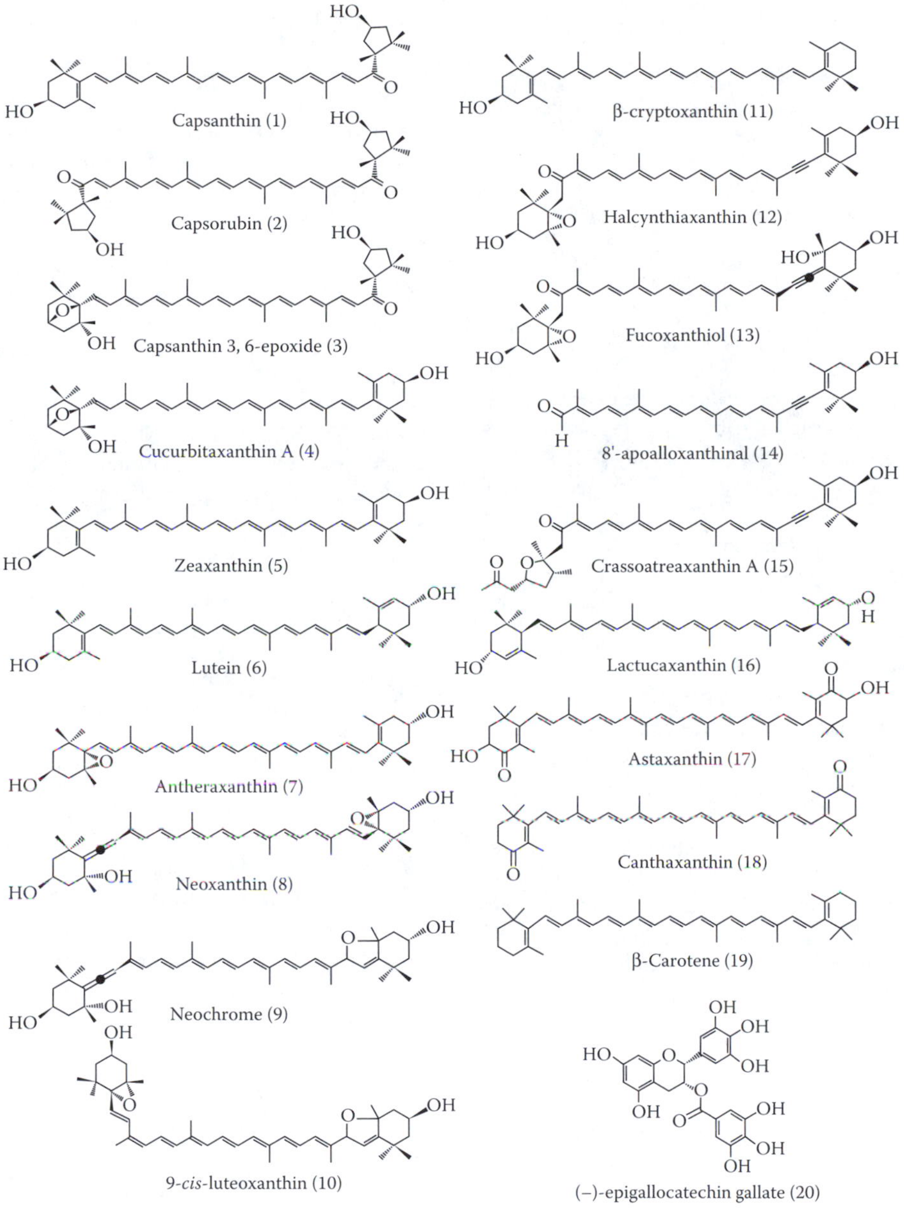

SCHEME C.14 Structure of carotenoids (1–19) and ECGC (20). (From Murakami et al., *Cancer Lett.,* 149:115–123, 2000. With permission.)

fastest singlet oxygen-quenching rate, while lutein the least, with astaxanthin and canthanxin intermediate.

Considerable variability between the efficacy of different carotenoids was also shown by Pool-Zobel and coworkers (1997). These researchers showed that carotenoid-rich plant products, such as tomato juice, carrot juice, and spinach powder, consumed by 23 healthy, non-smoking males between the ages of 27–40, all exerted cancer-protective effects. Using the Comet assay for DNA damage, which specifically measures oxidation of pyrimidines in DNA, only carrot juice reduced endogenous oxidative damage (Figure C.21).

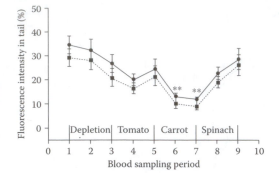

FIGURE C.21 Levels of DNA-strand breaks I peripheral blood lymphocytes from humans receiving different vegetable products. The extent of DNA damage is indicated by the percentage of fluorescence in the comet tail ("tail intensity"). Results are shown as means ± SEM, n = 21–23 subjects, means of three slides per subject. *Statistically significant in comparison to sampling time 1; two-sided Student's t-test, $p < 0.05$. (From Pool-Zobel et al., *Carcinogenesis,* 18:1847–1850, 1997. With permission.)

References

Albanes, D., Heinonen, O.P., Taylor, P.R., Virtano, J., Edwards, B.K., Rantalahti, M., Hartman, A.M., Palmgren, J., Freedman, L.S., Haapakoshi, J., Barret, M.J., Prietinen, P., Malila, N., Tala, E., Lippo, K., Salomaa, E.R., Tangrea, J.A., Teppo, L., Askin, F.B., Taskinen, E., Erozan, Y., Greenwald, P., and Huttumen, J.K., Alpha-tocopherol and beta-carotene supplement and lung cancer incidence in the alpha-tocopherol, beta-carotene cancer prevention study: Effects of base-line characteristics and study compliance, *J. Natl. Cancer Inst.,* 88:1560–1570, 1996.

Ames, B.N., Gold, L.S., and Willett, W.C., The causes and prevention of cancer, *Proc. Natl. Acad. Sci.,* 92:5258–5265, 1995.

Block, G., Patterson, B., and Subar, A., Fruit and vegetables, and cancer prevention: A review of the epidemiological evidence, *Nutr. Canc.,* 18:1–29, 1992.

Cantrell, A., McGarvey, D.J., Truscott, T.G., Rancan, F., and Bohm, F., Singlet oxygen quenching by dietary carotenoids in a model membrane environment, *Arch. Biochem Biophys.,* 412:47–54, 2003.

D'Odorico, A., Martines, D., Kiechl, S., Egger, G., Oberhollenzer, F., Bonvicini, P., Sturniolo, G.C., Naccarato, R., and Willett, J., *Atherosclerosis,* 153: 231–239, 2000.

Kozuki, Y., Miura, Y., and Yagasaki, K., Inhibitory effects of carotenoids on the invasion of rat ascites hepatoma cells in culture, *Cancer Lett.,* 151:111–115, 2000.

Mares-Perlman, J.A., Brady, W.E., Klein, R., Klein, B.E.K., Bowen, P., Stacewicz-Sapuintzakis, M., and Palta, M., *Arch. Ophthamol.,* 113:1518–1523, 1995.

Murakami, A., Nakashima, M., Koshiba, T., Maoka, T., Nishino, H., Yano, M., Sumida, T., Kim, A.K., Koshimizu, K., and Ohigashi, H., Modifying effects of carotenoids on superoxide and nitric oxide generation from stimulated leukocytes, *Cancer Lett.,* 149: 115–123, 2000.

Nishino, H., Tokuda, H., Murakoshi, M., Satomi, Y., Masuda, M., Onozuka, M., Yamaguchi, S., Takayasu, J., Tsuruta, J., Okuda, M., Khachik, F., Narisawa, T., Takasuka, N., and Yano, M., *Biofactors,* 13:89–94, 1995.

Pool-Zobel, B.L., Bub, A., Muller, H., Woloowski, I., and Rechkemmer, G., Consumption of vegetables reduces genetic damage in humans: First results of a human intervention trial with carotenoid-rich foods, *Carcinogenesis,* 18:1847–1850, 1997.

Willett, W.C., Diet and health: What should we eat? *Science,* 264:532–537, 1994.

Ziegler, R.G. and Vogt, T.M., Tomatoes, lycopene, and risk of prostate cancer, *Pharm. Biol.,* 40(Suppl.): 59–69, 2002.

Carrot   Carrot (*Daucus carota* L.), a biennial of the *Umbelliferae* family, is grown throughout the world. It is an excellent source of carotenoids, particularly β-carotene. Pool-Zobel et al. (1997) conducted a human-intervention study in which he fed healthy, young men 330 mL carrot juice, tomato juice, and dried-spinach powder. The carrot juice, containing 22.3 mg β-carotene and 15.7 mg α-carotene, was the only one to decrease base oxidation, an indicator of oxidative damage, which was attributed to the ability of α-carotene and β-carotene to quench free radicals *in vivo*.

However, in spite of carrots being high in β-carotene, there are conflicting data with respect to their health benefits. For example, supplementing well-nourished populations with β-carotene did not prevent cancers or other health disorders (The Alpha-Tocopherol, Beta-Carotene Cancer Prevention Study Group, 1994; Greenberg et al., 1996; Hennekens et al., 1996). In other cases, the incidence of cancer actually increased in smokers taking β-carotene supplements

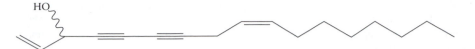

Falcarinol. (From Brandt et al., *Trends Food Sci. Technol.,* 15:384–393, 2004. With permission.)

C

(Omenn et al., 1996). The beneficial health effects associated with the consumption of β-carotene-rich vegetables seems contradictory and, in the case of carrots, may be due to the presence of other bioactive compounds. Such compounds may be polyacetylenes, falcarinol, and falcarindiol, found in vegetables such as carrots. Falcarinol or panaxynol, (9Z)-hepta-deca-1,9-dien-4,6-diyn-3-ol, is reported to be one the most bioactive components in carrots (Brandt and Christensen, 2000). While it has been shown to be cytotoxic against several human tumor cells (Saita et al., 1993; Bernart et al., 1996), falcarinol is also a potent skin sensitizer and irritant, as well as a neurotoxic at high concentrations (Hansen and Boll, 1986; Hansen et al., 1986). Recent work by Hansen and coworkers (2003) found falcarinol had biphasic activity, stimulating human cancer growth and cell proliferation between 0.01–0.05 µg/mL, while inhibiting cell proliferation at concentrations greater than 1 µg/mL. Thus, the effect of falcarinol on cell proliferation was concentration-dependent. In comparison, β-carotene had no effect as either a stimulator or inhibitor. Long-term storage, however, resulted in a 35 percent loss of falcarinol, while carrot pieces boiled in water suffered a 70 percent loss (Figure C.22). To maximize the health benefits derived from carrots, eating them raw was recommended.

Stoll et al. (2003) developed a pilot-plant scale process for recovering carotenoids from carrot pomace. The total carotene content (α- and β-carotene) of the concentrated hydrolysate was 64 g/kg, making it an excellent functional-food ingredient. Chau and coworkers (2004) showed carrot pomace was rich in insoluble fibers composed mainly of pectin material, hemicellulose, and cellulose. In particular, the water-insoluble solids exhibited significantly ($p < 0.05$) greater glucose absorption and amylase-inhibitory activities compared to cellulose. The hypoglycemic effects of some of these fractions could be useful in controlling postprandial glucose levels.

References

Alpha-tocopherol, Beta-Carotene Cancer Prevention Study Group, The effect of vitamin E and β-carotene on the incidence of lung cancer and other cancers in male smokers, *N. Engl. J. Med.,* 330:1029–1035, 1994.

Bernart, M.W., Cardellina, J.H., II, Balaschak, M.S., Alexander, M., Shoemaker, R.H., and Boyd, M.R., Cytotoxic falcarinol oxylips from *Dendropanax arboreus, J. Nat. Prod.,* 59:748–753, 1996.

Brandt, K. and Christensen, L.P., Vegetables as neutraceuticals-falcarinol in carrots and other root crops, in *Dietary Anticarcinogens and Antimutagens,* Johnson, I.T., and Fenwick, G.R., Eds., Royal Society of Chemistry, Cambridge, 2000, pp. 386–391.

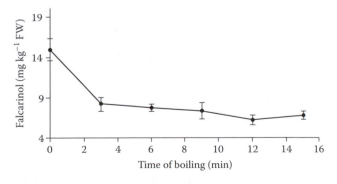

FIGURE C.22 Reduction in falcarinol content in carrot pieces during boiling in water. Values are mean ± SD of three processing replications. FW = fresh weight. (From Hansen et al., *J. Sci. Food Agric.,* 83:1010–1017, 2003.)

Brandt, K., Christensen, L.P., Hansen-Moller, J., Hansen, S.L., Heraldsdotter, J., Jesperen, L., Purups, S., Kharazmi, A., Barkholt, V., Frokiaer, H., and Kobaek-Larsen, M., Health promoting compounds in fruits and vegetables: A systematic approach for identifying plant components with impact on human health, *Trends Food Sci. Technol.*, 15:384–393, 2004.

Chau, C.-F., Chen, C.-H., and Lee, M.-H., Comparison of the characteristics, functional properties, and in vitro hypoglycemic effects of various carrot insoluble fiber-rich fractions, *Lebensm.-Wiss. u.-Technol.*, 37:155–160, 2004.

Greenberg, E.R., Baron, J.A., Karagas, M.R., Stukel, T.A., Niererberg, D.W., Stevens, M.M., Mandel, J.S., and Haile, R.W., Mortality associated with low plasma concentration of β-carotene and effect of oral supplementation, *J. Am. Med. Assoc.*, 275:699–703, 1996.

Hansen, S.L. and Boll, P.M., The polyacetylenic falcarinol as the major allergen in *Schefflera arboricola*, *Phytochemistry*, 25:529–530, 1986.

Hansen, S.L., Hammershoy, O., and Boll, P.M., Allergic contact dermatitis from falcarinol isolated from *Schefflera arboricola*, *Contact Derm.*, 14:91–93, 1986.

Hansen, S.L., Purup, S., and Christensen, L.P., Bioactivity of falcarinol and the influence of processing and storage on its content in carrots (*Daucus carota* L.), *J. Sci. Food Agric.*, 83:1010–1017, 2003.

Hennekens, C.H., Buring, J.E., Manson, J.E., Stampfer, M., Rosner, B., Cook, N.R., Belanger, C., LaMotte, F., Gaziano, J.M., Ridker, P.M., Willett, W., and Peto, R., Lack of effect of long-term supplementation with β-carotene on the incidence of malignant neoplasms and cardiovascular disease, *N. Eng. J. Med.*, 334:1145–1149, 1996.

Omenn, G.S., Goodman, G.E., Thornquist, M.D., Balmes, J., Cullen, M.R., Glass, A., Keogh, J.P., Meyskens, F.L., Jr., Valanis, B., and Williams, J.H., Jr., Effects of a combination of β-carotene and vitamin A on lung cancer and cardiovascular disease, *N. Engl. J. Med.*, 334:1150–1155, 1996.

Pool-Zobel, B.L., Bub, A., Muller, H., Wollowski, I., and Rechkemmer, G., Consumption of vegetable reduces genetic damage to humans: First results of a human intervention trial with carotenoid-rich foods, *Carcinogenesis*, 18:1847–1850, 1997.

Saita, T., Katano, M., Yamamoto, H., Fujito, H., and Mori, M., The first specific antibody against cytotoxic polyacetylenic alcohol, panaxynol, *Chem. Pharm. Bull.*, 41:549–552, 1993.

Stoll, T., Schweiggert, U., Schieber, A., and Carle, R., Process for the recovery of a carotene-rich functional food ingredient from carrot pommace by enzymatic liquefaction, *Innov. Food Sci. Emerging Technol.*, 4:415–423, 2003.

Casein   Casein is an important nutritional source of milk protein. Early studies showed that casein inhibited lipid oxidation by molecular encapsulation of the 1,4-pentadiene fatty acids (Laakso, 1984). To determine the primary sequence in casein responsible for its free-radical-scavenging activity, Suetsuna and coworkers (2000) examined peptides produced by peptic digestion of casein. A number of peptides exhibiting superoxide anion-scavenging activity (SOSA) were isolated in which the amino-acid sequence was Tyr-Phe-Tyr-Pro-Glu-leu (YFYPEL). Of the amino acids in the peptide, Glu-Leu appeared important for activity. Casein protein was also recognized as an important source of biologically active peptides (Chabance et al., 1998). Such peptides play an important role in the development of the immune system in newborns. Immunostimulating peptides identified in bovine casein were LLY (residues 191–193 β-casein), TTMPLW (C-terminal hexapeptide of α_{s1}-casein), and PGPIPN (residues 63–68 of β-casein) (Fiat et al., 1993). Xiao and coworkers (2000) investigated the effect of these three peptides on the production of tumor necrosis factor-α (TNF-α) and interleukine-6 (IL-6). The latter are multifunctional cytokines released by macrophages and play an important role in immunoregulation and host defenses (Akira et al., 1990). Xiao et al. (2000) also found that incubation of these three bovine-casein peptides with murine bone-marrow macrophages in the presence of lipopolysaccharide enhanced TNF-α and IL-6 production and nitric-oxide release. These changes could be important in the defense by the host against infection by pathogens.

References

Akira, S., Hirano, T., Taga, T., and Kishimoto, T., Biology of multifunctional cytokines: IL-6 and related molecules (IL-1 and TNF), *FASEB*, 4:2860–2867, 1990.

Chabance, B., Martean, P., Rambaud, J.C., Migliore-Samour, D., Boynard, M., Perrotin, P. Guillet, R., Jolles, P., and Fiat, A.M., Casein peptide release and passage to the blood in human during digestion of milk or yogurt, *Biochemie,* 80:155–165, 1998.

Fiat, A., Migliore-Samour, D., Jolles, P., Drouet, L., Sollier, C., and Caen, J., Biologically active peptides from milk proteins with emphasis on two examples concerning antithrombotic and immunomodulating activities, *J. Dairy Sci.,* 76:301–310, 1993.

Laakso, S., Inhibition of lipid peroxidation by casein: Evidence of molecular encapsulation of 1,4-pentadiene fatty acids, *Biochem. Biophys. Acta,* 792:11–15, 1984.

Suetsuna, K., Ukeda, H., and Ochi, H., Isolation and characterization of free radical scavenging activities of peptides derived from casein, *J. Nutr. Biochem.,* 11:128–131, 2000.

Xiao, C., Jin, L.Z., and Zhao, X., Bovine casein peptides co-stimulate naive macrophages with lipopoly-saccharides for proinflammatory cytokine production and nitric oxide release, *J. Sci. Food Agric.,* 81:300–304, 2000.

Catechins   Catechins are polyphenols widely distributed in fruits and vegetables, especially in tea (Scheme C.15). They have been shown to be anticarcinogenic, antiatherosclerotic, antimicrobial, and to act as antioxidants (Wang et al., 2000; Yang et al., 2000; Yang et al., 2001; McKay and Blumberg, 2002). In addition to scavenging free radicals, tea catechins may also modulate some cellular enzymes. Blache et al. (2002) studied the effect of (+)-catechin on acute iron-load-induced model of platelet hyperactivity. Beneficial effects were only observed in the iron-loaded animals and attributed to antioxidant properties of catechin or its metabolites. The presence of galloyl and gallate moieties in tea catechins, such as (–)-epicatechin gallate (ECG) and (–)-epigallocatechin gallate (EGCG), appears to enhance the antibacterial, anticancer, and radical-scavenging properties of catechin (Ikigai et al., 1993; Rice-Evans, 1995; Kitano et al., 1997). Caturla and coworkers (2003) examined the interaction of

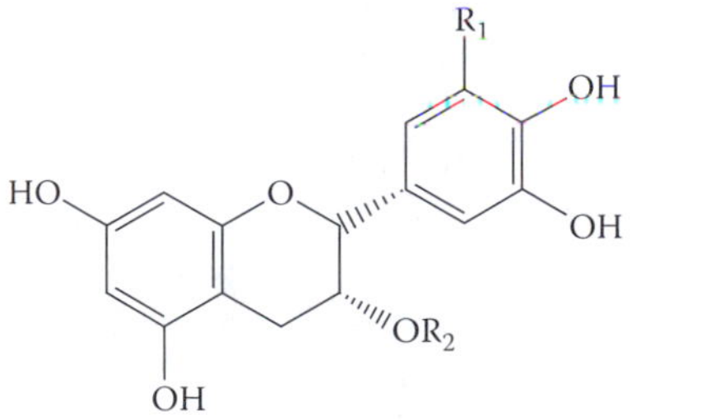

(–)-epigallocatechin 3-*O*-gallate ((–)-EGCg): R_1=OH, R_2=G
(–)-epigallocatechin ((–)-EGC): R_1=OH, R_2=H
(–)-epicatechin 3-*O*-gallate ((–)-ECg): R_1=H, R_2=G
(–)-epicatechin ((–)-EC): R_1=R_2=H

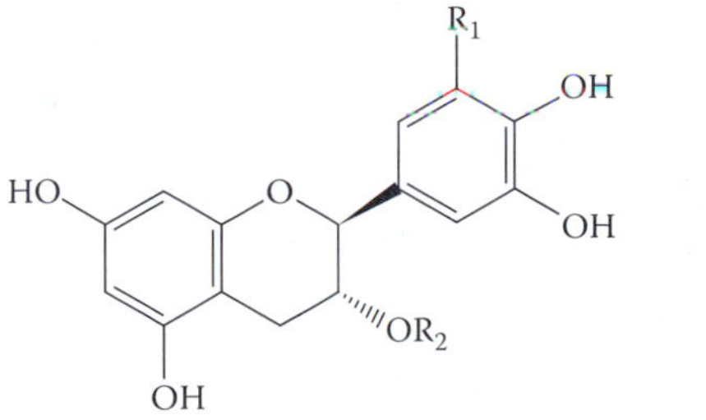

(–)-gallocatechin 3-*O*-gallate ((–)-GCg): R_1=OH, R_2=G
(–)-gallocatechin ((–)-GC): R_1=OH, R_2=H
(–)-catechin 3-*O*-gallate ((–)-Cg): R_1=H, R_2=G
(–)-catechin ((–)-C): R_1=R_2=H

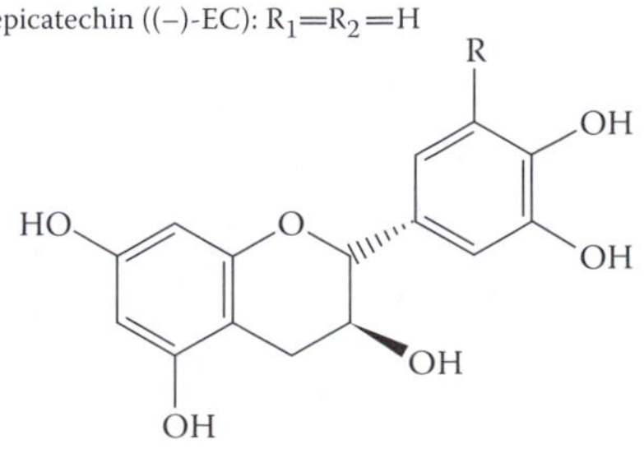

(+)-catechin ((+)-C): R=H
(+)-gallocatechin ((+)-GC): R=OH

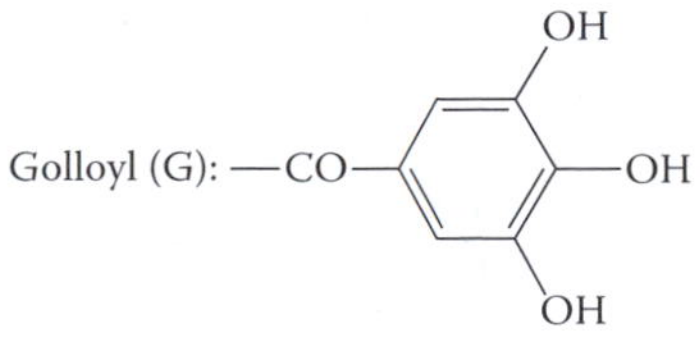

Golloyl (G): —CO—

SCHEME C.15 Tea catechin structures. (From Nishitani and Sagesaka, *J. Food. Comp. Anal.,* 17:675–685, 2004. With permission.)

four catechins from green tea and vegetables, (+)-catechin (C), (–)-epicatechin (EC), (–)-epicatechin gallate (ECG), and (–)epi-gallocatechin gallate (EGCG), with phospholipid-model membranes composed of 1,2-dimyristoyl-sn-glycero-3-phosphocholine (DMPC) or 1,2-dielaidoyl-sn-glycero-3-phosphoethanolamine (DEPE). Galloylated catechins, particularly ECG, affected the physical properties of phospholipid membranes by increasing lipid order and promoting the formation of detergent-resistant structures deep inside. In comparison, the nongalloylated catechins were located close to the phospholipid/water interface. ECG exhibited the highest antioxidant activity in this system, while EGCG produced leakage from $E.$ $coli$-isolated membranes via a specific interaction with phosphatidylethanolamine. The effects on the membranes by galloylated catechins could explain their multiple biological activities.

References

Blache, D., Durand, P., Prost, M., and Loreau, N., (+)-Catechin inhibits platelet hyperactivity induced by an acute iron load in $vivo$, $Free$ $Rad.$ $Biol.$ $Med.,$ 33:1670–1680, 2002.

Caturla, N., Vera-Samper, E., Villalain, J., Mateo, C.R., and Micol, V., The relationship between the antioxidant and the antibacterial properties of galloylated catechins and the structure of phospholipid model membranes, $Free$ $Rad.$ $Biol.$ $Med.,$ 34: 648–662, 2003.

Ikigai, H., Nakae, T., Hara, Y., and Shimamura, T., Bacteriacidal catechins damage the lipid bilayer, $Biochem.$ $Biophys.$ $Acta,$ 1147:132–136, 1993.

Kitano, K., Nam, K.Y., Kimura, S., Fujiki, H., and Imanishi, Y., Sealing effects of (–)epigallocatechin gallate on protein kinase C and protein phosphatase 2A, $Biophys.$ $Chem.,$ 65:157–164, 1997.

McKay, D.L. and Blumberg, J.B., The role of tea in human health, $J.$ $Am.$ $Coll.$ $Nutr.,$ 21:1–13, 2002.

Nishitani, E. and Sagesaka, Y.M., Simultaneous determination of catechins, caffeine and other phenolic compounds in tea using new HPLC method, $J.$ $Food.$ $Comp.$ $Anal.,$ 17:675–685, 2004.

Rice-Evans, C., Plant polyphenols: Free radical scavengers or chain-breaking antioxidants, $Biochem.$ $Soc.$ $Sym.,$ 61:103–116, 1995.

Wang, H., Provan, G.J. and Helliwell, K., Tea flavonoids: their functions, utilization, and analysis. $Trends$ $Food$ $Sci.$ $Technol.,$ 11:152–160, 2000.

Yang, C.S., Landau, J.M., Huang, M.T., and Newmark, H.L., Tea and tea polyphenols in cancer prevention, $J.$ $Nutr.,$ 130:472S–478S, 2000.

Yang, C.S., Landau, J.M., Huang, M.T., and Newmark, H.L., Inhibition of carcinogenesis by dietary polyphenolic compounds, $Ann.$ $Rev.$ $Nutr.,$ 21:381–406, 2001.

Cat's claw (*Uncaria tomentosa*) *see also* Quinic acid Cat's claw, a vine grown in Peru, has been used as a traditional medicine for treating a wide range of ailments, particularly digestive problems and arthritis. An in $vitro$ oxidant-induced stress study by Sandoval and coworkers (1998) showed Cat's claw acted as an anti-inflammatory agent by protecting the cells from oxidative stress, as well as inhibiting activation of NF-κB. Of the two species examined, *U. guianensis,* with much lower levels of oxindole or pentacyclic alkaloids, was far more potent. This suggested the latter compounds did not contribute to Cat's claw's antioxidant and anti-inflammatory properties. Further work by Sandoval et al. (2000) examined the effect of Cat's claw on other NF-κB-regulated genes implicated in inflammation as other examples of oxidative injury. Freeze-dried and micropulverized aqueous extracts from Cat's claw both inhibited DPPH in a dose-dependent manner. Of the two extracts, the freeze-dried one was far more effective (Figure C.23). In addition, there was a significant reduction in TNF-α, an NF-κB-dependent cytokine involved in chronic inflammation. The freeze-dried extract again proved to be the more potent inhibitor of TNF-α and was 1.5×10^4 more effective than its antioxidant activity. Ganzera et al. (2001) reported the alkaloid content of different samples of Cat's claw and its market products ranged from 0.156–0.962 percent. Anguilar and coworkers (2002) showed a spray-dried hydroalcoholic extract from Cat's claw had a significantly higher ($p < 0.05$) anti-inflammatory activity compared to an aqueous freeze-dried extract using the carrageenan-induced paw oedema model. The presence of pentacyclic oxindole alkaloids acting alone or synergistically with other metabolites were effective at concentrations as low as 0.001 μg/mL. Recent research,

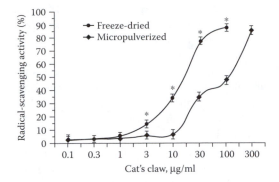

FIGURE C.23 Antioxidant activity of micropulverized and freeze-dried aqueous Cat's claw extracts, assessed by the DPPH radical method. Values are mean ± SEM of three experiments with three samples each. *Significant inhibition ($p < 0.001$) compared to same concentration of micropulverized Cat's claw. (From Sandoval et al., *Free Rad. Biol. Med.*, 29: 1–78, 2000. With permission.)

however, points to quinic-acid esters as active ingredients in Cat's claw water extracts (Sheng et al., 2005).

References

Anguilar, J.L., Rojas, P., Marcelo, A., Plaza, A., Bauer, R., Reininger, E., Klaas, A., and Merfort, I., Anti-inflammatory activity of two different extracts of *Uncaria tomentosa* (Rubiaceae), *J. Ethnopharmacol.*, 81:271–276, 2002.

Ganzera, M., Muhammad, I., Khan, R.A., and Khan, I.A., Improved method for the determination of oxindole alkaloids in *Uncaria tomentosa* by high performance liquid chromatography, *Planta Med.*, 67:447–450, 2001.

Sandoval, C.M., Thompson, J.H., Zhang, X.J., Liu, X., Mannick, E.E., Sadowska-Krowicka, H., Charbonnet, R.M., Clark, D.A., and Miller, M.J., Anti-inflammatory actions of Cat's claw: The role of NF-κB, *Aliment. Pharmacol. Ther.*, 12:1279–1289, 1998.

Sandoval, M., Charbonnet, R.M., Okuhama, N.N., Roberts, J., Krenova, Z., Trentacosti, A.M., and Miller, M.J.S., Cat's claw inhibits TNF-α production and scavenges free radicals: Role in cytoprotection, *Free Rad. Biol. Med.*, 29:1–78, 2000.

Sheng, Y., Akesson, C., Holmgren, K., Bryngelsson, C., Giamapa, V., and Pero, R.W., An active ingredient of Cat's claw water extracts, identification and efficacy of quinic acid, *J. Ethnopharmacol.*, 96: 577–584, 2005.

Cauliflower *see* **S-methylmethane thiosulfonate**

Cereal grains *see also* **Barley, Oats, Wheat, and Rice** Cereal grains contribute approximately 30 percent of the total dietary energy intake in adults in Britain and many other Western countries. Truswell (2002) reviewed the possible relationship between cereal-grain consumption and coronary heart disease (CHD). For example, in the scientific literature, oat fiber was far more effective in lowering total and LDL cholesterol compared to wheat fiber. Rice bran also lowers cholesterol. Based on his review, the author validates the health claim that whole-grain cereal foods and oat meal or bran lower cholesterol and the risk for CHD.

References

Truswell, A.S., Cereal grains and coronary heart disease, *Eur. J. Clin. Nutr.*, 56:1–14, 2002.

C

Chamomile Chamomile, a perennial flowering plant, grows well in the wild in Europe, particularly Croatia and Hungary. Many plants are called chamomile or have it as part of their common name. Five species in the United Kingdom and Europe include German chamomile (*Matricaria recucita*), Roman chamomile (*Chamaemelum nobile* or *Anthenis nobile*), foetid or stinking weed (*A. Cotula*), corn chamomile (*A. Arvensis*), and yellow chamomile. Roman chamomile (*Chamaemelum nobile* or *Anthenis nobile*) is the one most often referred to in English herbals. Commercially grown as a double-flowered form and, like chamomile, has an aromatic bitterness, the chamomile plant (*Matricaria chamomilla*), a member of the *Asteracea* family, is used as a medicinal tea for treating fever, diarrhea, menstrual pain, and inflammation, as well as intestinal and hepatic disorders (Mann and Staba, 1986). It is also the active principle in creams for atopic eczema (Patzelt-Wenczler and Ponce-Poschl, 2000).

One of the major components in chamomile is the flavonoid apigenin (see Apigenin), which

C

TABLE C.18
Main Components
in Chamomile Essential Oil

Component	%
(E)- β-Farnesene	28.8
α-Bisabolol oxide A	41.8
α-Bisabolol oxide B	4.3
α-Bisabolol oxide	5.3
β-Bisabolol oxide	2.3
Germacrene-D	2.2
Chamazulene	2.2
(Z,E)- α-Farnesene	1.6

Source: Adapted from Hernandez-Ceruelos et al., *Toxicol. Lett.*, 135:103–110, 2002.

was found to inhibit adhesion-molecular expression, prostaglandin, and cyclooxygenase, as well as the proinflammatory cytokine interleukin (IL)-6 in cell culture (Panes et al., 1986). Smolinski and Pestka (2003) showed chamomile apigenin inhibited LPS-induced IL-6 and TNF-α production in cell culture, further confirming its anti-inflammatory properties.

The oil component in chamomile, comprising less than 2 percent, contains the terpene bisabolol, and the sesquiterpenes matricine and chamazulene, both of which exhibit anti-inflammatory properties (Jakolev et al., 1983; Villegas et al., 2001). Hernandez-Ceruelos and coworkers (2002) identified 13 compounds in chamomile essential oil (Table C.18). α-Bisabolol oxide A and (E)-β-farnesene accounted for just under 70 percent of the total, while the remainder included smaller amounts of various bisabolol oxides, chamazulene and germacrene. These researchers clearly demonstrated the effectiveness of chamomile essential oil to inhibit sister chromatid exchanges induced by mutagens, daunorubicin and methyl methanesulfonate, in mouse bone-marrow cells. The antineoplastic daunorubicin acts on DNA through the production of free radicals, causing genotoxic damage, such as an increase in the rate of sister chromatid exchanges (Noviello et al.,1994). The results for daunorubicin, summarized in Table C.19, show Chamomile (CO) significantly reduced genotoxic damage in a

dose-dependent manner. Addition of 5, 50, and 500 mg/kg of CO, in the presence of 10 mg/kg of dauorubicin, resulted in an antigenotoxic response corresponding to 25.8 percent, 63.1 percent, and 75.6 percent, respectively. A similar effect was observed for methyl methanesulfonate (MMS), in which the corresponding antigenotic responses for 250, 500, and 1000 mg/kg of CO, in the presence of 25 mg/kg MMS, were 24.8 percent, 45.8 percent, and 60.6 percent, respectively. While consumption of green tea was reported to reduce human oxidative stress, the ability of chamomile tea to act in a similar manner requires further investigation.

References

Hernandez-Ceruelos, A., Madrigal-Bujaidar, E., and de la Cruz, C., Inhibitory effect of chamomile essential oil on the sister chromatide exchanges induced by daunorubicin and methyl methanesulfonate in mouse bone marrow, *Toxicol. Lett.*, 135:103–110, 2002.

Jakolev, V., Isaac, O., and Flaskamp, E., Pharmacological investigation with compounds of chamazulene and matricine, *Planta Med.*, 49:67–73, 1983.

Mann, C. and Staba, E., 1986. Herbs, spices and medicinal plants, in *Advances in Botany, Horticulture and Pharmacy,* vol. 1, Food Products Press, Binghamton, NY, 1986, pp. 235–280.

Noviello, E., Alnigi, M.G., Cimoli, G., Rovini, E., Mazzoni, A., Parodi, S., De Sessaf, F., and Russo, P., Sister chromatide exchanges, chromosomal aberrations and cytotoxicity produced by topoisomerase II-targeted drugs in sensitive (A2780) and resistant (A2780-DX-3) human ovarian cells: Correlation with the formation of DNA double-strand breaks, *Mutat. Res.*, 311:21–29, 1994.

Panes, J., Gerritsen, M.E., Anderson, D.C., Miyasaka, M., and Granger, D.N., Apigenin inhibits tumor necrosis factor-induced intercellular adhesion moecule-1 upregulation *in vivo*, *Microcirculation,* 3: 279–286, 1996.

Patzelt-Wenczler, R. and Ponce-Poschl, E., Proof of efficacy of Kamillos (R) cream in atopic cream, *Eur. J. Med. Res.*, 19:171–175, 2000.

Smolinski, A.T. and Pestka, J.J., Modulation of lipopolysaccharide-induced pro-inflammatory cytokine production *in vitro* and *in vivo* by herbal constituents apigenin (chamomile), ginseonide Rb_1

TABLE C.19
Effect of Chamomile Oil (CO) on Sister Chromatide Exchanges (SCEs) Induced by Dauorubicin (Dau) in Mouse Bone-Marrow Cells

	Dose (mg/kg)	Mice No.	SCE[1] X + E.D.	Inhibition (%)
Corn oil	0	5	1.57 + 0.31*	
CO	500	5	1.53 + 0.30*	
Dau	10	5	11.0 + 1.49	
CO + Dau	5 + 10	5	8.59 + 1.20*	25.79
CO + Dau	50 + 10	5	5.06 + 0.59*	63.1
CO + Dau	500 + 10	5	3.88 + 0.65*	75.58

[1] Each SCE value is the mean of 30 second-division cells per mouse. *Statistically significant difference with respect to the value of Dau.

Source: Adapted from Hernandez-Ceruelos et al., *Toxicol. Lett.,* 135:103–110, 2002.

C

(ginseng) and partenolide (feverfew), *Food Chem. Toxicol.,* 41:1381–1390, 2003.

Villegas, L.F., Marcalo, A., Martin, J., Fernandez, I.D., Maldonado, H., Vaisberg, A.J., and Hammond, G.B., (+)-*epi*-α-bisabolol is the wound-healing principle of *Peperomia galioides*: An investigation of the *in vivo* wound-healing activity of related terpenoids, *J. Nat. Prod.,* 64:1357–1358, 2001.

Chasteberry   The dried ripe fruit from the Chasteberry tree (*Vitex*) has been used to treat female reproductive problems since ancient Greece (Brown, 1994). It was also used to decrease sexual desire in men during medieval times, hence, the name chaste tree or monk's pepper (Snow, 1996). In Germany, it is a well-recognized treatment for menstrual irregularities and premenstrual syndrome (PMS) (Blumenthal et al., 1998). Extracts of chasteberry tree berries were shown to bind dopamine receptors in the anterior pituitary, decreasing the basal- and thyrotropin-release-hormone that secretes prolactin (Jarry et al., 1994; Sliutz et al., 1993). In the second and third week of their cycles, women suffering from PMS have markedly higher levels of prolactin (Halbreich, 1976). The successful treatment of PMS by *Vitex* was attributed to its ability to reduce prolactin (Bohnert, 1997; Mayo, 1997). The active ingredients in chasteberry are iridoid glycosides-agnuside (0.6 percent) and aucubin (0.3 percent), together with flavonoids and essential oils (Gomaa et al., 1978). Dittmar and coworkers (1992) treated 175 women suffering from PMS with *Vitex* or pyridoxine and evaluated them during the second half of their menstrual cycle with a Premenstrual Tension Scale and the CGI scale. The efficacy of the CGI score for *Vitex* was 77.1 percent compared to 60.6 percent for pyridoxine. While no drug interactions have been reported for *Vitex,* it could counteract the effectiveness of birth-control pills because of its effect on prolactin (Feldmann et al., 1990).

References

Blumenthal, M., Gruenwald, J., and Hall, T., *The Complete German Commission E. Monograph: Therapeutic Guide to Herbal Medicines*, Intergrative Medicine Communications, Boston, 1998.

Bohnert, K.J., The use of *Vitex agnus-castus* tincture, *Der Frauenartz,* 32:867–870, 1997.

Brown, D.J., Herbal research review: *Vitex agnus castus* clinical monograph, *Quarterly Rev. Natural Med.,* Summer:111–121, 1994.

Dittmar, F., Bohnert, J.J., and Peeters, M., Premenstrual syndrome: Treatment with a phytopharmaceutical, *Therapiewoche Gynakol.,* 5:867–870, 1992.

Feldmann, H.U., Abrecht, M., and Lamertz, M., Therapie bei Gelbkorschwache bzw. Pramenstruellem Syndrom mit vitex-agnus-castus Tinktur, *Gyne.,* 11:421–425, 1990.

Gomaa, C.S., El-Moghazy, M.A., and Halim, F.A., Flavonoids and iridoids from *Vitex agnus-castus, Planta Med.,* 33:277, 1978.

C

Halbreich, V., Serum prolactin in women with premenstrual syndrome, *Lancet*, 2:654–656, 1976.

Jarry, H., Leonhardt, S., and Gorkow, C., *In vitro* prolactin but not LH and FSH release is inhibited by compounds in extracts of *Agnus castus*: Direct evidence for dopaminergic principle by the dopamine receptor assay, *Exp. Clin. Endocrinol. Diabetes*, 102: 448–454, 1994.

Mayo, J., Premenstrual syndrome: A natural approach to management, *Clin. Nutr. Insights*, 5:1–8, 1997.

Sliutz, G., Speiser, P., and Schultz, A.M., *Agnus castus* extracts inhibit prolactin secretion of rat pituitary cells, *Horm. Metab. Res.*, 25:253–255, 1993.

Snow, J.M., *Vitex agnus-castus* L. (*Verbenaceae*), *Protocol J. Bot. Med.*, 1:20–23, 1996.

Cherries   Cherries are highly colored fruit rich in anthocyanins. For example, Wang and coworkers (1999a) showed that anthocyanins and cyanidin isolated from tart cherries had antioxidant and anti-inflammatory properties similar to commercial products. These researchers (Wang et al., 1999b) identified, in addition to chlorogenic acid methyl ester, three novel antioxidants in tart cherries, such as 2-hydroxy-3-(*o*-hydroxyphenyl) propanoic acid, 1-(3′,4′-dihydroxycinnamoyl)-cyclopenta-2,5-diol, and 1-(3′,4′-dihydroxycinnamoyl)-cyclopenta-2,3-diol. Tart-cherry anthocyanin extracts were shown by Tall et al. (2004) to be beneficial for treating inflammatory pain. Using an acute-inflammation rat model, an equivalent reduction in inflammation-induced thermal hyper-

algesia, mechanical hyperalgesia, and paw edema was evident with the highest dose of tart-cherry extract (400 mg/kg) compared to the drug indomethacin (5 mg/kg). The potential of tart-cherry anthocyanins to reduce persistent and chronic pain in patients is promising, but requires further clinical studies.

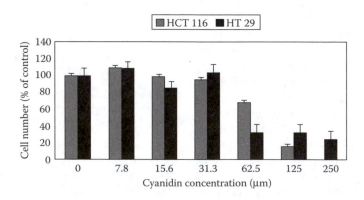

Cyanidin

(Adapted from Kang et al., *Cancer Lett.*, 194:13–19, 2003.)

Kang et al. (2003) showed tart-cherry anthocyanins and the aglycone cyanidin all inhibited the development of intestinal tumors in Apc[Min] mice, as well as the growth of colonic tumors in human colon-cancer cell lines HT29 and HCT 116. Cyanidin was far more effective than anthocyanins in inhibiting the growth of these human colon-cancer cells, as shown in Figure C.24.

This was evident by the IC_{50} values for cyanidin being 85 and 63 µM for the HCT 116 and HT 29 cells compared to 260 and 585 µM for the anthocyanins.

FIGURE C.24 Effect of cyanidin on the growth of human colon-cancer cells. Gray bars, HCT 116 cells; black bars, HT 29 cells. Error bars = Standard error of the mean. (From Kang et al., *Cancer Lett.*, 194:13–19, 2003. With permission.)

References

Kang, S.-Y., Seeram, N.P., Nair, G.M., and Bourquin, L.D., Tart cherry anthocyanins inhibit tumor development in Apc[Min] mice and reduce proliferation of human colon cancer cells, *Cancer Lett.*, 194:13–19, 2003.

Tall, J.M., Seeram, N.P., Zhao, C., Nair, G.M., Meyer, R.A., and Raja, S.N., Tart cherry anthocyanins suppress inflammation-induced pain behavior in rat, *Behav. Brain Res.*, 153:181–188, 2004.

Wang, H., Nair, M.G., Strasburg, G.M., Chang, Y.-C., Booren, A.M., Gray, J.I., and DeWitt, D., Antioxidant and anti-inflammatory activities of anthocyanins and their aglycon, cyanidin, from tart cherries, *J. Nat. Prod.*, 62:294–296, 1999a.

Wang, H., Nair, M.G., Strasburg, G.M., Booren, A.M., and Gray, J.I., Novel antioxidants from tart cherries (*Prunus cerasus*), *J. Nat. Prod.*, 62:86–88, 1999b.

TABLE C.20
Inhibition of ACE by Peptidic Fractions Obtained by Reverse-Phase Chromatography of a Chickpea Legumin Hydrolysate. Effluent from C_{18} HPLC Were Pooled in Six Fractions and Analyzed for ACE-Inhibitory Activity

Fractions (Elution Time, Min)	Inhibition of ACE (% Residual Activity)
0–10	97
10–15	90
15–20	92
20–25	78
25–30	76
35–40	58

Source: From Yust et al., *Food Chem.*, 81:363–369, 2003. With permission.

Chickpea   Chickpea (*Cicer arietinum* L.) is the third most important grain legume based on total production (FAO, 1994). It is a rich source of dietary protein because of its well-balanced amino-acid composition, bioavailability, and low levels of antinutritional factors compared to other legumes (Friedman, 1996). The importance of legumes such as chickpeas is related to it being one of the low-glycemic index (GI) foods. The importance of such foods is due to their ability to improve metabolic control of hyperlipidemia in diabetic and healthy individuals (Frost et al., 1999; Jenkins et al., 1994). The classification of GI is based on the postprandial blood-glucose response based on the rate of digestion and absorption of carbohydrates present in the food. Goni and Valentin-Gamazo (2003) prepared three test meals of 50 g carbohydrates, including a spaghetti, in which wheat was partially replaced with chickpea flour (25 percent), a wheat spaghetti, and white bread. While the two spaghettis had similar levels of resistant starch and dietary fiber, the indigestible fraction was significantly higher in the chickpea-containing product. When fed to 12 healthy volunteers, the postprandial rise in blood glucose was much smaller with the chickpea product with a GI of 58 ± 6 compared to 73 ± 5 for the corresponding 100 percent wheat pasta. The low glycemic response observed for the product containing chickpea could lead to its incorporation to produce other low-GI foods.

The main storage protein of chickpea is legumin, a globulin composed of six αβ subunits. Yust et al. (2003) examined the production of bioactive peptides by subjecting chickpea legumin to proteolytic digestion with alcalase, an inexpensive and nonspecific protease. Of the peptidic fractions isolated by reverse-phase chromatography, only those with the longest retention times (35–45 min) had high ACE-inhibitory activity (Table C.20). This is not unexpected, as ACE-inhibitory activity peptides usually contain hydrophobic amino acids, which interact more with the column, taking a longer time to be eluted. Further examination of these peptides confirmed the presence of hydrophobic amino acids, with methionine detected as the most abundant. Identification of chickpea peptides with ACE-inhibitory activity suggests their possible use in lowering blood pressure *in vivo*.

References

FAO, *FAO Yearbook Production*, FAO, Rome, 1994.

Friedman, M., Nutritional value of proteins from different food sources, a review, *J. Agric. Food Chem.*, 44:6–29, 1996.

Frost, G., Leeds, A.A., Dore, C.J., Madieros, S., Brading, S., and Dornhorst, A., Glycaemic index as a determinant of serum HDL-cholesterol concentration, *Lancet,* 353:1045–1048, 1999.

Goni, I. and Valentin-Gamazo, C., Chickpea flour ingredient slows glycemic response to pasta in healthy volunteers, *Food Chem.,*81:511–515, 2003.

Jenkins, D.J.A., Jenkins, A.L., Wolever, T.M.S., Vuksan, V., Rao, A.V., Thompson, L.U., and Joss, R.G., Low glycemic index: Lente carbohydrates and physiological effects of altered food frequency, *Am. J. Clin. Nutr.,* 54:S706–S709, 1994.

Yust, M.M., Pedroche, J., Giron-Calle, J., Alaiz, M., Millan, F., and Vioque, J., Production of ace inhibitory peptides by digestion of chickpea legumin with alcalase, *Food Chem.,* 81:363–369, 2003.

Chilean berry (*Aristotelia chilensis*)

Chilean berry (*ach*) is an edible, black-colored fruit with medicinal properties. *Ach* was found to contain six indole alkaloids (Kan et al., 1997). Recent studies by Miranda-Rottmann and coworkers (2002) showed *ach* was a much richer source of phenolic antioxidants compared to cranberry, blueberry, blackberry, strawberry, raspberry, and red wine. In addition, *ach* also had the highest scores for total radical-trapping potential and total antioxidant reactivity in *in vitro* antioxidant tests. Most of *ach's* antioxidant properties were in the anthocyanin-rich fraction of the juice. It was responsible for the effective inhibition of copper-induced LDL oxidation and the dose–response protection of hydrogen-peroxide-induced intracellular oxidative stress in human endothelial-cell cultures.

References

Kan, H., Valcic, S., Timmerman, B.N., and Montenegro, C., Indole alkaloids from *Aristotelia chilensis* (Mol.) Stuntz, *Int. J. Pharmacogn.,* 35:215–217, 1997.

Miranda-Rottmann, S., Aspillaga, A.A., Perez, D.D., Vasquez, L., Martinez, A.L.F., and Leighton, F., Juice and phenolic fractions of the berry *Aristotelia chilensis* inhibit LDL oxidation *in vitro* and protect human endothelial cells against oxidative stress, *J. Agric. Food Chem.,* 50:7542–7547, 2002.

Chili peppers *see also* **Capsaicin**   Chili peppers, a member of the *Capsicum* family, are consumed extensively as spices. The principal pungent and irritant ingredient in chili peppers is capsaicin. A discussion of the health-related properties of chili peppers can be found under capsaicin.

Chinese herbs   In China, the idea that food and medicine were equally important for preventing and curing diseases has been passed down to the present day from the ancient legend describing an herbalist, Shennong, who tasted many different types of herbs (Zhang, 1990). With the development of functional foods and nutraceuticals, attempts are being made to bridge the typical Chinese medicated diet and functional foods and nutraceuticals (Xu, 2001). Chinese herbal extracts have been used to treat a variety of cancers, but their efficacy on pancreatic cancer has not been reported. Schwartz and coworkers (2003) examined the effect of ethanol extracts of two quality-controlled, dried, encapsulated supplements of 15 (SPES) and eight (PC-SPES) Chinese herbs on eight human pancreatic-cancer-cell lines. Both extracts were significantly toxic to the pancreatic-cancer cells and induced apoptosis. Both extracts, however, need further evaluation as agents for the clinical treatment of pancreatic cancer. SPES could be combined with cell-cycle-independent cytotoxic drugs, while PC-SPES, because of its G2-blocking pattern, may be useful as a radiation sensitizer.

References

Schwartz, R.E., Donohue, C.A., Sadava, D., and Kane, S.E., Pancreatic cancer *in vitro* toxicity mediated by Chinese herbs SPES and PC-SPES: Implications for monotherapy and combination treatment, *Cancer Lett.,* 189:59–68, 2003.

Xu, Y., Perspectives on the 21st century development of functional foods: Bridging Chinese medicated diet and functional foods, *Inter. J. Food Sci. Technol.,* 36: 229–242, 2001.

Zhang, E.Q., *Chinese Medicated Diet*, Shangai Publishing House, Shangai College of Traditional Chinese Medicine, 1990, pp. 1–15.

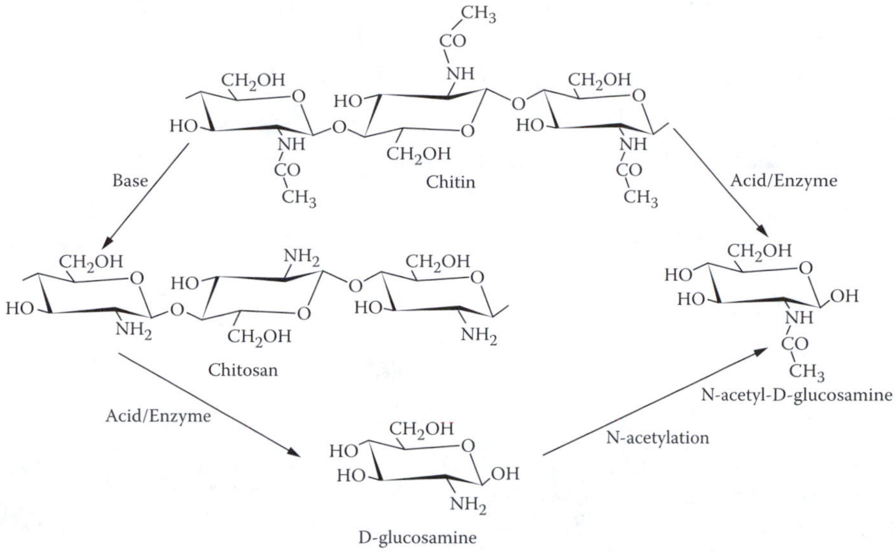

SCHEME C.16 Preparation of chitin derivatives. (From Shahidi et al., *Trends Food Sci. Technol.*, 10:97–105, 1999. With permission.)

Chitin and chitosan   Chitin is the next most abundant polysaccharide in nature after cellulose. It is a natural polymer composed of the aminosugar *N*-acetylglucosamine. The major deacylated form of chitin, chitosan, is found in crustaceans, such as crabs, lobsters, and shrimp. It is a versatile biopolymer with many derivatives formed, as shown in Scheme C.16 (Shahidi et al., 1999). Since chitin and chitosan are both capable of complexing transition metals, Kamil and coworkers (2002) examined its potential as an antioxidant. Using chitosans of different viscosity, these researchers found that lower-viscosity chitosan exhibited strong antioxidant activity and could be a potential source of natural antioxidant for stabilizing lipid-containing foods. Chitosan also appeared to enhance intestinal permeability, permitting the absorption of hydrophillic drugs (Kotze et al., 1997). Recent work by Ranaldi and coworkers (2002) suggested that chitosan ingestion altered intestinal-barrier function, permitting the entry of potentially toxic or allergenic substances. Taha and Swailam (2002) noted that 0.04 percent of chitosan suppressed the growth and hemolysin production of *Aeromonas hydrophilia*. Song and coworkers (2002) improved the solubility of chitosan by conjugating it with lysozyme *via* a Maillard-type reaction. The resulting chitosan–lysozyme conjugate had enhanced emulsifying properties and bactericidal action against *Escherichia coli* K-12.

Chitosan was also found to increase fat elimination in the stool of rats (Sugano et al., 1980; Ebihara and Schneeman, 1989). In addition, dietary chitosan reduced cholesterol in rats, suggesting it as a possible dietary supplement. Bokura and Kobayashi (2003) recently reported chitosan significantly reduced total cholesterol in female volunteers with mild to moderate hypercholesterolemia. In the subgroup, more than 60 years of age, there was a greater tendency for cholesterol reduction in the chitosan group compared to the placebo group (Table C.21). After eight weeks of treatment, total cholesterol in the chitosan group decreased from 241 to 226 mg/dL, while the placebo remained essentially the same. A significant reduction was also observed for LDL cholesterol in the chitosan group, while the placebo group remained unchanged.

References

Bokura, H. and Kobayashi, S., Chitosan decreases total cholesterol in women: A randomized, double-blind, placebo-controlled trial, *Eur. J. Clin. Nutr.*, 57: 721–725, 2003.

TABLE C.21
Values of Serum Lipids of Subjects with More Than 60 Y of Age[1,2]

Parameter	Baseline		Eight-Week Assessment	
	Chitosan	Placebo	Chitosan	Placebo
Total cholesterol (mg/dL)	241 + 30	237 + 26	226 + 29*	242 + 27
HDL cholesterol (mg/dL)	66 + 18	67 + 12	64 + 15	66 + 12
LDL cholesterol (mg/dL)	153 + 28	152 + 27	135 + 22**	151 + 24
Triglycerides (mg/dL)	130 + 62	95 + 38	110 + 55	94 + 35

[1] Chitosan, n = 16; placebo, n = 20

[2] * $p < 0.05$; ** $p < 0.01$ compared with the baseline,

Source: Adapted from Bokura and Kobayashi, *Eur. J. Clin. Nutr.,* 57:721–725, 2003.

Ebihara, K. and Schneeman, B.O., Interaction of bile acids, phospholipids, cholesterol and triglyceride with dietary fibres in the small intestine of rats, *J. Nutr.,* 119:1100–1106, 1989.

Kamil, Y.V.A., Jeon, Y.J., and Shahidi, F., Antioxidative activity of chitosans of different viscosity in cooked comminuted flesh of herring (*Clupea harengus*), *Food Chem.,* 79:69–77, 2002.

Kotze, A.F., de Leeuw, B.J., Lue Ben, H.L., de Boer, A.G., Verhoef, J.C., and Junginger, H.L., Chitosan for enhanced delivery of therapeutic peptides across intestinal epithelia: *In vitro* evaluation of Caco-2 cell monolyers, *Int. J. Pharm.,* 159:243–243, 1997.

Ranaldi, G., Marigliano, I., Vespignani, I., Perozzi, G., and Sambuy, Y., The effect of chitosan and other polycations on tight junction permeability in human intestinal Caco-2 cell line, *J. Nutr. Biochem.,* 13:157–167, 2002.

Shahidi, F., Kamil, J.Y.V.A., and Jeon, Y.J., Food applications of chitin and chitosans, *Trends Food Sci. Technol.,* 10:97–105, 1999.

Song, Y., Babiker, E.E., Usui, M., Saito, A., and Kato, A., Emulsifying properties and bacteriocidal action of chitosan-lysozyme conjugates, *Food Res. Inter.,* 35:459–466, 2002.

Sugano, M., Fujikama, T., Hiratsuji, Y., Nakashima, K., Fukuda, N., and Hasegawa, Y., A novel use of chitosan as a hypocholesterolemic agent in rats, *Am. J. Clin. Nutr.,* 33:787–793, 1980.

Taha, S.M.A. and Swailam, M.H., Antibacterial activity of chitosan against *Aeromonas hydrophilia, Nahrung,* 46:337–340, 2002.

Chlorogenic acid   Fruit and vegetable extracts, such as obtained from carrots, burdock (gobou), apricot, and prune, were found to inhibit the formation of 8-hydroxydeoxyguanosine (8-OH-dG) (Kasai et al., 2000). 8-OH-dG, a key marker of cellular oxidative stress during carcinogenesis, induces point mutations in mammalian cells (Kasai, 1997). A common inhibitor in these extracts was chlorogenic acid, which was shown to inhibit 8-OH-dG in a rat-tongue carcinogenesis model.

Chlorogenic acid. (From Wen et al., *Food Microbiol.,* 20:305–311, 2003. With permission.)

Chlorogenic acid (CGA), an esterified product of caffeic acid and quinic acid, was reported by Hemmerle and coworkers (1997) to modulate glucose-6-phosphatase, an enzyme involved in glucose metabolism. Nardini et al. (1995, 1997) also showed it decreased oxidation of LDL cholesterol and total cholesterol, thereby reducing the risk of cardiovascular disease. Rodrigues de Sotillo and Hadley (2002) found a significant reduction in plasma triacylglycerols, total cholesterol, and postprandial glucose in Zucker rats treated with chlorogenic acid.

References

Hemmerle, H., Burger, H.J., Below, P., Schubert, G., Rippel, R., Schindler, P.W., Paulus, E., and Herling, A.W., Chlorogenic acid and synthetic chlorogenic acid derivatives: Novel inhibitors of hepatic glucose-6-translocase, *J. Med. Chem.*, 40:137–145, 1997.

Kasai, H., Fukada, S., Yamaizume, Z., Sugie, S., and Mori, H., Action of chlorogenic acid in vegetables and fruits as an inhibitor of 8-hydroxydeoxy-gua-nosine, formation *in vitro* and in a rat carcinogenesis model, *Food Chem. Toxicol.*, 38:467–471, 2000.

Kasai, H., Analysis of a form of oxidative DNA damage, 8-hydroxy DNA damage, in *Antimutagenesis and Anticarcinogenesis Mechanisms III,* Brozetti, G., Ed., Plenum Press, New York, 1997, p. 257.

Nardini, M., D'Aquino, M., Tomassi, G., Gentili, V., Di Felice, M., and Scaccini, C., Inhibition of human low-density lipoprotein oxidation by caffeic acid and other hydroxycinnamic acid derivatives, *Free Rad. Biol. Med.*, 19:541–552, 1995.

Nardini, M., Natella, F., Gentili, V., Di Felice, M., and Scaccini, C., Effect of caffeic acid dietary supplementation on the antioxidant defense system in rat: An *in vivo* study, *Arch. Biochem. Biophys.*, 342:157–160, 1997.

Rodrigues de Sotillo, D.V. and Hadley, M., Chloro-genic acid modifies plasma and liver concentrations of cholesterol, triaylglycerol, and minerals in (*fa/fa*) Zucker rats, *J. Nutr. Biochem.*, 13:717–726, 2002.

Wen, A., Delaquis, P., Stanich, K., and Toivonen, P., Antilisterial activity of selected phenolic acids, *Food Microbiol.*, 20:305–311, 2003.

Chlorophyll and chlorophyllin *see also* **Pheophytin and Pheophorbide**   Epidemiological studies associated consumption of dark-green vegetables, rich sources of clorophyll pigments, with cancer protection. Antigenotoxic properties of chlorophylls were subsequently demonstrated using short-term genotoxicity assays (Dashwood, 1997; Negishi et al., 1997; Dashwood et al., 1998). Insolubility of chlorophyll in aqueous solutions, however, led to an investigation of the chemoprotective effects of its stable, water-soluble derivative, chlorophyllin (CHL). Porphyrin compounds, such as chlorophyll and CHL, were known to protect against a variety of direct- and indirect-acting mutagens, such as aflatoxin B1, heterocyclic amines, and nitrosamines (Dashwood et al., 1991; Guo et al, 1995; Romert et al., 1992; Hayatsu et al., 1999). Further studies confirmed the anticancer properties of CHL by its inhibition of induction of hepatocarcinogenesis by aflatoxin B1 and dibenzo[α,l]pyrene (DBP) in rainbow trout (Reddy et al., 1996). Xu and Dashwood (1999) found chlorophyllin was a very effective inhibitor of heterocyclic amine-induced colon carcinogenesis in male F344 rats. A clinical trial over 16 weeks involving 180 Chinese individuals living in an area known to have high exposure to dietary aflatoxins by Egner et al. (2003) examined the intervention of administering CHL three times a day. They

Chlorophyll *a* and chlorophyllin (Chung et al., *Cancer Lett.,* 145:57–64, 1999. With permission.)

C

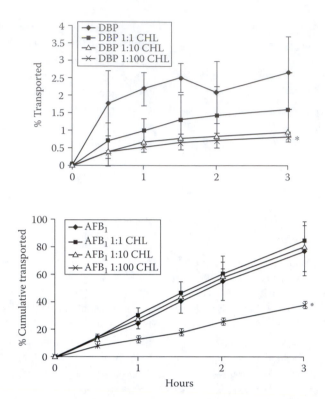

FIGURE C.25 The transport of carcinogens (DBP and AFB_1) from apical to basolateral across Caco-2 monolayers in the presence of increasing molar ratios of CHL. Panels A–B represent the transport of DBP and AFB_1 at concentrations of 1.0 μM with buffer alone (black diamond) and with CHL present in concentrations of 1.0 ( )m, 10.0 (Δ), and 100.0 (x) μM. Experiment in panel A was performed in "nonsink" conditions, while experiment in panel B was "in sink" conditions and is displaced as cumulative transport (*). Values for all timepoints within a treatment group are significantly different from the corresponding control value (Panel a, DBP with CHL at 10.0 and 100.0; Panel B, AFB_1 at 100 μMm $p < 0.05$). (From Mata et al., *Toxicol.*, 196:117–125, 2004. With permission.)

found CHL effectively reduced by 50 percent the median level of urinary excretion of afla-toxin-N^7-guanine, a DNA adduct biomarker associated with increased risk for liver cancer, compared to the placebo. This study demonstrated the safety and efficacy of using CHL to reduce the genotoxic and cytotoxic effects of aflatoxins in populations at high risk.

Using Caco-2 cell monolayers, Mata and coworkers (2004) suggested one mechanism for the chemopreventive effect of CHL against carcinogens involved reducing the bioavailability of aflatoxin B_1 and DBP. Directly binding CHL with these carcinogens in the intestinal tract could inhibit their transportation from the apical (AP) to the basolateral (BL), as seen in Figure C.25.

Increasing the molar ratios of CHL from 1 to 100 μM significantly reduced the percent of DBP transported, while 100 μM CHL was needed to reduce the transport of aflatoxin B_1 approximately 47 percent.

Using cultured fibroblast cells from Chinese hamster lung (V79), Bez et al. (2001) showed chlorophyll *a*, chlorophyll *b*, and chlorophyllin all protected V79 cells from DNA damage induced by methyl methanesulphonate (MMS) by desgenotoxic action and by bioantigenotoxic mechanisms with similar efficiency. Negraes and coworkers (2004) evaluated the anticlasto-genicity of chlorophyllin in different phases of the cell cycle by its ability to reverse DNA damage induced by ethyl methane sulfonate. A greater protective effect by CHL against ethyl methyl sulfonate (70–80 percent) was observed during the G2/S phase.

References

Bez, G.C., Jordao, B.Q., Vicentini, V.E.P., and Mantovani, M.S., Investigation of gentoxic and antigenotoxic activities of chlorophylls and chlorophyllin in cultured V79 cells, *Mutat. Res.,* 497:139–145, 2001.

Chung, W.-Y., Leew, J.-M., Park, M.-Y., Yook, J.-I., Kim, J., Chung, A.-S., Surh, Y.-S., and Park, K.-K., Inhibitory effects of chlorophyllin on 7,12-dimethylbenz[α]anthracene-induced bacterial mutagenesis and mouse skin carcinogenesis, *Cancer Lett.,* 145:57–64, 1999.

Dashwood, R.H., Chlorophylls as anticarcinogens (review), *Int. J. Oncol.,* 10:721–727, 1997.

Dashwood, R.H., Breinholt, V., and Bailey, G.S., Chemopreventive properties of chlorophyllin: Inhibition of aflatoxin B_1 (AFB1)-DNA binding *in vivo* and antimutagenic activity against AFB1 and two heterocyclic amines in *Salmonella* mutagenicity test, *Carcinogenesis,* 12:939–942, 1991.

Dashwood, R.H., Negishi, T., Hayatsu, H., Breinholt, V., Hendricks, J., and Bailey, G., Chemopreventive properties of chlorophylls towards aflatoxin B_1: A review of the antimutagenicity and anticarcinogenicity data in rainbow trout, *Mutat. Res.,* 399:245–253, 1998.

Egner, P.A., Munoz, A., and Kensler, T.W., Chemoprevention with chlorophyllin in individuals exposed to dietary aflatoxin, *Mutat. Res.,* 523–524:209–216, 2003.

Guo, D., Horio, D.T., Grove, J.S., and Dashwood, R.H., Inhibition by chlorophyllin of 2-amino-3-methylimidazo-[4,5-*f*]quinoline-induced tumorigenesis in the male F344 rat, *Cancer Lett.,* 95:161–165, 1995.

Hayatsu, H., Sugijama, C., Arimoto-Koboyashi, S., and Negishi, T., Porphyrins as possible preventions of heterocyclic amine carcinogens, *Cancer Lett.,* 143:185–187, 1999.

Mata, J.E., Yu, Z., Gray, J.C., Williams, D.E., and Rodrigues-Proteau, R., Effects of chlorophyllin on transport of dibenzo(α, *l*)pyrene, 2-amino-1-methyl-6-phenylimidazo-[4,5-*b*]pyridine, and aflatoxin B_1 across Caco-2 cell monolayers, *Toxicolology,* 196:117–125, 2004.

Nagraes, P.D., Jordao, B.Q., Vicentini, V.E.P., and Mantovani, M.S., Anticlastogenicity of chlorophyllin in the different cell cycle phases in cultured mammalian cells, *Mutat. Res.,* 557:177–182, 2004.

Negishi, T., Rai, H., and Hayatsu, H., Antigenotox activity of natural chlorophylls, *Mutagenesis,* 376:97–100, 1997.

Reddy, A., Coffing, S., Baird, W., Henticks, J., and Bailey, S., Chlorophyllin (CHL), indole-3-carbinol (13C) and β-naphthoflavone (BNF) chemoprevention against dibenzo[α, *l*]pyrene (DBP) in trout, *Proc. Am. Assoc. Cancer Res.,* 37:1883, 1996.

Romert, L., Curvall, M., and Jenssen, D., Chlorophyllin is both a positive and negative modifier of mutagenicity, *Mutat. Res.,* 7:349–355, 1992.

Xu, M. and Dashwood, R.H., Chemoprotective studies of heterocyclic amine-induced colon carcinogenesis, *Cancer Lett.,* 143:179–183, 1999.

Chocolate   Chocolate contains fats, sugars, and protein, together with small quantities of magnesium, potassium, calcium, iron, and riboflavin, as well as the stimulant caffeine. The main ingredient in all chocolates is cocoa, derived from beans cultivated in West Africa and Southeast Asia. Among the hundreds of compounds in cocoa are a group of polyphenolic compounds or flavonoids. One group of flavonoids, the procyanidins, account for 35 percent of all polyphenols in cocoa. Procyanidins consist of flavan-3-ol(–) epicatechin (epicatechin) and its polymers (Adamson et al., 1999). Evidence from epidemiological studies

Epicatechin. (Adapted from Babich et al., *Toxicology, in vitro.,* 19:231–242, 2005)

suggest that diets high in polyphenols reduce the risk of cardiovascular disease and related chronic diseases. Chocolate flavonoids are potent antioxidants capable of protecting LDL from oxidation. Richelle and coworkers (1999) demonstrated a physiologically significant increase in plasma levels of epicatechin (0.7 µmol/L) in eight healthy male volunteers after consuming 80 g of black chocolates. Wang and coworkers (2000) demonstrated a marked increase in plasma levels of epicatechin in healthy adults 2 h following the consumption of procyanidin-rich chocolates. Rein et al., (2000) showed that a polyphenolic-rich cocoa beverage exerted an aspirin-like effect in 30 healthy subjects by suppressing platelet activation and function, key factors in the development of coronary artery disease. A recent study by Mursu et al. (2004) showed that nonsmoking, healthy young volunteers consuming 75 g daily of dark chocolate and dark chocolate enriched with cocoa polyphenols increased their HDL-cholesterol levels by 11.4 percent and 13.7 percent, respectively. In comparison, the control group consuming white chocolate had a small but significant decrease in HDL cholesterol levels of –2.9 percent. No effect of cocoa polyphenols on lipid peroxidation was observed in the young subjects maintained on the study.

Cocoa procyanidins were found by Mao et al. (1999) to exhibit immunomodulatory effects by inhibiting proliferation and suppressing the production of interleukin-2 and human T-lymphocytes. Carnesecchi and coworkers (2002) further examined the antiproliferative effects of cocoa polyphenols using human colon-cancer cells. The cocoa flavonols and procyanidins caused nonapoptotic cell death and blocked the G2/M phase of the cell cycle. They suggested polyamine biosynthesis as one of the targets affected.

References

Adamson, G.E., Lazarus, S.A., Mitchell, A.E., Prior, R.L., Cao, G., Jacobs, P.H., Kramer, B.G., Hammerstone, J.F., Rucker, R.B., Ritter, K.A., and Schmidt, H.H., HPLC method for quantification of procyanidins in cocoa chocolate and correlation to total antioxidant activity, *J. Agric. Food Chem.,* 47:4168–4186, 1999.

Babich, H., Kruska, M.E., Nissim, H.A. and Zuckerbraun, H.L. Differential *in vitro* cytotoxicity of (–)-epicatechin gallate (ECG) to cancer and normal cells from human oral cavity. *Toxicol. in vitro.* 19:231–241, 2005.

Carnesecchi, S., Schneider, Y., Lazarus, S.A., Coehlo, D., Gosse, F., and Raul, F., Flavonols and procyanidins of cocoa and chocolate inhibit growth and polyamine biosynthesis of human colonic cancer cells, *Cancer Lett.,* 175:147–155, 2002.

Mao, T.U., Powell, J., Van De Water, J., Keenz, C.L., Schmitz, H.H., and Gershwin, M.E., The influence of procyanidins on the transcription of interleukin-2 in peripheral blood mononuclear cells, *Int. J. Immunother.,* 15:23–29, 1999.

Mursu, J., Voutilainen, S., Nurmi, T., Rissanen, T.H., Virtanen, J.K., Kaikkonen, J., Nyyssonen, K., and Salonen, J.T., Dark chocolate consumption increases HDL cholesterol concentration and chocolate fatty acids may inhibit lipid peroxidation in healthy humans, *Free Rad. Biol. Med.,* 37:1351–1359, 2004.

Rein, D., Paglieroni, T.G., Wun, T., Pearson, D.A., Schmitz, H.H., Gosselin, G., and Keen, C.L., Cocoa inhibits platelet activation and function, *Am. J. Clin. Nutr.,* 72:30–35, 2000.

Richelle, M., Tavazzi, I., Enslen, M., and Offord, E.A., Plasma kinetics in man of epicatechin from black chocolate, *Eur. J. Clin. Nutr.,* 53:22–26, 1999.

Wang, J.F., Schramm, D.D., Holt, R.R., Ensunsa, J.L., Fraga, C.G., Schmitz, H.H., and Keen, C.L., A dose–response effect from chocolate consumption on plasma epicatechin and oxidative damage, *J. Nutr.,* 130:2115S–2119S, 2000.

Choline Choline is a dietary component essential for normal cell functions. In addition to its incorporation into lecithin and sphingomyelin in cell membranes, it is required for the synthesis of the neurotransmitter, acetyl choline. Choline is also involved in methyl metabolism, as well as for lipid transport and metabolism (Zeisel and Blusztajn, 1994). Eggs are particularly high in choline (300 mg/egg),

$$H_3C - \overset{+}{\underset{H_3C}{\overset{H_3C}{N}}} - CH_2 - CH_2OH$$

mostly in the form of phosphatidylcholine or lecithin. Animal studies have found a choline diet may lead to mental retardation, renal dysfunction, and hemorrhage, as well as bone abnormalities (Fairbanks and Krider, 1945; Handler and Bernheim, 1949; Newberne and Rogers, 1986). During rodent-brain development, there are two periods where choline availability is important. The first is during embryonic days 12–17, and the second is during postnatal days 16–30. Supplementation with choline during these periods is associated with enhanced memory performance (Meck and Williams, 1997, 1999). While no human studies have been conducted so far, Zeisl (2000) suggested that the inclusion of two eggs a day in the diet of pregnant women would be a prudent measure to ensure the dietary requirements of choline are adequately met.

Since hypertension is considered a risk factor for impairments in memory, learning, and attention processes, De Bruin et al. (2003) examined the combined effect of uridine and choline on these cognitive deficits in 5- to 7-month-old spontaneously hypertensive rats (SHR). They found that SHR had significantly impaired visual attention processes based on the five-choice serial reaction time (5-CSRT), which were normalized following supplementation with uridine and choline. Using the Morris water maze as a measure of spatial learning and mnemonic capabilities, supplementation similarly improved these cognitive disorders in both SHR and normotensive Wistar-Kyoto rats.

This model could be used to screen compounds that may have therapeutic potential for treating these cognitive disorders.

References

De Bruin, N.M.W.J., Kiliaan, A.J., De Wilde, M.C., and Broersen, L.M., Combined uridine and choline administration improves cognitive deficits in spontaneously hypertensive rats, *Neurol. Learning Memory*, 80:63–79, 2003.

Fairbanks, B.W. and Krider, J.L., Significance of B-vitamins in swine nutrition, *N. Am. Vet.*, 26:18–23, 1945.

Handler, P. and Bernheim, F., Choline deficiency in the hamster, *Proc. Exptl. Med.*, 72:569, 1949.

Meck, W. and Williams, C., Simultaneous temporal processing is sensitive to prenatal choline availability in mature and aged rats, *Neuroreport*, 8:3045–3051, 1997.

Meck, W. and Williams, C., Choline supplementation during prenatal development reduces proactive interference in spatial memory, *Dev. Brain Res.*, 105:51–59, 1999.

Newberne, P.M. and Rogers, A.E., Labile methyl groups and the promotion of cancer, *Ann. Rev. Nutr.*, 6:407–432, 1986.

Zeisel, S.H., Choline: Needed for normal development of memory, *J. Am. Coll. Nutr.*, 19:528S–531S, 2000.

Zeisel, S.H. and Blusztajn, J.K., Choline and human nutrition, *Nutr. Rev.*, 14:269–296, 1994.

C

Chondroitin sulfate Chondroitin sulfate (CS) is a group of heteropolysaccharides that are integral components of articular cartilage. They consist of alternate sequences of sulfated or unsulfated D-glucuronic acid (GlcA) and N-acetyl-D-galactosamine (GalNAc) residues linked through alternating [β $(1{\to}3)$] and [β $(1{\to}4)$] bonds (Scheme C.17). It is used for the treatment of osteoarthritis, a condition in which destructive changes of the osteoarthritic joint leads to pain and functional disability. Current treatment is aimed at management via physical, pharmacological, and surgical approaches. Chondroitin sulfate allows the cartilage to resist tensile stresses by giving the cartilage resistance and elasticity (Muir, 1986). Osteoarthritis is characterized by the destruction of cartilage by degradative enzymes, which are completely inhibited by chondroitin sulfate (Bartolucci et al., 1991; Bassleer et al., 1992). In reviewing the literature, Deal and Moskowitz (1999) concluded there is a sufficient number of studies

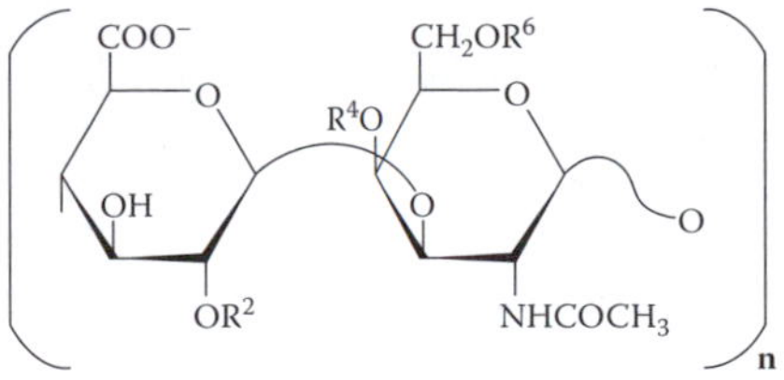

	R^2	R^4	R^6
Δ Di-0S	H	H	H
Δ Di-6S	H	H	SO_3^-
Δ Di-4S	H	SO_3^-	H
Δ Di-2, 6 di S	SO_3^-	H	SO_3^-
Δ Di-4, 6 di S	H	SO_3^-	SO_3^-
Δ Di-2, 4 di S	SO_3^-	SO_3^-	H
Δ Di-2, 4, 6 tri S	SO_3^-	SO_3^-	SO_3^-

SCHEME C.17 Structure of chondroitin sulfate disaccharides and compositional properties. (From Sim et al., *J. Chromatogr. B.*, 818:133–139, 2005. With permission.)

suggesting efficacy of glucosamine, chondroitin sulfate, and collagen sulfate equal to that seen in the symptomatic treatment of osteoarthritis using NSAIDs. The effectiveness of chondroitin sulfate and glucosamine was recently reviewed by Hungerford and Jones (2003).

References

Bartolucci, C., Cellai, L., Corrandini, C., Corradini, D., Lamba, D., and Velona, I., Chondroprotective action of chondroitin sulfate: Competitive action of chondroitin sulfate on the digestion of hyaluronan by bovine testicular hyaluronidase, *Int. J. Tiss. Reac.*, 13:311–317, 1991.

Bassleer, C., Henrotin, Y., and Franchiment, P., *In vitro* evaluation of drugs proposed as chondroprotective agents, *Int. J. Tiss. Reac.*, 14:231–241, 1992.

Deal, C.L. and Moskowitz, R.W., Nutraceuticals as therapeutic agents in osteoarthritis, the role of glucosamine, chondroitin sulfate, and collagen hydrolysate, *Rheum. Dis. Clin. North. Am.*, 25:379–395, 1999.

Hungerford, D.S. and Jones, L.C., Glucosamine and chondroitin sulfate are effective in the management of osteoarthritis, *J. Arthroplasty*, 18:5–9, 2003.

Muir, H., Current and future trends in articular cartilage research and osteoarthritis, in *Articular Cartilage and Osteoarthritis*, Kuettner, K.E., Schleyerbach, R., and Hascoll, V.C., Eds., Raven Press, New York, 1986, p. 423.

Sim, J.-S., Jun, G., Toida, T., Cho, S.Y., Choi, D.W., Chang, S.-Y., Linhardt, R.J., and Kim, Y.S., Quantitative analysis of chondroitin sulfate in raw materials, ophthalmic solutions, soft capsules and liquid preparations, *J. Chromatogr. B.*, 818:133–139, 2005.

Chromium   After calcium, chromium is the largest-selling mineral supplement in the United States. Around 10 million Americans use chromium supplements, some for the prevention or treatment of diabetes (Nielsen, 1996). Many studies suggested chromium alleviates severe symptoms associated with diabetes (Jeejeebhoy et al., 1977; Fox and Sabovic, 1998; Ravina et al., 1999). Althius and coworkers (2002) carried out a systematic review of the literature and a meta-analysis of randomized clinical trials that assessed the impact of dietary chromium supplements on glucose, insulin, and glycated hemoglobin (HbA$_{1c}$) in healthy subjects and in individuals with glucose intolerance or type 2 diabetes. No association was observed between chromium and glucose or insulin in nondiabetic patients. Only one study of 155 diabetic subjects in China found chromium reduced glucose and insulin and HbA$_{1c}$ levels (Anderson et al., 1997). Althuis and Wittes (2003) defended a number of criticisms made about their study, claiming they only summarized randomized clinical trials that assessed the impact of chromium on glucose, insulin, and Hb A$_{1c}$. Further studies, however, were recommended, using controlled, randomized clinical trials, to establish the efficacy of chromium in the treatment of diabetes.

References

Althius, M.D., Jordan, N.E., Ludington, E.A., and Wittes, J.T., Glucose and insulin responses to dietary chromium supplements: A meta-analysis, *Am. J. Clin. Nutr.*, 76:148–155, 2002.

Althius, M.D. and Wittes, J.T., Reply to D.S. Kalman, M.F. McCarty, V. Juturu and J.R. Komorinski, *Am. J. Clin. Nutr.*, 78:192–193, 2003.

Anderson, R.A., Cheng, N., Bryden, N.A., Polansky, M.M., Chi, J., and Feng, J., Elevated intakes of supplemented chromium improve glucose and insulin variables in individuals with type 2 diabetes, *Diabetes*, 46:1786–1791, 1997.

Fox, G. and Sabovic, Z., Chromium picolate supplementation for diabetes mellitus, *J. Fam. Pract.*, 46:83–86, 1998.

Jeejeebhoy, K., Chu, R., Marliss, E., Greenberg, G., and Bruce-Robertson, A., Chromium deficiency, glucose intolerance, and neuropathy reversed by chromium supplementation in a patient receiving long-term total perenteral nutrition, *Am. J. Clin. Nutr.*, 30:531–538, 1977.

Nielsen, F., Controversial chromium: Does the superstar mineral of the mountebanks receive appropriate attention from clinicians and nutritionists, *Nutr. Today*, 31:226–233, 1996.

Ravina, A., Slezak, L., Mirsky, N., Bryden, N., and Anderson, R., Reversal of corticosteroid-induced diabetes mellitus with supplemental chromium, *Diabet. Med.*, 16:164–167, 1999.

Cinnamaldehyde   Cinnamaldehyde (CNMA), a major component in cinnamon-bark oil, is used extensively as a flavoring agent in beverages, ice cream, sweets, and chewing gum. Because of its inhibitory effect on farnesyltransferase activity, cinnamaldehyde derivatives were screened as potential anticancer agents by Koh and associates (1998). CNMA has been detected in tobacco smoke so that a number of contradictory genotoxicity studies were reported (Neudecker, 1992; Mereto et al., 1994; Stammati et al., 1999). Imai et al. (2002) investigated the effects of CNMA on lung carcinogenesis using mice initiated with 4-(methyl-nitrosamino)-1-(3-pyridyl)-1-butanone (NNK).

Cinnamaldehyde (CNMA). (Adapted from Kim et al., *J. Stored Prod. Res.,* 40:55–63, 2004.)

They found CNMA significantly reduced the multiplicity of lung tumors in CB6F1-TgHras2 (rasH2) and non-Tg female mice. Using an oxidation-sensitive fluorescence probe, DCFH-DA, Ka and coworkers (2003) showed CNMA induced apoptosis in human promyelocytic leukemia HL-60 cells by generation of reactive-oxygen species (ROS). ROS induces mitochondrial permeability transition with the dissipation of the transmembrane potential ($\Delta_{\psi m}$), triggering the release of cytochrome *c* and the subsequent activation of caspase cascades needed for the onset of apoptosis. This work provided the first evidence on the mechanism of the anticancer effect of CNMA, with further work needed to establish CNMA as a chemopreventive agent for use in cancer treatment.

Jeong et al. (2003) examined the antitumor effect of a more stable synthetic cinnamaldehyde derivative, CB403, by chemically modifying 2′-hydroxycinnamaldehyde extracted from stem bark. CB403 inhibited the tumor growth of 20 human-cell tumor lines, with SW6720, a human colon-cancer line, being the most sensitive. Further work showed CB403 was cytostatic, inducing mitotic arrest in cancer cells with potential as an anticancer agent.

Structure of CB403. (From Jeong et al., *Biochem. Pharmacol.,* 65:1343–1350, 2003. With permission.)

References

Imai, T., Yasuhura, K., Tamura, T., Takizawa, T., Ueda, M., Hirose, M., and Mitsumori, K., Inhibitory effects of cinnamaldehyde on 4-(methyl nitrosamino)-1-(3-pyridyl)-1-butanone-induced lung carcinogenesis in raH2 mice, *Cancer Lett.,* 175:9–16, 2002.

Jeong, H.-W., Han, D.C., Son, K.-H., Han, M.Y., Lim, J.-S., Ha, J.-H., Lee, C.W., Kim, H.M., Kim, H.-C., and Kwon, H.K., Antitumor effect of the cinnamaldehyde derivative CB403 through the arrest of a cell cycle progression in the G_2/M phase, *Biochem. Pharmacol.,* 65:1343–1350, 2003.

Ka, H., Park, H.-J., Jung, H.-J., Choi, J.-W., Cho, K.-S., Ha, J., and Lee, K.-T., Cinnamaldehyde induces apoptosis by ROS-mediated mitochondrial permeability transition in human promyelocytic leukemia HL-60 cells, *Cancer Lett.,* 196:143–152, 2003.

Kim, H.-K., Kim, J.-R., and Ahn, Y.J., Acaricidal activity of cinnamaldehyde and its cogeners against *Tyrophagus putrescentiae* (Acri: Acaridae), *J. Stored Prod. Res.,* 40:55–63, 2004.

Koh, W.S., Yoon, S.Y., Kwon, B.M., Jeong, T.C., Nam, K.S., and Han, M.Y., Cinnamaldehyde inhibits lymphocyte proliferation and modulates T-cell differentiation, *Int. J. Immunopharmacol.,* 20:643–660, 1998.

Mereto, E., Brambilla-Campart, G., Ghia, M., Martelli, A., and Brambilla, G., Cinnamaldehyde-induced micronuclei in rodent liver, *Mutat. Res.,* 322:1–8, 1994.

Neudecker, T., The genetic toxicology of cinnamaldehyde, *Mutat. Res.,* 277:173–175, 1992.

Stammati, A., Bonsi, P., Zucco, F., Moezelaar, R., Alakomi, H.L., and von Wright, A., Toxicity of selected plant volatiles in microbial and mammalian short-term assays, *Food Chem. Toxicolol.,* 37:813–823, 1999.

Cinnamon *see also* **Cinnamaldehyde**   Cinnamon is a widely used flavoring agent in foods. Jarvill-Taylor et al. (2001) showed that methyl hydroxychalcone polymer (MHCP) isolated from cinnamon mimicked insulin by triggering glucose uptake, glycogen synthesis, phosphatidyl-3-kinase dependency, glycogen-synthase activation, and glycogen synthase kinase-3β activity. Dual treatment with insulin showed synergism was evident between these two compounds. Based on these results, MHCP appeared a good insulin mimetic, potentially useful in treating insulin resistance. A recent study by Schoene et al. (2005) found water-soluble, polymeric polyphenols from cinnamon inhibited proliferation of hematologic tumor-cell lines by altering the proliferative signals regulating progression through the cell cycles.

References

Jarvill-Taylor, K.J., Anderson, R.A., and Graves, D.J., A hydroxychalcone derived from cinnamon functions as a mimetic for insulin in 3T3-L1 adipocytes, *J. Am. Coll. Nutr.,* 20:327–336, 2001.

Schoene, N.W., Kelly, M.A., Polansky, M.M., and Anderson, R.A., Water-soluble polymeric polyphenols from cinnamon inhibit proliferation and alter cell cycle distribution patterns of hematologic tumor cell lines, *Cancer Lett.,* 2005 (in press).

Citrus flavonoids *see* **Hesperidin, Limonene, Naringenin, and Nobiletin**   Citrus fruit is a rich source of several groups of flavonoids, such as flavanone and flavone glycosides, as well as highly methoxylated flavones and polymethoxylated flavones (Horowitz and Gentili, 1977). The latter were found to exert antiproliferative activities against cancer cells (Kawaii et al., 1999; Iwase et al., 2001). Manthey and Guthrie (2002) isolated polmethoxylated flavones from orange peel and showed they had strong, antiproliferative activities toward human cancer-cell lines.

References

Horowitz, R.M. and Gentili, B., Flavonoid constituents in citrus, in *Citrus Science and Technology,* vol. 1, Nagy, S., Shaw, P.E., and Veldius, M.K., Eds., AVI Publishing, Westport, Connecticut, 1977, pp. 397–426.

Iwase, Y., Takemura, Y., Ju-ichi, M., Yano, M., Ito, C., Furikawa, H., Mukainaka, T., Kuchide, M., Tokuda, H., and Nishino, H., Cancer chemopreventative activity of 3,5,6,7,8,3′,4′-heptamethoxyflavone from the peel of citrus plants, *Cancer Lett.,* 163:7–9, 2001.

Kawaii, S., Yomono, Y., Katase, E., Ogawa, K., and Yano, M., Antiproliferative activity of flavonoids on several cancer cell lines, *Biosci. Biotechnol. Biochem.,* 63:896–899, 1999.

Manthey, J. and Guthrie, N., Antiproliferative activities of citrus flavonoids against six human cancer cell lines, *J. Agric. Food Chem.,* 50:5837–5843, 2002.

Citrus fruit *see also* **Grapefruit, Lemons, Limes, Mandarins, Oranges, and Tangerines**   Citrus fruits contain significant amounts of limonene in the peel and smaller amounts in the pulp. Limonene is a monocyclic monoterpene formed by the union of two isoprene molecules. Carbon-4 in limonene is assymetric so that it exists as two optically active forms, *d* and *l*. Limonene has been shown to block and suppress carcinogenic events due to its inhibitory action on certain biochemical pathways in tumor tissues (Elson and Yu, 1994). Monoterpenoids, such as limonene, have been reported to cause tumor regressions with limited toxicity. Limonene significantly reduced azoxymethane-induced colonic aberrant crypt foci in rats fed 5 percent limonene in their drinking water (Kawamori et al., 1996). Limonene is used as a flavor and fragrant agent and is listed as safe (GRAS) in food by the Food and Drug Administration. Manthey and Guthres (2002) showed that poly-methoxylated flavones in citrus exhibited strong antiproliferative activities against six human cell lines, suggesting their use as anticancer agents in humans.

References

Elson, C.E. and Yu, S.G., The chemoprevention of cancer by mevalonate-derived constituents of fruits and vegetables, *J. Nutr.,* 124:607–614, 1994.

Kawamori, T., Tanaka, T., Hirose, Y., Ohnishi, M., and Mori, H., Inhibitory effects of *d*-limonene on the development of colonic aberrant crypt foci induced by azoxymethane in F344 rats, *Carcinogenesis,* 17: 369–372, 1996.

Manthey, J.A. and Guthries, N., Antiproliferative activities of citrus flavonoids against six human cancer cell lines, *J. Agric. Food Chem.,* 50:5837–5843, 2002.

Club moss *see also* **Huperzine A**   An extract from Club moss (*Huperzia serrata*) has been used for centuries in Chinese medicine to treat swelling, fever, and blood disorders. The principal component extracted is a sesquiterpene alkaloid, huperzine A, shown in clinical trials to have neuroprotective properties, which may be beneficial in the treatment of Alzheimer's disease (Zangara, 2003). For further information consult the section on huperzine A.

References

Zangara, A., The psychopharmacology of huperzine A: An alkaloid with cognitive enhancing and neuroprotective properties of interest in the treatment of Alzheimer's disease, *Pharmacol. Biochem. Behav.,* 75:675–686, 2003.

Cocoa (*Theobroma cacao*) *see also* **Chocolate**
Cocoa is a very rich source of procyanidins, oligomeric flavonoids containing flavan-3-ol units. These compounds are extremely beneficial for their protection against cardiovascular disease by scavenging oxygen and nitrogen species (Rice-Evans et al., 1996). In addition, their ability to inhibit oxidant enzymes has also been reported (Middleton et al., 2000). A recent paper by Mursu et al. (2004) showed healthy, young volunteers consuming 73 g per day of dark chocolate or dark chocolate enriched with cocoa polyphenols had their HDL cholesterol increased by 11.4 percent and 13.7 percent. Schewe and coworkers (2001) reported that epicatechin and cocoa procyanidins inhibited mammalian 15-lipoxygenase, a key enzyme in lipid peroxidation of biomembranes and plasma lipoproteins. Recent research by Schewe et al. (2002) concluded that (–)-epicatechin and its low-molecular-weight procyanidins inhibited both dioxygenase and 5,6-leukotriene A_4 (LTA_4) synthase activities of human 5-lipoxygenase, which could account for the anti-inflammatory effects of cocoa products. Inhibition of growth and polyamine biosynthesis by human colonic cancer cells by cocoa powder and extracts was reported by Carnesecchi and coworkers (2002). The procyanidin-enriched extracts significantly decreased ornithine decarboxylase and *S*-adenosyl-methionine decarboxylase, two key enzymes of polyamine biosynthesis. These results suggested polyamine metabolism may be an important target in the antiproliferative effects of cocoa polyphenols. Yamagishi et al. (2002) reported cocoa liquor proanthocyanidins protected the lungs from 2-amino-1-methyl-6-phenylimidazo[4,5-*b*] pyridine (PhIP)-induced tumorigenesis, and rat pancreatic carcinogenesis in the initiation stage but not mammary carcinogenesis.

References

Carnesecchi, S., Schneider, Y., Lazarus, S.A., Coehlo, D., Gosse, F., and Raul, F., Flavonols and procyanidins of cocoa and chocolate inhibit growth and polyamine biosynthesis of human colonic cancer cells, *Cancer Lett.,* 175:147–155, 2002.

Middleton, E., Jr., Kandaswami, C., and Theoharides, T.C., The effects of plant flavonoids on mammalian cells: Implications for inflammation, heart disease and cancer, *Pharmacol. Rev.,* 52:673–751, 2000.

Mursu, J., Voutilainen, S., Nurmi, T., Rissanen, T.H., Virtanen, J.K., Kaikkonen, J., Nyyssonen, K., and Salonen, J.T., Dark chocolate consumption increases HDL cholesterol concentration and chocolate fatty acids may inhibit lipid peroxidation in healthy humans, *Free Rad. Biol. Med.,* 37:1351–1359, 2004.

Rice-Evans, C.A., Miller, N.J., and Pangana, G., Structure-antioxidant activity relationship of flavonoids and phenolic acids, *Free Rad. Biol. Med.,* 20:933–956, 1996.

C

Schewe, T., Sadik, C., Klotz, L.O., Yoshimoto, T., Kuhn, H., and Sies, H., Polyphenols in cocoa: Inhibition of mammalian 15-lipoxygenase, *Biol. Chem.*, 383:1687–1696, 2001.

Schewe, T., Kuhn, H., and Sies, H., Flavonoids of cocoa inhibit recombinant human 15-lipoxygenase, *J. Nutr.*, 132:1825–1829, 2002.

Yamagishi, M., Natsume, M., Osakabe, N., Okazaki, K., Nakamura, H., Furukawa, F., Imazawa, T., Nishikawa, A., and Hirose, M., Effects of cacao liquor proanthocyanidins on PhIP-induced mutagenesis *in vitro*, and *in vivo* mammary and pancreatic tumorigenesis in female Sprague–Dawley rats, *Cancer Lett.*, 185:123–130, 2002.

Coconut (*Cocos nucifera*)   Coconut is the seed of the coconut palm tree native to the Pacific region of the tropics. It is composed of a thick outer fibrous husk surrounding a hard, stony shell. The lining of the shell, or kernel, contains a white, fleshy, oily area called the meat.

Coconut oil is high in saturated fatty acids. Lauric acid, a 12-carbon saturated acid, accounts for almost 50 percent of the total fatty acids present. Feeding healthy Polynesians coconut oil, butter, and safflower diets, however, still showed cholesterol synthesis was lower on the coconut/safflower-oil diets compared to diets rich in butter (Cox et al., 1998). Padmakumaran Nair and coworkers (1999) reported that human volunteers fed a diet of coconut oil and coconut-kernel protein had lower serum-total- and LDL-cholesterol levels compared to feeding coconut oil alone. The beneficial effects of the kernel protein was attributed to its very low lysine/arginine ratio.

References

Cox, C., Sutherland, W., Mann, J., de Jong, S., Chisholm, A., and Skeaff, M., Effects of dietary coconut oil, butter, and safflower oil on plasma lipids, *Eur. J. Clin. Nutr.*, 52:650–654, 1998.

Padmakumaran Nair, K.G., Rajamohan, T., and Kurup, P.A., Coconut kernel protein modifies the effect of coconut oil on serum lipids, *Plant Foods Hum. Nutr.*, 53:133–144, 1999.

Pillai, M.G., Thampi, B.S.H., Menon, V.P., and Leelamma, S., Influence of dietary fiber from coconut kernel (*Cocos nucifera*) on the 1,2-dimethylhydrazine-induced lipid peroxidation, *J. Nutr. Biochem.*, 10:555–560, 1999.

Coenzyme Q$_{10}$ Coenzyme Q$_{10}$ (CoQ$_{10}$), a lipid-soluble ubiquinone found naturally in foods, boosts the immune system, enabling the body to defend against viruses and microorganisms. Beef heart and muscle are the richest sources of CoQ$_{10}$, although it is still present in other tissues. Plants provide varied amounts of CoQ compounds that can be converted to CoQ$_{10}$ by the liver. Almonds, pistachios, and peanuts are very good sources, providing 10–30 ppm of CoQ$_{10}$ (Hamid et al., 1995).

Coenzyme Q$_{10}$. (From Kommuru et al., *Int. J. Pharm.*, 212:233–246, 2001. With permission.)

Crude palm oil contains around 80 ppm but drops to around 10–30 ppm after processing. Shults et al. (2002) conducted the first placebo-controlled, multicenter clinical trial on CoQ$_{10}$ suggesting it slows down the progression of early-stage Parkinson's disease. The ability of CoQ$_{10}$ to enhance mitochondrial function and to act as a potent antioxidant and mop up harmful free radicals generated by normal metabolism appeared to be the underlying mechanism involved. Kwong and coworkers (2002) found that dietary supplementation of CoQ$_{10}$ to rats elevated CoQ homologues, selectively decreased protein oxidative damage, and increased antioxidative potential.

Several controlled studies showed CoQ$_{10}$ substantially lowered blood pressure in hypertensive patients (Singh et al., 1999; Burke et al., 2002). Hodgson et al. (2002) showed CoQ$_{10}$ improved both blood pressure and glycemic control in subjects with type 2 diabetes. The

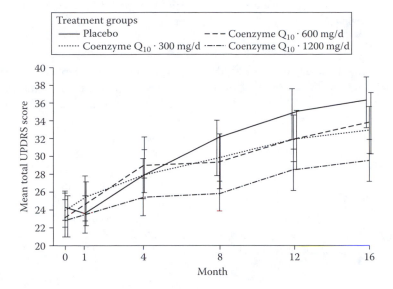

FIGURE C.26 Unified Parkinson's Disease Rating Scale (UPDRS) scores. The scores for the total UPDRS (last observation carried forward) are expressed as mean (SEM). Higher scores indicate more severe features of Parkinson's disease. Results of a test for a linear trend between the dosage and the mean change in the total UPDRS score indicated a trend for coenzyme Q$_{10}$ to reduce the increasing disability over time ($p = .09$). The score change for the 1200-mg/d coenzyme Q$_{10}$ group was significantly different from that of the placebo group ($p = .04$). (From Shults et al., *Arch. Neurol.,* 59:1541–1550, 2002. With permission.)

primary effect of CoQ$_{10}$ was to significantly decrease systolic and diastolic blood pressures and HbA$_{1C}$. None of these improvements were associated with reduced oxidative stress, as there was no change in the amount of F$_2$-isoprostanes.

Shults et al. (1997) reported lower levels of CoQ$_{10}$ in the mitochondria isolated from the plasma of patients suffering from Parkinson's disease (PD). These researchers later showed that oral consumption of dosages of CoQ$_{10}$ of 400, 600, and 800 mg/day were well-tolerated by patients with PD with significant elevations in blood-plasma levels (Shults et al., 1998). Further work by Shults et al. (2002) showed doses of up to 1200 mg/day were well-tolerated by PD subjects. At the highest dosage, a significant slowing down of PD was observed based on the lower tremor score using the Unified Parkinson's Disease Rating Scale (UPDRS), as shown in Figure C.26. Muller et al. (2003), using a double-blind study, fed much lower doses of CoQ$_{10}$ to PD patients of 360 mg/day over a four-week period. A moderate improvement in PD symptoms and visual function, as measured with the Farnsworth–Munsell 100 Hue test (FMT), with studies using higher dosages presently under way. Both these studies point to the potential of CoQ$_{10}$ in the treatment of PD.

References

Burke, B.E., Neuenschwander, R., and Olson, R.D., Randomised double-blind, placebo-controlled trial of coenzyme Q$_{10}$ in isolated systolic hypertension, *South. Med. J.,* 94:1112–1117, 2002.

Hamid, A.H., Choo, Y.M., Goh, S.H., and Khor, H.T., The uniquinones of palm oil, in *Nutrition, Lipids, Health, and Disease,* Ong, Niki, and Packer, Eds., AOCS Press, U.S.A., 1995, p. 122–128.

Hodgson, J.M., Watts, G.F., Playford, D.A., Burke, V., and Croft, K.D., Coenzyme Q$_{10}$ improves blood pressure and glycaemic control: A controlled trial in subjects with type 2 diabetes, *Eur. J. Clin. Nutr.,* 56: 1137–1142, 2002.

Kwong, L.K., Kamzalov, S., Rebrin, I., Bayne, A.-C., Jana, C.K., Morris, P., Forster, M.J., and Sohal, R.S., Effects of coenzyme Q$_{10}$ administration on its tissue concentrations, mitochondrial oxidant generation, and oxidative stress in the rat, *Free Rad. Biol. Med.,* 33:627–638, 2002.

Muller, T., Buttner, T., Gholipour, A.-F., and Kuhn, W., Coenzyme Q_{10} supplementation provides mild symptomatic benefit in patients with Parkinson's disease, *Neurosci. Lett.,* 341:201–204, 2003.

Kommuru, T.R., Gurley, B., Khan, M.A., and Reddy, I.K., Self-emulsifying drug delivery systems (SEDDS) of coenzyme Q_{10}: Formulation development and bioavailability assessment, *Int. J. Pharm.,* 212:233–246, 2001.

Shults, C.W., Haas, R.H., Passov, D., and Beal, M.F., Coenzyme Q_{10} levels correlate with the activities of complexes I and II/III in mitochondria from parkisonian and non-parkinsonian subjects, *Ann. Neurol.,* 42:261–264, 1997.

Shults, C.W., Beal, M.F., Fontaine, S., Nakano, K., and Haas, R.H., Absorption, tolerability and effects on mitochondrial activity of oral coenzyme Q_{10} in parkinsonian patients, *Neurology,* 50:793–795, 1998.

Shults, C.W., Oakes, D., Kieburtz, K., Beal, F., Haas, R., Plumb, S., Juncos, J.L., Nutt, J., Shoulson, I., Carter, J., Kompoliti, K., Perlmutter, J.S., Reich, S., Stern, M., Watts, R.L., Kurlan, R., Molho, E., Harrison, M., Lew, M., and the Parkinson's Study Group, Effects of coenzyme Q_{10} in early Parkinson's disease, *Arch. Neurol.,* 59:1541–1550, 2002.

Singh, R.B., Niaz, M.A., Rastogi, S.S., Shukla, P.K., and Thakur, A.S., Effect of hydrosoluble Coenzyme Q_{10} on blood pressures and insulin resistance in hypertensive patients with coronary artery disease, *J. Hum. Hypertens.,* 13:203–208, 1999.

Coffee   Coffee is a popular beverage that is consumed worldwide. Epidemiological studies on the relationship between coffee and cancer suggests that moderate coffee consumption (2–5 cups/day) does not represent a risk to humans (Schilter et al., 2001a). Many studies, in fact, showed an inverse relationship existed between certain cancer risks and coffee consumption (Nishi et al., 1996; Giovannucci, 1998; Inoue et al., 1998). Meta-analysis of five cohort and 12 case-control studies all pointed to a significant inverse relationship between coffee consumption and colorectal cancer (Giovannucci et al., 1998). The chemoprotective effect of coffee has been demonstrated in experimental animals by its inhibitory effects on carcinogens, nitrosamines, and 1,2-dimethylhydrazine (Gershbein, 1994; Nishikawa et al.,

1986). Anticarcinogenic effects were also demonstrated for green, as well as roasted, coffees in animal models treated with 7,12-dimethylbenz[α]anthacene (Miller et al., 1988, 1993).

Caffeine and polyphenols, such as chlorogenic acid and their degradation products, were considered to be among the compounds responsible for the chemoprotective properties of coffee (Stadler, 2001; Schilter et al., 2001b). A specific lipid fraction in coffee was associated with its ability to inhibit DMBA-induced cancer in rats, mice, and hamsters (Lam et al., 1982; Wattenberg et al., 1986; Miller et al., 1991). This fraction contained diterpenes, cafestol, and kahweol C + K.

Structures of coffee diterpenes cafestol (C) and kahweol (K). (From Cavin et al., *Food Chem. Toxicol.,* 40: 1155–1163, 2002. With permission.)

The difficulty in isolating these components separately, combined with the instability of kahweol, led to studies using a mixture of these two compounds. Cavin et al. (2002) showed the diterpene mixture prevented DNA binding with aflatoxin B1 and the environmental carcinogen, benzo[a]-pyrene(B[α])P in rat hepatocyte cultures in a dose-dependent response (Figure

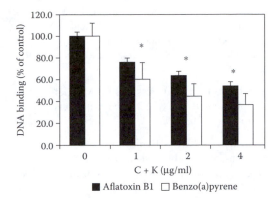

FIGURE C.27 Dose-dependent effect of cafestol and kahweol (C + K) on the formation of aflatoxin B_1 metabolites and benzo[α]pyrene-induced DNA adducts *in vitro*. Results presented are means obtained from five experiments with two independent cultures per treatment (± S.D.). These are expressed as the percentage of the mean value derived from control cultures. In control, the absolute binding rate (equal to 1005) were in average 6.5 pmol AFB1 and 4.5 pmol B[α]P/mg DNA, respectively. *Significantly different from control rat primary hepatocytes ($p < 0.05$) using the Student's t-test. (From Cavin et al., *Food Chem. Toxicol.,* 40:1155–1163, 2002. With permission.)

C.27). These diterpenes also reduced the genotoxicity of several other carcinogens, including 7,12-dimethylbenz[a]-anthracene (DMBA), aflatoxin B1, and 2-amino-1-methyl-6-phenylimidazo[4,5-b]pyridine (PhIP), using animal models and cell cultures. Chemoprotective effects were attributed to induction of conjugating enzymes (e.g., gluthione *S*-tranferases and glucuronyl *S*-transferases), increased protein expression involved in antioxidant defense (e.g., γ-glutamyl cysteine synthetase and heme oxygenase-1), and inhibition of expression or activation of cytochromes P450, the latter normally involved in activation of the carcinogen. The molecular mechanism appeared similar to many cancer-chemopreventive blocking agents and involves the Nrf2 transcription factor through regulation of *cis*-acting, antioxidant-responsive-element (ARE)-driven gene expression. Further work by Cavin and coworkers (2003) showed C + K inhibited B[a]P-DNA adduct formation in primary rat hepatocytes and human bronchial Beas-2B cells. Huber et al. (2003) showed that K/C and Turkish coffee

(cafestol alone) both increased hepatic DNA repair protein O6-methylguanine-DNA methyltransferase (MGMT) in a dose-dependent manner. The increase in MGMT expression provides new insight regarding the antimutagenic/anticarcinogenic potential of these coffee components.

Van Dam and Feskens (2002) reported coffee consumption may reduce the risk of type 2 diabetes mellitus. Of 17,111 Dutch men and women between the ages of 30–60, those drinking a minimum of seven cups of coffee a day were 0.50 (95 percent CI 0.35 = 0.72, p = 0.0002) times as likely to develop diabetes mellitus compared to those drinking two or fewer cups. Components in coffee that could contribute to this effect are caffeine, chlorogenic acid, and magnesium.

Tavani and coworkers (2003) observed an inverse relationship between coffee intake and risk of oral, pharyngeal, and esophageal cancers. A total of 749 and 395 cases were studied suffering from oral/pharyngeal and esophageal cancers, respectively. The multivariate odds ratio (OR) for those drinking more than three cups of coffee/day compared to one cup of coffee/day were 0.6 (95 percent CI 0.5–0.9) for oral/pharyngeal and 0.6 (95 percent CI 0.4–0.9) for esophageal cancer, irrespective of age, sex, education, and alcohol consumption. These results suggested coffee consumption may decrease the risk of oral/pharyngeal and esophageal cancers.

References

Cavin, C., Bezencon, C., Guignard, G., and Schilter, B., Coffee diterpenes prevent benzo[a]pyrene genotoxicity in rat and human culture systems, *Biochem. Biophys. Res. Commun.,* 306:488–495, 2003.

Cavin, C., Holzhaeuser, D., Scharf, G., Constable, A., Huber, W.W., and Schilter, B., Cafestol and kahweol, two coffee specific diterpenes with anticarcinogenic activity, *Food Chem. Toxicol.,* 40:1155–1163, 2002.

Gershbein, L.L., Action of dietary trypsin, pressed coffee oil, silmarin and iron salt on 1,2-dimethylhydrazine tumorigenesis by gavage, *Anticancer Res.,* 14:1113–1116, 1994.

Giovannucci, E., 1998. Meta-analysis of coffee consumption and risk of colorectal cancer, *Am. J. Epidemiol.,* 147:1043–1057, 1998.

C

Huber, W.W., Scharf, G., Nagel, G., Prustomersky, S., Schulte-Hermann, R., and Kaina, B., Coffee and its chemopreventive components kahweol and cafestol increase the activity of 60-methylguanine-DNA methyltransferase in rat liver-comparison with phase II xenobiotic metabolism, *Mutat. Res.*, 522:57–68, 2003.

Inoue, M., Tajima, K., and Hirose, K., Tea and coffee consumption and the risk of digestive tract cancers: Data from a comparative case-referent study in Japan, *Cancer Causes Control*, 9:209–216, 1998.

Lam, L.K.T., Sparnins, V.L., and Wattenberg, L.W., Isolation and identification of kahweol and cafestol palmitate as active constituents of green coffee beans that enhance glutathione *S*-transferase activity in the mouse, *Cancer Res.*, 42:1193–1198, 1982.

Miller, E.G., Formby, W.A., Rivera-Hidalgo, F., and Wright, J.M., Inhibition of hamster buccal pouch carcinogenesis by green coffee, *Oral Surg.*, 65:745–749, 1988.

Miller, E.G., Gonzales-Sanders, A.P., Couvillon, A.M., Binnie, W.H., Sunahara, G.I., and Bertholet, R., Inhibition of oral carcinogenesis by roasted beans and roasted coffee bean fractions, in *Association Scientific International du Café*, 15th ASIC International Colloquium on Coffee, Paris, 1993, pp. 420–425.

Miller, E.G., McWhorter, K., Rivera-Hidalgo, F., Wright, J.M., Hirsbrunner, P., and Sunahara, G.I., Kahweol and cafestol: Inhibitors of hamster buccal pouch carcinogenesis, *Nutr. Cancer*, 14:41–46, 1991.

Nishi, M., Ohba, S., Hirata, K., and Miyake, H., Dose-response relationship between coffee and the risk of pancreas cancer, *Jpn. J. Oncol.*, 26:42–48, 1996.

Nishikawa, A., Tanaka, T., and Mori, H., An inhibitory effect of coffee on nitrosamine-hepatocarcinogenesis with aminopyrine and sodium nitrite in rats, *J. Nutr. Growth Cancer*, 3:161–166, 1986.

Schilter, B., Cavin, C., Tritscher, A., and Constable, A., Coffee: Health and safety considerations, in *Coffee Recent Developments*, Clarke, R.J., and Vitzhthum, O.G., Eds., Blackwell Science, London, 2001a, pp. 165–183.

Schilter, B., Holzhaeuser, D., and Cavin, C., Health benefits of coffee, *Proceedings of the 19th International Scientific Colloquium on Coffee*, Trieste, May 14–18, 2001b.

Stadler, R.H., The use of chemical markers and model studies to assess the *in vitro* pro- and antioxidative properties of methyl xanthine-rich beverages, *Food Rev. Int.*, 17:385–418, 2001.

Tavani, A., Bertuzzi, M., Talamini, R., Gallus, S., Parpinel, M., Franceschi, S., Levi, F., and La Vecchia, C.L., Coffee and tea intake and risk of oral, pharyngeal and esophageal cancer, *Oral Oncol.*, 39:695–700, 2003.

Van Dam, R.M. and Feskens, E.J.M., Coffee consumption and risk of type 2 diabetes mellitus, *Lancet*, 360:1477–1478, 2002.

Wattenberg, L.W., Hanley, A.B., Barany, G., Sparnins, V.L., and Fenwick, G.R., Inhibition of carcinogenesis by some minor constituents, in *Diet, Nutrition and Cancer*, Hayashi, Y., Ed., Japan Science Society Press, Tokyo, 1986, pp. 193–203.

Colostrum   The first mammary gland fluid secreted by mammals during the first four days after birth is known as the colostrum. Besides the major nutritional components normally associated with milk, colostrum contains many minor bioactive components capable of treating many human diseases. For example, the presence of immunoglobulins in the colostrum is extremely important, as these antibodies play a crucial role in immune protection. Casswall et al. (1998) showed that oral immunoglobulins from bovine colostrum effectively treated *Helicobacter pylori* infections in infants in rural Bangladesh. Bovine colostrum, particularly I_g, could provide an immunological supplement in infant formula and other hyperimmune foods (Dominguez and coworkers, 1997). A range of growth factors present include insulin-like growth hormone (IGF) and transforming growth factor (TGF), as well as lactoferrin and lactoperoxidase. For a long time, breast-fed babies were known to be resistant to certain types of infections, particularly intestinal disorders (Jatsky and coworkers, 1985). Among the immune factors in colostrum is an iron-binding protein with antibacterial and antiviral properties, lactoferrin (Wilson, 1997). Purified lactoferrins were shown to inhibit the effects of HIV in cells and fibroblasts (Swart et al., 1998). Colostrum provides a wide range of benefits, including preventing gastrointestinal damage from nonsteroidal, anti-inflammatory drugs (NSAIDs). A number of commercial products are available. An excellent review of colostrum was published by Uruakpa and coworkers (2002).

References

Casswall, T., Sarker, S., Albert, et al., Treatment of *Heliobacter pylori* infection in infants in rural Bangladesh with oral immunoglobulins from hyperimmune bovine colostrum, *Aliment. Pharmacol. Therapies,* 12:563–568, 1998.

Dominguez, E., Perez, M.D., and Calvo, M., Effect of heat treatment on the antigen-binding activity of antiperoxidase immunoglobulins in bovine colostrum, *J. Dairy Sci.,* 80:182–187, 1997.

Jatsky, G.V., Kuvaeva, I.B., and Gribakin, S.G., Immunological protection of the neonatal gastointestinal tract: The importance of breast-feeding, *Acta Pediatr. Scand.,* 74:246–249, 1985.

Swart, P.J., Kuipers, E.M., Smit, C., Van-Der-Strate, B.W., Harmsen, M.C., and Meijer, D.K., Lactoferrin: Antiviral activity of lactoferrin, *Adv. Exp. Med. Biol.,* 443:205–213, 1998.

Wilson, J., Immune system breakthrough: Colostrum, *J. Longevity Res.,* 3:7–10, 1997.

Uruakpa, F.O., Ismond, M.A.H., and Aboundu, E.N.T., Colostrum and its benefits: A review, *Nutr. Res.,* 22:755–767, 2002.

Conjugated linoleic acid   Conjugated linoleic acid (CLA), a class of positional and geometrical conjugated isomers of linoleic acid containing two double bonds separated by a single bond was first reported in dairy products and beef (Pariza et al., 2001). The main isomers identified in foods are *cis*-9, *trans*-10 (c9,t11) and *trans*-10, *cis*-12 (t10,c12) CLA. CLA has some unique chemoprotective properties (Belury, 1995). For example, it has been reported that CLA lowered total body fat and increased lean body mass (Blankson et al., 2000; Delany et al., 1999). In addition, a number of other health benefits have been associated with CLA, including chemopreventative effects against tumors (Visonneau et al., 1996). CLA is also reported to lower cholesterol and to be antiatherogenic. Wilson and coworkers (2000) showed a diet containing conjugated linoleic acid fed to hypercholesterolemic hamsters over 12 weeks significantly reduced the development of early aortic atherogenesis more effectively than linoleic acid, due possibly to changes in the susceptibility of LDL cholesterol to oxidation. Subsequent work by Kritchevsky et al. (2002) showed that a diet containing as little as 0.05 percent CLA reduced the severity of atherosclerosis in the aortic arch of hamsters by 20 percent and in the thoracic aorta by 8 percent. Increasing the level of CLA in the diet was accompanied by a corresponding decrease in the severity of atherosclerosis. Based on the effectiveness in the hamster diet of 0.5 percent CLA level, these researchers felt that a normal human diet could contain an effective level of dietary CLA.

Using a 2-amino-1-methyl-6-phenylimidazo[4,5-*b*]pyridine (PhIP)-induced rat mammary carcinogenesis model, Futakuchi and coworkers (2002) reported conjugated linoleic acid from safflower or perilla oil decreased carcinogenesis in the postinitiation period, with inhibition of cell proliferation. The antiproliferative effects of two commercial preparations of CLA, containing isomers (c9,t11-CLA, c9,c11-CLA, and t10,c12-CLA), were examined by Palombo et al. (2002) using human colorectal (HT-29, MIP-101) and prostate (PC-3) carcinoma cells. Both the type and concentration of individual CLA isomers determined their antiproliferation effects. The greatest potency against proliferation of colorectal-cancer cells was observed for t10,c12-CLA, while c9,t11 and t10,c12 isomers were only moderately effective against prostate-cancer cells.

Cis-9, trans-11 CLA

Trans-10, cis-12 CLA

CLA isomers. (From Evans et al., *J. Nutr. Biochem.,* 13:508–516, 2002. With permission.)

C

TABLE C.22
Effect of CFA-S on Cell Proliferation of Mammary Adenocarcinoma and Colon Epithelium

Treatment DMH + DMBA		Number of Lesions Examined	PCNA[1] Positive Index (%) Mammary Adenocarcinoma	Colon Epithelium
(+)	Control	10	7.5 + 4.2	28.8 + 5.8
(+)	CFA-S 0.01%	10	5.7 + 2.5	21.7 + 5.7*
(+)	CFA-S 0.05%	10	6.3 + 3.4	22.3 + 4.7*
(+)	SFA-S 0.1%	10	6.4 + 2.8	22.4 + 6.0*
(+)	CFA-S 1%	10	4.7 + 2.4	19.7 + 5.5**
(+)	CFA-2%	10	6.9 + 3.6	23.4 + 5.6*

[1] PCNA-Proliferating cell nuclear antigen. *$p < 0.05$, ** $p < 0.01$ vs. control values.

Source: Cheng et al., *Cancer Lett.*, 196:161–168, 2003. With permission.

Kimoto et al. (2001) reported that 1 or 0.1 percent CLA safflower oil (CFA-S) suppressed mammary carcinogenesis in a two-stage model in female rats. Recent work by Cheng et al. (2003) showed that the optimal level for inhibiting carcinogenesis in rat mammary glands and colon, induced by 1,2-dimethyl-benz[α]-anthracene (DMBA) and 1,2-dimethylhydrazine (DMH), was 1 percent (Table C.22).

A recent study by Albers and coworkers (2003) showed that supplementation with a 50:50 CLA mixture (c9,t11 + t10,c12) enhanced the immune system of healthy males by increasing the sero-protection rate following hepatitis B vaccination. This could be beneficial to those individuals who are slow or low responders to the vaccination. Further research is needed, however, to determine whether similar effects are accrued following exposure to infection. A recent review on conjugated linoleic acid by Wahle et al. (2004) is recommended.

References

Albers, R., van der Wielen, R.P.J., Brink, E.J., Hendriks, H.F.J., Dorovska-Taran, V.N., and Mohede, I.C.M., Effects of cis-9, trans-11 and trans-10, cis-12 conjugated linoleic acid (CLA) isomers on immune function in healthy men, *Eur. J. Clin. Nutr.*, 57:595–60, 2003.

Belury, M.A., Conjugated dienoic linoleate: A polyunsaturated fatty acid with unique chemoprotective properties, *Nutr. Rev.*, 53:83–89, 1995.

Blankson, H., Stakkestad, J.A., Fagetun, H., Thom, E., Wadstein, J., and Gudmundsen, O., Conjugated linoleic acid reduces body fat in overweight and obese humans, *J. Nutr.*, 130:2370–2377, 2000.

Cheng, J.L., Futakuchi, M., Ogawa, K., Iwata, T., Kasai, M., Tokudome, S., Hirose, M., and Shirai, T., Dose response study of conjugated fatty acid derived from safflower oil on mammary and colon carcinogenesis pretreated with 7,12-dimethylbenzanthracene (DMBA) and 1,2-dimethylhydrazine (DMH) in female Sprague–Dawley rats, *Cancer Lett.*, 196:161–168, 2003.

Delany, J.P., Blohm, F., Truett, A.A., Scimeca, J.A., and West, D.B., Conjugated linoleic acid rapidly reduces body fat content in mice without affecting energy intake, *Am. J. Physiol.*, 276:1172–1179, 1999.

Evans, M.E., Brown, J.M., and McIntosh, M.K., Isomer-specific effects of conjugated linoleic acid (CLA) on adiposity and lipid metabolism, *J. Nutr. Biochem.*, 13:508–516, 2002.

Futakuchi, M., Cheng, J.L., Hirose, M., Kimoto, N., Cho, Y.-M., Iwata, T., Kasai, M., Tokudome, S., and Shirai, T., Inhibition of conjugated fatty acids derived from safflower or perilla oil of induction and development of mammary tumors in rats induced by 2-amino-1-methyl-6-phenylimidazo[4,5-b]pyridine (PhIP), *Cancer Lett.*, 178:131–139, 2002.

Kimoto, N., Hirose, M., Futakuchi, M., Iwata, T., Kasai, M., and Shirai, T., Site-dependent modulating effects of conjugated fatty acids from safflower oil in a rat two-stage carcinogenesis model in female Sprague–Dawley rats, *Cancer Lett.*, 168:15–21, 2001.

Kritchevsky, D., Tepper, S.A., Wright, S., and Czar-necki, S.K., Influence of graded levels of conjugated linoleic acid (CLA) on experimental atherosclerosis in rabbit, *Nutr. Res.*, 22:1275–1279, 2002.

Palombo, J.D., Ganguly, A., Bistrian, B.R., and Menard, M.P., The antiproliferative effects of biolog-ically active isomers of conjugated linoleic acid on human colorectal and prostatic cancer cells, *Cancer Lett.*, 177:163–177, 2002.

Pariza, M.W., Park, Y., and Cook, M.E., The biolog-ical active isomer of conjugated linoleic acid, *Prog. Lipid Res.*, 40:283–298, 2001.

Visonneau, S., Cesano, A., Tepper, S.A., Scimeca, J., Santoli, D., and Kritchevsky, D., Effect of different concentrations of conjugated linoleic acid (CLA) on tumor cell growth *in vitro*, *FASEB*, 9:A869, 1996.

Wahle, K.W.J., Heys, S.D., and Rotondo, D., Conju-gated linoleic acids: Are they beneficial or detrimen-tal to health? *Prog. Lipid Res.*, 43:553–587, 2004.

Wilson, T.A., Nicolosi, R.J., Chrysam, M., and Kritchevsky, D., Conjugated linoleic acid reduces early aortic athersclerosis greater than linoleic acid in hypercholesterolemic hamsters, *Nutr. Res.*, 20: 1795–1805, 2000.

Coriander (*Coriandrum sativum* L.)   Corian-der is an annual herb with delicate, bright leaves. Its seeds are used to flavor foods, while its aromatic oil is used in cream lotions and perfumes. Anilakumar et al. (2001) examined the effect of feeding 10 percent coriander-seed powder on hexachlorocyclohexane-induced oxidative stress in rat livers. The antioxidant properties of coriander-seed powder were evi-dent by a reduction in conjugated dienes, hydro-peroxides, and malondialdehyde in the liver. Prefeeding coriander-seed powder appeared to counteract the effect of hexachlorocyclohexane by enhancing the hepatic oxidant system. Guerra et al. (2005) recently isolated five car-otenoids, β-carotene, β-cryptoxanthin epoxide, lutein-5,6-epoxide, violaxanthin, and neoxan-thin, from an ether extract of coriander. Of these, β-carotene represented 61.4 percent of the total carotenoids isolated. The antioxidant activity of the crude fraction was much greater than the individual fractions, suggesting syner-gism between the individual fractions. Delaquis

et al. (2002) compared the antimicrobial activ-ity of a number of essential oils, including cori-ander. Distilled fractions of purified coriander oil proved far more effective in inhibiting test microorganisms compared to the crude oil. Sev-eral purified fractions were obtained, with the more potent fraction containing a mixture of α-pinene (89.4 percent) and camphene (8.5 per-cent).

References

Anilakumar, K.R., Nagaraj, N.S., and Santhanam, K., Effect of coriander seeds on hexachlorocyclohex-ane induced lipid peroxidation in rat liver, *Nutr. Res.*, 21:1455–1462, 2001.

Delaquis, P.J., Stanich, K., Girard, B., and Mazza, G., Antimicrobial activity of individual and mixed fractions of dill, cilantro, coriander and eucalyptus essential oils, *Int. J. Food Microbiol.*, 74:101–109, 2002.

Guerra, N.B., de Almeido Melo, E., and Filho, J.M., Antioxidant compounds from coriander (*Corian-drum sativum* L.) etheric extract, *J. Fd. Comp. Anal.*, 18:193–199, 2005.

Corn bran   Corn bran, produced by dry mill-ing, was shown by several researchers to lower cholesterol (Shane and Walker, 1995; Vidal-Quintanar et al., 1997). The particle size of corn bran was shown by Ebihara and Nakamoto (2001) to affect plasma cholesterol, fecal out-put, and cecal fermentation in rats. A fiber-free diet was compared to a corn-bran (50 g/kg) diet, ranging in different particle sizes, from 105 to 500 μm. A reduction in particle size was accom-panied by a decrease in plasma cholesterol, fecal wet weight, and fecal bulking effect in the rats. Examination of rat liver showed a corre-sponding increase in cholesterol concentration, cecal-wall weight, and wet weight of cecal con-tent, together with higher levels of total organic acids in the cecal, such as acetic and n-butyric acids.

References

Ebihara, K. and Nakamoto, Y., Effect of particle size of corn bran on the plasma and cholesterol concen-tration, cecal output and cecal fermentation in rats, *Nutr. Res.*, 21:1509–1518, 2001.

C

C

Shane, J.M. and Walker, P.M., Corn bran supplementation of low-fat controlled diet lowers serum lipids in men with hypercholesterolemia, *J. Am. Diet. Assoc.*, 95:40–45, 1995.

Vidal-Quintanar, R.L., Hernandez, L., Conde, K., Vergara-Jimenes, M. and Fernandez, M.L., Lime treated corn husks lower plasma LDL cholesterol in guinea pigs by altering hepatic cholesterol metabolism, *J. Nutr. Biochem.*, 8:479–486, 1997.

Corn-fiber oil   Corn-fiber oil is a by-product of dry milling of corn. Wilson and coworkers (2000) found that the oil extracted from corn-oil fiber reduced plasma and hepatic cholesterol and increased fecal cholesterol excretion in hamsters fed a hypercholesterolemic diet, to a much greater degree than corn oil. Corn-oil diets containing soy sterols or stanols exhibited similar effects on plasma cholesterol levels and cholesterol excretion to that of corn-fiber oil.

Reference

Wilson, T.A., DeSimone, A.P., Romano, A., and Nicolosi, R.J., Corn fiber oil lowers plasma cholesterol levels and increases cholesterol excretion greater than corn oil to diets containing soy sterols and soy stanols in hamsters, *J. Nutr. Biochem.*, 11: 443–449, 2000.

Corn oil   Corn oil is a premium-quality oil rich in ω-6 fatty acids. Linoleic acid (C18:2 ω-6) accounts for approximately 60 percent of the total fatty acids in corn oil, while oleic acid (C18:1 ω-9) comprises around 26 percent. Many studies have shown corn-oil diets fed over a long duration lower total and LDL cholesterol, while HDL-cholesterol remained unchanged (Iacono and Dougherty, 1991). The greater-than-expected lowering of cholesterol by corn oil was explained, in part, due to the presence of naturally occurring plant sterols in the oil (Mattson et al., 1982; Laraki et al., 1993). Corn oil has been shown to significantly lower elevated blood pressure (Iacono and Dougherty, 1993) and reduce the progression of diabetic angiopathy in adult onset diabetes mellitus (Houtsmuller et al., 1982). However, corn oil appears to increase the rate of growth

of established tumors. Rusyn and coworkers (1999) showed corn oil rapidly activated the nuclear factor-κB (NF-κB) in Kupffer cells through an oxidant-dependent mechanism. This is turn triggers the production of the tumor necrosis factor α (TNF-α). An earlier study by Gonzalez et al. in 1991compared corn oil (high in ω-6 fatty acids) with fish oil (high in ω-3 fatty acids) on the growth of human breast-carcinoma cell lines. Unlike fish oil, which significantly increased lipid peroxidation and decreased tumor volume, corn oil increased human breast-carcinoma volume.

References

Gonzalez, M.J., Schemmel, R.A., Gray, J.I., Dugan, L., Jr., Sheffield, L.G., and Welsch, C.W., Effect of dietary fat on growth of MCF-7 carcinomas in erythmic nude mice: Relationship between carcinoma growth and lipid peroxidation product levels, *Carcinogenesis*, 12:1231–1235, 1991.

Houtsmuller, A.J., van Hal-Ferwerds, J., Zahn, K.J., and Henkes, H.E., Favourable influences of linoleic acid as the progression of diabetic micro- and macroangiopathy in adult onset diabetes mellitus, *Prog. Lipid Res.*, 20:377–386, 1982.

Iacono, J.M. and Dougherty, R.M., Lack of effect of linoleic acid on the high-density lipoprotein-cholesterol fraction on plasma lipoproteins, *Am. J. Clin. Nutr.*, 53:660–664, 1991.

Laraki, L., Pelletier, X., Mourot, J., and Derby, G., Effects of dietary phytosterol on liver lipids and lipid metabolism enzymes, *Ann. Nutr. Metab.*, 37:129–133, 1993.

Mattson, F.H., Grundy, S.M., and Crouse, J.R., Optimising the effect of plant sterols on cholesterol absorption in man, *Am. J. Clin. Nutr.*, 35:697–700, 1982.

Rusyn, I., Bradham, C.A., Cohn, L., Schoonhoven, R., Swenberg, J.A., Brenner, D.A., and Thurman, R.G., Corn oil activates nuclear factor-κB on heptic Kupffer cells by oxidant-dependent reactions, *Carcinogenesis*, 20:2095–2100, 1999.

Cranberry fruit   Cranberry (*Vaccinium macrocarpon* Ait. Ericaceae), a native fruit in North America, has been reported to provide health benefits, such as preventing bacterial adhesion in urinary-tract infections of *Escherichia coli*

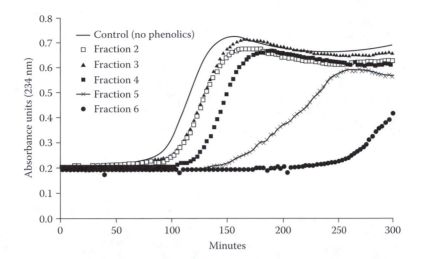

FIGURE C.28 Effect of cranberry flavonoid fractions on lag time of Cu^{2+}-induced LDL oxidation. Histograms show the mean (n = 3) and the error bars the SEM. Significant differences ($p < 0.05$) between treatment means are denoted by different letters above the error bars. Fraction 2 contained a hydroxycinnamic acid peak and several anthocyanins. Fractions 3 and 4 also contained flavonoids. Fraction 4 also contained a few low-molecular-weight proanthocyanidins. Fractions 5 and 6 both contained proanthocyanidins. (From Porter et al., *J. Sci. Food Agric.,* 81:1306–1313, 2001. With permission.)

and stomach ulcers (Burger et al., 2000; Foo et al., 2000), inhibiting lipoprotein oxidation (Wilson et al., 1998), and exhibiting anticancer properties (Bomser et al., 1996). Many of these health benefits are associated with its phenolic content, which was shown to be highest per serving among 20 fruits examined and ranked sixth in antioxidant capacity (Vinson et al., 2001). Yan and coworkers (2002) found the highest radical-scavenging activity was associated with cranberry extract. Their flavonol glycosides had similar or superior antioxidant activity to vitamin E when assayed using either the diphenyl-2-picrylhydrazyl radical-scavenging method or the low-density lipoprotein oxidation system. Cyanidin 3-galactoside stood out by its superior antioxidant activity to flavonoids and vitamin E using both methods.

Porter and coworkers (2001) showed six cranberry phenolic fractions inhibited Cu^{2+}-induced low-density (LDL) oxidation in human serum (Figure C.28). Only several fractions (5 and 6) that contained proanthocyanidins significantly increased the LDL-oxidation lag time. One of these fractions contained trimers through to heptamers, with the more potent fraction containing pentamers through to nonamers. The anticancer activity of cranberries

was attributed to inhibition of ornithine decarboxylase (ODC) by flavonol glycosides and proanthocyanidins (Kandil et al., 2002). This enzyme was previously shown to be involved in tumor proliferation. Two cranberry extracts were reported by Guthrie (2000) to inhibit the proliferation of breast-cancer cells. Yan et al. (2002) also reported the selective inhibition of two of seven tumor-cell lines by a methanolic extract from cranberry fruit ranging from 16–125 µg/mL. Murphy et al. (2003) identified several new triterpenoid hydroxycinnamates from a bioactive cranberry fruit fraction, *cis*-(1) and *trans*-(2) 3-*O*-*p*-hydroxycinnamoyl ursolic acids (Scheme C.18). Both were found to inhibit tumor-cell growth. The greatest antitumor activity, however, was associated with the s isomer(1), resulting in a 50 percent growth inhibition in MCF-7 breast, ME180 cervical, and PC3 prostate-tumor lines in the presence approximately 20 µM. Based on these results, cranberries clearly contain an array of compounds with potential health benefits.

References

Bomser, J., Madhavi, D.L., Singletary, K., and Smith, M.A., *In vitro* anticancer activity of fruit extracts from *Vaccinium* species, *Planta Med.,* 62:212–216, 1996.

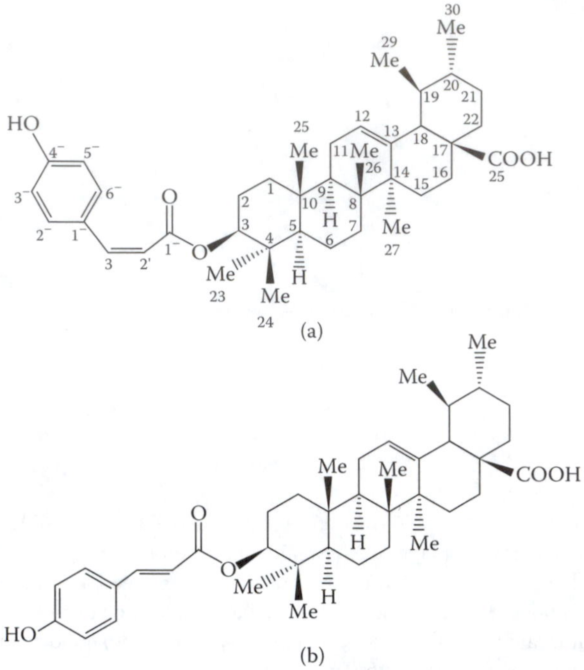

C

SCHEME C.18 Bioactive triterpenoids, *cis*- (a) and *trans*- (b) 3-*O*-p-hydroxycinnamoyl ursolic acids. (From Murphy et al., *J. Agric. Food Chem.,* 51:3541–3545, 2003. With permission.)

Burger, O., Ofek, I., Tabak, M., Weiss, E.I., Sharon, I., and Neeman, I., A high molecular mass constituent of cranberry juice inhibits *Heliobacter pylori* adhesion to human gastric mucus, *FEMS Immunol. Med. Microbiol.,* 29:295–301, 2000.

Foo, L.Y., Howell, A.B., and Vorsa, N., The structure of cranberry proanthocyanidins which inhibit adherence of uropathogenic P-fimbriated *Eschrichia coli in vitro. Phytochemistry,* 54:173–181, 2000.

Guthrie, N., Effect of cranberry juice and products on human breast cancer cell growth, *FASEB J.,* 14: A771, 2000.

Kandil, F.E., Smith, M.A.L., Rogers, R.B., Pepin, M.F., Song, L.L., Pezzuto, J.M., and Siegler, D.S., Composition of a chemopreventive proanthocyanidin-rich fraction from cranberry fruits responsible for the inhibition of 12-*O*-tetradecanoyl phorbol-13-acetate (TPA)-induced ornithine decarboxylase (ODC) activity, *J. Agric. Food Chem.,* 50:1063–1069, 2002.

Murphy, B.T., MacKinnon, S.L., Yan, X., Hammond, G.B., Vaisberg, A.J., and Neto, C.C., Identification of triterpene hydroxycinnamates with *in vitro* antitumor activity from whole cranberry fruit (*Vaccinium macrocarpon*), *J. Agric. Food Chem.,* 51:3541–3545, 2003.

Porter, M.L., Krueger, C.G., Wiebe, D.A., Cunningham, D.G., and Reed, J., Cranberry proanthocyanidins associate with low-density lipoprotein and inhibit *in vitro* Cu^{2+}-induced oxidation, *J. Sci. Food Agric.,* 81:1306–1313, 2001.

Vinson, J.A., Dabbagh, Y.A., Serry, M.M., and Jang, J., Plant flavonoids, especially tea flavonols, are powerful antioxidants using an *in vitro* oxidation model for heart disease, *J. Agric. Food Chem.,* 43:2800–2802, 1995.

Wilson, T., Porcari, J., and Harbin, D., Cranberry extract inhibits low density lipoprotein oxidation, *Life Sci.,* 62:381–386, 1998.

Yan, X., Murphy, B.T., Hammond, G.B., Vinson, J.A., and Neta, C.C., Antioxidant activities and antitumor screening of extracts from cranberry fruit (*Vaccinium macrocarpon*), *J. Agric. Food Chem.,* 50: 5844–5849, 2002.

Cranberry juice   Sobota (1984) first reported that fresh cranberry juice prevented bacterial adhesion, a prerequisite for the development of urinary-tract infection. Later studies by Ahuja et al. (1998) showed cranberry juice had no antibacterial activity but inhibited adhesion by *P. fimbriae*. The substances in cranberry juice responsible were shown to be the condensed tannins, proanthocyanidins. Howell et al. (1998) found cranberry proanthocyanidins prevented adherence of uropathogenic P-fimbriated *Escherichia coli* to the urinary tract. The effect was detectable in the presence of 10–50 µg/mL proanthocyanidins. Examination of senior residents (mean age 78.5 years) in a long-care facility by Avorn and coworkers (1994) found that consumption of 300 mL of a cranberry cocktail significantly decreased infections by bacteriuria and pyuria. The protective role of cranberry juice was further supported by Haverkorn and Mandigers (1994), who found fewer cases of bacteriuria in patients given cranberry juice (15 mL) diluted with water twice a day for a month. Based on clinical studies carried out to-date, Lowe and Fagelman (2001) encouraged supplementing cranberries, as juice, concentrate, or in cocktail formulations, because of its beneficial effect in preventing urinary-tract infections. Burger et al. (2000) also showed cranberry juice inhibited adhesion of *Helicobacter pylori*, a major cause of gastrointestinal infections in humans.

Pedersen and coworkers (2000) reported an increase in plasma antioxidant capacity following consumption of cranberry juice.

References

Ahuja. S., Kaack, B., and Roberts, J., Loss of fimbrial adhesion with the addition of *Vaccinium macrocarpon* to the growth medium of P-fimbriated *Escherichia coli*, *J. Urol.*, 159:559–562, 1998.

Avorn, J., Monane, M., Gruwitz, J.H., Glynn, R.J., Choodisovskiy, I., and Lipsitz, A., Reduction of bacteriuria and pyuria after ingestion of cranberry juice, *JAMA*, 271:751–754, 1994.

Burger, O., Ofek, I., Tabak, M., Weiss, E.I., Sharon, N., and Neeman, I., A high molecular mass constituent of cranberry juice inhibits *Helicobacter pylori* adhesion to human gastric mucus, *FEMS Immunol. Med. Microbiol.*, 29:295–301, 2000.

Haverkorn, M.J. and Mandigers, J., Reduction of bateriuria and pyuria using cranberry juice (letter), *JAMA*, 272:590, 1994.

Howell, A.B., Vorsa, N., Marderosian, A.D., and Foo, L.Y., Inhibition of the adherence of p-fimbriated *Escherichia coli* uroepithelial surfaces by proanthocyanidin extracts from cranberries, *N. Eng. J. Med.*, 339:1085–1089, 1998.

Lowe, F.C. and Fagelman, E., Cranberry juice and urinary infections, what is the evidence? *Urol.*, 57:407–413, 2001.

Pedersen, C.B., Kyle, J., Jenkinson, A. M., Garnder, P.T., McPhail, D.B., and Duthie, G.G., Effects of blueberry and cranberry juice consumption on the plasma antioxidant capacity of healthy female volunteers, *Eur. J. Clin. Nutr.*, 54:405–408, 2000.

Sobota, A.E., Inhibition of bacterial adherence by cranberry juice: Potential use for the treatment of urinary tract infections, *J. Urol.*, 131:563–568, 1984.

Crocin *see also* **Saffron**   The pistils of *Crocus sativus* L. have been used in traditional Chinese medicine to treat disorders of the central-nervous system. Extracts obtained from *Crocus sativus* were shown to prevent tumor

Crocin. (From Soeda et al., *Life Sci.*, 69:2887–2898, 2001. With permission.)

formation, atherosclerosis, and hepatic injury (Gainer and Jones, 1975; Salomi et al., 1991; Wang et al., 1991). Ethanol is well-known to impair brain functions, such as learning and memory. Research conducted on *Crocus sativus* L. showed that components in this extract antagonize ethanol-induced memory impairment. The component responsible was identified as crocin (crocetin di-gentiobiose) (Sagiura et al., 1995). Subsequent work by Abe and coworkers (1998) showed crocin selectively antagonized the inhibitory effect of ethanol on *N*-methyl-D-aspartate (NDMA) receptor-mediated responses in hippocampal neurons, suggesting it may be useful for treating brain disorders. The pathology of neurode-generative diseases is associated with unexpected neuron deaths occurring during a stroke (Crowe, 1997), trauma (Hill et al., 1995), or in the brains of Alzheimer's patients (Pettmann and Henderson, 1998). A possible therapeutic strategy for treating these disorders would be to prevent neuronal-cell death as overexpression of the tumor necrosis factor (TNF-α) has been implicated in the pathogenesis of Alzheimer's disease (Fillit et al., 1991) and Parkinson's disease (Boka et al., 1994). Using neuronally differentiated PC-12 cells, Soeda and coworkers (2001) showed that in cells treated with 10 µM crocin, the normal features of cell death were not evident due to suppression of TNF-α-induced expression Bcl-2 proteins, which triggers signals that activate caspase-3 and the development of apoptosis.

Escribano and coworkers (1996) compared the effectiveness of crocin, safranal, and picrocrocin, compounds present in saffron (*Crocus sativus* L.), on their ability to inhibit the growth of human cancer cells. A 50 percent inhibition of cell growth (LD_{50}) was observed with 3 mM crocin in which cells showed wide cytoplasmic vacuole-like areas, reduced cytoplasm, cell shrinkage, and pyknotic nuclei. These researchers viewed crocin as one of the more promising compounds in saffron as a cancer therapeutic agent.

References

Abe, K., Suguira, M., Shoyama, Y., and Saito, H., Crocin antagonizes ethanol inhibition of NMDA receptor-mediated responses in rat hippocampal neurons, *Brain Res.,* 787:132–138, 1998.

Boka, G., Anglade, P., Wallach, D., Javoy-Agid, F., Agid, Y., and Hirsch, E.C., Immunocytochemical analysis of tumor necrosis factor and its receptor in Parkinson's disease, *Neurosci. Lett.,* 172:151–154, 1994.

Crowe, M.J., Bresnahan, J.C., Shuman, S.L., Masters, J.N., and Beattie, M.S., Apoptosis and delayed degeneration after spinal cord injury in rats and monkeys, *Nat. Med.,* 3:73–76, 1997.

Escribano, J., Alonso, G.-L., Coca-Prados, M., and Fernandez, J.-A., Crocin, safranal and picrocrocin from saffron (*Crocus sativus* L.) inhibit the growth of human cancer cells *in vitro, Cancer Lett.,* 100:23–30, 1996.

Fillit, H., Ding, W.H., Buee, L., Kalman, L., Altstiel, L., Lawlor, B., and Wolf-Klein, G., Elevated circulating tumor necrosis factor and its receptor in Alzheimer's disease, *Neurosci. Lett.,* 129:318–320, 1991.

Gainer, J.L. and Jones, J.R., The use of crocetin in experimental atherosclerosis, *Experentia,* 31:548–549, 1975.

Hill, I.E., MacManus, J.P., Rasquinha, I., and Tuor, U.I., DNA fragmentation indicative of apoptosis following unilateral cerebral hypoxia-ischemia in the neonatal rat, *Brain Res.,* 676:398–403, 1995.

Pettmann, B. and Henderson, C.E., Neuronal cell death, *Neuron,* 20:633–647, 1998.

Salomi, M.J., Nair, S.C., and Panikkar, K.R., Inhibitory effect of *Nigella sativa* and saffron on chemical carcinogenesis, *Nutr. Cancer,* 16:67–72, 1991.

Soeda, S., Ochiai, T., Paopong, L., Tanaka, H., Shoyama, Y., and Shimeno, H., Crocin suppresses tumor necrosis factor-α-induced cell death of neuronally differentiated PC-12 cells, *Life Sci.,* 69:2887–2898, 2001.

Suguira, M., Shoyama, Y., Saito, H., and Nishiyama, N., Crocin improves the ethanol-induced impairment of learning behaviors of mice in passive avoidance tasks, *Proc. Jap. Acad.,* 71:319–324, 1995.

Wang, E., Norred, W.P., Bacon, C.W., Riley, R.T., and Merrill, A.H., Jr., Inhibition of sphingolipid biosynthesis by fumonisins: Implications for diseases associated with Fusarium moniforme, *J. Biol. Chem.,* 266:1486–1490, 1991.

Cruciferous vegetables *see also* **Brassica**
Cruciferous vegetables, including cabbages, broccoli, Brussels sprouts, radish, mustard, and cress, are all high in glucosinolates. When these vegetables are cut, ground, or damaged, the glucosinolates are hydrolyzed by an enzyme, myrosinase, producing biologically active isothiocyanates (ITC) and indoles. There appears to be an inverse relation between cruciferous vegetables and the risk of cancer (Verhoeven et al., 1997; Talalay and Fahey, 2001). Lampe and Peterson (2002) reviewed the chemoprotective effects of the high glucosinolate content of cruciferous vegetables and their metabolites, ITC and indoles, in relation to cancer prevention. Since isothiocyanates are strong inhibitors of phase I enzymes but inducers of phase II enzymes (Zhang and Talalay, 1998), cruciferous vegetables were considered cancer chemopreventors, which was confirmed in human-intervention studies (Bogaards et al., 1998; Nojhoff et al., 1995). Steinkeller et al. (2001) presented evidence that cruciferous vegetables and their constituents protect against bioactivation of DNA-reactive dietary carcinogens. Induction of uridinediphospho-glucuronsyl transferase (UDPGT) appeared the protective mechanism involved against heterocyclic amines by the cruciferous vegetables.

Isthiocyanates formed in the digestion of cruciferous vegetables are conjugated with glutathione and excreted in the urine as their corresponding mecapturic acids (Scheme C.19). Vermeulen and coworkers (2003) developed an efficient method for monitoring the intake and action of isothiocyanates by measuring the corresponding mercapturic acids as biomarkers.

References

Bogaards, J.J., Verhagen, H,., Willems, M.I., van Poppel, G., and van Bladeren, P.J., Consumption of Brussels sprouts results in elevated glutathione-S-transferase levels in human blood plasma, *Carcinogenesis*, 15:1073–1075, 1994.

Lampe, J.W. and Peterson, S., *Brassica* and cancer risk: Genetic polymorphisms alter the preventive effects of cruciferous vegetables, *J. Nutr.*, 132:2991–2992, 2002.

Nojhoff, W.A., Mulder, T.P., Verhagen, H., van Poppel, G., and Peters, W.H., Effects of consumption of Brussels sprouts on plasma and urinary glutathione-S-transferase class-alpha and pi in humans, *Carcinogenesis*, 16:955–957, 1995.

Steinkeller, H., Rabot, S., Freywald, C., Nobis, E., Scharf, G., Chabicovsky, M., Knasmuller, S., and Kassie, F., Effects of cruciferous vegetables and their constituents on drug metabolizing enzymes involved in the bioactivation of DNA-reactive dietary carcinogens, *Mutat. Res.*, 480–481:285–297, 2001.

Talalay, P. and Fahey, J.W., Phytochemicals from cruciferous plants protect against cancer by modulating carcinogen metabolism, *J. Nutr.*, 131:3027S–3033S, 2001.

Verhoeven, D.T.H., Verhagen, H., Goldbohm, P.A., Van den Brandt, P.A., and van Poppel, G., A review of mechanism underlying anticarcinogenicity by Brassica vegetables, *Chemico-Biol. Interact.*, 103:79–129, 1997.

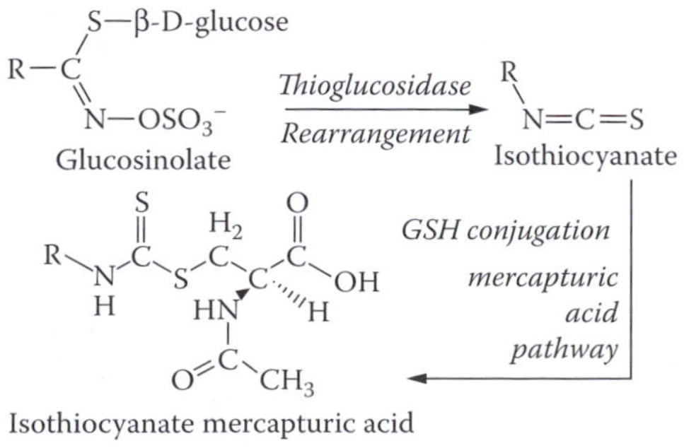

SCHEME C.19 Glucosinolates enzymatically hydrolyzed to isothiocyanates are then conjugated to glutathione, followed by excretion as mercapturic acids in the urine. (From Vermeulen et al., *J. Agric. Food Chem.*, 51:3554–3559, 2003. With permission.)

Vermeulen, M., van Roujen, H.J.M., and Vaes, W.H., Analysis of isothiocyanate mercapturic acids in urine: A biomarker for cruciferous vegetable intake, *J. Agric. Food Chem.*, 51:3554–3559, 2003.

Zhang, Y. and Talalay, P., Mechanism of differential potencies of isothiocyanates as inducers of anticarcinogenic Phase 2 enzymes, *Cancer Res.*, 58:4632–4639, 1998.

Curcumin Curcumin, the yellow pigment from turmeric, was shown to be a potent inhibitor of radiation-induced initiation of mammary tumors in rats (Inano et al., 2000). The inhibitory effect of curcumin on telomerase reverse-transcriptase (hHERT) activity was reported by Ramachandran and coworkers (2002) in MCF-7 breast-cancer cells. This effect was dose dependent, with 93.4 percent inhibition in the presence of 100 μM curcumin. The inhibition of telomerase activity appeared to involve

Curcumin. (From May et al., *Anal. Biochem.*, 337:62–69, 2005. With permission.)

down-regulating hHERT expression by the breast-cancer cells. The ability of curcumin to inhibit the formation of the Fos-Jun-DNA complex led Hahm and coworkers (2002) to synthesize 12 symmetrical cucurminoids. One of these, BJC005, proved to be 90 times more effective than curcumin and more potent than momordin, a potent Fos-Jun inhibitor.

References

Hahm, E-R., Cheon, G., Lee, J., Kim, B., Park, C., and Yang, C., New and known symmetrical curcumin derivatives inhibit the formation of Fos-Jun-DNA complex, *Cancer Lett.*, 184:89–96, 2002.

Inano, H., Onoda, M., Inafuku, N., Kubota, M., Kamada, Y., Osawa, T., Kobayashi, H., and Wakabayashi, K., Potent preventive action of curcumin on radiation-induced initiation of mammary tumorigenesis in rats, *Carcinogenesis,* 21:1835–1841, 2000.

May, L.A., Tourkina, E., Hoffman, S.P., and Dix, T.A., Detection and quantitation of curcumin mouse lung cell cultures by matrix-assisted laser desorption ionization time of flight mass spectrometry, *Anal. Biochem.*, 337:62–69, 2005.

Ramachandran, C., Fonseca, H.B., Jhabvala, P., Escalan, E.A., and Melnick, Curcumin inhibits telomerase activity through human telomerase reverse transcriptase in MCF-7 breast cancer cell line, *Cancer Lett.*, 184:1–6, 2002.

Cucurbita andreana In Latin America, the flowers, leaves, and vine tips of cucurbita spp. are widely consumed, because they exhibit a wide range of biological activities in plants and animals. Early work identified a group of terpenoid compounds or cucurbitacins present (Metcalf et al., 1982; Miro, 1995). These are highly oxygenated, tetracyclic triterpenes containing a cucirbitane skeleton characterized by a 19-(10→9β)abeo-10α-lanost-5-ene. Some of these cucurbitacins were shown to exhibit anti-inflammatory effects linked possibly to inhibition of cyclooxygenase (COX) enzymes.

A recent study by Jayaprakasam et al. (2003) showed these cucurbitacins (B, D, E, and I) exhibited potent anticancer activity, as well as

Curcurbitacins. (From Jayaprakasam et al., *Cancer Lett.,* 189:11–16, 2003. With permission.)

inhibited COX-2 enzyme. Further research is needed to determine the toxicity of these compounds.

References

Jayaprakasam, B., Seeram, N.P., and Nair, M.G., Anticancer and anti-inflammatory activities of cucurbitacins from *Cucurbita andreana, Cancer Lett.,* 189:11–16, 2003.

Metcalf, R.L., Rhodes, A.M., and Metcalf, R.A., Cucurbitacin cntent and diabroticites (*Coleoptera; Chrysomelidae*) feeding upon cucurbita spp., *Environ. Entomol.,* 11:931–937. 1982.

Miro, M., Cucurbitacins and their pharmacological effects, *Phytother. Res.,* 9:159–168, 1995.

Curdlan Curdlan, a β1,3-glucan synthesized by *Alcaligenes faecalis* var. *myxogenes,* was reported to have a number of health benefits (Jezequel, 1998). Shimizu et al. (1999) found rats fed a curdlan diet produced lower cecal pH accompanied by the release of large amounts of short-chain fatty acids (SCFA) and a lower ratio of fecal secondary bile acids. The anticancer properties of curdlan were further demonstrated by Shimizu and coworkers (2002), who showed a diet containing 5 percent curdlan significantly reduced dimethylhydrazine (DMH)-induced aberrant crypt foci development in Sprague–Dawley rats. Curdlan proved more effective than either cellulose or gellan gum in reducing the number of aberrant crypt foci (Figure C.29).

A search for antihuman immunodeficiency virus (HIV) agents to treat AIDS that did not have serious side effects led to the identification of a polysulphonated polysaccharide, curdlan sulfate (Molla et al., 1996). *In vitro* studies showed the anti-HIV activity in sulfated curdlan was due to its effects on viral replication by preventing binding to HIV virions to CD4+ lymphocyte cells and synctium formation (Baha et al., 1988). Further research showed a synthetic

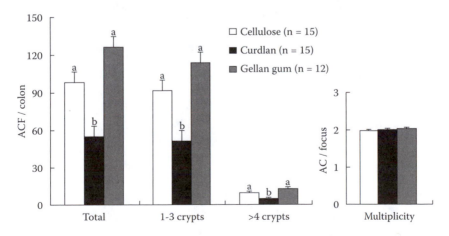

Curdlan. (From Jezequel, *Cereal Foods World*, 43:361–364, 1998. With permission.)

FIGURE C.29 Numbers of DMH-induced aberrant crypt foci (ACF) of rats fed experimental diets. Bars are means ±SEM. Each bar with different letters indicates differences from Tukey's test ($p < 0.05$). (From Shimizu et al., *Nutr. Res.,* 22:867–877, 2002. With permission.)

curdlan sulfate exhibited high anti-HIV activity and low toxicity. A series of phase I/II clinical tests conducted on curdlan sulfate in the U.S.A. between 1992 and 1996, however, found no significant improvements in patients given intravenous doses of 100 to 300 mg over the short term (Gordon et al., 1997). Jeon and coworkers (2000) analyzed NMR signals for polymeric interactions between curdlan sulfate and an HIV protein but obtained precipitates rather than gels, which did not yield any structural information. Further work is needed to establish the efficacy of curdlan sulfate, based on its anti-HIV properties, as a long-term therapy for AIDS.

A recent double-blind, placebo-controlled study on patients suffering from severe and severe/cerebral malaria by Havlik et al. (2005) examined the efficacy and safety of using curdlan sulfate as an adjunct medication with conventional therapy, artesunate. Curdlan sulfate was found to reduce the severity of cerebral malaria by shortening the fever-clearance period. No additional complications were observed with curdlan sulfate, such as renal failure or pulmonary oedema, as it appeared to be well-tolerated. However, the small number of patients in this study suggests further clinical trials with a larger number of patients is warranted.

References

Baba, M., Snoeck, R., Pauwels, R., and Declerq, S., Sulfated polysaccharides are potent and selective inhibitors of various enveloped virus, including herpes simplex virus, cytomegalvirus, vesicular stamatis virus and human immunodeficiency virus. *Antimicrob, Agents Chemother.,* 32:1742–1745, 1988.

Gordon, M., Guralnik, M., Kaneko, Y., Minura, T., Baker, M., and Lang, W., A phase 1 study of curdlan sulfate — an HIV inhibitor. Tolerance, pharmaco-kinetics and effects on coagulation and on CD4 lymphocytes. *J. Med.,* 25 (1–4): 163–180, 1994.

Gordon, M., Deeks, S., De Marzo, C., Goodgame, J., Guralink, M., Lang, W., Mimura, T., Pearce, D., and Kaneko, Y., Curdlan sulfate (CRDS) in a 21-day intravenous tolerance study in human immunodeficiency virus (HIV) and cytomealovirus (CMV) infected patients: Indication of anti-CMV activity with low toxicity, *J. Med.,* 28:108–128, 1994, 1997.

Havlik, I., Looareesuwan, S., Vannaphan, S., Wilairatana, P., Krudsood, S., Thuma, P.E., Kozbor, D., Watanabe, N., and Kaneko, Y., Curdlan sulfate in human severe/cerebral *Plasmodium falciparum* malaria, *Trans. Roy. Soc. Trop. Med. Hyg.,* 2005 (in press).

Jeon, K.-J., Katsuraya, K., Inazu, T., Kaneko, Y., Mimura, T., and Uryu, T., NMR spectroscopic detection of interactions between a HIV protein sequence and a highly anti-HIV active curdlan sulfate, *J. Am. Chem. Soc.,* 122:12536–12541, 2000.

Jezequel, V., Curdlan: A new functional β-glucan, *Cereal Foods World*, 43:361–364, 1998.

Molla, A., Korneyeva, M., Gao, O., Vasavonda, S., Schipper, P.J., Markowitz, M., Chernyavsky, T., Niu, P., Lyons, N., Hsu, A., Grannerman, G.R., Ho, D.D., Boucher, C.A.B., Leonard, J.M., Norbeck, D.W., and Kemf, D.J., Ordered accumulation of mutations in HIV proteases confers resistance to ritonavir. *Nature Med.,* 2:760–762, 1996.

Shimizu, J., Kudoh, K., Wada, M., Takita, T., Innami, S., Maekawa, A., and Tadokoro, T., Dietary curdlan suppresses dimethylhydrazine-induced aberrant crypt foci formation in Sprague–Dawley rat, *Nutr. Res.,* 22:867–877, 2002.

Shimizu, J., Wada, M., Takita, T., and Innami, S., Curdlan and gellan gum, bacterial gel-forming polysaccharides exhibit different effect on lipid metabolism, cecal formation and fecal bile excretion in man, *J. Nutr. Sci. Vitaminol.,* 45:251–262, 1999.

D

Daidzein Daidzein, one of the major isoflavone aglycones in soybean, is usually present in the form of its β-glucoside, daizin. While isoflavones are bitter and astringent, they all exhibit antihemolytic, antioxidative, antifungal, estrogenic, and antitumoral properties (Naim et al., 1976; Farmakaladis et al., 1985; Miyazawa et al., 1999). It is the antioxidant properties of isoflavones that are generally attributed for their anticancer properties (Ruiz-Larrea et al., 1997; Stoll, 1997). The free-radical-quenching properties of daidzen prevented the formation of oxidized DNA, 8-hydroxy-2'-deoxy-guanosine, in cells and DNA exposed to oxidants or in men

Diadzein. (From Peng et al., *Food Chem.*, 87:135–139, 2004. With permission.)

consuming 1 liter of soy milk daily over a four-week period (Giles and Zwei, 1997; Mitchell and Collins, 1999). Djuric et al. (2001) conducted a pilot study in which a combination of daidzein and genistein, in the form of a tablet, reduced endogenous oxidative DNA damage, as measured as 5-hydroxymethyl-2'-deoxyuridine (5OhmdU), in the blood cells of men and women kept on a twice-daily regimen of 50 mg isoflavone tablets for three weeks. After one week of supplementation, there was a 61 percent decrease in 5OhmdU in the blood cells of women, while it took three weeks before there was a corresponding decrease of 47 percent in men. This reduction in oxidative damage was considered a possible mechanism for its anticancer properties. Guo and coworkers (2004) showed daidzein had a biphasic effect on the cell growth of a human colon-cancer cell line LoVo. At low concentrations (< 1 µM) daidzein stimulated growth, while at high concentrations (> 10 µM) cell growth was inhibited in a dose-dependent manner. Inhibition of cell growth was characterized by cell-cycle arrest at G0/G1, DNA fragmentation, and enhanced caspase-3 activity.

Daidzein belongs to the family of diphenolic compounds with structural similarities to natural and synthetic estrogens and antiestrogens (Kurzer, 1999). It binds to estrogen receptors, although somewhat weakly compared to estradiol. The estrogenic properties of phytoestrogens, such as daidzein, are thought to prevent bone resorption and increase bone density. This is particularly important, as osteoporosis is generally linked to decrease in steroid production associated with menopause in women. Osteoblasts, the most important cells in bone tissues, are critical to bone formation and bone density. Daidzein was shown to stimulate protein synthesis, alkaline-phosphatase activity, and DNA content in an osteoblast MC3T3-E1 cell (Sugimoto and Yamaguchi, 2000), as well as significantly increase alkaline-phosphatase activity, DNA, and calcium content in bone tissues (Gaio and Yamaguchi, 1999). Jia et al. (2003) showed that daidzein stimulated osteoblast growth in newborn Wistar rats at various stages (from osteoprogenitors to terminally differentiated osteoblasts). For example, the production of osteocalcin, a specific marker protein for the terminal differentiation of osteoblasts, was significantly increased in the presence of daidzein in a concentration-dependent manner (Figure D.30). In addition, daidzein regulated bone-morphogenetic protein (BMP) by significantly increasing BMP2RNA and protein synthesis in osteoblastic cells cultured *in vitro*.

References

Djuric, Z., Chen, G., Doerge, D.R., Heilbrun, L.K., and Kucuk, O., Effect of soy isoflavone supplemen-

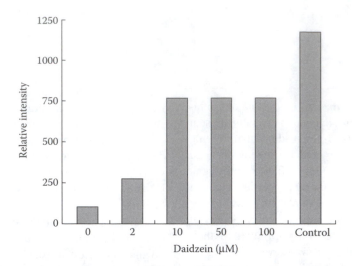

FIGURE D.30 Effect of daidzein on osteocalcin synthesis in osteoblastic cells incubated for two days. Each value is the mean ± of six dishes. (*) $p < 0.05$, compared to the control without daidzein. (Adapted from Jia et al., *Biochem. Pharmacol.*, 65:709–715, 2003. With permission.)

tation on markers of oxidative stress in men and women, *Cancer Lett.*, 172:1–6, 2001.

Farmakaladis, Hathock, J.N., and Murphy, P., Estrogenic potency of genistin and daidzin in mice, *J. Agric. Food Chem.*, 33:385–389, 1985.

Gaio, Y.H. and Yamaguchi, M., Anabolic effect of daidzein on cortical bone in tissue culture: Comparison with genistein effect., *Mol. Cell Biochem.*, 19: 93–97, 1999.

Giles, D. and Wei, H., Effect of structurally related flavones/isoflavones on hydrogen peroxide production and oxidative DNA damage in phorbol ester-stimulated HL-60 cells, *Nutr. Cancer.*, 29:77–82, 1997.

Guo, J.M., Xiao, B.X., Liu, D., Grant, M., Zhang, S., Lai, Y.F., Guo, Y.B., and Liu, Q., Biphasic effect of daidzein on cell growth of human colon cancer cells, *Food Chem. Toxicol.*, 42:1641–1646, 2004.

Jia, T.-L., Wang, H.-Z., Xie, L.-P., Wang, X.-Y., and Zhang, R.-Q., Daidzein enhances osteoblast growth that may be mediated by increased bone morphogenetic protein (BMP) production, *Biochem. Pharmacol.*, 65:709–715, 2003.

Kurzer, M.S. and Xu, X., Dietary phytoestrogens, *Ann. Rev. Nutr.*, 17:353–381, 1999.

Mitchell, J.H. and Collins, A.R., Effects of soy milk supplement on plasma cholesterol levels and oxidative DNA damage in men — a pilot study, *Eur. J. Nutr.*, 38:143–148, 1999.

Miyazawa, M., Sakano, K., Nakamura, S., and Kosaka, H., Antimutagenicity activity of isoflavones from soybean seeds (*Glycine max* Merril), *J. Agric. Food Chem.*, 47:1346–1349, 1999.

Naim, M., Gestetner, B., Birk, Y., and Bondi, A., Antioxidative and antihemolytic activity of soybean isoflavones. *J. Agric. Food Chem.*, 22: 806–810, 1976.

Peng, Y., Chu, Q., Liu, F., and Ye, J., Determination of isoflavones in soy products by capillary electrophoresis with electrochemical detection, *Food Chem.*, 87:135–139, 2004.

Ruiz-Larrea, M.B., Mohan, A.R., Paganga, G., Miller, N.J., Bolwell, G.P., and Rice-Evans, C.A., Antioxidant activity of phytoestrogenic isoflavone, *Free Rad. Res.*, 26:63–70, 1997.

Stoll, B.A., Eating to prevent breast cancer: Potential role for soy supplements, *Ann. Oncol.*, 8:223–225, 1997.

Sugimoto, E. and Yamaguchi, M., Stimulatory effect of daidzein in osteoblastic MC3T3-E1 cells, *Biochem. Pharmacol.*, 59:471–475, 2000.

Dairy products Epidemiological studies identified a close relationship between the intake of dairy products and blood pressure. This is related to such minerals as calcium and potassium, which are inversely linked to blood pressure and the incidence of hypertension (McCarron, 1989).

Since dairy products provide 70–75 percent of total dietary calcium intake, these studies identified higher arterial pressure or hypertension in populations or individuals with low dairy and low calcium, magnesium, and phosphorus intakes. A multicenter, randomized clinical trial by the National Heart, Lung, and Blood Institute of the United States entitled "Dietary Approaches to Stop Hypertension" (DASH) compared a typical American diet low in fruits, vegetables, and dairy products with the DASH diet, a low-fat dairy products and a high fruit-and-vegetable diet (Appel et al., 1997). This was a fairly definitive study, which showed those individuals with high blood pressure or hypertension clearly benefited from the DASH diet. Overall, at least three servings of low-fat dairy products were recommended per day by the Institute of Medicine for adults below 50 years of age taking 1000 mg calcium per day, while those over 50 needed four servings of low-fat dairy products and 1200 mg of calcium per day (Standing Committee on the Scientific Evaluation of Dietary References, 1997). A summary of the biomedical literature by Miller et al. (2000) covers the benefits of dairy products, particularly in relation to blood pressure. A recent paper by McCarron and Heany (2004) estimated that if Americans simply increased their intake of dairy foods to the current recommendation of three to four servings per day, the reduction in disease burden could result in a substantial medical savings of more than $200 billion over a five-year period.

References

Appel, L.J., Moore, T.J., Obarzaneck, E., Vollmer, V.M., Svetkey, L.P., Sacks, F.M., Bray, G.A., Vost, T.M., Cutler, J.A., Windhauser, M.M., Lin, P.H., and Karanja, N., A clinical trial of the effects of dietary patterns on blood pressure, *N. Eng. J. Med.,* 336: 1117–1124, 1997.

McCarron, D.A., Calcium metabolism and hypertension, *Kidney Int.,* 35:717–736, 1989.

McCarron, D.A. and Heany, R.P., Estimated health-care savings with adequate dairy intake, *Am. J. Hyperten.,* 17:88–97, 2004.

Miller, G.D., DiRienzo, D.D., Reusser, M.E., and McCarron, D.A., Benefits of dairy product consumption on blood pressure in humans: A summary of the biomedical literature, *J. Am. Coll. Nutr.,* 19:147S–164S, 2000.

Standing Committee on the Scientific Evaluation of Dietary References Intakes, Dietary Reference Intakes for Calcium, Phosphorus, Magnesium, Vitamin D and Fluoride, *Natl. Academy Press,* Washington, DC.

D

Dandelion   The dandelion (*Taraxacum officinale),* considered by most homeowners to be a nuisance plant, is a common plant grown commercially in Europe and the United States. Its choleretic, antirhematic, and diuretic properties have made dandelions an herbal medicine (Bradley, 1992; Bissett, 1994). The bitter substances identified in dandelion thought to be responsible for its therapeutic properties were sequiterpene lactones, taxacoside triterpenes, phytosterols, phenolic acids, flavonoids, vitamins, and minerals (Racz-Kotilla et al., 1974; Kuusi et al., 1985; Wichtl, 1994; Williams et al., 1996). Mascolo et al. (1974) reported leaf-dandelion extracts exhibited anti-inflammatory properties in experimental animals. Subsequent research by Cristinf and coworkers (1996) showed that aqueous dandelion extracts containing cinnamic acids and coumarins had anti-tumor activity. Cho et al. (2002) examined any possible diuretic effects exerted by aqueous extracts of dandelion leaves in streptozotocin-induced diabetic male Sprague–Dawley rats. Since diabetes-related complications are associated with oxidative stress, these researchers examined the effect of the dandelion-leaf extracts on hepatic antioxidant enzyme activities and lipid profiles in the experimental animals. The most notable differences were observed in serum and hepatic lipids, as shown in Table D.23.

Supplementation with dandelion extract (DWE) lowered total cholesterol and triglycerides, while raising HDL-cholesterol in the diabetic rats. In addition, treatment with DWE significantly lowered the atherogenic index. These results suggested that DWE treatment could be useful as antioxidant therapy to correct hyperglycemia and protect against free radicals. Further work is needed to identify the specific components responsible.

D

TABLE D.23
Effect of Dandelion Water-Extract Supplementation on Serum and Hepatic Lipids in Diabetic Rats[1]

	Nondiabetic	Diabetic	Diabetic-DWE
Serum			
Total Cholesterol (mmol/L)	2.41 ± 0.07^a	3.10 ± 0.15^b	2.44 ± 0.31^a
HDL Cholesterol (mmol/L)	0.81 ± 0.06^a	0.33 ± 0.04^c	0.67 ± 0.07^b
Triglyceride (mmol/L)	1.57 ± 0.12	2.85 ± 0.42^b	1.63 ± 0.08^a
Atherogenic index[2]	1.95 ± 0.28^a	8.44 ± 0.94^c	2.68 ± 0.50^b
Liver			
Cholesterol (mmol/g)	0.16 ± 0.01^a	0.28 ± 0.06^b	0.20 ± 0.03^a
Triglyceride	0.12 ± 0.02^a	0.23 ± 0.02^b	0.14 ± 0.02^a

[1,a,b,c] Means in the same row not sharing a common superscript are significantly different between groups ($p < 0.05$).

[2] Atherogenic index: total cholesterol–HDL cholesterol/HDL cholesterol.

Source: From Cho et al., *Clin. Chim. Acta,* 317:109–117, 2002. With permission.

Hu and Kitts (2003) demonstrated, for the first time, the antioxidant and cytotoxic properties of dandelion-flower fractions. The two fractions, a water extract (WF) and an ethyl acetate (EAF) extract, both had significant ($p < 0.05$) free-radical-scavenging activity for DPPH radical. EAF was a stronger scavenger than WF, although both had considerably less activity than TROLOX. Both fractions significantly ($p < 0.05$) reduced the viability of a human colon colorectal adenocarcinoma cell line (Caco-2), with WF exhibiting greater toxicity. The most abundant bioactive compound identified in both fractions was the flavone luteolin-7-glucoside. It was considered to be the primary antioxidant present in dandelion flowers responsible for the protective effects observed. In order to establish dandelions as a potential source of natural antioxidants and bioactives, further research using *in vivo* models is required.

Trojanova et al. (2004) showed an infusion prepared from dandelion root with boiling water enhanced the growth of bifidobacteria species isolated from fermented milk products and infant feces. They attributed this prebiotic effect to the high quantity of nondigestible oligofructans present in dandelion roots.

References

Bradley, P.R., *British Herbal Compenstium*, Vol. 1, British Herbal Medicine Association, Bournemouth, 1992, p. 73.

Bissett, N.G., *Herbal Drugs and Phytopharmaceuticals*, Medpharm, Stuttgart, 1994, p. 486.

Cho, S.-Y., Park, J.-K., Park, E.-M., Choi, M.-S., Lee, M.-K., Jeon, S.-M., Jang, M.K., Kim, M.-J., and Park, Y.B., Alternation of hepatic antioxidant enzyme activities and lipid profile in streptozotocin-induced diabetic rats by supplementation of dandelion water extract, *Clin. Chim. Acta,* 317:109–117, 2002.

Cristinf, A.W., Finoma, G., and Jenny, G., Flavonoids: Cinnamic acids and coumarins from the different tissues and medicinal preparations of *Taraxacum officinale, Phytochemistry,* 42:121–127, 1996.

Hu, C. and Kitts, D.D., Antioxidant, prooxidant, and cytotoxic activities of solvent-fractionated dandelion (*Taraxacum officinale*) flower extracts *in vitro, J. Agric. Food Chem.,* 51:301–310, 2003.

Kuusi, T., Pyysalo, H., and Autio, K., The bitterness properties of the dandelion II. Chemical investigations. *Lebensm-Wiss. Technol.* 18:347–349, 1985.

Mascolo, N., Autore, G., Capasso, F., Menghini, A., and Fasulo, M.P., Biological screening of Italian medicinal plants for anti-inflammatory activity, *Phytother. Res.,* 1:28–31, 1974.

Racz-Kotilla, E., Racz, G., and Solomon, A., The action of *Taraxacum officinale* extracts on body weight and diuresis of laboratory animals, *Planta Med.,* 26:212–217, 1974.

Trojanova, I., Rada, V., Kokoska, L., and Vlkova, E., The bifidogenic effect of Taraxacum officinale root, *Fitoterapia,* 75:760–763, 2004.

Wichtl, M., in *Herbal Drugs and Phytopharmaceuticals,* CRC Press, Boca Raton, Florida, 1994, pp. 486–489.

Williams, C.A., Goldstone, F., and Greenham, J., Flavonoids, cinnamic acids and coumarins from different tissues and medicinal preparations of *Taxacum officinale, Phytochemistry,* 42:121–, 1996.

Delphinidin   Delphinidinin is an aglycone (-glycosides) of one of the most abundant anthocyanins found in plant food sources. In addition to eliciting an endothelium-dependent relaxant

Delphinidin. (From Favot et al., *Cardiovasc. Res.,* 59:478–487, 2003. With permission.)

effect, it has been shown to inhibit the growth of human tumor-cell lines (Andriambeloson et al., 1998; Martin et al., 2002). Martin and coworkers (2003) showed delphinidin inhibited serum and vascular endothelium growth factor (VEGF), which normally induces proliferation of bovine aortic epithelial cells. The antiproliferation mechanism appeared to involve activation of ERK-1/2 pathway with overexpression of nitric-oxide synthase, shown previously to protect bovine aortic epithelial cells from apoptosis (Martin et al., 2001). This property of delphinidin should be important in atherosclerosis, as proliferation is crucial for the development and stability of atherosclerotic plaque. Using chicken embryos and human umbilical-vein endothelial cells (HUVECs), Favot et al. (2003) showed inhibition of angiogenesis by delphinidin affected two major steps, endothelial-cell migration and proliferation. At a minimal concentration of 10 µg/mL, delphinidin inhibited basal, as well as VEGF stimulation, of proliferation of HUVECs by 22 ± 3.9 percent and 21 ± 5.4 percent, respectively (Figure D.31). Inhibition of proliferation by delphinidin was correlated with blocking the cell cycle G_0/G_1 phase by reversing the VEGF-induced decrease of cyclin-dependent kinase inhibitor p27[kip1] and VEGF-induced increase of cyclin D1 and cyclin A. Since a major step in angiogenesis is proliferation, which facilitates tumor growth, delphinidin should be a useful cancer chemopreventive agent.

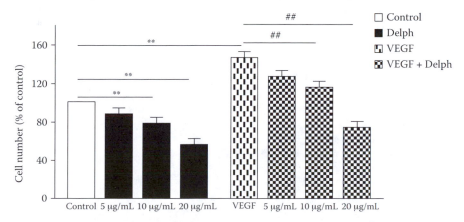

FIGURE D.31 Effect of delphinidin on basal- and VEGF-stimulated proliferation of HUVECs incubated for 72 h with or without 5, 10, and 20 µg/mL delphinidin without or with 10 ng/mL VEGF. Data represent four experiments. ** $p < 0.01$ versus control cells, ## $p < 0.01$ versus VEGF-treated cells. (From Favot et al., *Cardiovasc. Res.,* 59:478–487, 2003. With permission.)

D

References

Andriambeloson, E., Magnier, C., Haan-Archipoff, G., Lobstein, A., Anton, R., Beretz, A., and Stoclet, J.C., Natural dietary polyphenolic compounds cause endothelium-dependent vasorelaxation in rat thoracic aorta, *J. Nutr.,* 128:2324–2333, 1998.

Favot, L., Martin, S., Keravios, T., Adriantsitohaina, R., and Lugnier, C., Involvement of cyclin-dependent pathway in the inhibitory effect of delphinidin on angiogenesis, *Cardiovasc. Res.,* 59:478–487, 2003.

Martin, S., Favot, L., Matz, R., Lugnier, C., and Adriantsitohaina, R., Red wine polyphenols increase calcium in bovine aortic endothelial cells: A basis to elucidate signaling pathways leading to nitric oxide production, *Br. J. Pharmacol.,* 135:1579–1587, 2002.

Martin, S., Adrianbelosom, E., Takeda, K,. and Adriantsitohaina, R., Anti-apoptotic effect of an anthocyanin, delphinidin, is mediated on a cyclic-GMP increase and NO dependent pathway, *Thromb. Haemost.,* 86:446, 2001.

Martin, S., Favot, L., Matz, R., Lugnier, C., and Adriantsitohaina, R., Delphinidin inhibits endothelial cell proliferation and cell cycle progression through a transient activation of ERK-1/2, *Biochem. Pharmacol.,* 65:669–675, 2003.

Desert plant (*Retama raetum*)   Maghrani and coworkers (2003) show an aqueous extract from the desert plant, *Retama raetam*, significantly reduced the blood glucose in normal rats 6 hours after a single dose and two weeks after a second dose was administered. This hypoglycemic effect was found to be more pronounced in streptozotocin-induced diabetic rats. No effect was observed on plasma insulin levels, suggesting the mechanism was extra-pancreatic.

References

Magrhani, M., Lemhadri, A., Jouad, H., Michel, J.-M., and Eddouks, M., Effect of the desert plant *Retama raetam* on glycaemia in normal and streptozotocin-induced diabetic rats, *J. Ethnopharmacol.,* 87:21–25, 2003.

Devil's claw   Devil's claw (*Harpagophytum procumbens*), a tuber with large, hooked, claw-like fruit, is used medicinally in Africa and Germany. Chrubasik et al. (1996) found it was effective for treating acute low-back pain. Subsequent reports demonstrated the ability of Devil's claw to improve theumatic disorders (ESCOP, 1996; Wegener, 1998). Laudahn and Walper (2001) evaluated the clinical effectiveness and tolerance of an extract from Devil's claw in 117 patients suffering from nonradicular back pain over a six-month period. A film-coated tablet containing 480 mg *Harpagophytum* extract LI 174 was taken twice a day over the eight-week treatment period. A significant reduction in both the Arhus back-pain index and the multidimensional pain scale was recorded during over the treatment period. A significant increase in the mobility of the spinal column was observed, as measured by a significant reduction (p, 0.001) in the average finger–floor distance. This dropped from the initial 15.1 cm to 10.2 cm at the conclusion of the treatment and indicates a reduction in pain (Figure D.32).

This study reported that an alleviation of pain was experienced by 73.5 percent of all patients in this study to moderate to very good. The *Harpagophytum* extract was slow acting and could provide alternate treatment for those patients with known sensitivity to NSAIDs. The

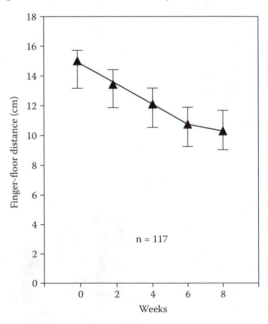

FIGURE D.32 Change in the average finger–floor distance (95 percent confidence interval, p, 0.01). (From Laudahn and Walper, *Phytother. Res.,* 15:621–624, 2001.)

mode of action appears to be anti-inflammatory and analgesic and may reflect the iroid glycosides present in the extract, particularly the main one, harpagoside. These studies suggest that Devil's claw may have considerable potential for the treatment of chronic back pain.

Harpagoside. (From Gunther and Schmidt, *J. Pharm. Biomed. Anal.,* 37:817–821, 2005. With permission.)

The anti-inflammatory properties of Devil's claw root extracts were demonstrated for the first time by Kaszkin and coworkers (2004) who showed two extracts high in harpagoside (8.9 percent and 27 percent) both attenuated IL-1β-stimulated nitric-oxide (NO) formation in rat mesangial cells by inhibition of iNOSmRNA expression due to inhibition of NF-κB activation. This inhibitory effect was not observed in extracts low in harpagoside so that its presence at high levels is required for the anti-inflammatory properties of Devil's claw. However, other unidentified constituents, in addition to harpagoside, also appeared to be involved.

References

Chrubasik, S., Zimper, C.H., Schutt, U., and Ziegler, R., Effectiveness of *Harpagophytum procumbens* in treatment of acute low back pain, *Phytomedicine,* 31–10, 1996.

ESCOP, Monograph *Harpagophytum radix,* in *ESCOP Monographs of the Medicinal Uses of Plant Drugs,* Biol. 2, Centre of Complementary Health Services, University of Exeter, Exeter, 1996, pp. 1–7.

Gobel, H., Heinze, A., Niederberger, U., and Gerber, D., Effekte von *Harpagophytum*-Extrakt LI 174 auf die sensoricsche, motorische und vaskularer Muskeilreagibiltat bei der Behandlung muskularer Ruckenshmerzen, 15:10–18, 2001.

Gunther, M. and Schmidt, P.C., Comparison between HPLC and HPTLC-densitometry for the determination of harpagoside from *Harpagophytum procumbens* CO$_2$-extracts, *J. Pharm. Biomed. Anal.,* 37:817–821, 2005.

Kaszkin, M., Beck, K.F., Koch, E., Erdelmeir, C., Kusch, S., Pfeilschifter, J., and Loew, D., Downregulation of iNOS expression in rat mesangial cells by special extracts of *Harpagophytum procumbens* derives from harpagoside-dependent and independent effects, *Phytomedicine,* 11:585–595, 2004.

Laudahn, D. and Walper, A., Efficacy and tolerance of *Harpagophytum* extract LI 174 in patients with chronic non-radicular back pain, *Phytother. Res.,* 15: 621–624, 2001.

Wegener, T., Die Teufelskralle (*Harpagophytum procumbens* DC.), In der Therapie rheumatischer Erkankungen, *Der Schmerz.,* 19:284–294, 1998.

Diacylglycerol (DAG)   The introduction of diacylglycerol (DAG) oil, an edible oil enriched in DAG (80 percent), has unique health benefits. Studies focused on the nutritional properties of 1,3- and 1,2 (or 2,3)-DAG, which account for around 10 percent of various dietary oils. Particular interest in DAG was related to its ability to significantly lower serum triacylglycerols in rats fed a diet composed mainly of 1,3-DAG compared to triacylglycerols (TAG). In addition, Nagao et al. (2000) associated dietary DAG with a decrease in body weight and visceral-fat mass. Murase and coworkers (2001) examined the effect of DAG on obesity, hyperinsulinemia, and hyperleptinemia in obese and diabetes-prone C57/6J mice. They found DAG suppressed body fat compared to TAG, even though they had similar fatty acids. The reduction in body fat, a recognized risk for diabetes and coronary heart disease, suggested a possible role for DAG in the management of obesity. Further work by Murase et al. (2002) on the long-term effects of dietary DAG on obesity in C57BL/6J rats showed marked changes in β-oxidation and related gene expression in the

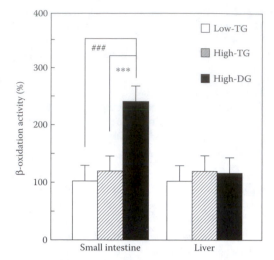

FIGURE D.33 β-Oxidation activity in the small intestine and livers of rats fed respective (TG, triacylglycerol; DG, diacylglycerol) diets for 10 days, as measured by palmitic-acid oxidation activities. Values expressed as means ± SD. *** $p < 0.001$ (From Murase et al., *J. Lipid Res.*, 43:1312–1319, 2002. With permission.)

small intestine (Figure D.33). Since the energy value per weight and digestibility for DAG and TAG were similar, the reduced body-fat accumulation effect by DAG had to involve another mechanism. DAG was shown to up-regulate mRNA levels in fatty-acid transport (fatty-acid transporter and liver fatty-acid-binding protein), β-oxidation (acetyl CoA oxidase and medium-chain acetyl CoA dehydrogenase), and thermogenesis (uncoupling protein) in the intestine. The potent stimulation of intestinal lipid metabolism by 1,3-DAG on overweight and obese men and women was shown by Maki et al. (2002) to reduce mean body weight by 3.6 percent compared to 2.5 percent for the TAG group. The weight loss and body-fat reduction promoted by the diet containing the DAG oil could be a useful addition to diet therapy for obesity. Kamphuis et al. (2003) showed the benefits associated with replacing modest amounts of TAG with DAG were decreased respiratory quotients and higher fat oxidation. In addition, several measures of appetite were significantly lower with DAG treatment, confirming its potential in diet therapy for obesity. Kasamatsu et al. (2005) recently reported that a diet incorporating

DAG oil was safe with no evidence of any genotoxic effects.

References

Kamphius, M.M.J.W., Mela, D.J., and Westerterp-Plantenga, M.S., Diacylglycerols affect substrate oxidation and appetite in humans, *Am. Clin. Nutr.*, 77:1133–1139, 2003.

Kasamatsu, T., Ogua, R., Ikeda, N., Morita, O., Saigo, K., Watabe, H., Saito, Y., and Suzuki, H., Genotoxicity studies on dietary diacylglycerol (DAG) oil, *Food. Chem. Toxicol.*, 43:253–260, 2005.

Maki, K.C., Davidson, M.H., Tsushima, R., Matsuo, N., Tokimitsu, I., Umporowicz, D.M., Dicklin, M.R., Foster, G.S., Ingram, K.A., Anderson, B.D., Frost, S.D., and Bell, M., Consumption of diacylglycerol oil as part of a reduced-energy diet enhances loss of body weight and fat in comparison with consumption of a triaylglycerol control oil, *Am. J. Clin. Nutr.*, 76:1230–1236, 2002.

Murase, T., Aoki, M., Wakisaka, T., Hase, T., and Toimitsu, I., Anti-obesity effect of diacylglycerol in C57BL/6J mice: Dietary diacylglycerol stimulates lipid metabolism, *J. Lipid Res.*, 43:1312–1319, 2002.

Murase, T., Mizuno, T., Omachi, T., Onizawa, K., Komine, Y., Kondo, H., Hase, T., and Tokimitsu, I., Dietary diacylglycerol suppresses high fat and high sucrose diet-induced body fat accumulation in C57BL/6J mice, *J. Lipid Res.*, 42:372–378, 2001.

Nagao, T., Watanabe, H., Goto, N., Onizawa, K., Taguchi, H., Matsuo, N., Yasukawa, T., Tsushima, R., Shimasaki, H, and Itakura, H., Dietary diacylglycerol suppresses accumulation of body fat compared to triacylglycerol in men in a double-blind controlled trial, *J. Nutr.*, 130:792–799, 2000.

Diallyl disulfide   Diallyl disulfide (DADS) is formed during the eating of garlic or as a major component of cooked garlic. It is an oil-soluble sulfur compound accounting for 60 percent of garlic oil, which inhibits the proliferation of human colon-, lung-, and skin-cancer cells in culture (Sundaram and Milner, 1996a).

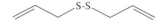

Diallyl disulfide. (Adapted from Tapiero et al., *Biomed. Pharmacother.*, 58:183–193, 2004.)

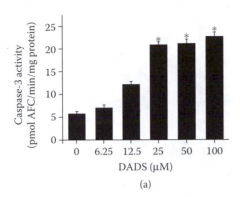
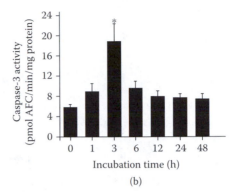

FIGURE D.34 DAD-induced apoptosis through activation of caspase-3 by treating HL-60 cells (5×10^6) with either (a) a range of concentrations (0–100 µM) of DAD for 3 h, or (b) 25 µM DAD for a period of 1, 3, 16, 24, and 48 h. Values represent means ± SEMS of six separate experiments. Key: (*) $p < 0.05$ when compared with control bu one-way ANOVA using Turkey's multicomparison procedures. (From Kwon et al., *Biochem. Pharmacol.*, 63:41–47, 2002. With permission.)

Sundaram and Milner (1996b) proposed that DADS induced apoptosis of human colon-tumor cells by enhancing the intracellular calcium concentration. Apoptosis, programmed cell death, can be initiated by oxidative stress through the production of reactive-oxygen species (ROS). These oxygen species then activate a family of cysteine proteases, caspases, involved in cell-death induction. Using human leukemia HL-60 cells, Kwon and coworkers (2002) examined the mechanism used by DADS to induce apoptosis. They provided evidence that incubating HL-60 cells with increasing levels of DADS stimulated the production of reactive-oxygen intermediates, with the subsequent activation of caspase-3 leading to the onset of apoptosis (Figure D.34).

DADS was also found to exert a chemoprotective effect against benzo[a]pyrene (BP)-induced forestomach carcinogenesis in mice, which correlated with the induction of the expression of Pi class glutathione (GSH) transferase *m*GSTP1-1. Further work by Bose and coworkers (2002) showed the ally group in DADS was critical for its induction of *m*GSTP1, although the oligosulfide chain was equally important.

Oncongenes are very important in the transformation of normal cells into tumors. For example, oncongenes, such as H-*ras,* play a role in development and maintenance of solid tumors so that targeting and inhibiting these oncongenes could be an effective way of inhibiting tumors. Using implanted experimental brain C6 glioma cells, Perkins et al. (2003) showed that expression of H-*ras* was significantly ($p < 0.05$) reduced in the brain-tumor tissue of rats treated with DADS prior to implantation.

References

Bose, C., Guo, J., Zimniak, L., Srivastava, S.K., Singh, S.P., Zimniak, P., and Singh, S.V., Critical role of ally groups and disulfide chain in induction of Pi class glutathione transferase in mouse tissue *in vivo* by dially disulfide, a naturally occurring chemopreventative agent in garlic, *Carcinogenesis,* 23:1661–1665, 2002.

Kwon, K.-B., Yoo, S.-J., Ryu, D.-G., Yang, J.-Y., Rho, H.-W., Kim, J.-S., Park, J.-W., Kim, H.-R., and Park, B.-H., Induction of apoptosis by diallyl disulfide through activation of caspase-3 in human leukemia HL-60 cells, *Biochem. Pharmacol.*, 63:41–47, 2002.

Perkins, E., Calvert, J., Lancon, J.A., Parent, A.D., and Zhang, J., Inhibition of H-*ras* as a treatment for experimental brain C6 glioma, *Mol. Brain Res.,* 111: 42–51, 2003.

Sundaram, S.G. and Milner, J.A., Diallyl disulfide inhibits proliferation of human tumor cells in culture, *Biochem. Biophys. Acta,* 1315:15–20, 1996a.

Sundaram, S.G. and Milner, J.A., Diallyl disulfide induces apoptosis of human colon tumor cells, *Carcinogenesis,* 17:669–673, 1996b.

Tapiero, A., Townsend, D.M., and Tew, K.D., Organosulfur compounds from alliceae in the prevention of human pathologies, *Biomed. Pharmacother.,* 58: 183–193, 2004.

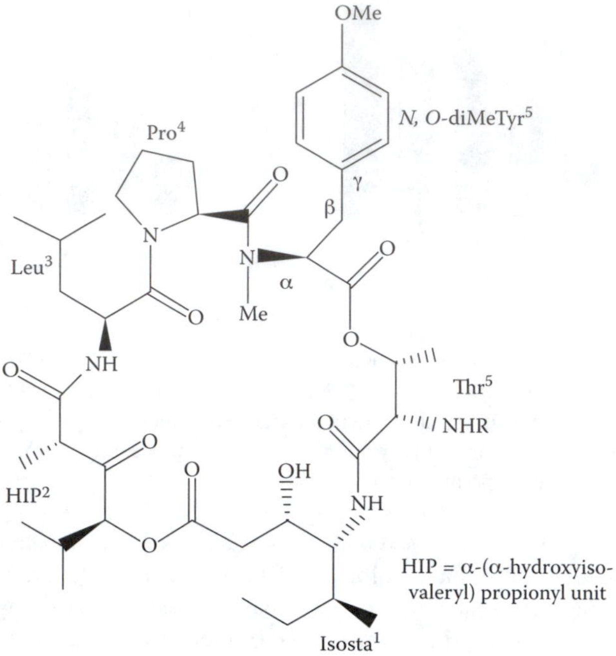

D

Didemnin B. (From Pfizenmayer et al., *Bioorg. Med. Chem. Lett.,* 8: 3653–3656, 1998. With permission.)

Didemnin B Didemnin B, a natural marine product, was first isolated from the Caribbean tunicate (sea squirt) (Reinhart et al., 1981). It is a cyclic depsipeptide that exhibits both antiviral and antitumor properties (Reinhart et al., 1981, 1983). Didemnin B was shown to induce apoptosis in human promycloid HL-60 cells at an optimum concentration of 1 µM (Grubb et al., 1995). Johnson and coworkers (1996) showed that didemnin B induced apoptosis via tyrosinase phosphorylation as it was inhibited by the addition of protein tyrosinase kinase inhibitors. Subsequent work by Beidler et al. (1999) showed induction of apoptosis in human breast-carcinoma cell MCF7 by didemnin involved activation of caspases. Apoptosis was only observed in the presence of 100 nM didemnin or higher, while inhibition of protein synthesis occurred at much lower levels with an IC_{50} of 12 nM. These researchers suggested the need for the development of didemnin B analogs that minimally affect protein synthesis while specifically targeting apoptosis of cancer cells.

Didemnin was shown to have promising preclinical antitumor activity at low concentrations (Crampton et al., 1984). A phase II study on didemnin B on advanced malignant melanoma by Hochster et al. (1999) showed some clinical activity, which needed further exploration. Other clinical trials on patients with recurrent or refractory anaplastic astrocytoma, Glioblastoma multiforme, or central nervous-system tumors, however, proved unsuccessful (Mettelman et al., 1999; Taylor et al., 1999). Aplidin®, a compound similar to didemnin B with oxidation of the hydroxylic group of the side chain to ketone, was shown to have a lower toxic effect and better therapeutic indexes than didemnin B. Successful phase I studies with Aplidin® has led to a phase II trial for studying its pharmacokinetics.

References

Beidler, D.R., Ahuja, D., Wicha, M.S., and Toogood, P.L., Inhibition of protein synthesis by didemnin B is not sufficient to induce apoptosis in human mammary carcinoma (MCF7) cells, *Biochem. Pharmacol.,* 58:1067–1074, 1999.

Crampton, S.L., Adams, E.G., Kuentzel, S.L., Li, L.H., Badiner, G., and Bhuyan, B.K., Biochemical and cellular effect of didemins A and B, *Cancer Res.*, 44:1796–1801, 1984.

Grubb, D.R., Wolvetang, E.J., and Lawen, A., Didemnin B induces cell death by apoptosis: The fastest induction of apoptosis ever described, *Biophys. Res. Commun.*, 215:1130–1136, 1995.

Hochster, H., Oratz, P., and Ettinger, D.S., A phase II study of didemnin B (NSC 325319) in advanced malignant melanoma: An Eastern Cooperative Oncology Group Study (PB3687), *Invest. New Drugs*, 16: 259–263, 1999.

Johnson, K.L., Vaillant, F., and Lawen, A., Protein tyrosinase kinase inhibitors prevent didemnin B-induced apoptosis in HL-60 cells, *FEBNS Lett.*, 383: 1–5, 1996.

Mittelman, A., Chun, H.G., Puccio, C., Coombe, N., Lansen, T., and Ahmed, T., Phase II clinical trial of didemnin B in patients with recurrent or refractory anaplastic astrocytoma or Glibioblastoma multiforme (NSC 325319), *Invest. New Drugs*, 17:179–182, 1969.

Pfizenmayer, A.J., Vera, M.D., Ding, X., Xiao, D., Chen, W.-C., Jouie, M., Tandon, D., and Toogood, P.L., Synthesis and biological activity of [Tic⁵] didemnin B, *Bioorg. Med. Chem. Lett.*, 8:3653–3656, 1998.S

Reinhardt, K.L., Jr., Gloer, J.B., Hughes, R.G., Jr., Renis, H.E., McGovern, R.P., Swynenberg, E.B., Stringfellow, D.A., Kuentzel, S.L., and Li, L.H., Didemnins: Antiviral and antitumor depsipeptides from a Caribbean tunicate, *Science*, 212:933–935, 1981.

Reinhart, K.L., Jr., Gloer, J.B., Wilson, G.R., Hughes, R.G., Jr., Li, L.H., Renis, H.E., and McGovern, J.P., Antiviral and antitumor compounds from tunicates, *Fedn/roc.*, 42:87–90, 1983.

Taylor, S.A., Giroux, D.J., Jaeckle, K.A., Panella, T.J., Dakhil, S.R., and Schold, S.C., Phase II study of didemnin B in central nervous system tumors: A southwest oncology group study, *Invest. New Drugs*, 16:331–332, 1999.

Williamson, S.K., Wolf, M.K., Esenberger, M.A., O'Rourke, M., Brannon, W., and Crawford, E.D., Phase II evaluation of didemnin B in hormonally refractory mestatic prostate cancer, *Invest. New Drugs*, 13:167–170, 1995.

3,3'-Diindoylmethane (DIM)

3,3'-Diindoylmethane (DIM) is produced by the autolytic breakdown of the glucosinolate, glucobrassicin. This glucosinolate is found in members of the *Brassica* genus, particularly broccoli, Brussels sprouts, cabbage, and kale. The enzyme involved,

D

13C (Indole-3-carbinol) and DIM (3,3″-Diindoylmethane). (From Hong et al., *Biochem. Pharmacol.*, 63:1085–1087, 2002. With permission.)

myrosinase, hydrolyzes glucobrassicin to indole-3-carbinol (13C) then condenses rapidly to form DIM. The 13C is a known inhibitor of breast cancer, with several *in vivo* and *in vitro* test studies showing it blocks the cell cycle (Sharma et al., 1994; Cover et al., 1998; Rahman et al., 2000). DIM also shows promise as an anticancer agent. Several studies found DIM inhibited DMBA-induced tumor growth in rodents by as much as 95 percent (Chen et al., 1998). Hong and coworkers (2002) examined the antiproliferative properties of DIM in human cancer cells. DIM was found to inhibit proliferation of estrogen-dependent and estrogen-independent human breast-cancer cells, inducing apoptosis by decreasing cellular Bcl-2 levels and increasing Bax levels and the Bax/Bcl-2 ratio. The Bcl-2-related family of proteins is involved in the final stage of apoptosis, or programmed cell death. This mechanism appeared identical to that reported previously for 13C, the precursor of DIM, which also induced apoptosis in human breast-cancer cells by regulating the Bcl-2 family (Rahman et al., 2000).

References

Chen, I., McDougal, A., Wang, F., and Safe, S., Aryl hydrocarbon receptor mediated antiestrogenic and antitumorigenic activity of diindoylmethane in human breast cells, *Carcinogenesis,* 19:1631–1639, 1998.

Cover, C.M., Hsieh, S.J., Tran, S.H., Hallden, G., Kim, G.S., Bjeldanes, L.F., and Firestone, G.I., Indole-3-carbinol inhibits expression of cyclin-dependent kinase-6 and induces G_1 cell cycle arrest of human breast cancer cells independent of estrogen receptor signaling, *J. Biol. Chem.,* 273:3838–3847, 1998.

Hong, C., Firestone, G.L., and Bjeldanes, L.F., Bcl-2 family-mediated apoptotic effects of 3,3′-diindoylmethane (DIM) in human breast cells, *Biochem. Pharmacol.,* 63:1085–1087, 2002.

Rahman, K.W., Aranha, O., Glazyrin, A., Chinni, S.R., and Sarkar, F.H., 2000. Translocation of Bax to mitochondria induces a apoptotic cell death in indole-3-carbinol (13C) treated breast cancer cells, *Oncology,* 19:5764–5771, 2000.

Sharma, S., Stutzman, J.D., Kelloff, G.J., and Steele, V.E., Screening potential chemopreventative agents using biochemical markers of carcinogenesis, *Cancer Res.,* 54:5848–5855, 1994.

Dill oil   The essential oil of dill (*Anethum graveolens* L.) was reported to inhibit a broad range of microorganisms (Deans and Ritchie, 1987; Nakatani, 1994). Delaquis et al. (2002) examined the antimicrobial activity of a number of spices, including dill. While dill oil exhibited the lowest activity against the test organisms, distilled-oil fractions, containing higher concentrations of active components, were more effective. The main active components responsible were D-limonene and carvone, which accounted for 97.5 percent of those identified by gas chromatography. While D-limonene inhibited both Gram-negative and Gram-positive bacteria present in the pure extract, the dill oil itself had little effect on Gram-negative bacteria.

Lazutka and coworkers (2001) studied the genotoxicity of a number of essential oils, including dill oil. Dill was reported to be the most clastogenic, with the seed oil slightly greater than oil from dill herbs. The growing market for essential oils, such as dill, suggests the need to identify the genotoxic components so they can be reduced or removed by breeding.

References

Delaquis, P.J., Stanich, K., Girard, B., and Mazza, G., Antimicrobial activity of individual and mixed fractions of dill, cilantro, coriander and eucalyptus essential oils, *Int. J. Food Microbiol.,* 74:101–109, 2002.

Deans, S.G. and Ritchie, G., Antibacterial properties of plant essential oils, *Int. J. Food Microbiol.,* 5:165–180, 1987.

Lazutka, J.R., Mierauskiene, J., Slapsyte, G., and Dedonyte, V., Genotoxicity of dill (*Anethum graveolens* L.), peppermint (*Menthax piperita* L.) and pine (*Pinus sylvestris* L.) essential oils in human lymphocytes and *Drosophila melanogaster, Food Chem. Toxicol.,* 39:485–492, 2001.

Nakatani, N., Antioxidative and antimicrobial constituents of herbs and spices, *Dev. Food Sci..* 34:251–271, 1994.

D1 : R = H
D2 : R = CH$_3$
D7 : R = C$_2$H$_5$

D3

Structures of diospyrins D1, D2, D3, and D7 (From Chakrabarty et al., *Cancer Lett.,* 188:85–93, 2002. With permission.)

Diospyrin Diospyrin, a bisnaphthoquinonoid isolated from the bark of *Diospyros montana* Roxb. in India, is a dimer of 7-methyljuglone linked together via C-2 to C-6 (Sidhu and Pardhasaradhi, 1967, 1976a,b). It was shown to inhibit Ehrlich ascites carcinoma in mice (Hazra and Banerjee, 1994). Norhanom and Hazra (1997) found diospyrin and its synthetic derivatives inhibited Epstein–Barr virus early antigen expression in Raji cells exposed to the carcinogen 12-*O*-tetradecanoylphorbol-13-acetate.

Adeniyi et al. (2000) later reported dimeric naphthoquinones, diospyrin and isodiospyrin, both exhibited antibacterial activity. Chakrabarty et al. (2002) examined possible anticancer properties of diospyrin (D1) and several derivatives, including diethyl ether diospyrin (D7). Using four human cancer lines (HL-60, K-562, MCF-7, and HeLa), the diethyl ether derivative was the most cytotoxic, while diospyrin the least (Figure D.35). Diethyl ether diospyrin appeared to induce apoptosis through activation of caspase-3 and caspase-8. While diospyrin induced apoptosis in human cancer-cell lines, diethyl ether diospyrin was a far more potent antitumor agent. The possibility of developing new diospyrin derivatives with stronger anti-cancer properties as chemopreventive agents requires further study.

References

Adeniyi, B.A., Fong, H.H.S., Pezzuto, J.M., Luyengi, L., and Odelola, H.A., Antiobacterial activity of diospyrin, isodiospyrin and bisisodiospyrin from the root of *Diospyros piscatoria* (Gurke)(Ebenaceae), *Phytother. Res.,* 14:112–117, 2000.

Chakrabarty, S., Roy, M., Hazra, B., and Bhattacharya, R.K., Induction of apoptosis in human cancer cell lines by diospyrin, a plant-derived bisnaphthoquinonoid, and its synthetic derivatives, *Cancer Lett.,* 188:85–93, 2002.

Hazra, B. and Banerjee, A., New diospyrin derivatives with improved inhibitory activity towards Ehrlich ascites carcinoma, *Med. Sci. Res.,* 22:351–353, 1994.

Norhanom, A.W. and Hazra, B., Inhibition of tumor promoter-induced Epstein–Barr virus activation by diospyrin, a plant-derived antitumor compound and its synthetic derivatives, *Phytother. Res.,* 11:588–590, 1997.

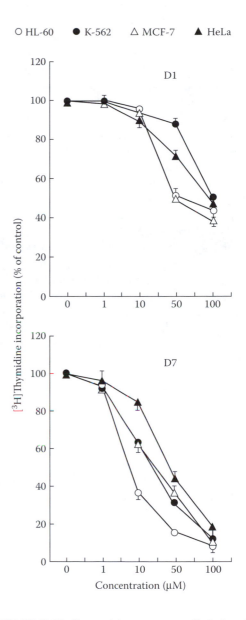

FIGURE D.35 Cytotoxicity on tumor cells induced by exposure for 48 h to different concentrations of diospyrin (D1) and diospyrin diethyl ether (D7) as assessed by MTT reduction. (From Chakrabarty et al., *Cancer Lett.,* 188:85–93, 2002. With permission.)

Sidhu, G.S. and Pardhasaradhi, M., Structure of diospyrin, *Tetrahedron Lett.,* 8:1313–1316, 1967a.

Sidhu, G.S. and Pardhasaradhi, M., Structure of the so-called red "methyl ester" of diospyrin, *Tetrahedron Lett.,* 8:4263–4267, 1967b.

Docosahexaenoic acid (DHA)   Docosahexaenoic acid (DHA, C22:6ω-3) is consumed primarily in fish oils. Epidemiological studies suggested that the levels of DHA in the blood were inversely associated with risk factors for cardiovascular disease. A study by Conquer and Holub (1998) showed that DHA supplementation in humans increased serum DHA as non-esterified fatty acid at levels that were potentially antithrombotic. Liu and coworkers (2001) found a significant increase in plasma omega-3 fatty acids and in HDL-cholesterol in 36 hyperlipidemic patients fed bread containing fish oil. Since omega-3 fatty acids appear to inhibit the proliferation of breast-cancer cells, Chen and Auborn (1999) examined the effect of DHA on the growth of human papillomavirus immortalized keratinocytes. DHA was found to inhibit the growth of these cells and was dose dependent. Park and coworkers (2000) reported that fish oil had a protective effect against cardiovascular disease by inhibiting hepatic HMG CoA reductase activity and increasing hepatic microsomal fluidity, leading to a reduction in plasma lipids.

References

Chen, D. and Auborn, K., Fish oil constituent docosahexaenoic acid selectively inhibits growth of human papillomavirus immortalized keratinocytes, *Carcinogenesis,* 20:249–254, 1999.

Conquer, J.A. and Holub, B.J., Effect of supplementation with different doses of DHA on the levels of circulating DHA as non-esterified fatty acids in subjects of Asian Indian background, *J. Lipid Res.,* 39:286–292, 1998.

Liu, M., Wallin, R., and Saldeen, T., Effect of bread containing fish oil on plasma phospholipid fatty acids, triglycerides, HDL-cholesterol, and malondialdehyde in subjects with hyperlipidemia, *Nutr. Res.,* 21:1403–1410, 2001.

Park, H.S., Choi, J.S., and Kim, K.H., Docosahexaenoic acid-rich fish oil and pectin have a hypolipidemic effect, but pectin increases risk factor for colon cancer in rats, *Nutr. Res.,* 20:1783–1794, 2000.

Echinacea (*Echinacea purpurea*) *Echinacea* (purple coneflower), a perennial, flowering plant indigenous to North America, is used to treat such conditions as bacterial/viral infections, cancer, seizures, and AIDS (O'Hara et al., 1998). However, evidence supporting its use as a therapeutic agent remains controversial. It is a popular herbal product in Europe and North America, where it is used to prevent upper-respiratory-tract infections. Variable results have been reported regarding the efficacy of *Echinacea* due, in large part, to the lack of standards defining the active ingredients. The suggested bioactive constituents of *Echinacea* include lipophyllic alkylamides polar caffeic acid derivatives, such as cichoric acid, glycoproteins, and polysaccharides (Bauer and Wagner, 1991). Goel and coworkers (2002) designed a study to examine the dose-related effects of *Echinacea* extracts with different levels of bioactive components on immunomodulation in rats. Their results indicated that extracts with optimal concentrations of cichoric acid, alkylamides, and polysaccharides were potentially effective in stimulating a nonspecific immune response, *in vivo*, in rats.

Gan et al. (2003) examined the mechanism of immunomodulation by *Echinacea* by studying its effect on natural-killer (NK) cells present in human peripheral blood mononuclear cells (PMBC). NK cells defend against human viral infections by producing cytokinins IFN-γ, TNF-α, and GM-CSF. *Echinacea* appeared to be a potent activator of NK cytoxicity, which explains, in part, its antiviral efficacy observed *in vivo*.

Carlo et al. (2003) compared the ability of *Echinacea* and St. John's Wort to modulate apoptosis in mice. Both exhibited significant, dose-related protection against apoptosis. For example, treatment of 30 mg/kg of *Echinacea* or St. John's Wort per day per mouse reduced apoptosis by 33 percent and 55 percent, respectively

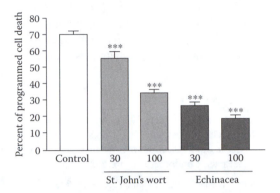

FIGURE E.36 Effect of St. John's Wort and *Echinacea* (30–100 mg/kg per day) on spontaneous apoptosis after 18 h *in vitro* cultivation. Values are means of at least seven determinations $\pm$ SEM. ***$p < 0.001$ versus control. (From Carlo et al., *Pharmacol. Res.*, 48:273–277, 2003. With permission.)

(Figure E.36). This reduction in apoptosis was accompanied by a corresponding decrease in Fas-Ag expression and an increase in Bcl-2 expression.

Echinacea products were used as adjuvants to reduce the side effects associated with cancer chemotherapy and radiotherapy (Bendel et al., 1988, 1989). The bioactive components involved are thought to be polysaccharide fractions containing neutral fucogalactoxyloglucans and arabino-galactans isolated from *Echinacea purpurea* cell cultures. Promising clinical and immunological effects were reported in patients with HIV-infection melanoma and leukemia who were injected with these polysaccharides (Emmendoerfer et al., 1999). A pilot study conducted in Germany by Melchart et al. (2002) showed injections of 2 mg of *Echinacea* polysaccharides in patients suffering from advanced gastric cancer slightly decreased leukopenia. The lack of a placebo-controlled group limited the outcome of this study, while production of adequate amounts of active and standardized *Echinacea purpurea* polysaccharide preparations remains a serious problem to be solved before further clinical trials can be carried out.

A novel diactylenic amide isolated from *Echinacea, N*-(2-methylpropyl)-2-*E*-undecene-8,10-diynamide, was recently synthesized by Kraus and Bae (2003). Such compounds were previously reported to be active against *A. aegyptii* larvae and *H. zea* neonates (Sun et al., 2002*).

References

Bauer, R. and Wagner, H., Echinacea species as potential immunostimulating drugs, in *Economic and Medicinal Plant Research,* Wagner, H., Ed., Academic Press, London, 1991, pp. 253–321.

Bendel, R., Bendel, V., Renner, K., Carstens, V., and Stolze, K., Zusatzbehandlung mit Esberitox bei Patientinnen mit cheo-strahlentherapeutischer Berhandlung eines fortgeschrittenen Mammakarzinoms, *Onkologie,* 12:32–38, 1989.

Bendel, R., Renner, K., and Stolze, K., Zusatzbehandlung mit Esberitox bei Patientinnen mit kurativer adjuvanter Bestrahlung nach Mammakarzinom, *Strahlenther Onkol.,* 164:278–283, 1988.

Carlo, G., Nuzzo, I., Capasso, R., Sanges, M.R., Galdiero, E., Capasso, F., and Carratelli, R., Modulation of apoptosis in mice treated with *Echinacea* and St. John's Wort, *Pharmacol. Res.,* 48:273–277, 2003.

Emmendoerfer, A.C., Wagner, H., and Lohmann-Matthes, M.L., Immunological active polysaccharides from *Echinacea purpurea* plant and cell cultures, in *Immunomodulatory Agents in Plants,* Wagner, H., Ed., Springer–Verlag, New York, 1999, pp. 89–104.

Gan, X.-H., Zhang, L., Heber, D., and Bonavida, B., Mechanism of activation of human peripheral blood NK cells at the single level of *Echinacea* water soluble extracts: Recruitment of lymphocyte-target conjugates and killer cells and activation of programming for lysis, *Int. J. Immunopharmacol.,* 13:931–941, 2003.

Goel, V., Chang, C., Slama, J.V., Barton, R., Bauer, R., Gahler, R., and Basu, T.K., Echinacea stimulates macrophage function in the lung and spleen of normal rats, *J. Nutr. Biochem.,* 13:487–492, 2002.

Kraus, G.A. and Bae, J., Synthesis of N-(2-methyl-propyl)-2E-undecene-8,10-diynamide, a novel constituent of *Echinacea angistofolia*, *Tetrahedron Lett.,* 44:5505–5506, 2003.

Melchart, D., Clemm, C., Weber, B., Draczynski, T., Worku, F., Linde, K., Widenhammer, W., Wagner, H.

and Saller, R., Polysaccharides isolated from *Echinacea purpurea herba* cultures to counteract undesired effects of chemotherapy — A pilot study, *Phytother. Res.,* 16:138–142, 2002.

O'Hara, M.A., Keifer, K., Farrelle, K., and Kemper, K., A review of the commonly used medicinal herbs, *Acta Family Med.,* 7:523–536, 1998.

Sun, L., Rezaei, K.A., Temelli, F., and Ooraikul, B., Supercritical fluid extraction of alkylamides from *Echinacea angustifolia*, *J. Agric. Food Chem.,* 50: 3947–3953, 2002.

Eggs The relatively high cholesterol content of eggs deflected from their nutritional quality and led to a decrease in per capita consumption. Reviewing the available epidemiological data, Kritchevsky and Kritchevsky (2000) found only a moderate increase in the risk of coronary heart disease was associated with cholesterol intake. However, when other dietary confounders were taken into consideration, no risk of cardiovascular disease was evident in nondiabetic men and women consuming one-plus eggs per day. A cross-sectional and population-based study by Song and Kerver (2000) showed no association between egg consumption and serum cholesterol. This was supported by other researchers, who found egg consumption did not increase the risk of cardiovascular disease (Hu et al., 1999). A meta-analysis by Weggemans et al. (2001) found dietary cholesterol from eggs increased the ratio of dietary cholesterol to high-density lipoproteins in humans. Using a randomized, controlled, crossover trial with 49 healthy adults, Katz et al. (2005) found that ingestion of two eggs daily over the short term had no adverse effect on endothelial function or cholesterol levels.

Feeding hens diets enriched with fish oils, vegetables oils, or algal sources of docosahexaenoic acid (DHA) produced eggs high in omega-3 fatty acids, which are now sold in the supermarkets. Human subjects fed seven enriched eggs a week had significantly higher level of blood omega-3 fatty acids and HDL cholesterol (Farrell, 1998). Makrides et al. (2002) reported that feeding both breast-fed and formula-fed infants 6 to 12 months of age four omega-3-enriched egg yolks a week increased DHA, hemoglobin, and ferritin without affecting

TABLE E.24
Effects of Dietary Casein and Ovomucin in Serum and Liver Lipids and Fecal Steroid Excretion in Rats[1]

	Diet Group	
	Casein	Ovomucin
Serum		
Total cholesterol (a)	2.83 ± 0.21	1.96 ± 0.07[a]
HDL cholesterol (b)	0.53 ± 0.04	0.66 ± 0.06
LDL + VLDL cholesterol	2.30 ± 0.22	1.30 ± 0.08[a]
Atherogenic index: (b)/(a)(mol/mol)	0.19 ± 0.02	0.34 ± 0.03[a]
TG	0.38 ± 0.04	0.37 ± 0.03
Phospholipids	1.13 ± 0.08	1.04 ± 0.05
Liver		
Total lipids (mg/g liver)	142.8 ± 4.41	124.0 ± 2.47[a]
Cholesterol (μmol/g liver)	70.8 ± 2.4	66.9 ± 3.2
TG (μmol/g liver)	26.8 ± 2.9	24.8 ± 2.1
Phospholipids μ/3d)	118.8 ± 3.2	98.7 ± 1.6
Feces		
Dry weight (g/3d)	2.42 ± 0.06	2.56 ± 0.10
Cholesterol (μmol/3d)	252.5 ± 6.7	281.3 ± 9.5[b]
Bile acids (μmol/3d)	126.5 ± 5.8	151.9 ± 7.2[b]

[1] Mean ± SEM of six rats. Significantly different from casein control at:
[a] $p < 0.01$; [b] $p < 0.05$.

From Nagoaka et al., *Lipids*, 37:267–272, 2002. With permission.

cholesterol levels. A recent study showed the potential health benefits associated with feeding CLA-enriched eggs to rats (Cherian and Goeger, 2003).

Despite its much-maligned image, eggs have always been considered to be a functional food. For example, egg white, the cholesterol-free protein, contains a number of protein fractions, including ovalbumin, ovomucin, ovotransferin, and lysozyme. Several studies have shown egg white is hypocholesterolemic (Yamamoto et al., 1993; Asato et al., 1996). Nagaoka et al. (2002) demonstrated, for the first time, the superior hypocholesterolemic properties of ovomucin compared to casein. *In vitro* studies with Caco-2 cultured cells showed ovomucin had greater bile-acid-binding capacity, inhibiting cholesterol absorption. *In vivo* studies further demonstrated the hypocholesterolemic effect of ovomucin compared to casein (Table E.24). Rats fed ovomucin had significantly lower levels of serum cholesterol and tended to have higher

levels of HDL cholesterol compared to casein. In addition, the atherogenic index [(b)/(a)], defined as the ratio of HDL cholesterol to serum total cholesterol, was significantly higher than in the casein-fed group. This study illustrates the health benefits derived from the egg-white protein, ovomucin.

References

Asato, L., Wang, M.F., Chan, Y.C., Yeh, S.H., Chung, H.M., Chida, Y.C., Uezato, T., Suzuki, I., and Yamagata, N., Effect of egg white on serum cholesterol concentrations in young women, *J. Nutr. Sci. Vitamol.*, 42:87–96, 1996.

Cherian, G. and Goeger, M.P., Conjugated linoleic acid-enriched chicken egg yolk powder alters tissue fatty acids and serum immunoglobulin in rats, *Fed. Am. Soc. Exp. Biol.*, 17(Abstr., 203.17), 2003.

Farrel, D.J., Enrichment of hen eggs with n-3 long chain fatty acids and evaluation of enriched eggs in humans, *Am. J. Clin. Nutr.*, 68:538–544, 1998.

Hu, F.B., Stampfer, M.J., and Rimm, E.B., A prospective study of egg consumption and risk of cardiovascular disease in men and women, *J. Am. Med. Assoc.,* 281:1387–1394, 1999.

Katz, D.L., Evans, M.A., Nawaz, H., Njike, V.Y., Chan, W., Comerford, B.P., and Hoxley, M.L., Egg consumption and endothelial function: A randomized controlled crossover trial, *Int. J. Cardiol.,* 99:65–70, 2005.

Kritchevsky, S.B. and Kritchevsky, D., Egg consumption and coronary heart disease: An epidemiologic overview, *J. Am. Coll. Nutr.,* 19:549S–555S, 2000.

Makrides, M., Hawkes, J.S., Neumann, M.A., and Gibson, R.A., Nutritional effect of including egg yolk in the weaning diet of breast-fed and formula-fed infants: A randomized control trial, *Am. J. Clin. Nutr.,* 75:1084–1092, 2002.

Nagoaka, S., Masoaka, M., Zhang, Q., Hasegawa, M., and Watanabe, K., Egg ovomucin attenuates hypercholesterolemia in rats and inhibits cholesterol absorption in Caco-2 cells, *Lipids,* 37:267–272, 2002.

Song, W.O. and Kerver, J.M., Nutritional contribution of eggs to the American diet, *J. Am. College Nutr.,* 19:556S–562S, 2000.

Weggmans, R.M., Zock, P.L., and Katan, M.B., Dietary cholesterol from eggs increases the ratio of total cholesterol to high-density lipoprotein cholesterol in humans: A meta analysis, *Am. J. Clin. Nutr.,* 73:881–891, 2001.

Yamamoto, S., Kina, T., Yamagata, N., Kokubu, T., Shinjo, S., and Asato, L., Favorable effects of egg white protein on lipid metabolism in rats and mice, *Nutr. Res.,* 13:1453–1457, 1993.

Eicosapentaenoic acid (EPA)   Eicosapentaenoic acid (EPA)(C20:5ω-3) is an ω-3 polyunsaturated fatty acid found primarily in sea and freshwater fish (Eskin, 2002). The extremely slow conversion of α-linolenic acid (C18:3ω-3) to EPA by the human body makes fish an important source of this fatty acid. Minami and coworkers (2002) showed supplementation with EPA lowered plasma lipids, hepatic triacylglycerol levels, and abdominal-fat deposits accumulation, as well as improved insulin resistance in type 2 Otsuka Long-Evans Tokushima Fatty (OLETF) diabetic model rats (Table E.25).

A significant ($p < 0.001$) correlation was observed between glucose-infusion rates and relative-weight abdominal fat in these animals, suggesting that the effect of EPA on insulin sensitivity was related to decreased abdominal-fat accumulation. Long-term feeding of EPA could help to prevent insulin resistance in diabetes-prone rats by improving hypertriacylglycerolemia.

The ability of ω-3 polyunsaturated fatty acids to modulate tumor-cell growth was demonstrated for EPA by Chiu and Wan (1999). They showed EPA arrested cell-cycle progression at G0/G1 phase, inducing necrosis in human leukemic HL-60 and K-562 cells *in vitro*. EPA, however, only induced apoptosis in HL-60 cells by down-regulation of Bcl-2. Gillis and coworkers (2002) found EPA, alone or in combination with gamma-linolenic acid (GLA: 18:3 ω-6), reduced cell survival by inducing

TABLE E.25
Effect of Dietary Supplementation with EPA for 25 Weeks on Fasting Plasma Lipids of Diabetic Rats[1]

	Control		EPA	
	Mean	SD	Mean	SD
Triacylglycerol (mmol/L)	1.75	0.28	0.88*	0.27
Cholesterol (mmol/L)	1.7	0.18	1.23*	0.16
Phospholipids (mmol/L)	2.08	0.32	1.50*	0.24
Free fatty acids (mmol/L)	0.8	0.15	0.75	0.17

[1] Eight rats per group. Mean values were significantly different from the control, *$p < 0.05$.

Source: Adapted from Minami et al., *Br. J. Nutr.,* 87:157–162, 2002.

apoptosis and secondary necrosis in human pro-myelocytic HL-60 cells. Incubation of cells with 100 µmol/L EPA reduced cell viability to 27 percent and increased apoptosis to 263 percent compared to the control.

References

Chiu, L.C.M. and Wan, J.M.F., Induction of apoptosis in HL-60 cells by eicosapentaenoic acid (EPA) is associated with downregulation of Bcl-2 expression, *Cancer Lett.,* 145:17–27, 1999.

Eskin, N.A.M., Authentication of evening primrose, borage and fish oils, Chapter 4, in *Oils and Fats Authentication,* Jee, M., Ed., Blackwell Publishing/CRC Press, Boca Raton, 2002, chap. 6, pp. 97–98.

Gillis, R.C., Daley, B.J., Enderson, B.L., and Karlsted, D.D., Eicosapentaenoic acid and gamma-linolenic acid induce apoptosis in HL-60 cells, *J. Surg. Res.,* 107:145–153, 2002.

Minami, A., Ishimura, N., Sakamoto, S., Takishita, E., Mawatari, K., Okada, K., and Nakaya, Y., Effect of eicosapentaenoic acid ethyl ester *v.* oleic acid-rich safflower oil on insulin resistance in type 2 diabetic model rats with hypertriacylglycerolemia, *Br. J. Nutr.,* 87:157–162, 2002.

Ellagic acid   Ellagic acid, a complex planar molecule, has been attributed for the chemopreventive properties of berries, such as strawberries and raspberries. Siglin and coworkers (1995) reported that ellagic acid inhibited esophageal cancer in rats induced by *N*-nitrosomethylbenzylamine. Ellagic acid appeared to block the metabolic activation of the carcinogen, interfering

OH

Ellagic acid. (Adapted from Mertens-Talcott and Percival, *Cancer Lett.,* 218:141–151, 2005)

with the binding of reactive carcinogen metabolites with DNA and by stimulating the detoxification enzymes (Teel et al., 1986; Ahn et al., 1996). Barch et al. (1996) demonstrated the anticarcinogenic properties of ellagic acid, including inhibiting CYZP1A1-dependent activation of

benzo[*a*]pyrene; binding and detoxifying the diolepoxide of benzo[*a*]pyrene; binding DNA and reducing the formation of O^6-methylguanine by methylating carcinogenes; and inducing phase II detoxifying enzymes, glutathione *S*-transferase (GST) Ya, and NAD(P)H:quinone reductase. Structural examination of ellagic acid showed the 3- and 4-hydroxyl and the lactone groups were responsible for some of the different activities observed. Barch and coworkers (1995) previously showed in the rat that ellagic acid significantly increased total hepatic GST activity, hepatic GST-Ya activity and hepatic GST-Yam-RNA. The latter increased due to transcription induction of the GST-Ya gene by ellagic acid.

In order to be effective, ellagic acid must be available, but animal studies suggested only a fraction is orally bioavailable (Teel et al., 1988). Using a human intestinal-cell line Caco-2, Whitley et al. (2003) showed ellagic acid accumulated selectively in the epithelial cells of the areodigestive tract. Their results, illustrated in Scheme E.20, show ellagic acid (EA) enters the cell via the apical and is intercalated or bound to DNA. Another large portion is oxidized, possibly involving reactive-oxygen species (ROS), probably to quinines, where they bind to proteins. Losso and coworkers (2004) found that ellagic acid expressed a selective cytotoxicity and antiproliferative activity, and induced apoptosis in Caco-2, MCF-7m Hs 578T, and DU 145 cancer

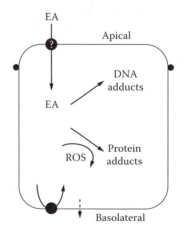

SCHEME E.20 Proposed schematic model of EA disposition in epithelial Caco-2 cells. ROS, Reactive-oxygen species. ? denotes potential transporters. (From Whitley et al., *Biochem. Pharmacol.,* 66:907–915, 2003. With permission.)

cells, showing no toxicity toward normal lung fibrblast cells. Induction of apoptosis in cancer cells by ellagic acid involved a decrease in ATP production, essential to the viability of the cancer cells.

References

Ahn, D., Putt, D., Kresty, L., Stoner, G.D., Fromm, D., and Hollenberg, P.F., The effects of dietary ellagic acid on rat hepatic and esophageal mucosal cytochromes P450 and phase II enzymes, *Carcinogenesis,* 17:821–828, 1996.

Barch, D.H., Rundhaugen, L.M., and Pillay, N.S., Ellagic acid induces transcription of the rat glutathione S-transferase-Ya gene, *Carcinogenesis,* 16:665–668, 1995.

Barch, D.H., Rundhaugen, L.M., Stoner, G.D., and Rosche, W.A., Structure-function relationships of the dietary anticarcinogen ellagic acid, *Carcinogenesis,* 17:265–269, 1996.

Clifford, M.N. and Scalbert, A., Ellagitannins — nature, occurrence and dietary burden, *J. Sci. Food Agric.,* 80:1118–1125, 2000.

Losso, J.N., Bansode, R.R., Trappey, A., II, Bawadi, H.A., and Truax, R., *In vitro* anti-proliferative activities of ellagic acid, *J. Nutr. Biochem.,* 15:672–678, 2004.

Mertens-Talcott, S.U. and Percival, S.S., Ellagic acid and quercetin interact synergistically with resveratrol in the induction of apoptosis and cause transient cell cycle arrest in human leukemia cells. *Cancer Lett.,* 218:141–151, 2005.

Siglin, J.C., Barch, D.H., and Stoner, G.D., Effects of dietary phenethyl isothiocyanate, ellagic acid, sunlidac and calcium on the induction and progression of *N*-nitrosomethylbenzylamine-induced esophageal carcinogenesis in rats, *Carcinogenesis,* 16:1101–1106, 1995.

Teel, R.W., Ellagic acid binding to DNA as a possible mechanism for is antimutagenic and anticarcinogenic action, *Cancer Lett.,* 30:329–336, 1986.

Whitley, A.C., Stoner, G.D., Darby, M.V., and Walle, T., Intestinal epithelial cell accumulation of the cancer preventive polyphenol ellagic acid-extensive binding to protein and DNA, *Biochem. Pharmacol.,* 66:907–915, 2003.

Ellagitannins Ellagic acid can also be complexed to form ellagitannins. These are water-soluble tannins, high-molecular-weight phenolic compounds capable of precipitating proteins and alkaloids (Santos-Beulga and Scalbert, 2000). They are structurally different from proanthocyanidins by being esters of hexahydroxydiphenic acid plus a polyol, glucose, or quinic acid (Scheme E.21). Acids and bases hydrolyze the ester bond, resulting in the formation of water-insoluble ellagic acid.

In Western diets, strawberries, raspberries, and blackberries are major sources of ellagitannins (Daniel et al., 1989). Ellagitannins are also in beverages produced from these fruit and loganberry (a hybrid of raspberry and blackberry) (Singleton et al., 1966), as well as in beer and tea (Nonaka et al., 1984). Ellagitannins appear to exert anticancer and antitumor properties. A study with transplantable tumors showed that number of ellagitannin oligomers (mainly dimers, but also a monomer, dimers, and tetramers) extended the life span of mice compared to the control (Yoshida et al., 1995). Castonguay and coworkers (1997) found raspberry ellagitannins containing sanguiin H6 and lambertianin inhibited TPA-stimulated DNA synthesis, TPA-induced ornithine decarboxylase, and TPA-stimulated hydroperoxide production by 42 percent, 30 percent, and 30 percent, respectively. However, no full autopsy report was given by Castonguay et al. (1997) or a control group receiving just ellagitannins.

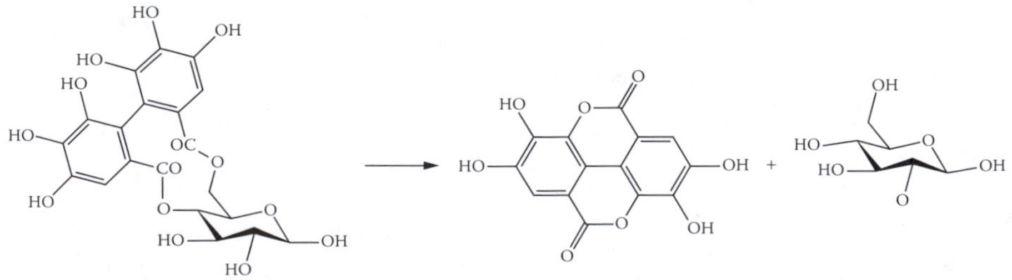

SCHEME E.21 Hydrolysis of ellagitannin to ellagic acid. (From Clifford and Scalbert, *J. Sci. Food Agric.,* 80:1118–1125, 2000. With permission.)

A number of reports have shown that some ellagitannins may be toxic to rodents and ruminants. Ellagitannin extracts were reported to inhibit a number of pathogenic bacteria (Scalbert, 1991; Silva et al., 1997). A recent review on ellagitannins by Clifford and Scalbert (2000), however, recommended that more work was needed to clarify their therapeutic benefits.

References

Castonguay, A., Gali, H.U., Perchellet, E.M., Gao, X.M., Boukharta, M., Jalbert, G., Okuda, T., Yoshida, T., Hatano, T., and Perchellet, J.P., Antitumorigenic and antipromoting activities of ellagic acid, ellagitannins, and oligomeric anthocyanin and proanthocyanin, *Int. J. Oncol.,* 10:367–373, 1997.

Clifford, M.N. and Scalbert, A., Ellagitannins — nature, occurrence and dietary burden, *J. Sci. Food Agric.,* 80:1118–1125, 2000.

Daniel, E.M., Krupnic, A.S., Heur, Y.-H., Blinzler, J.A., Nims, R.W., and Stoner, G.D., Extraction, stability, and quantitation of ellagic acid in various fruits and nuts, *J. Food Compos. Anal.,* 2:338–349, 1989.

Nonaka, G.-I., Sakai, R., and Nishioka, I., Hydrolysable tannins and proanthocyanidins from green tea, *Phytochemistry,* 23:1753–1755, 1984.

Santos-Buelga, C. and Scalbert, A., Proanthocyanidins and tannin-like compounds — nature, occurrence, dietary intake and affects on nutrition and health, *J. Sci. Food Agric.,* 80:1094–1117, 2000.

Scalbert, A., Antimicrobial properties of tannins, *Phytochemistry,* 30:3875–3883, 1991.

Silva, O., Duarte, A., Pimentel, M., Viegas, S., Barroso, H., Machado, J., Pires, I., Cabrita, J., and Gomes, E., Antimicrobial activity of *Taerminalia macroptera* root, *J. Ethnopharmacol.,* 57:203–207, 1997.

Singleton, V.L., Marsh, G.L., and Coven, M.J., Identification of ellagic acid as a precipitate from loganberry wine, *J. Agric. Food Chem.,* 14:5–8, 1966.

Yoshida, T., Hatano, T., Miyamoto, K., and Okuda, T., Antitumor and related activities of ellagitannin oligomers, in *Polyphenols 94,* Brouillard, R., Jay, M., and Scalbert, A., Eds., INRA Editions, Paris, 1995, pp. 123–132.

Emodin   Emodin (1,3,8-trihydroxy-6-methylanthraquinone), a naturally occurring constituent of many Chinese herbs, is known for antibacterial, anticancer, diuretic, immunosuppressive, and vasorelaxant properties (Muller et al., 1996; Wang et al., 1998; Lee, 2001). Koyama and coworkers (2002) showed emodin exhibited potent antitumor properties. Using a two-stage carcinogenesis test of mouse-skin tumors induced by topical application of 7,12-dimethyl-benz[*a*]-anthracene as an initiator and 12-*O*-tetradecanoylphorbol-13-acetate as a promotor, emodin inhibited the two-stage carcinogenesis test very effectively. Emodin was first shown to induce apoptosis in human kidney fibroblasts from lupus nephritis patients (Liu et al., 2000). Since then, other studies have shown

Emodin. (From Koyama et al., *Cancer Lett.,* 182: 135–139, 2002. With permission.)

apoptosis-inducing properties of emodin, including the structurally similar compound, aloe-emodin, on neurorectodermal cancer and lung-carcinoma cells (Lee et al., 2001; Pecere et al., 2000). Chen and coworkers (2002) showed emodin-induced apoptosis in human promyeloleukemic HL-60 cells via activation of the caspase-3 and not by its prooxidant activity. Srinivas et al. (2003) suggested the antiproliferative effects of emodin in human cervical-cancer cells was mediated through the induction of apoptosis. They also found that the induction of apoptosis by emodin was mediated by activation of caspase via the mitochondrial pathway.

References

Chen, Y.-C., Shen, S.-C., Lee, W.-R., Hsu, F.-L., Lin, H.-Y., Ko, C.-H., and Tseng, S.-W., Emodin induces apoptosis in human promyeloleukemic HL-60 cells accompanied by activation of caspase 3 cascade but independent of reactive oxygen species, *Biochem. Pharmacol.,* 64:1713–1724, 2002.

Koyama, J., Morita, I., Tagahara, K., Nobukuni, Y., Mukainaka, T., Kuchide, M., Tokuda, H., and Nishino, H., Chemopreventive effects of emodin and cassiamin B in mouse skin carcinogenesis, *Cancer Lett.,* 182:135–139, 2002.

E

Lee, H.Z., Effects and mechanisms of emodin on cell death in human lung squamous cell carcinoma, *Br. J. Pharmacol.,* 134:11–20, 2001.

Liu, C., Ye, R., and Tan, Z., Effect of emodin on fibroblasts in lupus mephritis, *Zhongguo Zhong Xi Yi Jei He Za Zhi,* 20:196–198, 2000.

Muller, S.O., Eckert, I., Lutz, W.K., and Stopper, H., Genotoxicity of the laxative drug components emodin, aloe emodin and danthron in mammalian cells: Topoisomerase II mediated? *Mutat. Res.,* 371:165–173, 1996.

Pecere, T., Gazzola, M.V., Mucignat, C., Parolin, C., Vecchia, F.D., Caaggioni, A., Basso, G., Diaspro, A., Salvato, B., Carli, M., and Palu, G., Aloe-emodin is a new type of anti-cancer agent with selective activity against neuroectodermal tumors, *Cancer Res.,* 60: 2800–2804, 2000.

Srinivas, G., Antoi, R.J., Srinivas, P., Vidhyalakshmi, S., Senan, V.P., and Karunagaran, D., Emodin induces apoptosis of human cervical cancer cells through poly(ADP-ribose) polymerase cleavage and activation of caspase-9, *Eur. J. Pharmacol.,* 473: 117–125, 2003.

Wang, H.H., Chung, J.G., Ho, C.C., Wu, L.T., and Chang, S.H., Aloe-emodin effects on arylamine N-acetyltransferase activity in the bacterium *Helicobacter pylori, Planta Med.,* 64:176–178, 1998.

Enterodiol and Enterolactone Enterodiol [2,3-*bis*(3-hydroxybenzyl)butane-1,4-diol] and enterolactone [*trans*-2,3-bis (3-hydroxy-ben-zyl)-γ-butyrolactone] are lignan-type phy-toestrogens produced by bacteria in the intestinal tract (Axelson et al., 1981, 1982) and from plant lignans matairesinol and seco-isolaricir-esinol (Borriello et al., 1985). These plant lig-nans are found in whole-grain cereals, seeds, nuts, legumes, and vegetables.

Enterodiol and enterolactone are both estro-gens and exert protective effects by their ability to compete with estradiol for the type II estro-gen receptor. Mousavi and Adlercreutz (1992) showed enterolactone at > 10 μM inhibited the growth of MCF-7 breast-cancer cells, while higher concentrations (> 50 μM) were found by Wang and Kurtzer (1997) to inhibit DNA synthe-sis. Other protective effects include the induction of the sex hormone-binding globulin as well as their inhibition of a number of steroid-metaboliz-ing enzymes, including aromatase, 5-α-reduc-tase, 7α-hydroxylase, and 17β-hydroxysteroid dehydrogenase. Aromatase appeared to play some role in the development of breast cancer and was moderately inhibited by enterolactone compared to enterodiol, a weaker inhibitor (Adlercreutz et al., 1993; Wang et al., 1994; Makeda et al., 2000). These phytoestrogens were also shown by Sanghvi et al. (1984) to signifi-cantly inhibit cholesterol 7α-hydroxylase (the rate-limiting enzyme for bile acids) *in vitro,* decreasing the formation of primary bile acids, thereby providing protection against colorectal cancer. The final, protective role of these phy-toestrogens is due to their antioxidant properties.

During the menstrual cycle these phytoestro-gens are excreted in large amounts, particularly during early pregnancy. Postmenopausal Japa-nese women who consumed large quantities of phytoestrogens in their diets were reported to have fewer complaints of hot flushes, night sweats, and other symptoms compared to women in other countries (Williams and Rut-ledge, 1998). Lignans, such as enterolactone, also appear to exert a chemoprotective effect against prostate cancer, as well coronary heart disease (Denmark-Wahnefried et al., 2001; Department of Health, 1994). An excellent review on enterodiol and enterolactone was published by Wang (2002).

Enterodiol, Enterolactone. (Adapted from Penalvo et al., *Anal. Biochem.,* 332:384–393, 2004.)

References

Adlercreutz, H., Bannnwart, C., Wahala, K., Makela, T., Brunow, G., Hase, T., Arosemena, P.J., Kellis, J.T., Jr., and Vickery, L.E., Inhibition of human aromatase by mammalian lignans and isoflavonoid phytoestrogens, *J. Steroid Biochem. Mol. Biol.*, 44:147–153, 1993.

Axelson, M. and Setchell, K.D.R., The excretion of lignans in rats — evidence for an intestinal bacterial source for this new group of compounds, *FEBS Lett.*, 123:337–342, 1981.

Axelson, M., Sjovall, J., Gustaffsen, B.E. and Setchell, K.D.R., Origin of lignans in mammals and identification of a precursor from plants, *Nature*, 298: 659–660, 1982.

Borrielo, S.P., Setchell, K.D.R., Axelson, M., and Lawson, A.M., Production and metabolism of lignans by the human fecal flora, *J. Appl. Bacterol.*, 58: 37–43, 1985.

Denmark-Wahnefried, W., Price, D.T., Polascik, T.J., Robertson, C.N., Anderson, E.E., Paulson, D.F., Walther, P.J., Gannon, M., and Vollmer, R.T., Pilot study of dietary fat restriction and flaxseed supplementation in men with prostate cancer before surgery: exploring the effects on hormonal levels, prostate-specific antigen, and histopathalogic features. *Urology*, 58:47–52, 2001.

Department of Health, Nutritional Aspects of Cardiovascular Disease, *Report on Health and Social Subjects*, N. 46, H.M. Stationary Office, London, 1994.

Makeda, T.H., Wahala, K.T., and Hase, T.A., Synthesis of enterolactone and enterodiol precursors as potential inhibitors of human estrogen synthetase (aromatase), *Steroids*, 65:437–441, 2000.

Mousavi, Y. and Adlercreutz, H., Enterolactone and estradiol inhibit each other's proliferation effect on MCF-7 breast cancer cells in culture, *J. Steroid Biochem. Mol. Biol.*, 41:615–619, 1992.

Penalvo, J.L., Nurmi, T., Haajanen, K., Al-Maharik, N., Botting, N., and Adlercreutz, H., Determination of lignans in human plasma by liquid chromatography with coulometric electrode array detection, *Anal. Biochem.*, 332:384–393, 2004.

Sanghvi, A., Diven, W.F., Seltman, H., Warty, V., Rizk, M., Kritchevsky, D., and Setchell, K.D.R., in *Drugs Affecting Lipid Metabolism*, Kritchevsky, D., Parletti, R., and Holmes, W.L., Eds., Plenum Press, New York, Vol. 8, p. 311.

Wang, L.-Q., Mammalian phytoestrogens: Enterodiol and enterolactone: A review, *J. Chromatogr. B.*, 777: 289–309, 2002.

Wang, C.F. and Kurzer, M.S., Phytoestrogen concentration determines effects on DNA synthesis in human breast cancer cells, *Nutr. Cancer*, 28:236–247, 1997.

Wang, C., Makela, T., Hase, T., Adlercreutz, H., and Kurzer, M., Lignans and flavonoids inhibit aromatase enzyme in human preadipocytes, *J. Steroid Biochem. Mol. Biol.*, 50:205–212, 1994.

Williams, R.L. and Rutledge, T., Recent phytoestrogen research, *Chem. Ind.*, 1:14–16, 1998.

(–)-Epicatechin (EC)   (–)-Epicatechin is a dietary flavonol present in many fruits, red wine, green teas, and cocoa products. *In vivo* studies showed that only small amounts of epicatechin are absorbed and converted to various

Epicatechin. (Adapted from Geetha et al., *Mutat. Res.*, 556:65–74, 2004.)

metabolites, including glucuronides, methyl derivatives, and sulfates. More than 60 µM of epicatechin and its metabolites were reported in the plasma of rats, following a single, intragastric dose of 100 mg (Scalbert and Williamson, 2000). Epicatechin was also reported in human plasma, following consumption of chocolate (Wang et al., 2000). Together with one of its *in vivo* metabolites, 3′-*O*-methyl epicatechin, epicatchin appeared to protect against neuronal cell death induced by oxidative stress (Schroeter et al., 2001). El-Mohsen et al. (2002) identified the presence of both epicatechin glucuronide and 3′-methyl epicatechin glucuronide in rat-brain tissue, following oral ingestion of (–)-epicatechin.

During inflammatory processes, peroxynitrite is formed by the action of superoxide and nitrogen monoxide, triggering activation of cellular stress-responsive signaling pathways, some of which may result in cell death (Radi et al., 2000; Klotz et al., 2002). (–)-Epicatechin appears capable of protecting biomolecules from oxidation and nitration by peroxynitrite (Pannala et al., 1997; Haenen et al., 1997; Schroeder et al., 2000). Schroeder and coworkers (2003) demonstrated the importance of the amphiphilic properties of (−)-epicatechin in protecting against peroxynitrite-induced nitration in both hydrophilic and lipophilic cellular phases. The removal or loading of (−)-epicatechin by murine endothelial cells from plasma suggests that under physiological conditions, it may be present to protect against damage from peroxynitrite.

References

El Mohsen, M.M.A., Kuhnle, G., Rchner, A.R., Schroeter, H., Rose, S., Jenner, P., and Rice-Evans, C.A., Uptake and metabolism of epicatechin and its access to the brain after oral ingestion, *Free Rad. Biol. Med.,* 33:1693–1702, 2002.

Geetha, T., Garg, A., Chopra, K., and Kaur, I.P., Delineation of antimutagenic activity of catechin, epicatechin and green tea extract, *Mutat. Res.,* 556: 65–74, 2004.

Haenen, G.R.M.M., Paquay, J.B.G., Korthouwer, R.E.M., and Bast, A., Peroxynitrite scavenging by flavonoids, *Biochem. Biophys. Res. Commun.,* 236: 591–593, 1997.

Klotz, L.O., Schroeder, P., and Sies, H., Peroxynitrite signaling: Receptor tyrosine kinases and activation of stress-responsive pathways, *Free Rad. Biol. Med.,* 33:737–743, 2002.

Pannala, A.S., Rice-Evans, C.A., Halliwell, B., and Singh, S., Inhibition of peroxynitrite-mediated tyrosine nitration by catechin polyphenols, *Biochem. Biophys. Res. Commun.,* 232:164–168, 1997.

Radi, P., Peluffo, G., Alvarez, M.N., Navilat, M., and Cayota, A., Unraveling peroxynitrite formation in biological systems, *Free Rad. Biol. Med.,* 30:463–468, 2001.

Scalbert, A. and Williamson, G., Dietary intake and bioavailability of polyphenols, *J. Nutr.,* 30:2073S–2085S, 2000.

Schroeder, P., Klots, L.O., and Sies, H., Amphiphilic properties of (−)-epicatechin and their significance for protection of cells against peroxynitrite, *Biochem. Biophys. Res. Commun.,* 307:69–73, 2003.

Schroeter, H., Spencer, J.P.E., Rice-Evans, C., and Williams, R.J., Flavonoids protect neurons from oxidized low-density-lipoprotein-induced apoptosis involving c-Jun, N-terminal kinase (JNK), c-Jun and caspase-3, *Biochem. J.,* 358:547–557, 2001.

Wang, J.F., Schramm, D.D., Holt, B.R., Ensunsa, J.L., Fraga, C.G., Schmitz, H.H., and Keen, C.L., A dose–response effect from chocolate consumption on epicatechin and indices of oxidative damage, *J. Nutr.,* 130:2109S–2114S, 2000.

Epigallocatechin gallate (EGCG) *see also* **Green tea** Epicatechin-3-gallate (EGCG) is one of the major water-soluble components in green tea. The antimutagenic properties of EGCG were shown by Muto et al. (1999) to

Epigallocatechin gallate. (Adapted from Furukawa et al., *Biochem. Pharmacol.,* 66:1769–1778, 2003.)

reduce benzo[*a*]pyrene (B[*a*]P)-induced mutations in the *rpsL* gene in the lung of 7-week-old mice by 60 percent. Pretreatment with EGCG was also found by Katiyar et al. (2001) to protect human skin from multiple exposures to UV light by inhibiting the production of hydrogen peroxide and nitric oxide in both the epidermis and dermis, as well as inflammatory leukocytes, CD11b+ (a surface marker of monocytes/macrophages and neutrophils), the major producers of reactive-oxygen species. EGCG protected the antioxidant enzyme, glutathione peroxidase, as well as restored total glutathione levels reduced by UV-exposed skin. Ohishi and coworkers (2002) reported EGCG acted synergistically with Sulindac, a well-established cancer-preventive agent, against colon cancer. The combination of EGCG and Sulindac significantly ($p < 0.01$) reduced the number of aberrant crypt foci (ACF)/colon to

10 ± 3.2 in AOM-induced rat-colon carcinogenesis compared to 21.4 ± 3.4 and 19.5 ± 5.8 for Sulindac and EGCG treatments, respectively. The synergistic effects of the combined treatment with Sulindak and EGCG enhanced apoptosis, suggesting EGCG could reduce the adverse side effects associated with such cancer-preventive agents as sulindak.

The antiatherosclerotic effects of EGCG were due to its inhibition of platelet function from inhibiting cytoplasmic calcium increase (Kang et al., 1999). Recent work by Lill and coworkers (2003) showed EGCG was the only active principle in green tea exerting platelet-inhibitory effects. EGCG was found to interrupt other signaling-transduction pathways, such as phosphorylation of p38 mitogen-activated protein kinase (MAPK) and extracellular signal-regulated kinase (ERK)-1/2. The presence and the location of the galloyl group appeared important for platelet aggregation. Catechin gallate (CG) and epicatechin gallate (ECG), with a galloyl group at the 3′ position, both stimulated platelet aggregation, while catechins without a galloyl group (catechin [C], epicatechin [EC]) or with the group in the 2′ position (epigallocatechin) were inactive.

References

Furukawa, A., Oikawa, S., Murata, M., Hiraku, Y., and Kawanishi, S., (–)-Epigallocatechin gallate causes oxidative damage to isolated and cellular DNA, *Biochem. Pharmacol.*, 66:1769–1778, 2003.

Kang, W.-S., Lim, I.-H., Yuk, D.-Y., Chung, K.-H., Park, J.-B., Yoo, H.-S. and Yun, Y.-P., Antithrombotic activities of green tea catechins and (–)-epigallocatechin gallate, *Thromb. Res.*, 96:229–237, 1999.

Katiyar, S.K., Afaq, F., Perez, A., and Mukhtar, H., Green tea polyphenol (–)-epigallocatechin-3-gallate treatment of human skin inhibits ultraviolet radiation-induced oxidative stress, *Carcinogenesis*, 22: 287–294, 2001.

Lill, G., Voit, S., Schror, K., and Weber, A.-A., Complex effects of different tea catechins on human platelets, *FEBS Lett.*, 546:265–270, 2003.

Muto, S., Yokoi, T., Gondo, Y., Katsuki, M., Shioyama, Y., Fujita, K., and Kamataki, T., Inhibition of benzo[a]pyrene-induced mutagenesis by (–)-epigallocatechin gallate in the lung of *rpsL* transgenic mice, *Carcinogenesis*, 20:421–424, 1999.

Ohishi, T., Kishimoto, Y., Miura, N., Shiota, G., Kohri, T., Hara, Y., Hasegawa, J., and Isemura, M., Synergistic effects of (–)-epigallocatechin gallate with sulindac against colon carcinogenesis of rats treated with azoxymethane, *Cancer Lett.*, 177:49–56, 2002.

Equol Equol (7-hydroxy-3-(4′-hydroxyphenyl-chroman), an estrogenic metabolite of daidzein, is a potent antioxidant formed in the intestinal tract by bacteria (Axelson et al., 1982). The ability to form and excrete equol appears to be linked to the beneficial effects of isoflavone

Equol. (Adapted from Muthyala et al., *Bioorg. Med. Chem.*, 12:1559–1567, 2004.)

intake and its regulation of endogenous hormones (Duncan et al., 2000). Equol excretors, with a more favorable hormone profile, were found to have a significantly lower risk of breast cancer. The more potent antioxidant properties of equol made it a far more effective inhibitor of LDL oxidation compared to daidzein or genistein (Yamakoshi et al., 2000). Hwang et al. (2003) showed equol inhibited LDL oxidation in J744 macrophage cells by reducing superoxide production, in part, by inhibiting NADPH oxidase activity. The overall effect was to prevent the modification of LDL to an atherogenic particle.

In addition to being one of the most biologically active metabolites of daidzein, equol had a significantly longer half-life in the body (Kelly et al., 1995). Equol was reported to have greater antiproliferative (Verma and Goldin, 1998; Dubey et al., 1999) and estrogenic (Markiewicz et al., 1993) activities in nonprostatic cells. The low incidence of prostate cancer in Asians because of the high levels of soy in their diet suggests equol may have a protective role against prostate cancer. Examination of prostatic fluids showed equol levels were present at much higher levels in Asians compared to Caucasians (Morton et al., 1997). Hedlund and coworkers (2003) treated benign and malignant prostatic epithelial human cells with equol, daizein, and genistein within concentration range found in prostatic fluids. Equol was found to be 10 times more potent than daidzein, inhibiting the growth of benign human prostatic epithelial cells by 37 percent and 80 percent in the presence of 10^{-6} and 10^{-5} M, respectively. It also exerted strong, antiproliferative effects against malignant cells at concentrations available in a normal soybean-containing diet.

References

Axelson, M., Kirk, D.N., Farrant, R.D., Cooley, G., Lawson, A.M., and Setcell, K.D.R., The identification of the weak estrogen equol in man and animals, *Biochem. J.,* 201:353–357, 1982.

Dubey, R.K., Gillespie, D.G., Imthurn, P., Rosselli, M., Jackson, E.K., and Keller, P.J., Phytoestrogens inhibit growth and MAP kinase activity in human aortic smooth muscle cells, *Hypertension,* 33(Part 2): 177–182, 1999.

Duncan, A.M., Merz-Demlow, B.E., Xu, X., and Phipps, W.R., Premenopausal equol excretors show plasma hormone profiles associated with lowered risk of breast cancer, *Cancer Epidemiol. Biomarkers Prev.,* 9:581–586, 2000.

Hedlund, T.E., Johannes, W.U., and Miller, G.J., Soy isoflavonoid equol modulates the growth of benign and malignant prostatic epithelial cells *in vitro, Prostate,* 54:68–78, 2003.

Hwang, J., Wang, J., Morazzoni, P., Hodis, H.N., and Sevanian, A., The phytoestrogen equol increases nitric oxide availability by inhibiting superoxide production: An antioxidant mechanism for cell-mediated LDL modification, *Free Rad. Biol. Med.,* 34: 1271–1282, 2003.

Kelly, G.E., Joannou, G.E., Reeder, A.Y., Nelson, C., and Waring, M.A., The variable metabolic response to dietary isoflavones in humans, *Proc. Soc. Exp. Biol. Med.,* 208:40–43, 1995.

Markiewicz, L., Garey, J., Adlecruet, H., and Gurpide, E., *In vitro* bioassays of non-steroidal phytoestrogens, *J. Steroid Biochem. Mol. Biol.,* 45:399–405, 1993.

Morton, M.S., Chan, P.S., Cheng, C., Blacklock, N., and Matos-Fereira, L., Lignans and isoflavonoids in plasma and prostatic fluid in men: Samples from Portugal, Hong Kong, and the United Kingdom, *Prostate,* 32:122–128, 1997.

Muthyala, R.S., Ju, Y.H., Sheng, S., Williams, L.D., Doerge, D.R., Katzenellenbogen, B.S., Helferich, W.G., and Katzenellenbogen, J.A., Equol, a natural estrogenic metabolite from soy isoflavones: Convenient preparation and resolution of R; and S-equols and their differing binding and biological activity through estrogen receptors alpha and beta, *Bioorg. Med. Chem.,* 12:1559–1567, 2004.

Verma, S.P. and Goldin, B.R., Effect of soy-derived isoflavonoids on the induced growth of MCF 7 cells by estrogenic environmental chemicals, *Nutr. Cancer,* 30:232–239, 1998.

Yamakoshi, J., Piskula, M.K., Izumi, T., Tobe, K., Saito, M., Kataoka, S., Obata, A., and Kikuchi, M., Isoflavone aglycone-rich extract without soy protein attenuates atherosclerosis development in cholesterol-fed rats, *J. Nutr.,* 130:1887–1893, 2000.

Esculentin   Esculentin, a coumarin derivative present in many plants, including the Chinese herb *Artemisia scoparia*, has been used for centuries in China as folk medicine. It has multiple biological activities, including inhibiting xanthine oxidase, platelet aggregation, and chemically induced mammary and lung carcinogenesis by *N*-methyl-*N*-nitrosourea and 4-(methylnitrosamino)-1-(3-pyridyl)-1-butanone, respectively (Egan et al., 1990; Okada et al., 1995; Matsunaga et al., 1998; Hecht et al., 1999). In addition to inhibiting soybean lipoxygenase (Neichi et al., 1983), esculentin is an antioxi-

Esculetin. (Pan et al., *Biochem. Pharmacol.,* 65: 1897–1905, 2003. With permission.)

dant (Lin et al., 2000), as well as inhibits the growth of human cancer cells (Noguchi et al., 1995). The antitumor property of esculentin was reported by Chu et al. (2001), as it induced apoptosis in human leukemia cells HL-60. The induction of apoptosis by esculentin was associated with cytochrome c translocation and caspase activation. Further work by Wang et al. (2002) showed esculentin inhibited the growth of human leukemia HL-60 cells in a time- and

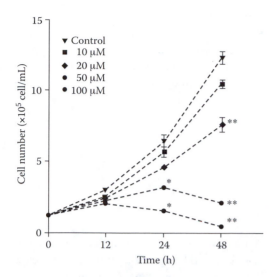

FIGURE E.37 Effect of esculentin on the growth of human leukemia HL-60 cells treated with different concentrations of esculentin for 12, 24, and 48 h. Cells were counted using the tryptan blue-dye exclusion assay. Results are the mean ± SD of three independent experiments, with levels of significance at * $p < 0.05$; ** $p < 0.01$ compared to a control group with DMSO (0.1 percent). (From Wang et al., *J. Cancer Lett.*, 188:163–168, 2002. With permission.)

dose-dependent manner (Figure E.37). A significant inhibition of growth was evident in the presence of 50 and 100 μM. The ability of esculentin to inhibit the growth of human leukemia HL-60 cells involved G1 phase cell-cycle arrest, as a result of inhibition of retinoblastoma protein (pRb) phosphorylation.

Vascular-proliferative disorders, such as atherosclerosis and restenosis, result from the proliferation of vascular smooth cells (VSMCs) induced by injury to the intima of the arteries. Recent studies by Pan et al. (2003) showed esculentin effectively inhibited VSMC proliferation and intima hyperplasia by blocking intima thickening in the artery of rats. Inhibition of cell proliferation by esculentin occurred via inhibition of an upstream effector of Ras and downstream events for three predominant signaling pathways, p42/44 MAPK activation, PI-3 activation, and early gene expression, as well as NK-κB and AP-1 activation. These results point to the potential therapeutic use of esculentin for treatment of restenosis following arterial injury.

References

Chu, C.-Y., Tsai, Y.-Y., Wang, C.-J., Lin, W.-L., and Tseng, T.-H., Induction of apoptosis by esculentin in human leukemia cells, *Eur. J. Pharmacol.*, 416:25–32, 2001.

Egan, D., O'Kennedy, R., Moran, E., Cox, D., Prosser, E., and Thornes, R.D., The pharmacology, metabolism, analysis and applications of coumarin and coumarin-related compounds, *Drug. Metab. Rev.*, 22:503–529, 1990.

Hecht, S.S., Kenney, P.M.J., Wang, M., Trushin, N., Angarwal, S., Rao, A.V., and Upadhyaya, P., Evaluation of butylated hydroxyanisole, myo-inositol, curcumin, esculentin, resveratrol and lycopene as inhibitors of benzo[a]pyrene plus 4-(methylnitrosamino)-1-(3-pyridyl)-1-butanone-induced lung tumorogenesis in A/J mice, *Cancer Lett.*, 137:123–130, 1999.

Lin, W.L., Wang, C.J., Tsai, Y.Y., Liu, C.L., Hwang, J.M., and Tseng, T.H., Inhibitory effect of esculentin on oxidative damage induced by *t*-butyl hydroperoxide, *Arch. Toxicol.*, 74:467–472, 2000.

Matsunaga, K., Yoshimi, N., Yamada, Y., Shimizu, M., Kawabata, K., Ozawa, Y., Hara, A., and Mori, H., Inhibitory effects of Nabumetone, a cyclooxygenase-2 inhibitor, and esculentin, a lipoxygenase inhibitor, on *N*-methyl-*N*-nitroso- urea-induced mammary carcinogenesis in rats, *Jpn. J. Cancer Res.*, 89:496–501, 1998.

Neichi, T., Koshihara, Y., and Murota, S.I., Inhibitory effect of esculentin on 5-lipoxygenase and leukotriene biosynthesis, *Biochem. Biophys. Acta*, 753: 130–132, 1983.

Noguchi, M., Earashi, M., Minami, M., Miyazaki, I., Tanaka, M., and Sasaki, T., Effects of piroxicam and esculentin on the MDA-MB-231 human, *Prostaglands Leukotrienes Ess. Fatty Acids*, 53:325–329, 1995.

Okada, Y., Miyauchi, N., Suzuki, K., Kobayashi, T., Tsutsui, C., Mayuzumi, K., Nishibe, S., and Okuyama, T., Search for naturally occurring substances to prevent the complications of diabetes: II. Inhibitory effect of coumarin and flavonoid derivatives on bovine lens aldose reductase and rabbit platelet aggregation, *Chem. Pharm. Bull.*, 43:1385–1387, 1995.

Pan, S.-L., Huang, Y.-W., Guh, J.-H., Chang, Y.-L., Peng, C.-Y., and Teng, C.-M., Esculentin inhibits Ras-mediated cell proliferation and attenuates vascular restenosis following angioplasty in rats, *Biochem. Pharmacol.*, 65:1897–1905, 2003.

E

Wang, C.-J., Hsieh, Y.-J., Chu, C.-Y., Lin, Y.-L., and Tseng, T.-H., Inhibition of cell cycle progression in human leukemia HL-60 cells by esculentin, *Cancer Lett.*, 183:163–168, 2002.

Ethanol *see also* **Alcohol**   Overall epidemiological evidence points to an association between alcohol consumption and increased risk of breast cancer (Smith-Warner et al., 1998). The association between alcohol consumption and circulating levels of steroid hormones, such as estradiol (Ginsberg, 1999), impaired immune systems, greater proliferation of mammary glands, and altered carcinogen metabolism (Singletary, 1997) are among the mechanisms proposed. Alcohol intake has also been linked to greater risks for breast tumors, depending on their hormone-receptor status. Singletary et al. (2003) showed increased cell proliferation, and cellular cAMP content only occurred when ethanol was added to human breast-cancer cell lines supplemented with estrogen receptors (ER+). Thus, the ability of ethanol to only stimulate proliferation of human breast-cancer cells with specific hormone-receptor characteristics may explain the modest increase in breast-cancer risk observed in epidemiological studies.

References

Ginsberg, E., Estrogen, alcohol and breast cancer risk, *J. Steroid Biochem. Mol. Biochem.*, 69:131–137, 1999.

Singletary, K., Ethanol and experimental breast cancer: A review, *Alcohol. Clin. Exp. Res.*, 21:334–339, 1997.

Singletary, K., Frey, R.S., and Yan, W., Effect of ethanol on proliferation and estrogen receptor-α expression in human breast cancer cells, *Cancer Lett.*, 165:131–137, 2001.

Smith-Warner, S., Spiegelman, D., Yaun, S., Vanden-Brandt, P., Folsom, A., Goldbohm, A., Graham, S.F., Holmberg, L., Howe, G., Marshall, J., Miller, A., Potter, J., Speizer, F., Willett, W., Wolk, A., and Hunder, D., Alcohol and breast cancer: A pooled analysis of cohort studies, *J. Am. Med. Assoc.*, 279:535–540, 1998.

Eugenol   Eugenol (4-allyl-1-hydroxy-2-methoxybenzene), a naturally occurring alkenylbenzene, is found in cloves, as well as in cinnamon, basil, and nutmeg (Rompelberg et al., 1993).

Eugenol. (Yoo et al., *Cancer Lett.*, 225:41–52, 2005. With permission.)

While it is used mainly as a flavoring agent, it was shown to be an effective inducer of detoxifying phase II enzyme (Rompelberg et al., 1993; Newberne et al., 1999). Eugenol also behaves as a chain-breaking antioxidant and inhibits lipid peroxidation (Nagababu and Lakshmaiah, 1992). The antimutagenic properties of eugenol were confirmed in a number of different studies (Rompelberg et al., 1995, 1996 a, b, c). Abraham (2001) examined the antigenotoxic effects of *trans*-anethole and eugenol in male Swiss albino mice treated with genotoxins, cyclophosphamide (CPH), ethyl methane sulfonate (EMS), *N*-methyl-*N*-nitro-*N*-nitrosoguanidine (MNNG), micronucleated polychromatic erythrocytes (Mn PCEs), procarbazine (PCB), polychromatic erythrocytes (PCEs), and urethane (URE). No antigenotoxic effects were observed when mice were administered eugenol and *trans*-anethole separately. However, pretreatment with both of these flavoring agents resulted in significant antigenotoxic effects against CPH, MNNG, and EMS. Dose-related antigenotoxic effects were also reported for both eugenol and *trans*-anethole against PCB and URE. A moderate, protective effect against these genotoxins was only observed in the combined presence of eugenol and *trans*-anethole.

The antiviral activity of eugenol was demonstrated by Benencia and Courreges (2000), who found it delayed the development of herpetic keratitis in the cornea of HSV-1 mice. *In vitro* studies showed eugenol inhibited the replication of the human herpesvirus and behaved synergistically with the drug acycloivir.

E

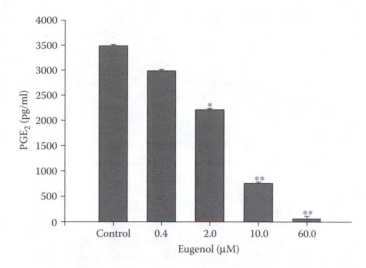

FIGURE E.38 Effects of eugenol on COX-2 enzyme activity in RAW264.7 cells stimulated with LPS (1 μg/mL) for 24 h and pretreated with eugenol for 30 min prior to adding exogenous arachidonic acid. After 15 min, the supernatant was removed and analyzed for PGE_2. Values significantly different from the control are shown by; *, $p < 0.05$, **, $p < 0.01$). (Kim et al., *Life Sci.,* 73:337–348, 2003. With permission.)

Kim et al. (2003) studied the effect of eugenol, isolated from clove (*Eugenia caryophyllata*), on COX-2 and gene expression of lipopolysaccharide (LPS)-activated mouse macrophages. Since COX-2 is implicated in inflammatory and carcinogenic processes, inhibition of this enzyme could help to prevent these processes. The direct inhibition of COX-2 by eugenol was demonstrated by its inhibition of PGE_2 formation in a dose-dependent manner in intact cells where the enzyme was induced by LPS and exogenous arachidonic acid as substrate (Figure E.38). Eugenol also inhibited the growth of human cancer cells by suppression of COX-2 gene expression, suggesting a possible role in cancer prevention.

An *ortho* dimer of eugenol, *bis*-eugenol, was shown by Murakami et al. (2003) to be a more potent antioxidant than eugenol and less cytotoxic. It inhibited lipopolysaccharide-stimulated activation of NF-κB, a transcriptional factor regulating inflammatory responses and cytokine expression. These researchers suggested *bis*-eugenol could be used in preventing oral diseases, as inhibition of NF-κB may prevent bacterium-stimulated alveolar bone resorption associated with adult periodontal diseases.

bis-Eugenol. (Murakami et al., *Biochem. Pharmacol.,* 66:1061–1066, 2003. With permission.)

References

Abraham, S.K., Anti-genotoxicity of *trans*-anethole and eugenol in mice, *Food Chem. Toxicol.,* 39:493–498, 2001.

Benencia, F. and Courreges, M.C., *In vitro* and *in vivo* activity of eugenol on human herpesvirus, *Phytother. Res.,* 14:495–500, 2000.

Kim, S.S., Oh, O.-J., Min, Y., Park, E.-J., Kim, Y., Park, H.J., Han, Y.N., and Lee, S.K., Eugenol suppresses cyclooxygenase-2 expression in lipopolysaccharide-stimulated mouse macrophage RAW264.7 cell, *Life Sci.,* 73:337–348, 2003.

Murakami, Y., Shoji, M., Hanazawa, S., Tanaka, S., and Fujisawa, S., Prevention effect of *bis*-eugenol, a *eugenol ortho dimer,* on lipolysaccharide-stimulated nuclear factor κB activation and inflammatory cytokine expression in macrophages, *Biochem. Pharmacol.,* 66:1061–1066, 2003.

Nagababu, E. and Lakshmaiah, N., Inhibitory effect of eugenol on non-enzymatic lipid peroxidation in rat liver mitochondria, *Biochem. Pharmacol.*, 43: 2393–2400, 1992.

Newberne, P., Smith, R.L., Doull, J., Goodman, J.L., Munro, I.C., Portoghese, P.S., Wagner, B.M., Weil, C.S., Woods, L.A., Adams, T.B., Lucas, C.D., and Ford, R.A., The FEMA GRAS assessment of *trans*-anethole used as a flavouring agent, *Food Chem. Toxicol.*, 37:789–811, 1999.

Rompelberg, C.J.M., Verhagen, H., and van Bladeren, P.J., Effects of the naturally occurring alkenyl-benzenes eugenol and *trans*-anethole on drug-metabolizing enzymes in the rat liver, *Food Chem. Toxicol.*, 31:637–645, 1993.

Rompelberg, C.J.M., Stenhuis, W.H., de Vogel, N., van Osenbruggen, W.A., Schouten, A., and Verhagen, H., Antimutagenicity of eugenol in the rodent bone marrow micronucleus test, *Mutat. Res.*, 346:69–75, 1995.

Rompelberg, C.J.M., Evertz, S.J.C.J., Bruijntjes-rozier, G.C.D.M., van den Heuvel, P.D., and Verhagen, H., Effect of eugenol on the genotoxicity of established mutagens in the liver, *Food Chem. Toxicol.*, 34:33–42, 1996a.

Rompelberg, C.J.M., Steenwinkel, S.T., van Asten, J.G., van Deft, J.H., Baan, R.A., and Verhagen, H., Effect of eugenol on the mutagenicity of benz(a)pyrene and the formation of benz(a)pyrene-DNA adducts in the λ-*lac* Z-transgenic mouse, *Mutat. Res.*, 369:87–96, 1996b.

Rompelberg, C.J.M., Vogels, J.T., de Vogel, N., Bruijntjes-Rozier, G.C., Stenhuis, W.H., Bogaards, J.J., and Verhagen, H., Effect of short term dietary administration of eugenol in humans, *Human Expt. Toxicol.*, 15:129–135, 1996c.

Yoo, C.-B., Han, K.-T., Cho, K.-S., Ha, J., Park, H.-J., Nam, J.-H., Kil, U.-H., and Lee, K.-T., Eugenol isolated from the essential oil of *Eugenia caryphyllata* induces a reactive oxygen species-mediated apoptosis in HL-60 human promyelocytic leukemia cells, *Cancer Lett.*, 225:41–52, 2005.

Evening primrose Evening primrose (*Oenothera biennis* L.) is a biennial plant belonging to the family *Onagracea*, a common weed native to North America. The oil content of the seeds is in range 17–25 percent, of which 7–10 percent is gamma linolenic acid (GLA, C18:3ω-6).

There is a growing demand for evening primrose oil because of the clinical and pharmaceutical applications associated with GLA. Oral administration of evening primrose, attributed to GLA, was found to substantially inhibit the growth of implanted human tumors in rats. High doses of oral GLA in the form of evening primrose oil elicited a response that prolonged life, without side effects, of patients suffering from liver, breast, brain, and esophageal cancers (Horrobin, 1994). The British Department of Health licensed evening primrose oil for the treatment of breast pain and premenstrual disease because of the effectiveness of GLA in relieving these symptoms (Horrobin, 1992).

Diabetes impairs the conversion of linoleic acid to its ω6-desaturated metabolites in humans, which is associated with renal, retinal, and neurological damage. In alcoholics, GLA appears to accelerate recovery of the liver, as well as reduce the severity of withdrawal symptoms. Other studies have shown GLA significantly reduced skin roughness in atopic eczema, as well as some clinical benefits on rheumatoid arthritis (Belch and Hill, 2000). Hamburger and coworkers (2002) recently found lipophilic radical scavengers in cold-pressed, nonraffinated evening primrose oil. Three esters exhibiting the most pronounced radical-scavenging activities and potent inhibitors of neutophil elastase and cyclooxygenase 1 and 2 *in vitro* were 3-*O*-*trans*-caffeoyl derivatives of betulinic, morolic, and oleanolic acids. In addition to GLA, evening primrose also contains antioxidative phenolic compounds (Shahidi et al., 1997). Subsequent work by Amarowicz et al. (1999) found pronounced antioxidative activity in the ethanol extracts of evening primrose, as well as its hydrophilic and hydrophobic fractions.

References

Amarowicz, R., Raab, B., and Karamac, M., Antioxidative activity of an ethanolic extract of evening primrose, *Nahrung*, 43:216–217, 1999.

Belch, J.J.F. and Hill, A., Evening primrose and borage oil in rheumatological conditions, *Am. J. Clin. Nutr.*, 71:352S–356S, 2000.

Hamburger, M., Riese, U., Graf, H., Melzig, M.F., Ciesielski, S., Baumann, D., Dittman, K. and Wagner, C., Constituents in evening primrose oil with radical scavenging cyclooxygenase and nutrophil elastase inhibitory activities, *J. Agric. Food. Chem.,* 50:5533–5538, 2002.

Horrobin, D.F., Nutritional and medical importance of gamma-linolenic acid, *Prog. Lipid Res.,* 31:163–194, 1992.

Horrobin, D.F., Unsaturated lipids: A new approach to the treatment of cancer, in *Effect of Fatty Acids and Lipids in Health and Medicine,* Diplock, A.T., Gutteridge, J.M.C., and Shukla, V.K.S., Eds., International Food Science Centre, Lystrup, Denmark, 1994, pp. 181–198.

Shahidi, F., Amarowicz, R., He, Y., and Wettasinghe, M., Antioxidant activity of phenolic extracts of evening primrose (*Oenothera biennis*): a preliminary study, *Food Lip.,* 4:75–86, 1997.

E

F

Farnesol Farnesol, a nonsteroid isoprenoid intermediate formed from mevalonate, is found in orange-peel oil and lemon-grass oil. In mammalian cells, farnesol is metabolized to farnesal, farnesoic acid, and prenyldicarboxylic acids (Bostedor et al., 1997). Isoprenoids, such as farnesol, are involved in cell-signaling transduction, as its phosphorylated form, farnesyl

Farnesol. (Adapted from Rao et al., *Cancer Det. Prev.*, 26:419–425, 2002.)

pyrophosphate, is needed for protein prenylation (Gelb,1997). Terpenoids, such as farnesol, with hydroxyl groups appear more active than terpene hydrocarbons by inhibiting MIA ZpaCa2 pancreatic-tumor cells (Burke et al., 1997). Farnesol was reported to inhibit the proliferation of some cell lines and induce apoptosis in a number of tumor-derived cell lines (Burke et al., 1997; Yasugi et al.,1994). Rioja et al. (2000) showed farnesol preferentially inhibited proliferation and induced apoptosis of leukemic cells without affecting normal, nontransformed cell lines.

Raner et al. (2002) observed that only farnesol, and not related isoprenoids, geranylgeraniol, geranylgeranyl pyroposphate (GGPP), and farnesyl pyrophosphate (FPP), inhibited certain rabbit-liver microsomal cytochrome P450 enzymes (Table F.26). Since cytochrome P450 plays a prominent role in the metabolism of pharmaceuticals and activation of potential carcinogens, its inhibition has important health benefits. Studies on AOM-induced colon carcinogenesis in rats by Rao et al. (2002) noted the chemopreventive properties of farnesol as it inhibited the formation of preneoplastic lesions in rats fed a diet containing 1.5 percent farnesol. Farnesol significantly inhibited ACF formation by 34 percent, while reducing multiplicity by 44 percent.

TABLE F.26
Percent Inhibition of Different P450 Activities in Rabbit-Liver Microsomes and a Reconstituted P450$_{2E1}$ System By Four Different Isoprenoids[1,2]

Activity	Farnesol	Geranylgeraniol	FPP	GGPP
In rabbit-liver microsomes				
p-Nitrophenol hydroxylation (30 μm)	60 ± 5	0 ± 1	0 ± 2	10 ± 5
Diclofenac-4-hydroxylation (0.20 mM)	45 ± 2	2 ± 1	0 ± 1	1 ± 1
Caffeine-N-demethylation (2.0 mM)	35 ± 2	0 ± 1	0 ± 1	0 ± 1
In reconstituted P450$_{2e1}$-3-27				
p-Nitrophenol hydroxylation (45 μM)	43 ± 3	2 ± 2	5 ± 3	3 ± 1

[1] Concentration of each isoprenoid was 80 μM.

[2] Errors based on the average deviation from the mean for three or more trials.

Source: From Raner et al., *Biochem. Biophys. Res. Commun.*, 293:1–6, 2002. With permission.

F

References

Bostedor, R.G., Karkas, J.D., Arison, B.H., Bansai, V.S., Vaidya, S., Gemershausen, J.I., Kurtz, M.M., and Bergstrom, J.D., Farnesol-derived dicarboxylic acids in the urine of animals treated with zaragozic acid A or with farnesol, *J. Biol. Chem.,* 272:9197–9203, 1997.

Burke, Y.D., Stark, M.J., Roach, S.L., Sen, S.E., and Crowell, P.L., Inhibition of pancreatic cancer growth by the dietary isoprenoids farnesol and geraniol, *Lipids*, 32:151–156, 1997.

Gelb, M.H., Protein prenylation, et cetera: Signal transduction in two dimensions, *Science,* 275:1750–1751, 1997.

Raner, G.M., Muir, A.Q., Lowry, C.W., and Davis, B.A., Farnesol as an inhibitor and substrate for rabbit liver microsomal P450 enzymes, *Biochem. Biophys. Res. Commun.,* 293:1–6, 2002.

Rao, C.V., Newmark, H.L., and Reddy, B.S., Chemo-preventive effect of farnesol and lanosterol on colon carcinogenesis, *Cancer Det. Prev.,* 26:419–425, 2002.

Rioja, A., Pizzey, A.R., Marson, C.M., and Thomas, N.S.B., Preferential induction of apoptosis of leukemic cells by farnesol, *FEBS Lett.,* 467:291–295, 2000.

Yasugi, E., Yokoyama, Y., Seyama, Y., Kano, K., Hayashi, Y., and Oshima, M., Dolichyl phosphate, a potent inducer of apoptosis in rat glioma C6 cells, *Biochem. Biophys. Res. Commun.,* 216:848–853, 1995.

Fennel   Fennel (*Foeniculum vulgare* Mill.) is an aromatic herb grown in Europe and Asia. The essential oil from the seeds of fennel has been used in foods, cosmetics, and pharmaceuticals. The major constituent of fennel oil is (E)-anethole (80 percent), followed by methyl chavicol (10 percent) and fenchone (7.5 percent) (Brand, 1993). Minor constituents include γ-pinene, limonene, β-pinene, α-myrcene, and

Arethole chavical. (Adapted from Gross et al., *Plant Sci.,* 163:1047–1053, 2002.)

para-cymene (Brand, 1993; Toth, 1967; Trenkle, 1972). The essential oil of *Foeniculum vulgare* was found by Ozbeck et al. (2003) to exert a potent hepatoprotective effect against carbon tetrachloride (CCl_4)-induced liver damage in rats.

Fennel seeds have been reported to promote menstruation, alleviate female climacteric, as well as increase libido (Albert-Puelo, 1980). Because of its antispasmodic effects, it has been used to treat some respiratory disorders (Reynolds, 1982). In folk medicine, fennel has been used to treat a number of gynecological complaints, such as dysmenorrhea, a condition of severe pain during menstruation. One of the major reasons for primary dysmenorrhea is increased ectopic uterine motility. Ostad et al. (2001) showed fennel essential oil significantly reduced the intensity of oxytocin- and PGE_2-induced uterine contractions obtained from virgin Wistar rats. Subsequent work by Namavar Jahromi et al. (2003) compared the effectiveness of sweet fennel (*Foeniculum vulgare* var. *duice*) and mefenamic acid in the treatment of primary dysmenorrhea in 70 women 15–24 years old, suffering from this problem. The results in Table F.27 show mefenamic acid was more effective in reducing pain intensity on the second and third days of menstruation, but there were no significant differences on any of the other days. This study corroborates earlier studies confirming the effectiveness of fennel extract in treating primary dysmenorrhea.

References

Albert-Puleo, M., Fennel and anise as estrogenic agent, *J. Ethonopharmacol.,* 2:337–344, 1980.

Brand, N., 1993. *Hagers handbuch der pharmazeutischen praxis,* in Hansel, R., Keller, K., Rimpler, H., and Schneider, G., Eds., Springer-Verlag, Berlin/Heidelberg, 5, 1993, pp. 156–181.

Gross, M., Friedman, J., Dudai, N., Larkov, O., Cohen, Y., Bar, E., Ravid, U., Putievsky, E., and Lewinsohn, E., Biosynthesis of estragole and *t*-anethole in bitter fennel (*Foeniculum vulgare* Mill. Var. *vulgare*) chemotypes, Changes in SAM: phenylpropene *O*-methyltransferase activities during development, *Plant Sci.,* 163:1047–1053, 2002.

TABLE F.27
Mean Intensity of Pain Reported By the Subjects and *P*-Values Measured Using the Paired *T*-Test for the Treated Cycles

Days	Control Cycles	Mefanamic-Acid-Treated Cycles	Fennel-Extract-Treated Cycles	*P*-Values
Day 1	9.9667	9.4167	9.5833	0.382
Day 2	7.0667	4.4167	5.4167	0.024
Day 3	4.2333	2.1667	3.125	0.052
Day 4	1.8667	0.5833	0.9583	0.384
Day 5	0.2759	0.167	0.1167	0.184

Source: From Namavar Jahromi et al., *Inter. J. Gynecol. Obstr.,* 80:153–157, 2003. With permission.

Namavar Jahromi, B.N., Tartifizadeh, A., and Khabnadideh, S., Comparison of fennel and mefenamic acid for the treatment of primary dysmenorrhea, *Inter. J. Gynecol. Obstr.,* 80:153–157, 2003.

Ozbek, H., Ugras, S., Dulger, H., Bayram, I., Tuncer, I., Ozturk, G., and Ozturk, A., Hepatoprotective effect of *Foeniculum vulgare* essential oil, *Fitoterapia,* 74:317–319, 2003.

Reynolds, E.F.J.F., Essential oils and aromatic carminatives, *The Extra Pharmacopeia* 28th edition. *Royal Pharmaceutical Soc.,* Martindale, Lond. 1982, p. 670–676.

Toth, L., Studies on the etheric oil of *Foeniculum vulgare,* II. Changes of different fennel oils before and after harvest, *Planta Med.,* 15:371, 1967.

Trenkle, K., Recent studies on fennel (*Foeniculum vulgare* M.), 2. The volatile oil of the fruit, herbs and roots of fruit-bearing plants, *Pharmazie,* 27:319–324, 1972.

Fenugreek   Fenugreek (*Trigonella foenum graecum*) seeds, widely used as a condiment, have also proved beneficial in India for the treatment of gastric disorders (Puri, 1968). They were shown to be beneficial in treating diabetics and hypercholesterolemic patients (Sharma et al., 1996). Pandian and coworkers (2002) reported that several fenugreek fractions were effective in treating an HCl-ethanol-induced gastric ulcer in rats compared to one of the commonly prescribed drugs, omeprazole. Fenugreek seeds were extracted with water and centrifuged with the supernatant used as the aqueous extract. A gel fraction was also prepared, following the procedure of Madar and Shomer (1990), which represented the polysaccharides of the seed coat. The severity of the ulcers was reduced markedly, following pretreatment of the rats with the fenugreek fractions prior to HCl-ethanol treatment. Maximum inhibition was observed with doses of 3 mL of the aqueous fractions and 700 mg of the gel fraction, with the results summarized in Table F.28. The fenugreek fraction proved to be as effective as omeprazole against the ulcerogenic effects of ethanol. Lipid peroxidation, as measured by TBARS, was found to be significantly lower in the pretreated rats compared to ethanol-treated rats, suggesting antioxidant activity in the fenugreek extracts, due possibly to the presence of flavonoids.

Al-Habouri and Raman (1998) reviewed the literature related to antidiabetic and hypocholesterolemic effects of fenugreek. While the antidiabetic effects were attributed to the gum fiber, the hypolipidemic effects were due to the saponins and sapogenins confined fiber. The lack of toxicity associated with fenugreek makes it excellent for management of diabetes and hypercholesterolemia. Recent work by Bin-Hafeez et al. (2003) showed fenugreek also had appreciable immunostimulatory activity.

Concern was raised regarding the potential of fenugreek to react with medications, such as warfarin (Lambert and Cormier, 2001; Heck et al., 2000). In addition, fenugreek may also potentiate antihypertensive and antidiabetic medication, as well as increase the risk of bleeding in women taking nonsteroidal anti-inflammatories, such as aspirin (Abebe, 2002).

TABLE F.28

Effect of Pretreatment with Fenugreek-Aqueous Extract (3 mL/rat), Gel Fraction (700 mg/rat), and Omeprazole (10 mg/rat) on the Volume of Gastric Secretion, Total Acidity, Pepsin Activity, and Protein Content in Ethanol-Treated Rats

	Normal	HCl-EtOH	Fenugreek-Aqueous Extract + HCl-EtOH	Fenugreek Gel + HCl-EtOH	Omeprazole + HCl-EtOH
Volume	3.38 ± 0.16	$5.73 \pm 1.9^*$	$4.00 \pm 1.77^{**}$	$4.8 \pm 0.23^{**}$	$4.2 \pm 0.20^{**}$
Total acidity[1]	121.0 ± 10	$74.4 \pm 15.5^*$	$60.43 \pm 6.8^{**}$	$68.5 \pm 4.8^{**}$	76.6 ± 1.8
Pepsin activity[2]	1.56 ± 0.2	$2.56 \pm 0.6^*$	$1.64 \pm 0.04^{**}$	$1.65 \pm 0.2^{**}$	$1.64 \pm 0.03^{**}$
Protein (mg/mL)	0.96 ± 0.2	$3.78 \pm 0.05^*$	$2.35 \pm 0.07^{**}$	$2.38 \pm 0.7^{**}$	$1.83 \pm 0.05^{**}$
Ulcer score	0	25.8 ± 0.75	11.16 ± 0.75	$9.14 \pm 1.27^{**}$	$17.6 \pm 1.5^{**}$

[1] mEq/3 h.

[2] µg tyrosine liberated/mg protein/h. Values are means $\pm$ S.D. from six rats in each group. *As compared to normal $p < 0.05$ (Student's t-test). **As compared to ethanol-treated, $p < 0.05$ (Student's t-test).

Source: From Suja Pandian et al., *J. Ethnopharmacol.*, 81:393–397, 2002. With permission.

Tiran (2003) cautioned women with such pre-existing conditions as gastrointestinal upset, diabetes, hypertensive disease, and cardiac disease or who are breast-feeding against using fenugreek.

References

Abebe, W., Herbal medication: Potential for adverse interactions with analgesic drugs, *J. Clin. Pharm. Ther.*, 27:391–401, 2002.

Al-Habori, M. and Raman, A., Antidiabetic and hypocholesterolemic effects of fenugreek, *Phytother. Res.*, 12:233–242, 1998.

Bin-Hafeez, B., Haque, R., Parvez, S., Pandey, S., Sayeed, I., and Raisuddin, S., Immunomodulatory effects of fenugreek (*Trigonella foenum graecum* L.) extract in mice, *Inter. Immunopharmacol.*, 3:257–265, 2003.

Heck, A.M., De Witt, B.A., and Lukes, A.L., Potential interactions between alternative therapies and warfarin, *Am. J. Health System Pharm.*, 17:1221–1227, 2000.

Lambert, J.P. and Cormier, A., Potential interaction between warfarin and boldo-fenugreek, *Pharmacotherapy*, 21:509–512, 2001.

Madar, Z. and Shomer, I., Polysaccharide composition of a gel fraction derived from fenugreek and its effect on starch digestion and bile acid absorption in rats, *J. Agric. Food Chem.*, 38:1535–1539, 1990.

Pandian, R., Anuradha, C.V., and Viswanathan, P., Gastroprotective effect of fenugreek seeds (*Trigonella foenum graecum*) on experimental gastric ulcer in rats, *J. Ethnopharmacol.*, 81:393–397, 2002.

Puri, D., Therapeutic potentials of fenugreek, *Indian J. Physiol. Pharmacol.*, 42:423–424, 1998.

Sharma, R.D., Sarkar, A., Hazra, D.K., and Misra, B., Hypolipidaemic effect of fenugreek seeds: A chronic study in non-insulin dependent diabetic patients, *Phytotherapy Res.*, 10:332–334, 1996.

Tiran, D., The use of fenugreek for breast feeding women, *Compl. Ther in Nurs. Midwif.*, 9:155–156, 2003.

Ferulic acid   Ferulic acid, found widely in fruits and vegetables, has strong antioxidant properties against peroxynitrite (Pannala et al., 1998) and oxidized low-density lipoprotein *in vitro* (Schroeder et al., 2000). Kanski and coworkers (2002) showed ferulic greatly reduced free-radical damage in neuronal-cell systems without causing cell death by protecting them against oxidative stress from hydroxyl and peroxyl radicals. This study pointed to the importance of natural antioxidants, such as ferulic acid,

Ferulic acid. (Adapted from Pannala et al., *Free Rad. Biol. Med.*, 24:594–606, 1998.)

TABLE F.29
Incidence and Multiplicity of Intestinal Tumors in Each Group[1]

Treatment	No. of Rats	Incidence[2] (%) and Multiplicity (Number in Parentheses)		
		Entire Intestine	Small Intestine	Large Intestine
(1) AOM alone	22	68(1.00 ± 0.90)	23(0.32 ± 0.63)	59(0.68 ± 0.63)
(2) AOM + 250 ppm FA[3]	22	32[5](0.36 ± 0.57)	5(0.05 ± 0.21)	32(0.32 ± 0.47)[6]
(3) AOM + 500 ppm FA[3]	22	36[6](0.45 ± 0.72)[5]	5(0.05 ± 0.21)	32(0.41 ± 0.72)
(4) AOM + 250 ppm FA[4]	22	55(0.64 ± 0.64)	23(0.23 ± 0.42)	41(0.41 ± 0.49)
(5) AOM + 500 ppm FA[4]	22	11(0.68 ± 0.76)	27(0.27 ± 0.45)	36(0.41 ± 0.58)
(6) 500 ppm FA alone	16	0	0	0
(7) No treatment	16	0	0	0

[1] AOM given once a week for three weeks at a dose of 15 mg/kg.
[2] No. of rats with colonic tumors/no. of rats examined.
[3] FA (Ferulic acid) exposure during initiation of the phase.
[4] FA (Ferulic acid) exposure during the postinitiation phase.
[5] Significantly different from AOM alone; $p < 0.03$.
[6] Significantly different from AOM alone; $p < 0.01$.
[7] Significantly different from AOM alone; $p < 0.05$.

Source: From Kawabata et al., *Cancer Lett.*, 157:15–21, 2000. With permission.

as a therapeutic agent against neurodegenerative disorders, such as Alzheimer's disease. A novel chemical derivative of ferulic acid (FA15) made by Murakami et al. (2000) to suppress phorbol ester-induced Epstein–Barr virus activation and superoxide anion generation *in vitro*. Murakami and coworkers (2002) later showed that, unlike ferulic acid, FA15 significantly attenuated phorbol ester-triggered hydrogen-peroxide production, edema formation, and papilloma development in ICR mouse skin. The ferulic-acid derivative, FA15, appeared to be a novel chemopreventive agent.

Ferulic acid was also a potent inhibitor of mutagenesis and carcinogenesis induced by polycyclic aromatic hydrocarbon. For example, ferulic acid prevented 4-nitroquinoline 1-oxide (4-QO)-induced tongue carcinogenesis in rats (Tanaka et al., 1993) and depressed TPA-induced skin tumorigenesis and pulmonary cancers in mice (Asanoma et al., 1994; Lesca, 1983). Kawabata et al. (2000) reported dietary ferulic acid significantly reduced the total number of aberrant crypt foci (ACF) in the colon of azoxymethane-treated (AOM) male rats. The incidence and multiplicity of intestinal neoplasms were also significantly reduced, as shown in Table F.29. The values obtained in the intestine, in the presence of ferulic acid, tended to be lower compared to treatment with AOM alone. The multiplicity of tumors in the entire intestine was significantly reduced in groups 2 and 3, in the large intestine in group, compared to group 1. The blocking effect of ferulic acid on AOM-induced colon carcinogenesis appeared to be related to its significant elevation of phase II detoxifying enzymes, glutathione *S*-transferase in the liver, and quinone reductase in the liver and colinic mucosa.

Rouau and coworkers (2003) recently detected a trimer of ferulic acid in alkali extracts of maize bran. Using 1D and 2D NMR, the structure of the trimer was identified as 4-*O*-8′, 5′-dehydrotriferulic acid.

References

Asanoma, M., Takahashi, K., Miyabe, M., Yamanoto, K., Yoshimi, N., Mori, H., and Kawazoe, Y., Inhibitory effect of topical application of polymerized ferulic acid, a synthetic lignin, on tumor promotion in mouse skin two-stage tumorigenesis, *Carcinogenesis*, 15:2069–2071, 1994.

Kawabata, K., Yamanoto, T., Hara, A., Shimizu, M., Yamada, Y., Matsunaga, K., Tanaka, T., and Mori, H., Modifying effects of ferulic acid on azoxymethane-induced colon carcinogenesis, *Cancer Lett.*, 157:15–21, 2000.

Kanski, J., Aksenova, M., Stoyanova, A., and But-terfield, D.A., Ferulic acid antioxidant protection against hydroxyl and peroxyl radical oxidation in synaptosomal and neuronal cell culture systems *in vitro*: Structure-activity studies, *J. Nutr. Biochem.,* 13:273–281, 2002.

Lesca, P., Protective effects of ellagic acid and other plant phenols on benzo[s]pyrene-induced neoplasia in mice, *Carcinogenesis,* 4:1651–1653, 1983.

Murakami, A., Kadota, M., Takahashi, D., Taniguchi, H., Nomura, E., Hosoda, A., Tsuno, T., Maruta, Y., Ohogashi, H., and Koshimizu, K., Suppressive effects of novel ferulic acid derivatives on cellular responses induced by phorbol ester by combined lipolysaccharide and interferon-gamma, *Cancer Lett.,* 157:77–85, 2000.

Murakami, A., Nakamura, Y., Koshimizu, K., Taka-hashi, D., Matsumoto, K., Hagihara, K., Taniguchi, H., Nomura, E., Hosoda, A., Tsuno, T., Maruta, Y., Kim, H.W., Kawabata, K., and Ohigashi, H., FA15, a hydro-phobic derivative of ferulic acid, suppresses inflamma-tory responses and skin tumor promotion: Comparison with ferulic acid, *Cancer Lett.,* 180:121–129, 2002.

Pannala, R., Razaq, B., Halliwell, S., Singh, C.A., and Rice-Evans, C.A., Inhibition of peroxynitrite dependent tyrosine nitration by hydroxycinnamates: Nitration or electron donation? *Free Rad. Biol. Med.,* 24:594–606, 1998.

Rouau, X., Cheynier, V., Surget, A., Gloux, D., Bar-ron, C., Meudec, E., Louis-Montero, J., and Criton, M., A dehydrotrimer of ferulic acid from maize bran, *Phytochemistry,* 63:899–903, 2003.

Schroeder, H., Williams, R.J., Martin, R., Iversen, L., and Rice-Evans, C.A., Phenolic antioxidants attenuate neuronal cell death following uptake of oxidized low-density lipoproteins, *Free Rad. Biol. Med.,* 29:1222–1233, 2000.

Tanaka, T., Kojina, T., Kawamori, T., Wang, A., Suzui, M., Okamoto, K., and Mori, H., Inhibition of 4-nitroquinoline-1-oxide induced rat tongue carcino-genesis by the naturally occurring plant phenolics caffeic, ellagic, chlorogenic and ferulic acids, *Car-cinogenesis,* 14:1321–1325, 1993.

Feverfew   Feverfew (*Tanacetum parthenium* L.), an aromatic herb, has been used as folk medicine for the treatment of migraine and arthritis (Berry, 1984; Johnson, 1984). Biolog-ical activity reported in the crude extracts from feverfew leaves may explain its therapeutic and anti-inflammatory properties. Such activity includes inhibition of platelet aggregation (Groenewegen and Heptinstall, 1990) and release of histamine from mast cells (Hayes and Foreman, 1987), as well as antinociceptive and anti-inflammatory activities in mice and rats (Jain and Kulkarni, 1999). Several sesquiter-pene ά-methylene butyrolactones in feverfew extracts, exhibiting these properties, were iden-tified as parthenolide and canin. Piela-Smith and Liu (2001) attributed the anti-inflammatory properties of feverfew extracts and parthenolid

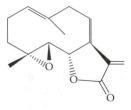

Parthenolide. (From Miglietta et al., *Chemico-Biol. Interactions*, 149:165–173, 2004. With permission.)

to their ability to inhibit the expression of proin-flammatory cellular-adhesion molecules in cul-tured synovial fibroblasts obtained from rheu-matoid-arthritis patients. Figure F.39 shows feverfew extract and parthenolide both inhib-ited the expression of an inflammation-related adhesion molecule, VCAM-1, induced by TNF. Kwok et al. (2001) examined the molecular basis for parthenolide's ability to inhibit the proinflammatory signaling pathway. They found it bound and inhibited the IκB kinase, a multisubunit complex responsible for cytokine-mediated stimulation of genes involved in the inflammation process. Smolinski and Pestka (2003) confirmed the anti-inflammatory prop-erties of three herbal constituents, including parthenolide on lipopolysaccharide-induced (LPS), proinflammatory cytokine production. They found that the data from cell culture could not accurately predict the effect in animals so that animal models were still needed for con-firmation. Fiebich and coworkers (2002) were the first to report parthenolide-inhibited activa-tion of p42/44 mitogen-activated protein kinase (MAPK), which reduced the production of induc-ible nitric-oxide synthase (iNOS) synthesis and nitric-oxide release. Since nitric oxide is impli-cated in the etiology of central-nervous system (CNS) diseases, such as multiple sclerosis, their

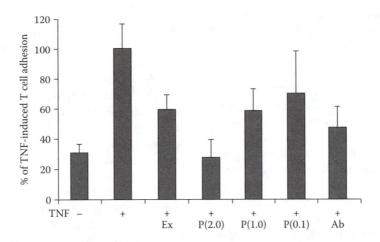

FIGURE F.39 Feverfew and parthenolide inhibition of synovial VCAM-1. Synovial FB was pretreated with feverfew extract (Ex) (1:80) or parthenolide (P) (2.0 and 1.5 μg/mL) for 4 h prior to treatment with TNF (500 μ/mL). (From Piela-Smith and Liu, *Cell Immunol.,* 209:89–96, 2001. With permission.)

results suggested parthenolide may have potential for treating CNS diseases where NO is part of the pathophysiology.

Pittler and coworkers (2000) systematically reviewed evidence for feverfew's efficacy to treat migraine. They concluded that the prevention of migraine by feverfew was still to be established. Nelson et al. (2002) showed that while the quantity of feverfew leaves in each capsule sold to consumers was similar, the parthenolide content per dosage form varied by as much as 150-fold and the percent parthenolide by 5.3-fold. The lack of standardization of feverfew products could explain the variability in efficacy.

References

Berry, M.I., Feverfew faces the future, *Pharm. J.,* 232:611–614, 1984.

Fiebich, B.L., Lieb, K., Engels, S., and Heinrich, M., Inhibition of LPS-induced p42/44 MAP kinase activation and iNOS/NO synthesis by parthenolide in rat primary microglial cells, *J. Neuroimmunol.,* 132:18–24, 2002.

Groenewegen, W.A. and Heptinstall, S., A comparison of the effects of an extract of feverfew and parthenolide, a component of feverfew, on human platelet activity *in vitro, J. Pharm. Pharmacol.,* 42:553–557, 1990.

Hayes, N.A. and Foreman, J.C., The activity of compounds extracted from feverfew on histamine release from rat mast cells, *J. Pharm. Pharmacol.,* 39:466–470, 1987.

Jain, N.K. and Kulkarni, S.K., Antinociceptive and anti-inflammatory effects of *Tanacetum parthenium* L. extract in mice and rats, *J. Ethnopharmacol.,* 68:251–259, 1999.

Johnson, E.S., *Feverfew: A Traditional Herbal Remedy for Migraine and Arthritis,* Sheldon Press, London, 1984.

Kwok, B.H.B., Koh, B., Ndubuisio, M.I., Elofsson, M., and Crews, C.M., The anti-inflammatory natural product parthenolide from the medicinal herb Feverfew directly binds to and inhibits IκB kinase, *Chem. Biol.,* 8:759–766, 2001.

Miglietta, A., Bozzo, F., Gabriel, L., and Bocca, C., Microtubule-interfering activity of parthenolide, *Chemico-Biol. Interactions,* 149:165–173, 2004.

Nelson, M.H., Cobb, S.E., and Shelton, J., Variations in parthenolide content and daily dose of feverfew products, *Am. J. Health Syst. Pharm.,* 15:1527–1531, 2002.

Piela-Smith, T.H. and Liu, X., Feverfew extracts and the sesquiterpene lactone parthenolide inhibit intercellular adhesion molecule-1 expression in human synovial fibroblasts, *Cell Immunol.,* 209:89–96, 2001.

Pittler, M.H., Vogler, B.K., and Ernst, E., Feverfew for preventing migraine, *Cochrane Database Syst. Rev.,* CD002286, 2000.

Smolinksi, A.T. and Pestka, J.J., Modulation of lipopolysaccharide-induced proinflammatory cytokine production *in vitro* and *in vivo* by the herbal constituents apigenin (chamomile), ginsenoside Rb_1 (ginseng) and paryhenolide (feverfew), *Food Chem. Toxicol.,* 41:1381–1390, 2003.

Fish There have been some reported studies of an inverse relationship between fish consumption and cardiovascular disease (Kromhout et al., 1985). Ecological studies suggest an inverse relationship between the incidence and mortality from cancer and fish consumption (Caygill et al., 1996; Kaizer et al., 1989). A recent panel report that reviewed epidemiological studies concluded that fish may protect against colon, rectal, and ovarian cancers (World Cancer Research Fund, American Institute for Cancer Research, 1997). Fernandez and coworkers (1999) examined the relation between the frequency of fish consumption and the risk of certain selected types of cancers in patients in northern Italy between 1983 and 1996. Their study suggested that even a small amount of fish reduced the risk particular of digestive-tract cancers.

References

Caygill, C.P.J., Charlett, A., and Hill, M.J., Fat, fish, fish oil and cancer, *Br. J. Cancer,* 74:159–164, 1996.

Fernandez, E., Chatenoud, L., La Vecchia, C., Negri, E., and Franceschi, S., Fish consumption and cancer risk, *Am. J. Clin. Nutr.,* 70:85–90, 1999.

Kaizer, L., Boyd, L., Kriukov, V., and Tritchler, D., Fish consumption and breast cancer risk: an ecological study, *Nutr. Cancer,* 1:61–68, 1989.

Kromhout, D., Bosschieter, E.B., and de Lezenne, C.C., The inverse relation between fish consumption and 20-year mortality from coronary heart disease, *N. Engl. J. Med.,* 312:1205–1209, 1985.

World Cancer Research Fund, American Institute for Cancer Research, *Food, Nutrition and the Prevention of Cancer: A Global Perspective,* American Institute for Cancer Research, Washington, D.C., pp. 452–459, 1997.

Fish oil *see also* **Docoahexaenoic and Eicosopentaenoic acids** Fish oils are rich in polyunsaturated fatty acids (PUFAs), particularly ω-3 fatty acids, which are known to reduce cholesterol. Chen and Auborn (1999) showed docosahexaenoic acid (DHA) in fish oil selectively inhibited the growth of human papillomarvirus (HPV) type 16 compared to eicosapentaenoic acid (EPA). These inhibitory effects were mediated via lipid peroxidation as α-tocopherol abrogated the effects of DHA. Liu et al. (2001) showed that a daily intake of a small amount of fish oil in bread fed to hyperlipidemic subjects significantly increased omega-3 fatty acids and HDL cholesterol levels, while decreasing triglycerides and malondialdehyde levels, reducing the risk of cardiovascular disease. A single-center, eight-month, randomized, double-blind, placebo-controlled study of 206 healthy nonsmoking subjects by Khan et al. (2003) showed the beneficial effects of fish oil on endothelial function. An increase of 6 percent EPA and 27 percent DHA in the diet, equivalent to eating oily fish two to three times per week, may significantly improve cardiovascular function and health.

In vitro studies with PUFAs from fish oil were found to enhance the efficacy of chemotherapeutic drugs against different cancer-cell types, such as MDA-MB 231 breast-cancer cells (Hardman et al., 1997), leukemic cells (De Salis and Meckling-Gill, 1995), and THKE tumorigenic human kidney epithelial cells (Maehle et al., 1995). The growth of human A549 lung-cancer cells, implanted subcutaneously on the backs of nude mice, was studied by Hardman and coworkers (2000a), who examined the change in the diet to 20 percent corn oil or 19 percent fish oil/1 percent corn oil on tumor growth. The growth of tumors was divided into two phases: phase I included the first 10 days on corn oil or fish diets plus four days for initiation of treatment with doxorubicin (DOX), commonly used in chemotherapy. Phase II commenced on the 14th day to allow sufficient time for DOX treatment to effect tumor size. No significant differences were observed in the rate of tumor growth in phase I, irrespective of the diets. During phase II, however, the tumors in animals consuming the fish-oil diet treated with iron and DOX were significantly regressed (Table F.30). In sharp contrast, the tumors in animals fed corn oil and treated with iron and DOX continued to grow. This study confirmed the potential benefit of

TABLE F.30
Growth Rate of A549 Human Lung Tumors (Mean mm³ Per Day + SD of Slope)

Final Diet/Treatment Group (n = 5)	Phase I[a]	Phase II
1) Corn oil; DOX	14.8 ± 1.9	−1.5 ± 1.8[b]
2) Fish oil; DOX	16.2 ± 1.8	−11.1 ± 1.5[c]
3) Corn oil + iron; DOX	15.9 ± 1.3	34.1 ± 4.2[d]
4) Fish oil + iron; DOX	11.2 ± 2.3	−13.1 ± 4.2[c]
5) Corn oil; no DOX	14.9 ± 2.0	14.9 ± 2.0[e]

[a] Linear-regression analyses showed that during phase I, all slopes were significantly different from 0. ANOVA of the slopes showed that the growth rates of the tumors (slopes) were not significantly different from each other during phase I, when mice were consuming either a corn-oil or a fish-oil diet without added iron and without DOX treatment.

[b,c,d,e] Linear-regression analyses showed that the tumor-growth rate (slope of the regression line) of the group of mice that consumed corn oil and was treated with DOX was not significantly different from a slope of 0. The tumor-growth rate of all other groups was a significant positive or negative slope. ANOVA, followed by Tukey's multiple comparisons test of the slopes, showed that growth rates (slopes) with the same letter are not significantly different, while growth rates with different letters are significantly different.

Source: From Hardman et al., *Cancer Lett.*, 158:109, 2000b. With permission.

F

fish oil as an adjuvant in the treatment of cancer. A combination of fish oil and butyrate-producing fiber pectin was shown by Hong and coworkers (2002) to upregulate apoptosis in colon cells exposed to the carcinogen azoxymethane. This effect was attributed to the oxidation of unsaturated mitochondrial lipids in fish, leading to an in increase in reactive-oxygen species.

A recent study by Pedersen and coworkers (2003) showed fish oil increased *in vivo* oxidation and *in vitro* susceptibility of LDL particles to oxidation in type 2 diabetic patients, characteristic of proatherogenic behavior. This contrasts with the beneficial effects that fish oil has on inflammation and heart disease, requiring more studies to establish its clinical significance.

References

Chen, D. and Auborn, K., Fish oil constituent docosahexaenoic acid selectively inhibits growth of human papillomavirus immortalized keratinocytes, *Carcinogenesis*, 20:249–254, 1999.

De Salis, H.M. and Meckling-Gill, K.A., EPA and DHA alter nucleoside drug and doxorubicin toxicity in L1210 cells but not in normal murine S1 macrophages, *Cell Pharmacol.*, 2:69–74, 1995.

Hardman, W.E., Barnes, C.J., Knight, C.W., and Cameron, I.L., Effects of iron supplementation and ET-18-OCH₃ on MDA-MB 231 breast carcinomas in nude mice consuming a fish oil diet, *Br. J. Cancer,* 76:347–354, 1997.

Hardman, W.E., Moyer, M.P., and Cameron, I.L., Dietary fish oil sensitizes A549 lung xenografts to doxorubicin chemotherapy, *Cancer Lett.*, 151:145–151, 2000a.

Hardman, W.E., Moyer, M.P., and Cameron, I.L., Erratum to dietary fish oil sensitizes A549 lung xenografts to doxorubicin chemotherapy, *Cancer Lett.*, 158:109, 2000b.

Hong, M.Y., Chapkin, R.S., Barhoumi, R., Burghardt, R.C., Turner, N.D., Henderson, C.E., Sanders, L.M., Fan, Y.-Y., Davidson, L.A., Murphy, M.E., Spinka, C.M., Carroll, R.J., and Lupton, J.R., Fish oil increases mitochondrial phospholipid unsaturation, upregulating reactive oxygen species and apoptosis in rat colonocytes, *Carcinogenesis,* 23: 1919–1926, 2002.

Khan, F., Elherik, K., Bolton-Smith, C., Barr, R., Hill, A., Murrie, I., and Belch, J.J.F., The effects of dietary fatty acid supplementation on endothelial function and vascular tone in healthy subjects, *Cardiovasc. Res.,* 59:955–962, 2003.

Liu, M., Wallin, R., and Saldeen, T., Effect of bread containing stable fish oil on plasma phospholipid fatty acids, triglycerides, HDL-cholesterol, and malondialdehyde in subjects with hyperlipidemia, *Nutr. Res.,* 21:1403–1410, 2001.

Maehle, L., Eilertsen, E., Mollerup, S., Schonberg, S., Krokan, H.E., and Haugen, A., Effects of n-3 fatty acids during neoplastic progression and comparison of *in vitro* and *in vivo* sensitivity of two human tumor cell lines, *Br. J. Cancer,* 71:691–696, 1995.

Pedersen, H., Petersen, M., Major-Pedersen, A., Jensen, T., Nielsen, N.S., Lauridsen, S.T., and Marckmann, P., Influence of fish oil supplementation on *in vivo* and *in vitro* oxidation resistance of low-density lipoprotein in type 2 diabetes, *Eur. J. Clin. Nutr.,* 57:713–720, 2003.

F

Flavonoids Flavonoids include a diverse group of more than 8000 polyphenolic compounds responsible for the antioxidant properties of fruits, vegetables, and herbs. The average daily intake of flavonoids in our diet was estimated to be around 1 g (Pierpoint, 1986). Flavonoids can be classified into eight groups, shown by their different basic skeleton structures, shown in Scheme F.22.

Examples of flavonoids are quercetin, myricetin, kempferol, and morin, characterized by a common ring structure, or flavone, but differing in the number and location of hydroxyl groups (Scheme F.23).

Zhu et al. (1999) found quercetin was most effective in protecting LDL from oxidation, followed by myricetin. Kampferol and morin exerted similar but much-less-protective effects, while ascorbic showed little or no effect (Figure F.40). Differences in efficacy among various flavonoids appeared to be related to the number and location of hydroxyl groups on the B ring and their stability in sodium-phosphate

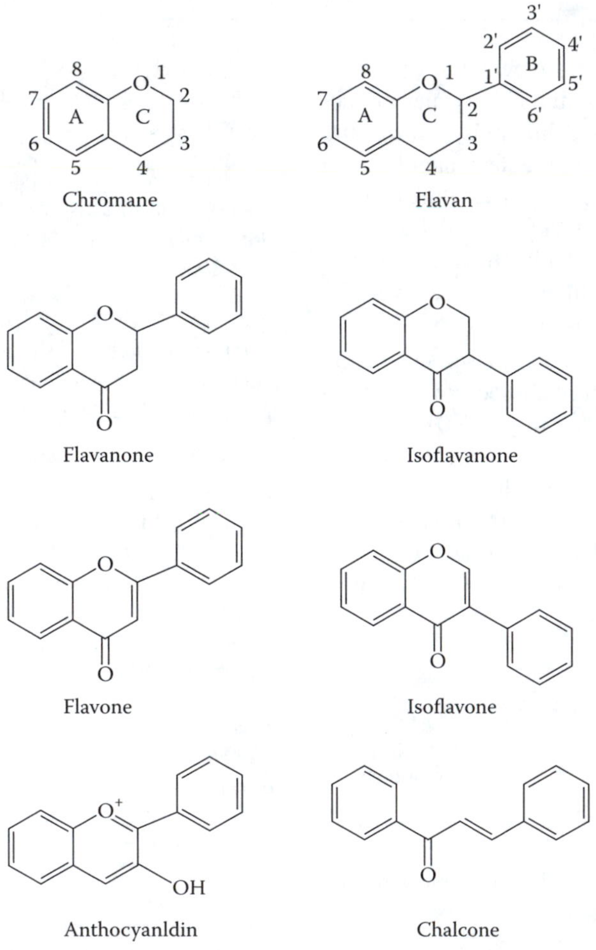

SCHEME F.22 Structures of basic flavonoid skeletons. (From Hodak, et al., *Chem. Biol. Interact,* 139:1–21, 2002. With permission.)

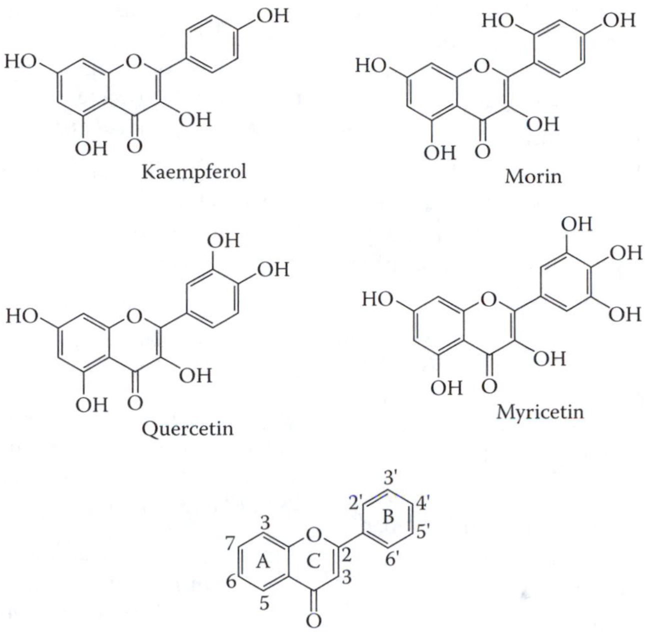

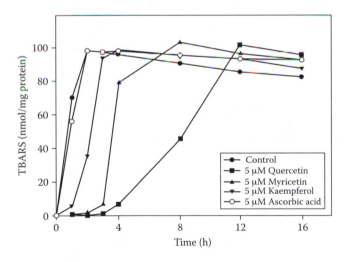

SCHEME F.23 Structures of kaemferol, morin, quercetin, and myricetin. (From Zhu et al., *J. Nutr. Biochem.*, 11:14–21, 2000. With permission.)

FIGURE F.40 Inhibitory effect of four flavonoids on the production of TBARS in Cu^{2+}-mediated oxidation of human low-density lipoprotein (LDL). Data expressed as means ± SD of five samples. (Zhu et al., *J. Nutr. Biochem.*, 11:14–21, 2000. With permission.)

buffer. This was confirmed in a recent study by Peng and Kuo (2003), which also found anti-oxidant activity was much stronger in quercetin and myricetin because of their *o*-dihydroxyl or vicinal-trihydroxyl groups. Kampferol, with a single hydroxyl in the B ring, did not protect Caco-2 cells from lipid peroxidation. The ability of flavonoids to scavenge peroxynitrite, a cyto-toxic intermediate formed from superoxide anion and nitric oxide, was also shown by Choi et al. (2002) to be dependent on the position of the hydroxyl group. Quercetin with an *ortho*-hydroxyl structure was the most potent scaven-ger, with an IC_{50} of 0.93 μM.

The neuroinflammatory disease multiple sclerosis (MS) is characterized by demyelination. A recent study by Hendriks et al. (2003) showed flavonoids had therapeutic potential because of their ability to limit the demyelination process in the myelin of adult mice brain tissue. The most effective flavonoids were quercetin, luteolin, and fisetin, with hydroxyl groups at the B-3 and B-4 positions in combination with a C-2,3 double bond.

Kobayashi and coworkers (2002) showed flavonoids were potent regulators of cyclin B and p21 for cell-cycle progression in human LNCaP prostate-cancer cells, and could play a preventative role in carcinogenesis.

In a review of flavonoids, Hodek et al. (2002) pointed out that while many of them exert beneficial effects, some may have mutagenic and prooxidant effects. Interaction of some flavonoids with cytochrome P450 (CYP) can result in enhanced activation of carcinogens or influence drug metabolism. In contrast, however, other flavonoids may have a beneficial effect by inhibiting activation of carcinogens by CYPs. Interaction of some flavonoids with prescribed drugs can lead to altered pharmacokinetics by either increasing their toxicity or reducing their therapeutic effects, depending on their structure (Tang and Stearns, 2001). For example, naringenin and bergamottin in grapefruit juice can lead to impaired hepatic metabolism of certain drugs (He et al., 1998; Bailey et al., 2000). The indiscriminate use of herbal products containing a wide range of flavonoids can similarly affect the efficacy and toxicity of drugs.

References

Bailey, D.G., Dresser, G.R., Kreeft, J.H., Munoz, C., Freeman, D.J., and Bend, J.R., Grapefruit-felodipine interaction: Effect of unprocessed fruit and probable active ingredients, *Clin. Pharmacol. Ther.,* 68:468–477, 2000.

Choi, J.S., Chung, H.Y., Kang, S.S., Jung, M.J., Kim, J.W., No, J.K., and Jung, H.A., The structure-activity relationship of flavonoids as scavengers of peroxynitrite, *Phytother. Res.,* 16:232–235, 2002.

He, K., Iyer, K.R., Hayes, R.N., Sinz, M.W., Woolf, T.F., and Hollenberg, P.F., Inactivation of cytochrome p450 3A4 by bergamottin, a component of grapefruit juice, *Chem. Res. Toxicol.,* 11:252–259, 1998.

Hendriks, J.J.A., de Vries, H.E., van der Pol, S.M.A., van den Berg, T.K., van Tol, E.A.F., and Dijkstra, C.D., Flavonoids inhibit myelin phagocytosis by macrophages; a structure-activity relationship study, *Biochem. Pharmacol.,* 65:877–885, 2003.

Hodek, P., Trefil, P., and Stiborova, M., Flavonoids — potent and versatile biologically active compounds interacting with cytochromes P450, *Chem. Biol. Interact.,* 139:1–21, 2002.

Kobayashi, T., Nakata, T., and Kuzumaki, T., Effect of flavonoids on cell cycle progression in prostate cancer cells, *Cancer Lett.,* 176:17–23, 2002.

Peng, I.W. and Kuo, S.M., Flavonoid structure affects the inhibition of lipid peroxidation in Caco-2 intestinal cells at physiological concentrations, *J. Nutr.,* 133:2184–2187, 2003.

Pierpoint, W.S., Flavonoids in the human diet, in *Progress in Clinical and Biological Research,* Vol. 213, Cody, V., Middleton, E., Jr., and Harborne, J.B., Eds., Alan R. Liss, New York, 1986, pp. 125–140.

Tang, W. and Stearns, R.A., Heterotropic cooperativity of cytochrome P450 3A4 and potential drug-drug interactions, *Curr. Drug. Metab.,* 2:185–188, 2001.

Zhu, Q.Y., Huang, Y., and Chen, Z.-Y., Interaction between flavonoids and α-tocopherol in human low density lipoprotein, *J. Nutr. Biochem.,* 11:14–21, 1999.

Flaxseed Flaxseed is obtained from flax (*Linum usitatissimum),* a versatile, blue-flowered crop. The seed, flat and oval with a pointed tip, is rich in protein, fat, and dietary fiber. Flaxseeds are one of the richest sources of the omega-3 fatty acid α-linolenic acid (ALA) (Oomah and Mazza, 2000). In addition, flaxseeds are also rich in phenolic compounds, particularly lignans, and dimers with a 2,3-dibenzylbutane structure (Harris and Haggerty, 1993). The lignan precursor in flaxseed is secoisolariciresinol diglycoside, or SDG, which appears to have some important health benefits. Yan et al. (1998) showed that supplementation of flaxseed in the diet reduced metastasis, the spread of malignant cells, in experimental mice with melanoma cells. Further work by Li et al. (1999) showed that dietary supplementation with SDG significantly decreased the number of lung tumors (Table F.31). In the control group, 59 percent (16 out of 27) of the mice had > 50 tumors compared to 30, 21, and 22 percent of mice fed diets containing 73, 147, and 293 μmol/kg SDG. A significant decrease in tumor cross-sectional area and volume were also observed with SDG-fed mice in a dose-dependent manner. Dabrosin and coworkers (2002) found that the addition of 10 percent flaxseed in the diet of nude mice with human breast-cancer xenografts showed a reduction in tumor growth and metastasis.

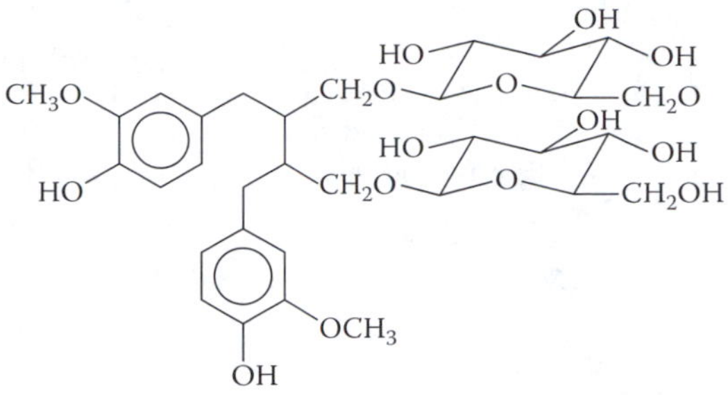

Secoisolariciresinol diglycoside. (From Rickard et al., *Cancer Lett.*, 161:47–55, 2000. With permission.)

F

TABLE F.31
Effect of Dietary Supplementation with SDG on Pulmonary Metastasis Cells in Mice

	Control					
	Mice with Lung Tumors			Tumors/Mouse		
	N	1–50 tumors	> 50 tumors	Median[a]	Mean + SE	Range
Control	27	11	16	62	64 ± 8	10–180
SDG						
73 μmol/kg	27	19	8	38	43 ± 5	8–117
147 μmol/kg	28	22	6[a]	36	42 ± 4	9–96
293 μmol/kg	27	21	6[a]	29[b]	33 ± 4	4–86

[a] Significantly different from the control, $p \leq 0.05$. Data analyzed using Fisher's exact test.

[b] Significantly different from the control, $p \leq 0.01$. Data analyzed using Kruskal-Wallis nonparametic and Duncan's multiple-comparison tests.

Source: From Li et al., *Cancer Lett.*, 142:91–96, 1999. With permission.

The presence of ALA in flaxseed appeared to protect against cardiovascular disease (Allman et al., 1995; Ferretti and Flanagan, 1996). Consumption of flaxseed either raw or defatted was shown to reduce total and LDL cholesterol in human subjects (Cunnane et al., 1993; Jenkins et al., 1999). Flaxseed oil was also found to be a potent inhibitor of proinflammatory mediators (Caughey et al., 1996; James et al., 2000). Flaxseed gum reduced blood-glucose response, as it behaved like a viscous fiber, while flaxseed protein interacted with the gums, as well as stimulated insulin secretion, reducing the glycemic response. Studies clearly showed flaxseed was an important functional food capable of slowing down the progression of many degenerative diseases (Oomah, 2001). A recent study by Bhathena and coworkers (2003) found flaxseed was more hypotriglyceridemic and hypocholesterolemic than soybean-protein concentrate. Consequently, flaxseed could provide an alternative, therapeutic treatment for individuals suffering from hypertriglyceridemia and hypercholesterolemia.

References

Allman, M.A., Pena, M.M., and Pang, D., Supplementation with flaxseed oil versus sunflower seed oil in healthy young men consuming a low fat diet: Effects on platelet composition and function, *Eur. J. Clin. Nutr.*, 49:168–178, 1995.

Bhathena, S.J., Ali, A.A., Haudenschild, C., Latham, P., Ranich, T., Mohamed, A.I., Hansen, C.T., and Velasquez, M.T., Dietary flaxseed meal is more protective than soy protein concentrate against hypertriglyceridemia and steatosis of the liver in an animal model of obesity, *J. Am. Coll. Nutr.*, 22:157–164, 2003.

Caughey, G.E., Mantzioris, E., Gibson, R.A., Cleland, L.G., and James, M.J., The effect on human tumor necrosis factor alpha and interlukin-1 beta production of diets enriched in n-3 fatty acids from vegetable oil or fish oil, *Am. J. Clin. Nutr.,* 63:116–122, 1996.

Cunnane, S.C., Ganguli, S., Menard, C., Liede, A.C., Hamadeh, M.J., Chen, Z.Y., Wolever, T., and Jenkins, D.J., High alpha-linolenic acid flaxseed (*Linum usitatissimum*): Some nutritional properties in humans, *Br. J. Nutr.,* 69:443–453, 1993.

Dabrosin, C., Chen, J., Wang, L., and Thompson, L.U., Flaxseed inhibits metastasis and decreases extracellular vascular endothelial growth in human breast cancer xenografts, *Cancer Lett.,* 185:31–37, 2002.

Ferretti, A. and Flanagan, V.P., Antithromboxane activity of dietary alpha-linolenic acid: A pilot study, *Prostaglandins Leukot Essent. Fatty Acids,* 54:451–455, 1996.

Harris, R.K. and Haggerty, W.J., Assays for potentially anticarcinogenic phytochemicals in flaxseed, *Cereal Foods World,* 38:147–151, 1993.

James, M.J., Gibson, R.A., and Cleland, L.G., Dietary polyunsaturated fatty acids and inflammatory mediator production, *Am. J. Clin. Nutr.,* 71: 343S–348S, 2000.

Jenkins, D.J., Kendall, C.W., Vidgen, E., Agarwal, S., Rao, A.V., Rosenberg, R.S., Diamandis, E.P., Novokmet, R., Mehling, C.C., Perera, T., Graffin, L.C., and Cunnane, S.C., Health aspects of partially defatted flaxseed including effects on serum lipids, oxidative measures, and *ex vivo* androgen and progestin activity: A controlled crossover trial, *Am. J. Clin. Nutr.,* 69:395–402, 1999.

Li, D., Yee, J.A., Thompson, L.U., and Yan, L., Dietary supplementation with secoisolariciresinol diglycoside (SDG) reduces experimental metastasis of melanoma cells in mice, *Cancer Lett.,* 142:91–96, 1999.

Oomah, D., Flaxseed as a functional food source, *J. Sci. Food Agric.,* 81:889–894, 2001.

Rickard, S.E., Yuan, Y.V., and Thompson, L.U., Plasma insulin-like growth factor I levels in rats are reduced by dietary supplementation of flaxseed or its lignan secoisolariciresinol diglycoside, *Cancer Lett.,* 161:47–55, 2000.

Yan, L., Yee, J.A., Li, D., McGuire, M.H., and Thompson, L.U., Dietary flaxseed supplementation and experimental metastasis of melanoma cells in mice, *Cancer Lett.,* 124:181–186, 1998.

Folic acid   An important therapy for treating advanced colorectal and other cancers involves a combination of leucovorin and fluorouracil (Mini et al., 1990; Buroker et al., 1994; Trave et al., 1988). The potentiation between leucovorin and fluorouracil is associated with the formation of the metabolite methylenetetrahydrofolate (CH_2FH_4) (Dohden et al., 1993; Raghunathan et al., 1997) Since folic acid, an

Folate. (Adapted from Park et al., *Biomaterials*, 26: 1053–1061, 2005.)

important B vitamin, can also elevate CH_2FH_4 levels, Raghunathan and Priest (1999) examined its ability to modulate the antitumor activity of fluorouracil. Implanted mouse mammary adenocarcinoma tumors were allowed to grow in mice maintained on a folic acid-depleted diet for 10 days. Folic acid (45 mg/kg) or fluorouracil (10 mg/kg) diluted in sterile saline solution were then injected i.p. The results in Table F.32 show that fluorouracil alone inhibited tumor growth by around 25 percent. In contrast, folic acid enhanced tumor growth almost twofold.

TABLE F.32
Folic-Acid Potentiation of Flourouracil Antitumor Activity[1]

Folic Acid (mg/kg)	Flourouracil (mg/kg)	Tumor Growth (mg/kg)
0	0	920 ± 69
0	10	694 ± 55
45	10	259 ± 16
45	0	1829 ± 218

[1] Values represent the means ± SEM from five mice.

Source: From Raghunathan and Priest, *Biochem. Pharmacol.,* 58:835–839, 1999. With permission.

However, when folic acid was administered 4 h prior to fluorouracil, to maximize accumulation of CH_2FH_4 and tetrahydrofolate (FH_4), tumor growth was significantly ($p < 0.001$) reduced by more than 70 percent. This study confirmed the ability of folic acid to potentiate the antitumor effects of fluorouracil. Folate status is now recognized as a factor in the prevention of carcinogenesis (Kim, 1999). A deficiency in folate is thought to increase the risk of malignancy by either DNA hypomethylation and proto-oncongene activation or by inducing uracil misincorporation, resulting in DNA breakage and chromosomal damage (Duthie, 1999). Recent studies pointed to an association between higher dietary folate and reduced breast-cancer risk in women with high alcohol intake (Zhang et al., 1999; Rohan et al., 2000; Negri et al., 2000; Sellers et al., 2001). The primary circulating form of folate is 5-methylenetetrahydrofolate, which is produced from 5,10-methylenetetrahydrofolate by the enzyme 5,10-methylenetetrahydrofolate reductase (MTHFR). In a case-control study with 62 women, Sharp et al. (2002) showed MTHFR polymorphisms may be modifiers of the relationship between dietary folate and breast cancer. While the number of subjects in this study was small, there was a trend between increasing folate intake and decrease in the risk of breast cancer. A recent study by Plaschke et al. (2003), however, was unable to find a similar association between high MTHFR activity and colorectal cancer.

References

Buroker, T.R., O'Connell, M.J., Wieand, H.S., Krook, J.E., Gerstner, J.B., Mailliard, J.A., Schaefer, P.L., Levitt, R., Kardinal, C.G., and Gesme, D.H., Jr., Randomized comparison of two schedules of fluorouracil and leucovorin in the treatment of advanced colorectal cancer, *J. Clin. Oncol.*, 12:14–20, 1994.

Dohden, K., Ohmura, K., and Watanabe, Y., Ternary complex formation and reduced folate in surgical specimens of human adenocarcinoma tissues, *Cancer*, 71:471–480, 1993.

Duthie, S.J., Folic acid instability and cancer: Mechanisms of DNA stability. *Br. Med. Bull.* 55: 578-592, 1999.

Kim, Y.I., Folate and cancer prevention: A new medical application of folate beyond hyperhomocysteinemia and neural tube defects, *Nutr. Rev.*, 57:314–321, 1999.

Mini, E., Trave, F., Rustum, Y.M., and Bertino, J.R., Enhancement of the antitumor effects of 5-fluorouracil by folinic acid, *Pharmacol. Ther.*, 47:1–19, 1990.

Negri, E., La Vecchia, C., and Franceschi, S., Re: Dietary folate consumption and breast cancer risk, *J. Natl. Cancer Inst.*, 92:1270–1271, 2000.

Park, E.K., Lee, S.B., and Lee, Y.M., Preparation and characterization of methoxy poly(ethylene glycol)/ poly(ε-coprolactone) amphiphilic block copolymeric nanospheres for tumor specific folate-mediated targeting of anticancer drugs, *Biomaterials*, 26:1053–1061, 2005.

Plaschke, J., Schwanebeck, U., Pistorius, S., Saeger, H.D., and Schackert, H.K., Methylenetetrahydrofolate reductase polymorphisms and risk of sporadic and hereditary colorectal cancer with or without microsatellite instability, *Cancer Lett.*, 191:179–185, 2003.

Raghunathan, K. and Priest, D.G., Modulation of fluorouracil antitumor activity by folic acid in a murine model system, *Biochem. Pharmacol.*, 58: 835–839, 1999.

Raghunathan, K., Schmitz, J.C., and Priest, D.G., Impact of schedule on leucovorin potentiation of fluorouracil antitumor activity in dietary folic acid depleted mice, *Biochem. Pharmacol.*, 53:1197–1202, 1997.

Rohan, T.E., Jain, M.G., Howe, G.R., and Miller, A.B., Dietary folate consumption and breast cancer risk, *J. Natl. Cancer Inst.*, 92:266–269, 2000.

Sellers, T.A., Kushi, L.H., Cerhan, J.R., Vierkant, R.A., Gapstur, S.M., Vachon, C.M., Olson, J.E., Therneau, T.M., and Folsom, A.R., Dietary folate intake, alcohol, and risk of breast cancer in a study of postmenopausal women, *Epidemiology*, 12:420–428, 2001.

Sharp, L., Little, J., Schofield, A.C., Pavlidou, E., Cotton, S.C., Miedzybrodzka, Z., Baird, J.O.C., Haites, N.E., Heys, S.D., and Grubb, D.A., Folate and breast cancer: Role of polymorphisms in methylenetetrahydrofolate reductase (MTHFR), *Cancer Lett.*, 181:65–71, 2003.

F

Trave, F., Rustum, Y.M., Petrelli, N.J., Herrera, L., Mittleman, A., Frank, C., and Creaven, P.J., Plasma and tumor tissue pharmacology of high-dose intravenous leucovorin calcium in combination with fluorouracil in patients with advanced colorectal carcinoma, *J. Clin. Oncol.,* 6:1184–1191, 1988.

Zhang, S., Hunter, D.J., Hankinson, S.E., Giovannucci, E.L., Rosner, B.A., Colditz, G.A., Speizer, F.E., and Willett, W.C., A prospective study of folate intake and the risk of breast cancer, *J. Am. Med. Assoc.,* 281:1632–1637, 1999.

Foxglove (*Digitalis purpurea*)   Foxglove first came into prominence more than 200 years ago when William Withering reported the efficacy of its leaves in treating congestive heart failure. Subsequent work, using the flouometric microculture cytoxicity assay, isolated a relatively high-molecular-weight fraction in the ethanolic extract of foxglove with potent antitumor activity (FMCA) (Larsson et al., 1992). This fraction was identified as digitoxin, a steroidal compound characterized by a five-membered, unsaturated lactone ring, belonging to a group of cardiac glycosides known as cardenolides. Another member of this group is digoxin. A second group of cardiac glycosides containing a six-membered, unsaturated lactone ring was also identified and referred to as bufadienolides. Of the latter, the therapeutically most important one is proscillardin A. Digitalis, or cardiac glycosides, refer to any steroidal glycoside compounds that cause characteristic positively inotropic (increase in maximum and velocity of myocardial contractile force associated with prolongation of relaxation period) and electrophysiological effects on the heart. Evidence strongly suggests that cardiac glycosides induce increases in intracellular Na^+ concentration or activity in which digitalis induces a positive inotropic effect.

The first large-scale, placebo-controlled mortality study to examine the effect of digoxin on 7788 patients suffering from chronic heart failure was conducted by Gheorghiade (1997). While digoxin had no effect on their survival, over 37 months of follow-up, the incidences of hospitalization due to worsening of heart failure were significantly lower in patients receiving digoxin compared to the placebo. Digoxin, the most commonly prescribed of the various cardiac glycoside preparations, was reported by Hauptman (1999) to be still useful for treating heart failure. Using primary cultures of tumor cells from patients and a human cell-line panel, Johansson et al. (2001) evaluated the cytotoxicity of five cardiac glycosides plus the saponin digitoxin and its aglycone digitoxigenin. Marked differences were observed among the different cardiac glycosides, with respect to their toxicities. Proscillaridin A proved to be the most potent in 9 of 10 human tumor lines, confirming the literature that cardenolides are

Structure of digitoxin. (From Hage and Sengupta, *J. Chromatogr. B.,* 724:91–100, 1999. With permission.)

weaker than the corresponding bufadienolides. The order of potency, after proscillaridin A, was digitoxin, ouabain, digoxin, lanatoside C, digitoxigenin, and digitonin, which paralleled their inhibitory potency on Na^+/K^+-transporting ATPase from human cardiac muscle reported previously for cardiac glycosides by Schonfeld et al. (1986). Reviewing the use of digitoxin as a treatment of congestive heart failure, Beltz et al. (2001) showed digitoxin exerted the same pharmacodynamic kinetics as digoxin. However, digitoxin was more lipophilic than digoxin, giving it a more stable pharmacokinetic profile and a lower incidence of toxic side effects. Roever and coworkers (2000) had shown previously that digitoxin had a lower rate of toxicity compared to digoxin when used by elderly patients. Patients taking digoxin had three times the odds of experiencing toxicity compared to digitoxin.

Cardiac glycosides can interact with other drugs, so caution must be exercised when introducing new pharmaceuticals. For example, quinidine inhibited the transport of digoxin across the cell membranes, particularly in the kidneys (Fromm et al., 2002), while amiodarone increased the steady state of digoxin so that dosages could be decreased by as much as 50 percent.

References

Beltz, G.G., Breithaupt-Grogler, K., and Osowski, U., Treatment of congestive heart failure — current status of use of digitoxin, *Eur. J. Clin. Inv.,* 31(Suppl. 2):10–17, 2001.

Fromm, M.F., Kim, R.B., Stein, C.M., Wilkinson, G.R., and Roden, D.M., Inhibition of P-glycoprotein-mediated drug transport: A unifying mechanism to explain the interaction between digoxin and quinidine, *Circulation,* 2002 (in press).

Gheorghiade, M., Digitoxin therapy in chronic heart disease, *Cardiovasc. Drugs Ther.,* 11:279–283, 1997.

Hage, D.S. and Sengupta, A., Characterisation of the binding of digitoxin and acetyldigitoxin to human serum albumin by high-performance affinity chromatography, *J. Chromatogr. B.,* 724:91–100, 1999.

Hauptmann, P.J., Digitalis, *Circulation,* 99:1265–1270, 1999.

Johansson, S., Lindholm, P., Gullbo, J., Larsson, R., Bohlin, L., and Claeson, P., Cytotoxicity of digitoxin and related glycosides in human tumor cells, *Anticanc. Drugs,* 12:475–483, 2001.

Larsson, R., Kristensen, J., Sandberg, C., and Nygren, P., Laboratory determination of chemotherapeutic drug resistance in tumor cells from patients with leukemias using a fluorescent microculture cytoxicity assay (FMCA), *Int. J. Cancer,* 50:177–185, 1992.

Roever, C., Ferrante, J., Gonzalez, E.C., and Roetzheim, R.G., Comparing the toxicity of digoxin and digitoxin in a geriatric population: Should an old drug be rediscovered, *South. Med. J.,* 93:5–15, 2000.

Schonfeld, W., Schonfeld, R., Menke, K.H., Weiland, J., and Repke, K.R.H., Origin of differences of inhibitory potency of cardiac glycosides in Na^+/K^+ transporting ATPase from human cardiac muscle, human brain cortex and guinea-pig cardiac muscles, *Anticacer. Drugs,* 12:475–483, 1986.

Fruits *see also* **Individual fruits**   A large number of epidemiological studies have associated the low incidence of common cancers, cardiovascular disease, and other chronic diseases to the high consumption of fruits and vegetables (Ness and Powles, 1997; Steinmetz and Potter, 1996). Lampe (1999) reviewed the many human studies in which phytochemicals identified in fruits and vegetables were investigated in an effort to assess their mechanisms of action. A large, prospective, cohort study of 39,876 female health professionals over a five-year period by Liu and coworkers (2000) indicated that a higher intake of fruits and vegetables may have a protective effect against cardiovascular disease. This is attributed to the naturally occurring antioxidants scavenging free radicals and preventing degenerative diseases, such as cancer, atherosclerosis, diabetes, and arthritis (Kaur and Kapoor, 2001). Thompson and coworkers (1999) showed that increased consumption of fruits and vegetables by a group of women significantly decreased the levels of urinary 8-hydroxydeoxy-guanosine (8 OhdG), malondialdehyde (MDA), and 8-isoprostane F-2α, all markers of oxidative cellular damage. The data generated by this study showed that increased fruit and vegetable consumption did in fact reduce cellular injury, as measured by these biomarkers. Broekmans et al. (2000) were the first to demonstrate that fruits and vegetables with moderate folate levels decrease plasma homocysteine, a risk factor for cardiovascular disease.

References

Broekmans, W.M.R., Klopping-Ketelaars, I.A.A., Shuurman, C.R., Verhagen, H., vab den Berg, H., Kok, F.J., and van Poppel, G., Fruits and vegetables increase plasma carotenoids and vitamins and decrease homocysteine in humans, *J. Nutr.,* 130: 1578–1583, 2000.

Kaur, C. and Kapoor, H.C., Antioxidants in fruits and vegetables — the millennium's health, *Int. J. Food Sci. Technol.,* 36:703–725, 2001.

Lampe, J.W., Health effects of vegetables and fruit: Assessing mechanisms of action in human experimental studies, *Am. J. Clin. Nutr.,* 70:475S–490S, 1999.

Liu, S., Manson, J.E., Lee, I.-M., Cole, S.R., Hennekens, C.H., Willett, W.C., and Buring, J.E., Fruit and vegetable intake and risk of cardiovascular disease: The Women's Health Study, *Am. J. Clin. Nutr.,* 72:922–928, 2000.

Ness, A.R. and Powles, J.W., Fruit and vegetables, and cardiovascular disease: A review, *Int. J. Epidemiol.,* 26:1–13, 1997.

Steinmetz, K.A. and Potter, J.D., Vegetable, fruit, and cancer prevention: A review, *J. Am. Diet. Assoc.,* 96: 1027–1039, 1996.

Thompson, H.J., Heimendinger, J., Haegele, A., Sedlacek, S.M., Gillete, C., O'Neille, C., Wolfe, P., and Conry, C., Effect of increased vegetable and fruit consumption on markers of oxidative cellular damage, *Carcinogenesis,* 20:2261–2266, 1999.

G

Gambieric acids Gambieric acids A–D are potent, antifungal compounds obtained from the marine dinoflagellate *Gambierdiscus toxicus* (Nagai et al., 1992). The antifungal activity of these ladder-shaped polyethers against *Aspergillus niger* is 2000 times greater than that of amphotericin B. Morohashi et al. (2000) determined the absolute configuration of gambieric acids A–D as shown in Scheme G.24.

Gambierdiscus toxicus also produces other polyethers, such as brevetoxins and ciguatoxins, which are highly toxic. These compounds exert their neurotoxicity by binding to a specific site on the voltage-gated sodium channels of excitable membranes (Catterall, 2000), refered to as site 5. Inoue and coworkers (2003) recently showed that gambieric acid-A, a nontoxic polyether, inhibited the binding of brevetoxin to site 5.

References

Catterall, W.A., From ionic currents to molecular mechanisms: The structure and function of voltage-gated sodium channels, *Neuron,* 26:13–25, 2000.

Inoue, M., Hirama, M., Satake, M., Sugiyama, K., and Yasumoto, T., Inhibition of brevetoxin binding to the voltage-gated sodium channel by gambierol and gambieric acid-A, *Toxicon,* 41:469–474, 2003.

Morohashi, A., Satake, M., Nagai, H., Oshima, Y., and Yasumoto, T., The absolute configuration of gambieric acids A-D, potent antifungal polyethers, isolated from the marine dinoflagellate *Gambierdiscus toxicus, Tetrahedron Lett.,* 56:8995–9001, 2000.

Nagai, H., Murata, M., Torigoe, K., Satake, M., and Yasumoto, T., Gambieric acids, new potent antifungal substances with unprecedented polyether structures from a marine dinoflagellate *Gambierdiscus toxicus, J. Org. Chem.,* 57:5448–5453, 1992.

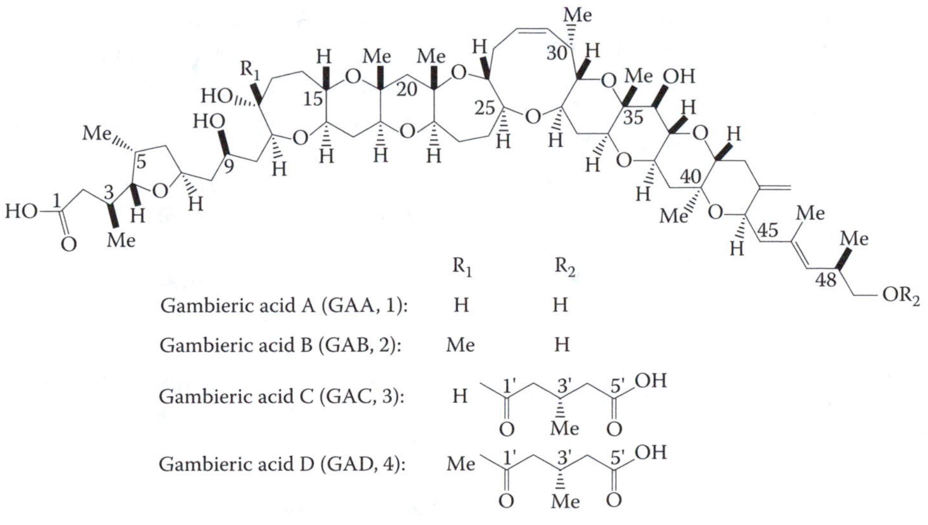

	R_1	R_2
Gambieric acid A (GAA, 1):	H	H
Gambieric acid B (GAB, 2):	Me	H
Gambieric acid C (GAC, 3):	H	
Gambieric acid D (GAD, 4):	Me	

SCHEME G.24 Structures of gambieric acids A–D. (From Morohashi et al., *Tetrahendron*, 56:8995–9001, 2000. With permission.)

Gamma amino butyric acid (GABA) The amino acid γ-amino butyric acid (GABA) is produced primarily by decarboxylation of glutamate by glutamate decarboxylase, a vitamin B_6-dependent enzyme. Found in many fruits and vegetables, GABA was reported

Gamma amino butyric acid (GABA). (From Mohorashi et al., *Tetrahendron*, 56:8995–9001, 2000. With permission.)

almost 50 years ago to reduce blood pressure in animals and man (Takahashi et al., 1953; Elliott and Hobbiger, 1959). This property was due, in part, to its ability to block peripheral ganglia (Stanton, 1963). Using hypertensive rats, Hayakawa and coworkers (2002) showed the antihypertensive effect of GABA involved possible inhibition of noradrenaline release from sympathetic nerve endings. Recent work by Inoue et al. (2003) examined the effect of a new, fermented-milk product containing GABA on mildly hypertensive patients. A randomized, placebo-controlled, single-blind trial on 39 mildly hypertensive patents (16 women and 23 men), ranging in age from 28–81 years, were fed the fermented milk product over a 12-week period. A significant ($p < 0.05$) decrease in systolic, diastolic, and mean blood pressure was observed after four weeks for the group fed the fermented-milk product (Figure G.41). The reduction in systolic and mean blood pressures were significantly lower for the treated group over the entire 12 weeks of the study. No side effects were observed from the intake of the fermented product, suggesting the potential of GABA-containing products for controlling blood pressure in patients suffering from mild hypertension.

References

Elliott, K.A.C. and Hobbinger, F., Gamma aminobutyric acid: Circulatory and respiratory effects in different species: Re-investigation of the anti-strychnine action in mice, *J. Physiol.*, 146:70–84, 1959.

Hayakawa, K., Kimura, M., and Kamata, K., Mechanism underlying gamma-aminobutyric acid-induced antihypertensive effect in spontaneously hypertensive rats, *Eur. J. Pharmacol.*, 438:107–113, 2002.

Inoue, K., Shirai, T., Ochiai, H., Kaso, M., Hayakawa, H., Kimura, M., and Sansawa, H., Blood-pressure-lowering effect of a novel fermented milk product containing γ-aminobutyric acid (GABA) in mild hypertensives, *Eur. J. Clin. Nutr.*, 57:490–495, 2003.

Stanton, H.C., Mode of action of gamma aminobutyric acid on the cardiovascular system, *Arch. Int. Pharmacodyn.*, 143:195–204, 1963.

Takahashi, H., Tiba, M., Iino, M., and Takayasu, T., The effect of γ-aminobutyric acid on blood pressure, *Jpn. J. Physiol.*, 5:334–341, 1955.

Gamma linolenic acid (GLA) Gamma linolenic acid (GLA, C18:3 ω-6) occurs abundantly in such plant seeds as borage, evening primrose, and black currants (Eskin, 2002). The conversion of GLA from dietary linoleic acid (C18:2 ω-6) in humans is impaired, as the enzyme involved, Δ 6-desaturase, is either blocked or saturated. Consequently oral GLA has been shown to treat a number of inflammatory disorders, such as rheumatoid arthritis (Leventhal et al., 1993; Zurrier et al., 1996) and atopic dermatitis (Horrobin, 1993; Andreassi et al., 1997). The benefits associated with GLA are attributed to its interference in AA metabolism to bioactive eicosanoids (Miller and Ziboh, 1988). This appears paradoxical, as GLA is a precursor of AA, which can bring about proinflammatory events. However, Peterson et al. (1999) reported dietary GLA exerted immunoregulatory fuctions. These anti-inflammatory effects were found by Kaku et al. (2001) to be due to the suppression of leukotriene B_4 production by high doses of GLA.

Gillis et al. (2002) showed GLA alone, or in combination with EPA, significantly induced neutrophil apoptosis and reduced cell viability in human promyelocytic leukemia HL-60 cells. This effect was attributed to GLA's ability to attenuate the production of leukotriene B_4 (LTB_4) by inhibiting 5-lipoxygenase (Ziboh and Fletcher, 1992). LTB_4 is crucial for neutrophil viability and chemotaxis. Using a rat-infusion glioma model, Leaver and coworkers (2002)

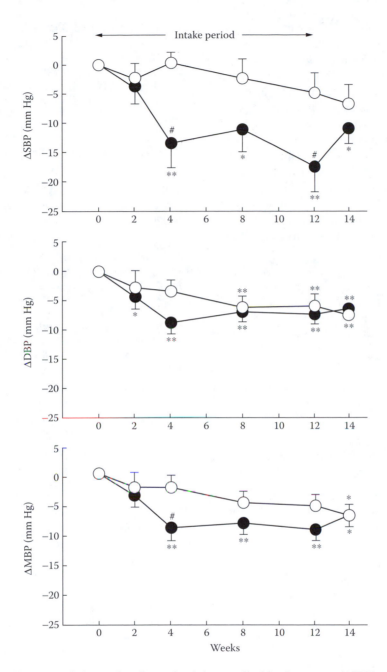

G

FIGURE G.41 Changes (relative to baseline values) in systolic blood pressure (ΔSBP), diastolic blood pressure (ΔDBP), and mean blood pressure (MBP) after intake of fermented-milk product with GABA (●) or placebo (○). (From Inoue et al., *Eur. J. Clin. Nutr.,* 57:490–495, 2003. With permission.)

found slow infusion of GLA of 2 mM/L over seven days stimulated regression in tumor size and cell death in tumor implants. The potential therapeutic, safe use of γ-linolenic acid for treating human gliomas was further verified by Bakshi et al. (2003). GLA (1 mg) was administered for seven days to nine patients via a cerebral reservoir or by direct, intratumoral delivery, with grade four disease and recurrent glioma. Some improvement in patient survival was observed, with no side effects reported.

GLA has also been studied as a novel, intravesical cytotoxic agent against superficial bladder cancer (Crook et al., 2000). The instability of GLA led to its coupling with a number of agents to enhance its half-life. Harris and coworkers (2003) used the formulation of meglumine GLA (MeGLA), as meglumine is a nontoxic compound used in radiological-contrast media, to assess its efficacy in 30 patients with recurrent transitional-cell carcinoma. No local or systemic side effects were observed following treatment of 15 patients with 50 mL of either 50 mg (1 mg/mL) or 125 mg (2.5 mg/mL) of MeGLA in water. The safety and tolerability of MeGLA were confirmed, and the 43 percent response rate indicated significant cytotoxic effects against transitional-cell carcinoma.

References

Andreassi, M., Forleo, P., Di Lorio, A., Masci, S., Abate, G., and Amerio, P., Efficacy of γ-linolenic acid in the treatment of patients with atopic dermatitis, *J. Int. Med. Res.,* 25:266–274, 1997.

Bakshi, A., Mukherjee, D., Bakshi, A., Banerji, A.K., and Das, U.N., γ-Linolenic acid therapy of human gliomas, *Nutrition,* 19:305–309, 2003.

Crook, T., Hall, S., Solomon, L., Bass, P., Cooper, A., and Birch, B., Intravesical meglumine gamma linolenic acid, phase 1 tolerability studies in patients undergoing cystetomy, *Urooncol.,* 1:39–42, 2000.

Eskin, N.A.M., Authentication of evening primrose, borage and fish oils, in *Oils and Fats Authentication,* Jee, M., Ed., Blackwell Publishing and CRC Press, 2002, chap. 4, pp. 95–107.

Gillis, R.C., Daley, B.J., Enderson, B.L., and Karlstad, M.D., Eicosapentaenoic acid and γ-linolenic acid induce apoptosis in HL-60 lines, *J. Surg. Res.,* 107:145–153, 2002.

Harris, N.M., Crook, T.J., Dyer, J.P., Cooper, A.J., and Birch, B.R., Intravesicular meglumine gamma-linolenic acid in superficial bladder cancer: An efficacy study, *Eur. Urol.,* 42:39–42, 2002.

Horrobin, D.F., Fatty acid metabolism in health and disease: the role of delta-6-desaturase, *Am. J. Clin. Nutr.,* 57:732S–736S, 736S–737S, 1993.

Kaku, S., Ohkura, K., Yunoki, S., Nonaka, M., Tachibana, H., Sugano, M., and Yamada, K., Dietary γ-linolenic acid dose-dependently modifies fatty acid composition and immune parameters in rats, *Prostaglandins Leukot. Essent. Fatty Acids,* 65:205–210, 2001.

Leaver, H.A., Wharton, S.B., Bell, H.S., Leaver-Yap, M.M., and Whittle, I.R., Highly unsaturated fatty acid induced tumor regression in glioma pharmacodynamics and bioavailability of gamma linolenic acid in an implantation glioma model: Effects on tumor biomass, apoptosis and neuronal tissue histology, *Prostaglandins,* 67:283–292, 2002.

Leventhal, L.J., Boyce, E.G., and Zurrier, R.B., Treatment of rheumatoid arthritris with gamma linolenic acid, *Ann. Intern. Med.,* 119:867–873, 1993.

Miller, C.C. and Ziboh, V.A., Gammalinolenic acid-enriched diet alters cutaneous eicosanoids, *Biochem. Biophys. Res. Commun.,* 154:967–974, 1988.

Peterson, L.D., Thies, F., and Calder, P.C., Dose-dependent effcts of dietary γ-linolenic acid on rat spleen lymphocyte functions, *Prostaglandins Leukot. Essent. Fatty Acids,* 61:19–24, 1999.

Ziboh, V.A. and Fletcher, M.P., Dose-response effects of dietary gamma linolenic acid-enriched oils on human polymorphonuclear-neutrophil biosynthesis of leukotriene B4, *Am. J. Clin. Nutr.,* 55:39–45, 1992.

Zurier, R.B., Rosseti, R.G., Jacobson, E.W., DeMarco, D.M., Liu, N.Y., Temming, J.E., White, B.M., and Laposata, M., Gamma-linolenic acid treatment of rheumatoid arthritis, a randomized, placebo-controlled trial, *Arthritis Rheum.,* 39:1808–1817, 1996.

***

Ganorderma   *Ganorderma* is a mushroom used in Oriental traditional medicine for treating many chronic diseases (Gao and Zhou, 2003). Polysaccharides present its fruit body, mycelia, or spores of *Ganordema* are pharmacologically active and include β-D-glucans, heteropolysaccharides, and glycoproteins. A fucose-containing glycoprotein isolated from *Ganordema lucidum* was shown to stimulate spleen-cell proliferation and cytokine expression (Wang et al., 2002). Over 100 triterpenoids were isolated from *Ganordema lucidum* including the highly oxidized lanostane-type triterpenoids, such as ganoderic and lucidenic acids. Cancer-preventive action by *Ganordema* was attributed to the antiproliferative properties of its triterpenoids by inducing apoptosis (Birt et al., 2001; Gan et al., 1998).

Ganordema products are sold as a single agent or with other herbal medicines. Clinical studies on prostate cancer patients using a combination of *Ganordema* and eight herbs (PC-SPES) showed a significant reduction in the prostate-specific antigen (PSA) levels (Small et al., 2000). *In vitro* and *in vivo* studies on *Ganordema* attributed its anticancer effects to antioxidative, free-radical scavenging, enhancement of the immune system, cell-cycle arrest, and apoptosis.

References

Birt, D.F., Hendrich, S., and Wang, W., Dietary agents in cancer prevention: Flavonoids and isoflavonoids, *Pharmacol. Ther.,* 90:157–177, 2001.

Gan, K.H., Fann, Y.F., Hsu, S-H., Kuo, K.W., and Lin, C.N., Mediation of the cytotoxicity of lanostanoids and steroids of *Ganordema tsugae* through apoptosis and cell cycle, *J. Nat. Prod.,* 61: 485–487, 1998.

Gao, Y. and Zhou, S., Cancer prevention and treatment by *Ganordema*, a mushroom with medicinal properties, *Food Rev. Inter.,* 19:275–325, 2003.

Small, E.J., Frohlich, M.W., Bok, R., Shinohara, K., Grossfeld, G., Rozenblat, Z., Kelly, W.K., Corry, M., and Reese, D.M., Prospective trial of the herbal supplement PC-SPES in patients with progressive prostate cancer, *J. Clin. Oncol.,* 18:3595–3603, 2000.

Wang, Y.Y., Khoo, K.H., Chen, S.T., Lin, C.C., Wong, C.H., and Lin, C.H., Stidies on the immunomodulating and antitumor activities *Ganordema lucidum* (Reishi) polysaccharides: Functional and proteomic analyses of a fucose-containing glycoprotein fraction responsible for the activities, *Bioorg. Med. Chem.,* 10:1057–1062, 2002.

Garden cress (*Lepidium sativum*)   Garden cress is fairly unique among the *Brassica* vegetables, as it contains only one glucosinolate, namely glucotropaeolin (GT) (Fenwick et al., 1983). This glucosinolate is then hydrolyzed by the enzyme myrosinase to yield the corresponding isothiocyanate, benzylisothiocyanate (BITC) (Scheme G.25). Glucosinolates have been shown to protect laboratory animals from chemically induced cancers by inhibition of phase I enzymes or by induction of glutathione *S*-transferase (Chung et al., 1992; Knasmuller et al., 1996; Zhang and Talalay, 1994).

Kassie and coworkers (2002) examined the chemoprotective properties of garden cress toward the genotoxic effects of the heterocyclic aromatic amine, 2-amino-3-methyl-imidazo[4,5-*f*] quinoline (IQ), in F344 rats. Garden-cress juice reduced the IQ-induced genotoxic effects and colonic-preneoplastic lesions by the induction of UDP-glucurononsyltransferase (UDPGT), a key enzyme in the detoxification of heterocyclic aromatic amines. Kassie et al. (2002) found that the amount of juice needed to produce these changes was quite small but similar to the level of glucosinolates consumed in a regular salad.

References

Chung, F.L., Chemoprevention of lung carcinogenesis by aromatic isothiocyanates, in *Cancer Chemoprevention,* Wattenberg, L.W., Lipkin, M., Boone, C.W., and Kelloff, G.J., Eds., CRC Press, Boca Raton, Florida, 1992, pp. 227–245.

Fenwick, G.R., Heaney, R.K., and Mullin, W.J., Glucosinolates and their breakdown products in food and food plants, *Crit. Rev. Food Sci. Nutr.,* 18:123–201, 1983.

Ishimoto, H., Fukushi, Y., and Tahara, S., Non-pathogenic *Fusarum* strains protect seedlings of *Lepidium sativum* and *Pythium ultimum*, *Soil Biol. Biochem.,* 36:409–414, 2004.

Glucotropaeolin   Benzyl isothiocyanate

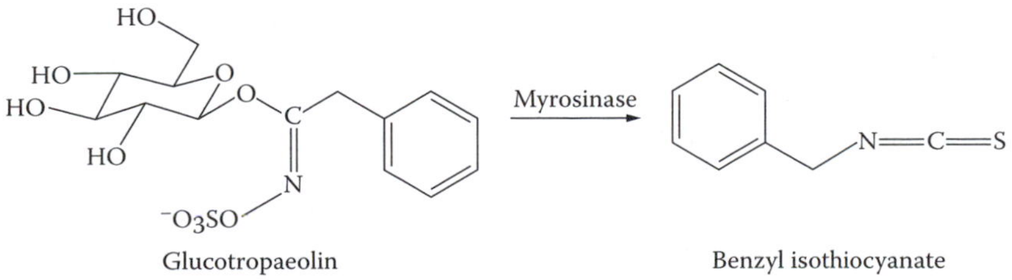

SCHEME G.25 Enzymic hydrolysis of glucotropaeolin to benzyl isothiocyanate. (From Ishimoto et al., *Soil Biol. Biochem.,* 36:409–414, 2004. With permission.)

Kassie, F., Rabot, S., Uhl, M., Huber, W., Qin, H.M., Helma, C., Schulte-Hermann, R.S., and Knasmuller, S., Chemoprotective effects of garden cress (*Lepidium sativum*) and its constituents towards 2-amino-3-methyl-imidazo [4,5-*f*]quinoline (IQ)-induced genotoxic effects and colonic preneoplastic lesions, *Carcinogenesis,* 23:1155–1161, 2002.

Knasmuller, S., Friesen, M.D., Holme, J.A., Alexander, J., Sanyal, R., Kassie, F., and Bartsch, H., Effects of phenethyl isothiocyanate on metabolism and on genotoxicity of dimethylnitrosamine and 2-amino-1-methyl-6-phenylimidazo[4,5-*b*]pyridine (PhIP), *Mutat. Res.,* 350:93–102, 1996.

Zhang, Y. and Talalay, P., Anticarcinogenic activities of organic isothiocyanates: Chemistry and mechanisms, *Cancer Res.,* 54:1976S–1981S, 1994.

G

Garlic   In addition to being a flavoring agent, garlic (*Allium sativum* L.) is also pharmacologically active against microbial infection, thrombosis, hypertension, hyperglycemia, hyperlipidemia, and cancer. The pharmacological properties of garlic, such as lipid-lowering effects, appear to be related to sulfur-rich compounds, particularly allicin. Shukla and Taneja (2002) clearly showed the antimutagenic effects of garlic extract (GE) in Swiss albino mice using an "*in vivo* chromosomal aberration assay." Pretreatment with 2.5 percent and 5 percent GE significantly suppressed chromosomal aberrations in cyclophosphamide (CP)-treated (a well-known mutagen) mice. The anticytoxic effects of GE were demonstrated by a significant increase in mitotoxic idex, as well as reduction in CP-induced clastogenicity. Sengupta et al. (2002) also showed that garlic constituents protected Swiss mice from DMBA-induced clastogenicity by significantly reducing chromosomal aberrations in the bone marrow. Iimuro and coworkers (2002) found that a garlic extract suppressed *Helicobacter pylori*-induced gastritis in Mongolian gerbils. Infection by this organism has been associated with the development of stomach cancer so that garlic extract appeared to be useful for reducing the risk of gastric cancer. Patients with benign prostate hyperplasia and prostate cancer showed significant improvements after consuming an aqueous garlic extract (1 mL/kg weight) for a month (Durak et al., 2003). In addition to reducing the mass of prostate, the urinary frequency was decreased, while maximum and average rates of urine flow increased. Cancer patients had significantly lower PSA values after consumption of the garlic extract.

Epidemiological data showed an inverse relationship between garlic consumption and reduced risk of cardiovascular disease (Kendler, 1987; Keys, 1980). In their review of garlic and cardiovascular disease, Banerjee and Maulik (2002) pointed to the need to identify specific components responsible for its cardioprotective effects. Ozturk et al. (1994) observed the beneficial effects of garlic extract on vascular responsiveness in normal rats. A recent study by Baluchnejadmojarad et al. (2003) showed an aqueous garlic extract significantly improved impaired endothelium-dependent relaxations, as well as decreased the enhanced contractile response to phenyl epinephrine in diabetic rats.

Fresh garlic was reported to lower blood pressure in spontaneously hypertensive rats (Foushee et al., 1982). Further researchers confirmed the ability of garlic to control mild hypertension. Al-Quattan et al. (1999) examined the effectiveness of garlic in treating more severe hypertension, such as in unilateral renovascular hypertension (URVH). Using a 2K1C hypertensive rat, they showed that a single dose had a maximum antihypertensive effect 2–6 h after administration, continuing for up to 24 h (Table G.33). Multiple doses of garlic also controlled the rise in blood pressure in these hypertensive rats. Sharif et al. (2003) showed a negative correlation between garlic, blood pressure, and angiotensin-converting enzyme (ACE) using the same 2K1C hypertensive model. An enteric-coated garlic-powder supplement suggested that the ability of garlic to lower blood pressure was attributed, in part, to a reduction in ACE activity.

References

Al-Quattan, K.K., Alnaqeeb, M.A., and Ali, M., The antihypertensive effect of garlic (*Allium sativum*) in the rat two-kidney-one-clip Goldblatt model, *J. Ethnopharmacol.,* 66:217–222, 1999.

Baluchnejadmojarad, T., Roghani, M., Homayounfar, H., and Hosseini, M., Beneficial effect of aqueous garlic extract on the vascular reactivity of

TABLE G.33
Effect of a Single Dose of Garlic (50 mg/kg)
on the Systolic Blood Pressure of Clipped Rats

Time	Water-Fed[1] control (mmHg ± SD)	Garlic-Fed[1] (mmHg ± SD)
Preclipping	123 ± 19	121 ± 15
Postclipping (preadministration)	135 ± 18	132 ± 8
30 min	141 ± 21	128 ± 9
2 h	140 ± 20	117 ± 9
6 h	139 ± 16	117 ± 5[*]
24 h	140 ± 17	131 ± 6
48 h	147 ± 13	141 ± 15

[1] Five rats were used in each group. [*] $p \leq 0.05$ compared with water-treated animals at the same time.

Source: From Al-Quattan et al., *J. Ethnopharmacol.*, 66:217–222, 1999. With permission.

G

streptozoticin-diabetic rats, *J. Ethnopharmacol.*, 85:139–144, 2003.

Banerjee, S.K. and Maulik, S.K., Effect of garlic on cardiovascular disorders: A review, *Nutr. J.*, 1:4, 2002.

Durak, I., Yllmaz, E., Devrim, E., Perk, H., and Kacmaz, M., Consumption of aqueous garlic extract leads to significant improvement in patients with benign prostate hyperplasia and prostate cancer, *Nutr. Res.*, 23:199–204, 2003.

Foushee, D.B., Ruffn, J., and Banerjee, U., Garlic as a natural agent for the treatment of hypertension: A preliminary report, *Cytobios*, 34:142–152, 1982.

Iimuro, M., Shibata, H., Kawamori, T., Matsumoto, T., Arakawa, T., Sugimura, T., and Wakabayashi, K., Suppressive effects of garlic extract on *Helicobacter pylori*-induced gastritis in Mongolian gerbils, *Cancer Lett.*, 187:61–68, 2002.

Kendler, B.S., Garlic (*Allium sativum*) and onion (*Alliuim cepa*): A review of their relationship to cardiovascular disease, *Prev. Med.*, 16:670–685, 1987.

Keys, A., Wine, garlic and CHD in seven countries. *Lancet*, 1:145–146, 1980.

Ozturk, Y., Aydin, S., Kosar, M., and Baser, K.H.C., Endothelium-dependent and independent effects of garlic and rat aorta, *J. Ethnopharmacol.*, 44:109–116, 1994.

Sengupta, A., Ghosh, S., and Das, S., Administration of garlic and tomato can protect from carcinogen induced clastogenicity, *Nutr. Res.*, 22:859–866, 2002.

Sharifi, A.M., Darabi, R., and Akbarloo, N., Investigation of antihypertensive mechanism of garlic in 2K1C hypertensive rat, *J. Ethnopharmacol.*, 86:219–224, 2003.

Shukla, Y. and Taneja, P., Antimutagenic effects of garlic extract on chromosomal aberrations, *Cancer Lett.*, 176:31–36, 2002.

Zhang, X.-H., Lowe, D., Giles, P., Fell, S., Connock, M.J., and Maslin, D.J., Gender may affect the action of garlic oil on plasma cholesterol and glucose levels of normal subjects, *J. Nutr.*, 131:1471–1478, 2001.

Genistein   One of the main isoflavone components in soy is genistein. It is a phytoestrogen and an antioxidant and acts on osteoblast-like cells, increasing cellular proliferation. Lee and coworkers (2001) found genistein stimulated cell proliferation, as well as protected against oxidative damage to osteoblast-like cells from the action of free radicals. Epidemiological evidence suggests the low incidence of prostate cancer among Asians is associated with a high intake of soy. Studies conducted by Wang et al. (2002) showed that dietary genistein suppressed chemically induced prostate cancer in Lobund Wistar rats. Po and coworkers (2002a) found genistein was not as effective in suppressing estrogen-receptor sites or inducing apoptosis

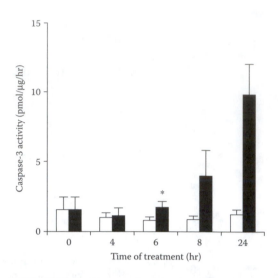

Genistein. (Adapted from Xu et al., *Structure*, 12: 2197–2207, 2004.)

using a transient transfection mouse model. Confirmation of the inability of soybean genistein to exert its chemoprotective effect through antagonizing the estrogen receptor was provided by Po et al. (2002b). Soybean genistein was also found by Hewitt and Singletary (2003) to inhibit adenocarcinoma tumor growth in a syngeneic mouse model. However, the greater inhibition by the soy extract compared to genistein suggested the presence of other components besides genistein.

The induction of apoptosis in a variety of cancer-cell lines by genistein is well-established (Lian et al., 1998; Shao et al., 1998). Recent research by Baxa and and Yoshimura (2003) showed that genistein induced inhibition of NF-κB by cleaving IκBα (Figure G.42). The latter is a protein residing in the cytosol, where it associates with NF-κB. These researchers also showed that caspase activity was involved in cleaving IκBα in genistein-treated cells. This was evident by a significant elevation of caspase-3 activity observed in genistein-treated T lymphoma 92316T cells after 6 h compared to the untreated cells. Other possible activities by genistein, such as inhibition of tyrosine kinase, which also reduces NF-κB, cannot be ruled out.

References

Baxa, D.M. and Yoshimura, F.K., Genistein reduces NF-κB in T lymphoma cells via a caspase-mediated cleavage of IκBα, *Biochem. Pharmacol.*, 66:1009–1018, 2003.

Hewitt, A.L. and Singletary, K.W., Soy extracts inhibits mammary adenocarcinoma growth in a syngeneic mouse model, *Cancer Lett.*, 192:133–143, 2003.

FIGURE G.42 Caspase-3 activation in genistein-treated cells. 92316T cells untreated (white bar) or treated with 60 μM genistein (black) assayed at 0, 4, 6, 8, and 24 h. $*p < 0.004$ compared to untreated cells, as determined by Student's t-test. (Baxa and Yoshimura, *Biochem. Pharmacol.*, 66:1009–1018, 2003. With permission.)

Lee, Y.-S., Chen, X., and Anderson, J.J.B., Physiological concentrations of genistein stimulate the proliferation and protect against free radical-induced oxidative damage of MC3T3-E1 osteoblast-like cells, *Nutr. Res.*, 21:1287–1298, 2001.

Lian, F., Bhuiyan, M., Li, Y., Wall, N., Kraut, M., and Sarker, F.H., Genistein-induced G2-M arrest, p21WAFI upregulation, and apoptosis in a non-small cell lung cancer cell line, *Nutr. Cancer*, 31:184–191, 1998.

Po, L.S., Chen, Z.-Y., Tsang, D.S.C., and Leung, L.K., Baicalein and genistein display differential actions on estrogen receptor (ER) transactivation and apoptosis in MCF-7 cells, *Cancer Lett.*, 187:33–40, 2002a.

Po, L.S., Wang, T.T., Chen, Z.-Y., and Leung, L.K., Genistein-induced apoptosis in MCF-7 cells involves changes in Bak and Bol-x without evidence of anti-oestrogenic effects, *Br. J. Nutr.*, 88:463–469, 2002b.

Shao, Z.M., Alpaugh, M.L., Fontina, J.A., and Barsky, S.H., Genistein inhibits proliferation similarly in estrogen receptor-positive and negative human breast carcinoma cell lines characterized by p21WAF1/CIP1 induction, G2.M arrest, and apoptosis, *J. Cell Biochem.*, 69:44–54, 1998.

Wang, J.M., Eltoum, I.-E., and Lamartiniere, C.A., Dietary genistein suppresses chemically induced prostate cancer in Lobund-Wistar rats, *Cancer Lett.,* 186:11–18, 2002.

Geraniol   Geraniol is an acyclic monoterpene alcohol found in the essential oils of fruits and herbs. Like many monoterpenes, geraniol has been reported to exert chemopreventive effects, including *in vivo* and *in vitro* antitumor activity against leukemia, hepatoma, and melanoma

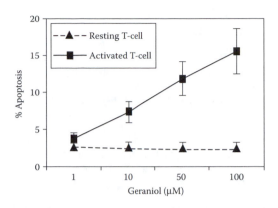

Geraniol. (From Duncan et al., *Biochem. Pharmacol.,* 68:1739–1747, 2004. With permission.)

cells in experimental animals (Shoff et al., 1991; Yu et al., 1995; Burke et al., 1997). Carnesecchi and coworkers (2001) demonstrated for the first time that geraniol (400 µM) inhibited the growth of a human colon cancer-cell line (Caco-2) by 70 percent. No cytotoxic effects or apoptosis were observed. The potent, antiproliferative effects of geraniol were attributed, in part, to a 50 percent decrease in ornithine decarboxylase activity, a key enzyme in polyamine biosynthesis, which is normally enhanced during carcinogenesis. Further research by these researchers (Carnesecchi and coworkers, 2002) showed that the antiproliferative effect of geraniol on Caco-2 cells was directly linked to perturbation of cell-membrane function, resulting in a 60 percent reduction of protein kinase C (PKC) activity. In addition, there was a 50 percent decrease in the active forms of p44/p42 extracellular signal-regulated protein kinases (ERK), suggesting perturbation in signal-transduction pathways.

FIGURE G.43   The rat T-cells apoptosis assay, resting and activated T-cells were treated with varying concentrations of geraniol (between 1 µmol/L and 100 µmol/L), and the activated T-cells showed higher apoptosis compared to resting cells. (From Ji et al., *Transpl. Proc.,* 34:1418–1419, 2002. With permission.)

The anticancer properties of monoterpenes were attributed to their ability to prevent isoprenylation of GTPases (Steinmetz et al., 1991). Ji and coworkers (2003) demonstrated geraniol exhibited modest immunosuppressive activity both *in vitro* and *in vivo*. This study provided the first evidence that geraniol induced apoptosis preferentially in activated T-cells (Figure G.43). Because of its suppressive property, geraniol was able to prolong graft survival in a cardiac allograft transplant model.

References

Burke, Y.D., Stark, M.J., Roach, S.L., Sen, S.E., and Crowell, P.L., Inhibition of pancreatic cancer growth by the dietary isoprenoids farnesol and geraniol, *Lipids,* 32:151–156, 1997.

Carnesecchi, S., Bradaia, A., Fischer, B., Coelho, D., Scholler-Guinard, M., Gosse, F., and Raul, F., Perturbation by geraniol of cell membrane permeability and signal transduction pathways in human colon cancer cells, *J. Pharmacol. Exp. Ther.,* 303:711–715, 2002.

Carnesecchi, S., Schneider, Y., Ceraline, J., Duranton, B., Gosse, F., Seiler, N., and Raul, F., Geraniol, a component of plant essential oils, inhibits growth and polyamine biosynthesis in human colon cancer cells, *J. Pharmacol. Exp. Ther.,* 298:197–200, 2001.

Duncan, R.E., Lau, D., El-Sohemy, A., and Archer, M.C., Geraniol and β-ionone inhibit proliferation, cell cycle progression, and cyclin-dependent kinase

G

2 activity in MCF-7 breast cancer cells independent of effects on HMG-CoA reductase activity, *Biochem. Pharmacol.*, 68:1739–1747, 2004.

Ji, P., Si, M.-S., Podnos, Y., and Imagawa, D.K., Monoterpene geraniol prevents acute allograft rejection, *Transpl. Proc.*, 34:1418–1419, 2002.

Shoff, S.M., Grummer., M., Yatvin, M.B., and Elson, C.E., Concentration-dependent increase of murine P388 and B16 population doubling time by the acyclic monoterpene geraniol, *Cancer Res.*, 51:37–42, 1991.

Steinmetz, K.A. and Potter, J.D., Vegetables, fruit, and cancer, I. Epidemiology, *Cancer Causes Cont.*, 2:325–327, 1991.

Yu, S.G., Hildebrandt, L.A., and Elson, C.E., Geraniol, an inhibitor of mevalonate biosynthesis, suppresses the growth of hepatomas and melanomas transplanted to rats and mice, *J. Nutr.*, 125:2763–2767, 1995.

(6)-gingerol
(Zingiber officinale, roscoe, zinglberaceae)

(6)-paradol
(Aframomum melegueta roscoe, zinglberaceae)

(From Lee and Suhr, *Cancer Lett.*, 134:163–168, 1998. With permission.)

Ginger   Ginger (*Zingiber officinale* Roscoe, Zingiberaceae) is used worldwide as a spice in the preparation of foods. In addition, the rhizome of ginger is a recognized treatment in traditional Oriental medicine for inflammation and rheumatism, as well as gastrointestinal problems. Koshimizu et al. (1988) found that the rhizome of ginger exerted antitumor properties by inhibiting 12-*O*-tetra-decanoylphorbol-13-acetate (TPA)-induced Epstein–Barr virus activation in Raji cells. A later study by Katiyar and coworkers (1996) showed topical application of an ethanol extract of ginger suppressed TPA-mediated induction of ornithine decarboxylase and its mRNA expression in SENCAR mouse skin. These workers also reported that the ginger extract protected the mouse skin from 7,12-dimethylbenz[*a*]-anthracene (DMBA)-induced carcinogenesis. The protective effects of ginger have been attributed to the presence of several phenolic compounds, or vanilloids, gingerol and paradol (Locksley et al., 1972; Lee and Surh, 1998; Park et al., 1998).

Abe et al. (2002) isolated a pungent principle present in Japanese ginger (*Zingiber mioga* Roscoe) as a labdane-type dialdehyde identified as galanals A and B. Miyoshi et al. (2003)

Galanal A; R = ◀OH
Galanal B; R = ·⁙⁙|OH

Structure of galanal A and B. (Adapted from Miyoshi et al., *Cancer Lett.*, 199:113–119, 2003.)

recently showed galanals A and B both significantly inhibited cell proliferation of human T lymphoma Jurkat cells in a dose-dependent manner (IC_{50} of 18 and 32 µMm, respectively) (Figure G.44). The mechanism of apoptosis involved reduction of the Bcl-2:Bax ratio and caspase-3 activation, suggesting their potential as anticancer agents.

A recent study by Hori and coworkers (2003) isolated five sulfonated compounds from *Zingiberis rhizome* (Shokyo), 4-gingesulfonic acid, and shogasulfonic acids A, B, C, and D, together with 6-gingesulfonic acid. Their potential bioactivity remains to be examined.

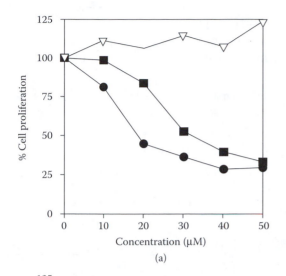

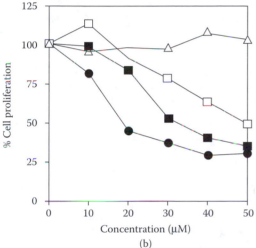

FIGURE G.44 Effect of compounds isolated from ginger plants on the cell growth of Jurkat cells. (A) Geranal A (●), galanal B (■), curcumin (□), or 6-gingerol (△). (Adapted from Miyoshi et al., *Cancer Lett.,* 199:113–119, 2003. With permission.)

References

Abe, M., Ozawa, Y., Uda, Y., Yamada, Y., Morimitsu, Y., Nakamura, Y., and Osawa, T. Labdane-type dialdehyde, pungent principle of myoga, *Zingiber mioga* Roscoe, *Biosci. Biotechnol. Biochem.,* 66:2698–2700, 2002.

Hori, Y., Miura, T., Hirai, Y., Fukumura, M., Nemoto, Y., Toriizuka, K., and Ida, Y., Pharmacognosticx studies on giner and related drugs-part 1: five sulfonated compounds from *Zingiberis rhizome* (Shokyo), *Phytochemistry,* 62:613–617, 2003.

Katiyar, S.K., Agarwal, R., and Mukhtar, H., Inhibition of tumor promotion in SENCAR mouse skin by ethanol extract of *Zingiber officinale* rhizome, *Cancer Res.,* 56:1023–1030, 1996.

Koshimizu, K., Ohigashi, H., Tokuda, H., Kondo, A., and Yamaguchi, K., Screening of edible plants against possible anti-tumor promoting activity, *Cancer Lett.,* 39:247–257, 1988.

Lee, E. and Surh, Y.-J., Induction of apoptosis in HL-60 cells by pungent vanilloids, [6]-generol and [6]-paradol, *Cancer Lett.,* 134:163–168, 1998.

Locksley, H.D., Rainey, D.K., and Rohan, T.A., Pungent compounds, part 1, an improved synthesis of paradols (alkyl 4-hydroxy-3-methoxyphenyethyl ketones) and an assessment of their pungency, *J. Chem. Soc. Perkin,* I:3001–3006, 1972.

Miyoshi, N., Nakamura, Y., Ueda, Y., Abe, M., Ozawa, Y., Uchida, K., and Osawa, T., Dietary ginger constituents, galanals A and B, are potent apoptosis inducers in human T lymphoma Jurkat cells, *Cancer Lett.,* 199:113–119, 2003.

Park, K.-K., Chun, K.-S., Lee, J.-M., Lee, S.S., and Surh, Y.-J., Inhibitory effects of [6]-gingerol, a major pungent principle of ginger, on phorbol ester-induced inflammation, epidermal ornithine decarboxylase activity and skin tumor promotion in ICR mice, *Cancer Lett.,* 129:139–144, 1998.

G

Gingerol Gingerols are the pungent oleoresin constituents present in ginger. The major gingerol component is [6]-gingerol (1-[4′-hydroxy-3′-methoxyphenyl]-5-hydroxy-3-decanone). Isolated [6]-gingerol appeared to be

(6)-gingerol

Tjendraputra, E., et al., *Bioorg. Chem.,* 29:156–163, 2001. With permission.

the active principle responsible for inhibiting secondary platelet activation and ATP release from platelets in human platelet-rich plasma. This inhibition is reversible, as it involves inhibition of arachidonic-acid metabolism and cyclooxygenase (COX) activity (Kiuchi et al., 1982; Guh et al., 1995). Koo and coworkers

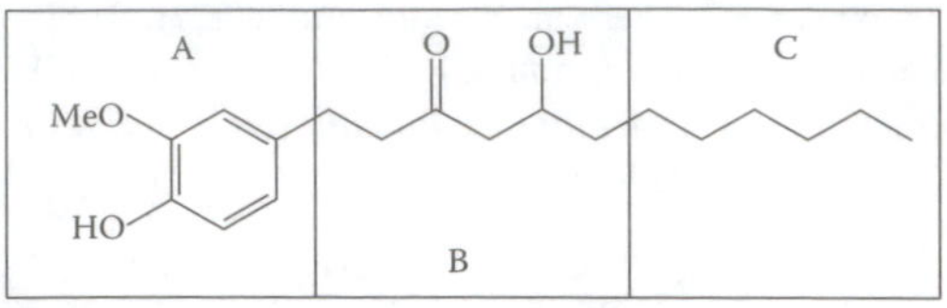

SCHEME G.26 Structural features of gingerol and synthetic analogues required for COX-2 inhibition. (A) Substitution pattern on the aromatic moiety, (B) functional group substitution pattern on the side chain, and (C) the lipophilic alkyl side chain. (From Tjendraputra et al., *Bioorg. Chem.*, 29:156–163, 2001. With permission.)

(2001) showed gingerols inhibited the arachidonic acid-induced platelet serotonin release reaction in a similar dose range as aspirin. Tjendraputra et al. (2001) examined 17 oleoresin principles of ginger (*Zingiber officinale,* Roscoe) together with synthetic analogues of gingerol. They all proved potent inhibitors of COX-2 and effective for treating inflammation. Based on their relative rates of inhibition, three important structural features were required for COX-2 inhibition: (1) lipophilicity of the alkyl side chain, (2) substitution pattern of hydroxy and carbonyl groups on the side chain, and (3) substitution of hydroxy and methoxy groups on the aromatic ring (Scheme G.26).

[6]-Gingerol is a strong antioxidant, as evident by its ability to inhibit $FeCl_3$-ascorbate-induced peroxidation of phospholipids (Aeschbach et al., 1994) or prevent the generation of reactive-oxygen species by xanthine oxidase (Chang et al., 1994). Park et al. (1998) demonstrated the antitumor activity of [6]-gingerol by its ability to significantly inhibit 7,12-dimethylbenz[*a*]-anthracene (DMBA)-induced skin papillomagenesis. This is shown in Table G.34 by its suppression of the tumor promoter-induced inflammation by reduction in mouse-ear edema. While [6]-gingerol reduced ear edema by 61 percent, it was much less than curcumin's 91 percent reduction at the same concentration of 10 μmol.

References

Aesbach, R., Loliger, J., Scott, B.C., Murcia, A., Butler, J., Halliwell, B., and Aruoma, O.I., Antioxidant actions of thymol, carvacrol, 6-gingerol, zingerone and hydroxytyrosol, *Food Chem. Toxicol.*, 32:31–36, 1994.

TABLE G.34
Inhibition of Tumor Promoter-Induced Inflammation in Mouse Ear by [6]-Gingerol[a]

Test compound	Increased ear weight (g)[a]	% Inhibition
None	5.26 ± 1.39[b]	0
[6]-Gingerol	1.84 ± 0.92[c]	61
Curcumin	0.46 ± 0.30[c]	91

[a] Values with [c] are significantly different from the control ($p < 0.005$).

[b] Values represent the mean ±SD (n=5)

Source: From Park et al., *Cancer Lett.*, 129:139–144, 1998. With permission.

Chang, W.-S., Chang, Y.-H., Lu, F.-L., and Chiang, H.-C., Inhibitory effects of phenolics on xanthine oxidase, *Anticancer Res.*, 14:501–506, 1994.

Guh, J.H., Ko, F.N., Jong, T.T., and Teng, C.M., Antiplatelet effect of gingerol isolated from *Zingiber officinale, J. Pharm. Pharmacol.*, 47:329–332, 1995.

Kiuchi, F., Shibuya, M., and Sankawa, U., Inhibitors of prostaglandin biosynthesis from ginger, *Chem. Pharm. Bull.*, 30:754–757, 1982.

Koo, K.L.K., Ammit, A.J., Tran, V.H., Duke, C.C., and Roufogalis, B.D., Gingerols and related analogues inhibit arachidonic acid-induced human platelet serotonin release and aggregation, *Thromb. Res.*, 103:387–397, 2001.

Park, K.-K., Chun, K.-S., Lee, J.-M., Lee, S.S., and Surh, Y.-J., Inhibitory effects of [6]-gingerol, a major pungent principle of ginger, on phosbol ester-induced inflammation, epidermal ornithine decarboxylase activity and skin tumor promotion in ICR mice, *Cancer Lett.*, 129:139–144, 1998.

Tjendraputra, E., Tran, V.H., Liu-Brennan, D., Roufogalis, B.D., and Duke, C.C., Effect of ginger constituents and synthetic analogues on cyclooxygenase-2 enzyme in intact cells, *Bioor. Chem.*, 29:156–163, 2001.

Ginkgo biloba   Extracts from the leaves of *Ginkgo biloba* L., one of the oldest phytomedicines in China, is still used extensively in therapy. The dry extract EGb 761, the essential component of *Ginkgo biloba*, is based on the content of flavonoids (24 percent) and terpenoids (6 percent). These preparations are used to treat diseases associated with advanced age, such as cerebrovascular and peripheral circulatory insufficiences and memory disturbances (Newall et al., 1996). The extract is an effective free-radical scavenger, with antioxidant activity capable of protecting against free-radical damage associated with such diseases as arteriosclerosis, rheumatism, and cancer. The action of EGb 761 on the human brain was confirmed by electroencephalography with enhancement of the α-wave component (Itil and Martorano, 1995; Luthringer et al., 1995). Animal studies showed EGb 761 facilitated acquisition and retention of memory (Cohen-Salmon et al., 1997; Winter, 1998) through protection of the hippocampus (Barkats et al., 1995). Since Alzheimer's disease is associated with a severely atrophied hippocampus, EGb 761 appeared to have potential as a treatment. The free-radical-scavenging effect of EGb 761 was demonstrated by the reduction of lipid peroxidation in a mouse-model brain with experimental cerebral ischemia (Pierre et al., 2002). EGb 761 prevents oxidative stress from destroying neurons, particularly by apoptosis, induced by glutamate, nitric oxide, and β-amyloid (Aβ) (Bastianetto and Quirion, 2002; Luo et al., 2002). Treatment of Wistar male rats with a *Ginkgo biloba* extract (GK 501) was shown by Hadjiivanova and Petkov (2002) to induce a significant decrease in the density (B_{max}) of β-adrenoreceptors in the frontal cortex and hippocampus regions of the brain (Table G.35). Since both of these areas are involved in cognition, it suggests that treatment with *Ginkgo biloba* extract may have a beneficial effect on learning and memory.

Brayboy and coworkers (2001) showed EGb 761 protected osteoblast-like bone cells (MC3T3-E1) from free-radical damage, as well as enhanced the proliferation of these cells. Ellnain-Wojtaszek and coworkers (2002) recommended that the leaves of *Ginkgo biloba* be stored for as short time as possible to prevent loss of free-radical-scavenging activity. Several excellent reviews on *Ginkgo biloba* were recently published in a new journal on nutraceuticals (Christen, 2003; Luo, 2003).

TABLE G.35
Effect of *In Vivo* Administration of *Ginkgo Biloba* Extract on β-Adrenergic Receptors in Different Rat Brain Regions[a,b,c]

Brain area	B_{max} (fmol/mg pr.)	
	Control	GK 501
Cortex	322.8 ± 21.4	228.1 ± 29.0[c]
Hippocampus	209.0 ± 20.1	162.8 ± 23.5[c]
Hypothalamus	119.6 ± 28.4	166.9 ± 26.0
Stratium	209.3 ± 23.0	226.7 ± 21.2

[a] *Ginkgo biloba* extract (90 mg/kg per day per os) or vehicle were administered for seven days.

[b] Results expressed as the mean ± SE for 5–10 rats.

[c] Significant difference between control and treated rats at $p < 0.05$.

Source: Adapted from Hadjiivanova and Petkov, *Phytother. Res.*, 16:488–492, 2002.

References

Barkats, M., Venault, P., Christen, Y., and Cohen-Salmon, C., Effects of long term treatment with EGb 761 on age-dependent structural changes in the hippocampi of three inbred mouse strains, *Life Sci.*, 56:213–222, 1995.

Bastianetto, S. and Quirion, R., EGb 761 is a neuroprotective agent against β-amyloid toxicity, *Cell. Mol. Biol.*, 48:693–697, 2002.

Brayboy, J.R., Chen, X.W., Lee, Y.S., and Anderson, J.J.B., The protective effects of Ginkgo biloba extract (EGb761) against free radical damage to osteoblast-like bone cells (MC3T3-E1) and the proliferative effects of Egb 761 on these cells, *Nutr. Res.*, 21:275–1285, 2001.

Cohen-Salmon, C., Venault, P., Martin, B., Rafalli-Sebille, M.J., Barkats, M., Clostre, F., Pardon, M.-C., Christen, Y., and Chapouthier, G., Effects of Ginkgo biloba extract EGb 761 on learning and memory, *J. Physiol.*, 91:91–300, 1997.

Christen, Y., From clinical observations to molecular biology: Ginkgo biloba extract EGB 761, a success for reverse pharmacology, *Curr. Top. Nutraceut. Res.*, 1:59–72, 2003.

Ellnain-Wojtaszek, M., Kruczynski, Z., and Kasprzak, J., Variations in the free radical scavenging activity of *Ginkgo biloba* L. leaves in the period of complete development of green leaves to fall of yellow ones, *Food Chem.*, 79:79–84, 2002.

Hadjiivanova, Ch.I. and Petkov, V.V., Effect of *Ginkgo biloba* extract on β-adrenergic receptors in different rat brain regions, *Phytother. Res.,* 16:488–492, 2002.

Itil, T. and Martirano, D., Natural substances in psychiatry (*Ginkgo biloba* in dementia), *Psychopharmacol. Bull.,* 31:147–158, 1995.

Luo, Y., Contemporary neuroscience meets traditional medicine — towards understanding *ginkgo biloba* neuroprotection, *Curr. Top. Nutraceut. Res.,* 1:49–58, 2003.

Lutheringer, R., d'Arbigny, P., and Macher, J.P., *Ginkgo biloba* extract (EGb 761), EEG and event-related potentials mapping profile, in *Advances in Ginkgo Biloba Extract Research*, Vol. A, Effects of Age-related Disorder, Christen, Y., Courtois, Y., and Droy-Lefaix, M.-T., Eds., Elsevier, Paris, 1995, pp. 107–118.

Newall, C.A., Anderson, L.A., and Phillipson, J.D., *Herbal Medicines,* The Pharmaceuticals Press, London, 1996.

Pierre, S., Jamme, I., Robert, K., Gerbi, A., Duran, M.-J., Sennoune, S., Droy-Lefaix, M.-T., Nouvelot, A., and Maixent, J.-M., *Ginkgo biloba* extract (EGb 761) protects Na, K-ATPase isoenzymes during cerebral ischemia, *Cell. Mol. Biol.,* 48:671–679, 2002.

Winter, J.C., The effect of an extract of Ginkgo biloba EGb761, on cognitive behavior and longevity in the rat, *Physiol. Behav.,* 63:425–433, 1998.

Ginseng   Ginseng, the root of *Panax ginseng*, has been used in Oriental medicine for many centuries to treat a wide range of ailments. In Europe, it is sold over the counter to enhance physical and mental performance. Ginseng products are either white or red. White ginseng is the dried root with the skin peeled off, whereas red ginseng is the steamed root, which is caramel-colored. White ginseng (includes lateral roots and root hairs) is commonly used in the European market, while red ginseng is the preferred form in Asia. The unique constituents identified in ginseng include several classes of compounds: triterpene saponins; essential oil-containing polyacetylenes and sesquiterpenes; polysaccharides; peptidoglycans; and nitrogen-containing compounds (Tang and Eisenbrand 1992). Triterpene saponins are referred to as ginsenosides, as their property appears to be a function of the number of monosaccharide residues in the sugar chain (Hostettmann and Marston, 1995). Thirty-one ginsenosides have been isolated from the roots of white and red ginseng that can be categorized into three groups, based on their aglycones, as protopanaxadiol-type, protopanaxatriol-type, and oleanolic acid-type saponins (Sticher, 1998). Ginseng is specified in the Swiss and German pharmacopeias on the total ginsensoside content, calculated as ginsenoside R_{g1}, as not less than 2.0 percent and 1.5 percent, respectively. The European pharmacopeia requires that the ginsenoside R_{ga} and R_{b1} content in ginseng must not be less than 0.3 percent.

Research on ginseng suggests ginsenosides have antiaging properties by enhancing the immune system by increasing serum-specific antibodies and I_gG content and protective B-lymphocytes (Nah et al., 1995; Liu et al., 1995; Yamada et al., 1995). In addition to ginsenosides other isolated components, such as polyacetylenes, panaxytriol, panaxynol, and panaxydol have cytotoxic, antiplatelet, and anti-inflammatory properties, respectively (Deng and Zhang, 1991; Matsunaga et al., 1995; Kobayashi et al., 1995). The hypoglycemic effect of ginseng is attributed to its polysaccharides, the panaxans, which are themselves peptidoglycans. Immunological activity is also associated with some of its polysaccharides, the ginsenans. While the precise structures of these polysaccharides are not fully known, their backbone chain is mainly β-1,3-linked D-galactoside (Tomoda et al., 1993).

References

Deng, H. and Zhang, J., Anti-lipid peroxidative effect of ginsenoside Rb1 and Rg1, *Chin. Med. J.,* 104:395–398, 1991.

Hostettmann, K. and Marston, A., *Saponins.* Cambridge University Press, Cambridge, U.K., 1995, p. 50.

Kobayashi, M., Mahmud, T., Umezome, T., and Kitgawa, I., The absolute stereostructure of panaxytriol, a biologically active diacetylenic acetogenin, from *Ginseng Radix* Rubra, *Chem. Pharm. Bull.,* 43:1595–1597, 1995.

Liu, J., Wang, S., Liu, H., Yang, L., and Nan, G., Stimulatory effect of saponin from Panax ginseng on immune function of lymphocytes in the elderly, *Mech. Ageing Dev.,* 83:43–53, 1995.

Matsunaga, H., Saita, T., Nagumo, F., Mori, M., and Katano, M., A possible mechanism for the cytoxicity of a polyacetylenic alcohol, panaxtriol, inhibition of mitochondrial respiration, *Cancer Chemother. Pharmacol.,* 35:291–296, 1995.

Nah, S., Park, H., and McCleskey, E.W., A trace component of ginseng that inhibits Ca^{2+} channels through a pertussis toxin-sensitive G-protein, *Proc. Natl. Acad. Sci.,* 92:8739–8743, 1995.

Sticher, O., Getting to the root of ginseng, *Chemtech,* (April):26–32, 1998.

Tang, W. and Eisenbrand, G., *Chinese Drugs of Plant Origin,* Springer Verlag, Berlin, 1992, pp. 711–737.

Yamada, H., Otsuka, H., and Kiyohra, H., Fractionation and characterization of anticomplimentary and mitogenic substances from Panax ginseng extract G-115, *Phytother. Res.,* 9:264–269, 1995.

Glabridin   Glabridin is the major isoflavan in licorice root (*Glycyrrhiza glabra*) with two hydroxyl groups at the 2′ and 4′ positions, a 2,2-dimethyl-γ-pyran ring fused to the B ring with a double bond between carbon 3 and 4 in the C ring. The conjugated double-bond system present in glabridin appeared to enhance its

Glabridin. (From Fukai et al., *Fitoterapia,* 74:624–629, 2003. With permission.)

antioxidant properties, which accounted for it being the most active compound isolated from licorice that inhibited LDL oxidation (Vaya et al., 1997: Belinsky et al., 1998). Tamir et al. (2000) demonstrated the estrogenic properties of glabridin, as well as its antiproliferative properties against human breast-cancer cells. Further research by Tamir and coworkers (2001) confirmed the estrogen-like properties of glabridin but also identified a new

phytoestrogen, glabrene, an isoflavene in licorice roots exhibiting stronger estrogenic agonist activity. Glabridin also affects the skin, as Yokota and coworkers (1998) found it inhibited melanogenesis and inflammation in cultured B16 murine-melanoma cells.

References

Belinsky, P.A., Aviram, M., Mahmood, S., and Vaya, J., Structural aspects of the inhibitory effect of glabridin on LDL oxidation, *Free Rad. Biol. Med.,* 24: 1419–1429, 1998.

Fuai, T., Satoh, K., Nomura, T., and Sakagami, T., Preliminary evaluation of antinephritis and radical scavenging activities of glabridin from *Glycyrrhiza glabra, Fitoterapia,* 74:624–629, 2003.

Tamir, S., Eizenberg, M., Somjen, D., Israel, S., and Vaya, J., Estrogen-like activity of glabrene and other constituents isolated from licorice root, *J. Steroid Biochem. Mol. Biol.,* 78:291–298, 2001.

Tamir, S., Eizenberg, M., Somjen, D., Stern, N., Shelach, R., Kiaye, A., and Vaya, J., Estrogenic and antiproliferative properties of glabridin from licorice in human breast cancer cells, *Cancer Res.,* 60:5704–5709, 2000.

Vaya, J., Belinsky, P.A., and Aviram, M., Antioxidant constituents from licorice roots: Isolation, structure elucidation and antioxidative capacity toward LDL oxidation, *Free Rad. Biol. Med.,* 23:302–313, 1997.

Yokota, T., Nishi, H., Kubota, Y., and Mizoguchi, M., The inhibitory effect of glabridin from licorice extracts on melanogenesis and inflammation, *Pigment Cell Res.,* 11:355–361, 1998.

Glucosamine sulfate   Glucosamine sulfate is a commonly used treatment for osteoarthritis. A three-year, randomized, placebo-controlled, double-blind study of 202 patients with knee osteoarthritis by Pavelka and coworkers (2002) showed that long-term treatment with glucosamine sulfate retarded the progression of the disease. Unlike systemic inflammatory diseases, such as rheumatoid arthritis, osteoarthritis is characterized by local inflammatory activity. A recent review by Amin et al. (1999) pointed to a local increase in the proinflammatory cytokine, interleukin-1β (IL-1β) during progression of osteoarthritis. IL-β initiates a whole series of events leading to cartillage damage, including activation of nuclear factor kappa B (NfκB). Using cell cultures of human osteoarthritic chondrocytes, Largo and coworkers (2003) showed glucosamine significantly inhibited NfκB activity, as well as the nuclear translocation of p50 and p65 proteins involved in the inflammatory process. The use of glucosamine and chondroitin sulfate for the symptomatic treatment of osteoarthritis has been controversial. Nevertheless, a recent review by Hungerford and Jones (2003) pointed to the many *in vitro* and *in vivo* animal clinical and human clinical studies that confirm both the efficacy and safety of their treatment of osteoarthritis.

References

Amine, A.R., Attur, M.G., and Abramson, S.B., Regulation of nitric oxide and inflammatory mediators in human osteoarthritis-affected cartilage: Implication for pharmacological intervention, in *The Pathophysiology and Clinical Applications of Nitric Oxide,* Rubanyi, Ed., Harwood Academic Publishers, Newark, New Jersey, 1999, pp. 397–413.

Hungerford, D.S. and Jones, L.C., Glucosamine and chondroitin sulfate are effective in the management of osteoarthritis, *J. Arthroplasty,* 18:5–9, 2003.

Largo, R., Alvarez-Soria, M.A., Diez-Ortego, I., Calvo, E., Sanchez-Pernaute, O., Egido, J., and Herrero-Beaumont, G., Glucosamine inhibits IL-1β-induced NFκB activation in human osteoarthritic chondrocytes, *Osteoarth. Cart.,* 11:290–298, 2003.

Pavelka, K., Gatterova, J., Olejarova, M., Machacek, S., Giacovelli, G., and Rovati, L.C., Glucosamine use and delay of progression of knee osteoarthritis, a 3 year, randomized, placebo-controlled, double-blind study, *Arch. Intern. Med.,* 162:2113–2123, 2002.

Glucosinolates   The reduced risk of colorectal cancer associated with the consumption of cruciferous vegetables is attributed to the presence of a group of secondary plant metabolites known as glucosinolates (Verhoeven et al., 1996). These bioactive, sulfur-containing components are hydrolyzed by an endogenous plant enzyme myrosinase (thioglucoside glucohydrolase EC 3.2.3.1) to isothiocyanates. This only occurs when the cells are broken or damaged by cutting or chewing, as myrosinase and glucosinolates are separated from each other in the intact plant. Glucosinolates are broken down into isothiocyanates, nitriles, thiocyanates, indoles, and oxazolidinethiones (Scheme G.27). Some of these degradation products, particularly the isothiocyanates (ITCs) and some indolic compounds, have health-protective effects. A typical glucosinolate is singrin, which was shown to reduce the number of precancerous lesions in a dimethylhydrazine (DMH)-induced rat colon cancer model (Smith et al., 1998). Lund and coworkers (2001) compared the ability of four isothiocyanates (ITC), benzyl-ITC, allyl-ITC

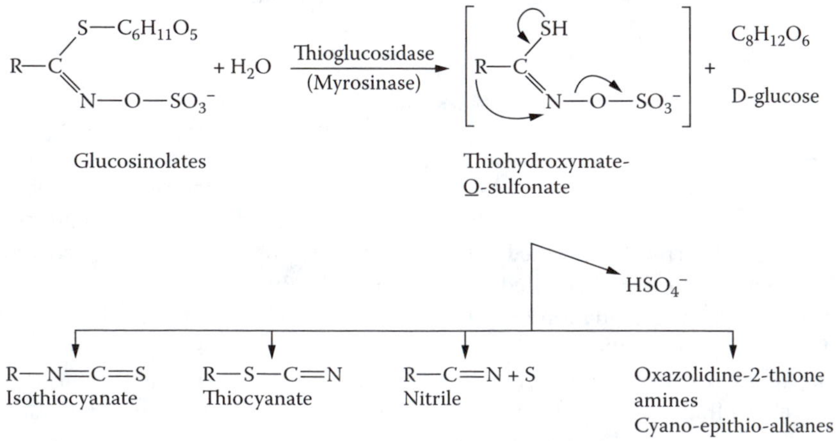

SCHEME G.27 Chemical structures of glucosinolates and their breakdown products following enzymic hydrolysis by myrosinase (Adapted from Pessina et al., *Arch. Biochem. Biophys.,* 280:383–389, 1990, by Steinkeller et al., *Mutat. Res.,* 480–481:285–287, 2001. With permission.)

(AITC), phenylethyl-ITC (PEITC), and methyl-sulphinylbutyl-ITC (sulforaphane), to induce apoptosis in colorectal adenocarcinoma cells (HT9). The relative potency of these compounds to reduce adherent cell number was BITC = AITC> PEITC>>sulforaphane. The primary action of these ITCs was to block rapidly proliferating cancer cells at G2/M. These researchers commented that reducing the levels of glucosinolates by breeding to reduce the hot and bitter flavors associated with their degradation products might impair the health benefits associated with these vegetables.

Glucosinolates are activators of liver-detoxification enzymes; their mode of protection appears to involve modulation of carcinogen metabolism by inducing phase II detoxification enzymes, while inhibiting phase I detoxification enzymes (Hecht, 1999). Shapiro et al. (1980) showed substantial amounts of isothiocyanates were converted to dithiocarbamates. Smith and coworkers (1998) observed that the purified glucosinolate, sinigrin, reduced the number of precancerous lesions in rat colon induced by dimethylhydrazine (DMH) and was associated with an increase in apoptosis within 48 hours of exposure to DMH. The underlying mechanism responsible for cell death induced by four isothiocyanates (ITCs), benzyl-ITC, allyl-ITC, phenylethyl-ITC, and methylsulphinylbutyl-ITC (sulforaphane), was studied by Lund et al. (2001). The primary mechanism involved blocking the rapidly proliferating colorectal adenocarcinoma (HT29) cancer cells in G2/M.

References

Hecht, S.S., Chemoprevention of cancer by isothiocyanates, modifiers of carcinogen metabolism, *J. Nutr.*, 129:768S–774S, 1999.

Lund, E.K., Smith, T.K., Clarke, R.G., and Johnson, I.T., Cell death in the colorectal cancer cell line HT29 in response to glucosinolate metabolites, *J. Sci. Food Agric.*, 81:959–961, 2001.

Pessina, A., Thomas, R.M., Palmieri, S., and Lussi, P.L., An improved method for purification of myrosinase and its physicochemical characterization, *Arch. Biochem. Biophys.*, 280:383–389, 1990.

Smith, T.K., Lund, E.K., and Johnson, I.T., Inhibition of dimethylhydrazine-induced aberrant crypt foci and induction of apoptosis in rat colon following oral administration of the glucosinolate sinigrin, *Carcinogenesis*, 19:267–273, 1998.

Steinkeller, H., Rabot, S., Freyald, C., Nobis, E., Scharf, G., Chabicovsky, M., Knasmuller, S., and Kassie, F., Effects of cruciferous vegetables and their constituents on drug metabolizing enzymes involved in the bioactivation of DNA-reactive dietary carcinogens, *Mutat. Res.*, 480–481:285–297, 2001.

Verhoeven, D.T., Goldbohm, R.A., Poppel, G., Verhagen, H., and van den Brandt, P.A., Epidemiological studies on brassica vegetables and cancer risk, *Cancer Epidemiol. Biomarkers Prevention*, 5:733–748, 1996.

G

Glycyrrhin and 18β-Glycyrrhetinic acid

Glycyrrhin, a pentacyclic triterpene derivative, is the main, water-soluble constituent of licorice roots (*Glycyrrhizza glabra* L.). Besides being a sweetening and flavoring agent in foods, glycyrrhin has been used in Asia and Europe for many years as an antidote, demulcent, and folk medicine. Glycyrrhin is hydrolyzed by the intestinal bacterial glucuronidase to the corresponding aglycone, 18β-glycyrrhetinic acid,

Glycyrrhetinic acid. (From Wang et al., *J. Chromatogr. A.*, 811:219–224, 1998. With permission.)

which is then absorbed by the body. Both glycyrrhin and its aglycone have been associated with a number of health benefits, including antiulcerative (Doll et al., 1962), anti-inflammatory (Ohuchi et al., 1981), antiviral (Ito et al., 1988), antihepatitis (Kiso et al., 1984), and antitumor (Suzuki et al., 1992) properties. Jeong and coworkers (2002) recently showed that the potent hepatoprotective properties of 18β-glycerrhetinic acid were due to its ability to block bioactivation of carbon tetrachloride by inhibiting cytochrome P450 2E1 expression.

References

Doll, R., Hill, I.D., Hutton, C., and Underwood, D.J., Clinical trial of a triterpenoid licorice compound in gastric and duodenal ulcer, *Lancet*, 2:793–796, 1962.

Itoh, M., Sato, A., Hirabayashi, K., Tanabe, F., Shigeta, S., Baba, M., De Clercq, E., Nakashima, H., and Yamamoto, N., Mechanism of inhibitory effect of glycyrrhizin on replication of human immunodeficiency virus (HIV), *Antiviral Res.,* 10:289–298, 1988.

Jeong, H.G., You, H.J., Park, S.J., Moon, A.R., Chung, Y.C., Kang, S.K., and Chun, H.Y., Hepatoprotective effects of 18-glycyrrhetinic acid on carbon tetrachloride-induced liver injury: Inhibition of cytochrome P450 2E1 expression, *Pharmacol. Res.*, 46: 221–227, 2002.

Kiso, Y., Tohkin, M., Hikino, H., Hattori, M., Sakamoto, T., and Namba, T., Mechanism of antihepatotoxic activity of glycyrrhizin. I. Effect of free radical generation and lipid peroxidation, *Planta Med.*, 50: 298–302, 1984.

Ohuchi, K., Kamada, Y., Levine, L., and Tsurufuji, S., Glycyrrhizin inhibits prostaglandin E2 production by activated peritoneal macrophages from rats, *Prostaglandin Med.*, 7:457–463, 1981.

Suzuki, F., Schmitt, D.A., Utsunomiya, T., and Pollard, R.B., Stimulation of host resistance against tumors by glycyrrhin, an active component of licorice roots, *In-Vivo*, 6:589–596, 1992.

Vaya, J. Bellinky, P.A., and Aviram, M., Antioxidant constituents from licorice roots: Isolation, structure elucidation and antioxidative capacity towards LDL oxidation, *Free Rad. Biol. Med.*, 23:302–313, 1997.

Glycyrrhizic acid Glycyrrhizic acid, another component of licorice root, was found to be active against a number of viruses, such as herpes simplex type 1, varicella-zoster virus, human cytomegalovirus, hepatitis A, B, and C viruses, human immunodeficiency virus-1, and influenza virus (Crance et al., 1994; Sato et al., 1996; Arase et al., 1997; Utsunomiya et al., 1997). Recently, Lin and coworkers (2003) showed glycyrrhizic acid inhibited the replication of the Epstein–Barr virus, which differed from

Glycyrrhizic acid. (From Wang et al., *J. Chromatogr. A.,* 811:219–224, 1998. With permission.)

mode of action of nucleoside analogues, which inhibit DNA polymerase. The ability of glycyrrhizic acid to protect against aflatoxin-induced oxidative stress in hepatoma cells was recently reported by Chan and coworkers (2003).

References

Arase, Y., Ikeda, K., Murashima, N., Chayama, K., Tsubota, A., Koida, I., Suzuki, Y., Saitoh, S., Kobayashi, M., and Kumada, H., The long term efficacy of glycyrrhizin in chronic hepatitis C patients, *Cancer*, 79:1494–1500, 1997.

Chan, H., Chan, C., and Ho, J.W., Inhibition of glycyrrhizic on aflatoxin B_1-induced cytoxicity in hepatoma cells, *Toxicology*, 188:211–217, 2003.

Crance, J.M., Leveque, F., Biziagos, E., van Cuyck-Gandre, H., Jouan, A., and Deloince, R., Studies on mechanism of action of glycyrrhizin against hepatitis A virus replication *in vitro*, *Antiviral Res.*, 23:63–76, 1994.

Lin, J.-C., Mechanism of action of glycyrrhizic acid in inhibition of Epstein–Barr virus replication *in vitro*, *Antiviral Res.*, 59:41–47, 2003.

Sato, H., Goto, W., Yamamura, J., Kurokawa, M., Kageyama, S., Takahara, T., Watanabe, A., and Shiraki, K., Therapeutic basis of glycyrrhizin on chronic hepatitis B, *Antiviral Res.*, 30:171–177, 1996.

Utsunomiya, T., Kobayashi, M., Pollard, R.B., and Suzuki, F., Glycyrrhizin an active component of licorice roots, reduces morbidity and mortality of mice infected with lethal doses of influenza virus, *Antimicrob. Agents Chemother.*, 41:551–556, 1997.

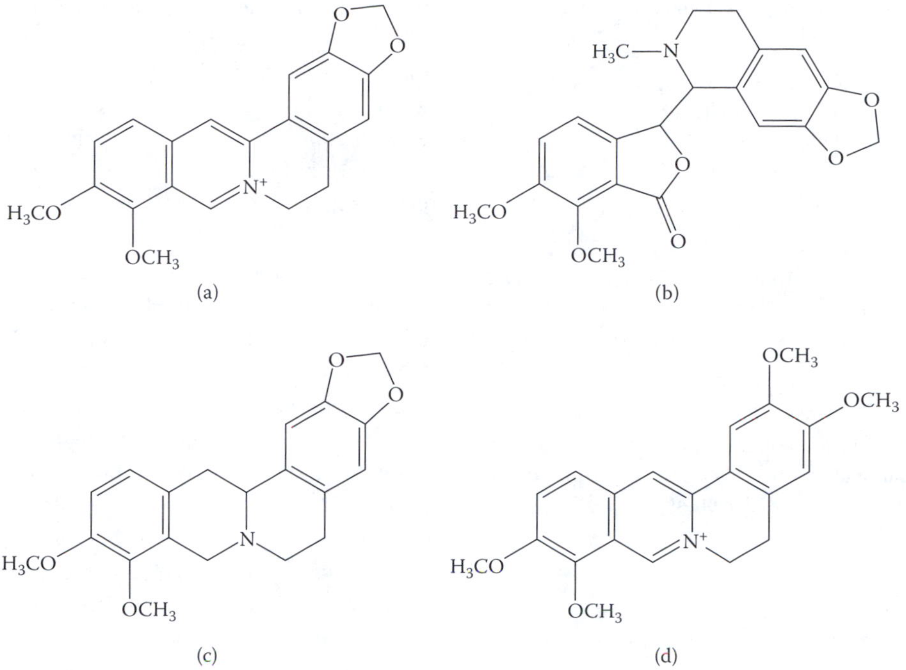

SCHEME G.28 Goldenseal isoquinoline alkalioids: berberine (a); hydrastine (b); canadine (c); palmatine (d). (From Weber et al., *J. Agric. Food Chem.*, 51:7352–7358, 2003. With permission.)

Goldenseal (*Hydrastis canadensis* L.)

Goldenseal (*Hydrastis canadensis* L.) is a perennial, herbaceous plant native to eastern North America. It is a medicinal herb used primarily for its antimicrobial properties (Diamond and Towers, 1999; Upton, 2001). Goldenseal is a very popular supplement and is often sold together with *Echinacea.* The dried roots or rhizome of goldenseal contain a number of isoquinoline alkaloids, the major ones being hydrastine and berberine, together with smaller amounts of canadine and palmatine (Scheme G.28). The American Herbal Pharmacopoeai states that fresh or dried roots from goldenseal should not contain less than 2.5 percent berberine and 2.0 percent hydrastine, on a dryweight basis (Upton, 2001). Berberine has been used to treat psoriasis and eye infections (Sabir et al., 1978; Muller et al., 1995).

Since goldenseal is used extensively in eyewashes and in skin lotions, Inbaraj and coworkers (2001) examined possible adverse interactions with light. In the presence of 50 μM berberine, UVA irradiation of transformed epidermal human-cell line, HaCaT keratinocytes, resulted in a decrease in cell viability of 80 percent, while tripling the amount of DNA damage. Based on these results, avoiding sunlight or artificial-light sources emitting UVA was recommended when using preparations containing goldenseal or berberine. However, these researchers pointed out that antiseptic properties associated with such topical preparations could be due to such interactions.

Rehman et al. (1999) showed that both *Echinacea* and goldenseal enhanced antibody production in rats, each acting on a different immunoglobulin subtype. *Echinacea* treatment improved the IgG immune response in rats one or two weeks after treatment with KLH, a novel antigen, keyhole limpet hemocyanin, while goldenseal augmented IgM response during the first two weeks of treatment. Such augmentation in antibody response could lead to identification of novel immune adjuvants.

References

Diamond, S. and Towers, G.H.N., in *Herbs, Botanicals and Teas,* Mazza, G. and Oomah, B.D., Eds.,

Technomic Publishing Co., Lancaster, Pennsylvania, 1999, pp. 177–211.

Inbaraj, J.J., Kukielczak, B.M., Bilski, Sandvik, S.L., and Chignell, C.F., Photochemistry and photocytotoxicity of alkaloids from goldenseal (*Hydrastis Canadensis* L.), 1. Berberine, *Chem. Res. Toxicol.,* 14:1529–1534, 2001.

Muller, K., Ziereis, K. and Gawlik, I., The antipsoriatic Mahonia aquifolium and its active constituents, II. Antiproliferative activity against cell growth of human keratinocytes, *Planta Med.,* 61:74–75, 1995.

Rehman, J., Dillow, J.M., Carter, S.M., Chou, J., Le, B., and Maisel, A.S., Increased production of antigen-specific immunoglobulins G and M following *in vivo* treatment with *Echinacea augustifolia* and *Hydrastis canadensis*, *Immunol. Lett.,* 68:391–395, 1999.

Sabir, M., Akhter, M.H., and Bhide, N.K., Further studies on the pharmacology of berberine, *Ind. J. Physiol. Pharmacol.,* 22:9–23, 1978.

Upton, R., Goldseal root, *Hydrastis canadensis*, in *Standards of Analysis, Quality Control and Therapeutics*, American Herbal Pharmacopoeia, Santa Cruz, California, 2001.

Weber, H.A., Zart, M.K., Hodges, A.E., Molloy, H.M., O'Brien, B.M., Moody, L.A., Clark, A.P., Harris, R.K., Overstreet, J.D., and Smith, C.S., Chemical comparison of goldenseal (*Hydrastis canadensis* L.) root powder from three commercial suppliers, *J. Agric. Food Chem.,* 51:7352–7358, 2003.

Grapefruit   Grapefruit juice has been reported to interact and elevate the pharmacological efficacy of a number of medications, including cyclosporine (Ducharme et al., 1995), midazolam (Kupferschmidt et al., 1995), felodipine (Bailey et al., 1990), and lovastatin (Kantola et al., 1998). The bioavailability of these drugs was enhanced 1.5- to 15-fold following ingestion of grapefruit juice. The lipophilic nature of these drugs necessitates their oxidative transformation by cytochrome P450 (CYP3A4) prior to excretion. The major flavonoid in grapefruit is naringin, which, together with its aglycone naringenin, both inhibit CYP3A4, although naringenin was found to be the more potent inhibitor *in vitro* (Miniscalo et al., 1992). However, Schmiedlin-Ren et al. (1997)

reported that the furanocoumarin derivative, dihydroxybergapten, was a far more potent inhibitor, which was later shown to have a very low IC$_{40}$ (Ho et al., 1998). The marked differences between the levels of naringin, naringenin, and bergapten (5-methoxypsoralen) in grapefruit and grapefruit-juice products were attributed by Ho et al. (2000) to the contradictory drug-interaction results reported in the literature. Tassaneeyakul et al. (2000) showed that, in addition to the human microsomal CYP3A4, CYP2C19 was also inhibited by grapefruit extract or its isolated furancoumarins. Using the carageenan-induced paw oedema model, Mahgoub (2001) also reported grapefruit juice potentiated the effects of the nonsteroidal, anti-inflammatory drug diclofenac to inhibit other cytochrome P450 isoenzymes. A new CYP3A4 inhibitor, a furanocoumarin derivative, paradisin C, was recently identified by Ohta and coworkers (2002) in grapefruit juice (Scheme G.29).

In vitro studies by Goff-Klein et al. (2003) on human liver microsomes and rat hepatocytes and microsomes showed interspecies differences involved different CYP450 isoenzymes in the metabolism of simvastatin (SV), a drug used to treat hypercholesterolemia, in the presence of bergamottin, a grapefruit component. Inhibition of CPY450 isoenzymes by bergamottin can lead to prolonged exposure to SV with high serum simastavin-acid concentrations, increasing the risk of skeletal-muscle toxicity (Bogman et al., 2001). Prolonged exposure to some drugs may be beneficial, while drugs, such as simastavin, could be harmful. As a result, grapefruit is no longer served in hospitals.

Miyata et al. (2002) examined the effect of grapefruit juice on the heterocyclic amine, 2-amino-1-methyl-6-phenylimidazo[4,5-b]pyridine (PhIP), a component in cooked meat and fish implicated in the etiology of colon cancer. They showed that pretreatment of rats with grapefruit juice suppressed colon DNA damage using the comet assay. A 6.2-fold and 5.4-fold increase in migration of DNA and frequency of tailed nuclei were observed in colon nuclei of PhIP-treated rats compared to vehicle-treated rats (Figure G.45). In contrast, a reduction of

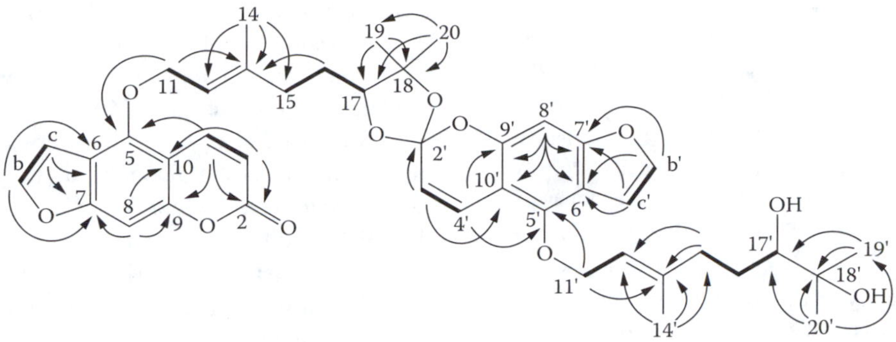

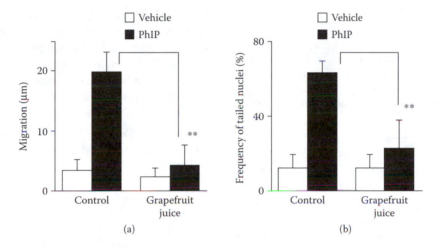

SCHEME G.29 COSY (bold lines) and HMC (arrows) NMR Spectral data correlations observed for paradisin C. (From Ohta et al., *Tetrahedron,* 58:6631–6635, 2002. With permission.)

FIGURE G.45 Effect of pretreatment with grapefruit juice on PhIP-induced DNA damage in rat colon. (a) Migration. (b) Frequency of tailed nuclei. Rats had free access to grapefruit juice five days prior to administration of PhIP (60 mg/kg). Colon nuclei were isolated 3 h after PhIP treatment. Migration measured as the difference between the length of the whole comet and the diameter of the head. Values represent the mean ± SD ($n = 3$ in each group). $**p < 0.01$, significant differences from corresponding control group. (From Miyata et al., *Cancer Lett.,* 183:17–22, 2002. With permission.)

20 percent and 36 percent in DNA migration and frequency of tailed nuclei was evident in grapefruit juice-treated rats compared to the control rats, respectively.

References

Bailey, D.G., Arnold, J.M.O., and Spence, J.D., Grapefruit juice-drug interaction, *Br. J. Clin. Pharmacol.,* 46:101–110, 1998.

Bogmann, K., Peyer, A.K., Torok, M., Kusters, E., and Drewe, J., HMG-CoA reductase inhibitors and P-glycoprotein modulation, *Br. J. Pharmacol.,* 132:1183–1192, 2001.

Ducharme, M.P., Warbasse, L.H., and Edwards, D.J, Disposition of intravenous and oral cyclosporine after administration with grapefruit juice, *Clin. Pharmacol. Ther.,* 57:485–491, 1995.

Goff-Klein, N.L., Koffell, J.-C., Jung, L., and Ubeaud, G., *in vitro* inhibition of simvastatin metabolism, an HMG-CoA reductase inhibitor in human and rat liver by bergamottin, a component of grapefruit juice, *Eur. J. Pharm. Sci.,* 18:31–35, 2003.

Ho, P.C., Saville, D.J., Coville, P.F., and Wanwimolruk, S., Content of CYP3A4 inhibitors, naringin, naringenin and bergapten in grapefruit and grapefruit juice products, *Pharm. Acta Helv.,* 74:379–385, 2000.

Ho, P.C., Wanwimolruk, S., and Saville, D.J., Inhibition of CYP3A4 in human liver microsomes by bioflavonoids and coumarin derivatives found in grapefruit juice, *Pharmacol. Sci.,* 1:S38, 1998.

Kantola, T., Kivisto, K.T., and Neuvonen, P.J., Grapefruit juice greatly increases serum concentration of lovastatin and lovastatin acid, *Clin. Pharmacol. Ther.,* 63:397–402, 1998.

Kupferschmidt, H.H.T., Ha, H.R., Ziegler, W.H., Meier, P.J., and Krahenbuhl, S., Interaction between grapefruit juice and oral midazolam in humans, *Clin. Pharmacol. Ther.,* 58:20–28, 1995.

Mahgoub, A.A., Grapefruit juice potentiates the anti-inflammatory effects of diclofenac on the carrageenan-induced rat's paw model, *Pharmacol. Res.,* 45: 1–4, 2002.

Miniscalco, A., Lundahl, J., Regardh, C.G., Edgar, B., and Eriksson, U.G., Inhibition of dihydropyridine metabolism in rat and human liver microsomes by flavonoids found in grapefruit juice, *J. Pharmacol. Exp. Ther.,* 261:1195–1199, 1992.

Miyata, M., Takano, H., Takahashi, K., Sasaki, Y.F., and Yamazoe, Y., Suppression of 2-amino-1-methyl-6-phenylimidazo[4,5-*b*]pyridine-induced DNA damage in rat colon after grapefruit juice intake, *Cancer Lett.,* 183:17–22, 2002.

Ohta, T., Maruyama, T., Nagahashi, M., Miyamoto, Y., Hosoi, S., Kiuchi, F., Yamagoe, Y., and Tsukamoto, S., Paradisin C: A new CYP3A4 inhibitor from grapefruit juice, *Tetrahedron,* 58:6631–6635, 2002.

Schmiedlin-Ren, P., Edwards, D.J., Fitzsimmons, M.E., He, K., Lown, K.S., Woster, P.M., Rahman, A., Thummel, K.E., Fisher, J.M., Hollenberg, P.F., and Watkins, P.B., Mechanisms of enhanced oral availability of CYP3A4 substrates by grapefruit constituents — decreased enterocyte CYP3A4 concentration and mechanism-based inactivation by furanocoumarins, *Drug Metab. Dispos.,* 25:1228–1233, 1997.

Tassaneeyakul, W., Guo, L-Q, Fukuda, K., Ohta, T., and Yamazoe, Y., Inhibition selectivity of grapefruit juice components on human cytochrome P450. *Arch. Biochem. Biophys.,* 378:356–363, 2000.

Grape juice

Grapes are one of the richest sources of phenolic compounds compared to other fruit (Machiex et al., 1990). They contribute flavonoids and polyphenolic tannins, in addition to nonflavonoid hydroxy-cinnamic acids, hydroxybenzoic acids, and stilbene. Many of these compounds were found to be potent antioxidants inhibiting the *in vitro* oxidation of LDL cholesterol. Frankel and coworkers (1998) found the commercial Concord and blends of grape juices had comparable inhibitory activity to that of red wine, with respect to the *in vitro* oxidation of human low-density lipoproteins. Using a hamster model of atherosclerosis, Vinson et al. (2001) showed grape juice was twice as effective in lowering cholesterol compared to dealcoholized wine or red wine, two to six times more effective in decreasing LDL, and twice as effective as red wine in preventing atherosclerosis (Figure G.46). Grape juice was a more efficient *ex vivo* antioxidant, as it was more effective in increasing the lag time by four times compared to either dealcoholized wine or red wine. Park et al. (2003) showed grape juice reduced total free-radical levels and DNA damage in 67 healthy Koreans (16 women and 51 men) maintained on a daily grape-juice regime of 480 mL pure grape juice twice a day for eight weeks. The results from this study combined, with antiplatelet and antioxidant benefits reported previously for grape consumption (O'Byrne et al., 2002; Vinson et al., 2000), suggests grape juice should become a regular part of a healthy diet.

References

Frankel, E.N., Bosanek, C.A., Meyer, A.S., Silliman, K., and Kirk, L.L., Commercial grape juices inhibit the *in vitro* oxidation of human low-density lipoproteins, *J. Agric. Food Chem.,* 46:834–838, 1998.

Machiex, J.J., Fleuriet, A., and Billot, J., The main phenolics of fruits, in *Fruit Phenolics*, CRC Press, Boca Raton, Florida, pp. 1–98, 1990.

O'Byrne, D.J., Devaraj, S., Grundy, S.M., and Jialal, I., Comparison of the antioxidant effects of concord grape juice flavonoids and α-tocopherol on markers of oxidative stress in healthy adults, *Am. J. Clin. Nutr.,* 76:1367–1374, 2002.

Park, Y.K., Park, E., Kim, J.-S., and Kang, M.-H., Daily grape juice consumption reduces oxidative DNA damage and plasma free radical levels in healthy Koreans, *Mutat. Res.,* 529:77–86, 2003.

Vinson, J.A., Teufel, K., and Wu, N., Red wine, dealcoholized red wine, and especially grape juice, inhibit atherosclerosis in a hamster model, *Atherosclerosis,* 156:67–72, 2001.

Vinson, J.A., Yang, J., Proch, J., and Liang, X., Grape juice, but not orange juice, has *in vitro*, *ex vivi*, and *ex vivo* antioxidant properties, *J. Med. Food,* 2:167–171, 2000.

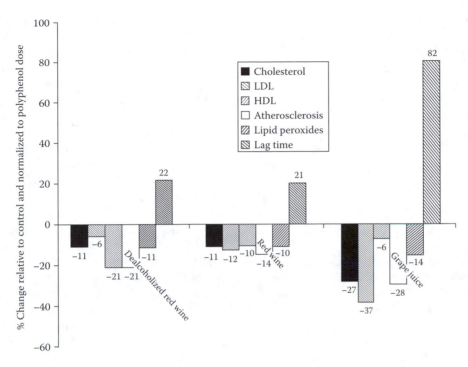

FIGURE G.46 Comparative polyphenol efficiency of beverages with respect to atherosclerosis, lipid, and antioxidant parameters. (Vinson et al., *Atherosclerosis,* 156:67–72, 2003. With permission.)

Grape seeds   Grape-seed extract is widely consumed in the United States as a dietary supplement because of a number of related health benefits associated with its bioflavonoids or procyanidins. Zhao et al. (1999) showed that a polyphenolic fraction from grape seeds exhibited antitumor-promoting activity by reducing tumor incidence in a 7,12-dimethylbenz-[*a*]anthracene (DMBA)-initiated and 12-*O*-tetradecanoylphorbol 13 acetate (TPA)-promoted SENCAR mouse skin two-stage carcinogenesis model system. The antitumor-promoting activity was attributed to the potent antioxidant properties of the grape-seed polyphenols. Procyanidin B5-3′ gallate was identified with the most potent antioxidant activity and potential as a cancer chemopreventive and anticarcinogenic agent. Agarwal and coworkers (2000) also showed grape-seed extract inhibited growth and induced apoptosis in human prostate-cancer cells, both in culture and in nude mice. These researchers (Agawal et al., 2002) found grape-seed extract induced apoptosis in human-

prostate carcinoma DU145 cells by activation of caspases.

Yamakoshi and coworkers (1999) showed that feeding a proanthocyanidin-rich grape-seed extract to cholesterol-fed rabbits significantly reduced severe atherosclerosis in the aorta. It decreased the number of oxidized LDL-positive, macrophage-derived foam cells in athertosclerotic lesions in the aorta of cholesterol-fed rabbits, as a result of its ability to trap reactive-oxygen species in aqueous solution. Shao et al. (2003) confirmed the cardioprotective activity of grape-seed proanthocyanidin by its ability to attenuate oxidant injury in chick embryonic ventricular myocytes. The molecular mechanisms involved in cardioprotection by a novel grape-seed proanthocyanidin extract (IH636) were shown by Bagchi et al. (2003) to include:

potent hydroxyl and other free-radical-
  scavenging activities
antiapoptotic, antinecrotic, and antien-
  donucleolytic potentials
modulation of apoptotic regulators, *bcl-*
  X_L, p53, and *c-myc* genes

inhibition of cytochrome P450 2E1
inhibition of adhesion molecules
modulation of proapoptotic and cardio-
    regulatory genes, *c-JUN*, *JNK-1*, and
    CD36.

References

Argawal, C., Sharma, Y., and Argawal, R., Anticarcinogenic effect of a polyphenolic fraction isolated
from grape seeds in human protate carcinoma
DU145 cells: Modulation of mitogenic signaling and
cell cycle regulators and induction of G1 arrest and
apoptosis, *Mol. Carcinog.,* 28:129–138, 2000.

Agarwal, C., Singh, R.P., and Agarwal, R., Grape
seed extract induces apoptotic death of human prostate carcinoma DU145 cells via caspases activation
accompanied by dissipation of mitochondrial membrane potential and cytochrome *c* release, *Carcinogenesis,* 23:1869–1876, 2002.

Bagchi, D., Sen, C.K., Ray, S.D., Das, D.K., Bagchi,
M., Preuss, H.G., and Vinson, J.A., Molecular mechanisms of cardioprotection by a novel grape seed
proanthocyanidin extract, *Mutat. Res.,* 523–524:87–
97, 2003.

Shao, Z.-H., Becker, L.B., Vanden Hoek, T.L., Schu-
macker, P.T., Li, C.-Q., Zhao, D., Wojcik, K., Anderson, T., Qin, Y., Dey, L., and Yuan, C.-S., Grape seed
proanthocyanidin extract attenuates oxidant injury in
cardiomyocytes, *Pharmacol. Res.,* 47:463–469, 2003.

Yamakoshi, J., Kataoka, S., Koga, T., and Ariga, T.,
Proanthocyanidin-rich extract from grape seeds
attenuates the development of aortic atherosclerosis
in cholesterol-fed rabbits, *Atherosclerosis,* 142:139–
149, 1999.

Zhao, J., Wang, J., Chen, Y., and Agarwal, R., Antitumor promoting activity of a polyphenolic fraction
isolated from grape seeds in the mouse skin two-
stage initiation-promotion protocol, and identification of procyanidin B5-3′-gallate as the most effective antioxidant constituent, *Carcinogenesis,* 20:
1737–1745, 1999.

Green tea   Green tea, a popular beverage in
Japan made from the leaves of *Camellia sinensis,* is recognized for its health benefits. It is a
nonfermented product obtained by leaf dessica-
tion that contains potent, polyphenolic antioxidants, with a flavan-3-olic structure, referred to
as green-tea catechins. They include seven

types, (–)-gallocatechin (GC), (–)-epigallocat-
echin (EGC), (+)-catechin (C), (–)-epigallocat-
echin-3-gallate (EGCG), (–)-epigallocatechin
(EC), (–)-gallocatechingallate (GCG), and (–)-
epicatechingallate (ECG) (Bonoli et al., 2003).

Many studies have shown that drinking EGCG
and green tea prevents carcinogenesis in rodent
organs (Wang et al., 1992; Fujiki, 2002).
Kavanagh et al. (2001) showed green tea had a
significant chemoprotective effect against 7,12-
dimethyl(*a*)anthracene (DMBA)-induced mammary tumorigenesis in Sprague–Dawley rats.
Inhibition of human breast cancer Hs578T cell
proliferation by green tea appeared to be mediated, in part, by induction of $p27^{Kip}$ cyclin-
dependent kinase inhibitor (CKI) expression.
Gupta et al. (2002) summarized the antimutagenic and anticlastogenic properties of green
and black teas. Green tea inhibited mutagenesis
at concentration levels equivalent to human
daily consumption. Using human umbilical-
vein endothelial cells, Kojima-Yuasa et al.
(2003) demonstrated, for the first time, that
green-tea extracts reduced expression of vascular endothelial growth factor (VEGF) receptors
fms-like tyrosine kinase (Flt-1) and fetal liver
kinase-1/Kinase insert domain containing
receptor (Flk-1/KDR). The antiangiogenic
property of green-tea extracts has therapeutic
potential in preventing the development of new
microvascular networks (angiogenesis) needed
for tumor growth. Maiti and coworkers (2003)
also found green-tea polyphenols inhibited
angiogenesis by reducing vascularization of
chicken chorioallantoic membrane (CAM) by
an angiogenin-like protein isolated from goat
serum. Kemberling et al. (2003) showed green-
tea EGCG effectively inhibited bladder-tumor
implantation growth in a Fischer 344 rat model,
pointing to its potential as an intravesical chemotherapeutic agent.

Reducing the risk of coronary artery disease
is associated with a number of factors, including inhibition of platelet function. EGCG was
reported to inhibit platelet aggregation, possibly
by involving inhibition of cytoplasmic calcium
increase (Kang et al., 1999). Lill and coworkers
(2003) found that only those green catechins
with a galloyl group in the 3′ position inhibited
platelet aggregation, while those without a galloyl group (catechin and epicatechin) or with

TABLE G.36
The Antiviral Effect of EGCG and Green Tea

Agent	IC$_{50}$ (µM)	
	Inactivation of Adenovirus	Effect on Infectious Virus Production
Epigallocatechin gallate (EGCG)	250	25
Green tea infusions[a] (GT-20)		
Gunpowder	245	34
Uncle Lee's	2840	N.D.
Celestial Seasonings	3095	45
Tetley	490	45

[a] Expressed in terms of estimated EGCG concentration in the tea.

Source: From Weber et al., *Antiviral Res.,* 58:167–173, 2003. With permission.

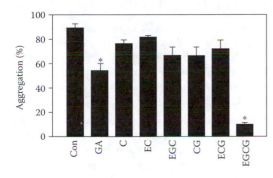

FIGURE G.47 Effect of various green-tea catechins (100 µmol/L) on thrombrin-induced platelet aggregation (means ± S.E.M., n = 5, *p < 0.05 versus control). (From Lill et al., *FEBS Lett.,* 546:265–270, 2003. With permission.)

the galloyl group in the 2′ position (epigallocatechin) did not. EGCG proved to be the most effective in reducing thrombrin-induced aggregation of washed human platelets (Figure G.47).

The ability of green-tea catechins to inhibit adenovirus infection and adenain, the human adenovirus 2 endopeptidase, was reported by Weber and coworkers (2003). EGCG proved the most potent inhibitor of four green-tea catechins tested with a IC$_{50}$ of 200 µM (Table G.36). Since the viral protease, adenain, appeared to be the target of EGCG, it is possible that all adenoviruses are sensitive to its action.

References

Bono, M., Colabufalo, P., Pelillo, M., Toschi, T.G. and Lerker, G., First determination of catechins and xanthines in tea beverage by micellar electrokinetic chromatograph, *J Agric. Food Chem.,* 51:1141–1147, 2003.

Fujiki, H., Two stages of cancer prevention with green tea, *J. Cancer Res. Clin. Oncol.,* 125:589–597, 1999.

Fujiki, H., Suganuma, M., Imai, K., and Nakachi, K., Green tea: Cancer preventive beverage and/or drug, *Cancer Lett.,* 188:1–2, 9–13, 2002.

Gupta, S., Saha, B. and Giri, A.K., Comparative antimutagenic and anticlastogenic effects of green tea and black tea. *Mutat. Res.,* 412:37–65, 2002.

Kang, W.S., Lim, I.H., Yuk, D.Y., Chung, K.H., Park, J.B., Yoo, H.S. and Yu, Y.P., Antithrombotic activities of green tea catechins and C-1-epigallocatechin gallate, *Thromb. Res.,* 96:229–237, 1999.

Kavanagh, K.T., Hafer, L.J., Kim, D.W., Mann, K.K., Sherr, D.H., Rogers, A.E. and Sonenshein, G.E., Green tea extracts decrease carcinogen-induced mammary tumor burden in rats and rate of breast cancer cell proliferation in culture, *J. Cell Biochem.,* 82:387–398, 2001.

Kemberling, J.K., Hampton, J.A., Keck, R.W., Gomez, M.A. and Selman, S.H., Inhibition of bladder tumor growth by the green tea derivative epigallocatechin-3-gallate, *J. Urol.,* 170:773–776, 2003.

Lill, G., Voit, S., Schror, K., and Weber, A.-A., Complex effects of different green tea catechins on human platelets, *FEBS Lett.,* 546:265–270, 2003.

Maiti, T.K., Chatterjee, J. and Dasgupta, S., Effect of green tea polyphenols on angiogenesis induced by an angiogenin-like protein, *Biochem. Biophys. Res. Commun.,* 308:64–67, 2003.

Toschi, T.G., Bordoni, A., Hrelia, S., Bendini, A., Lercker, G., and Biagi, P.L., The protective role of different green tea extracts after oxidative damage is related to their catechin composition, *J. Agric. Food Chem.,* 48:3973–3978, 2000.

Wang, Z.Y., Hong, J.-Y., Huang, M.T., Ruehl, K.R., Conney, A.H., and Yang, C.S., Inhibition of *N*-nitros-odiethylamine and 4-(methylnitrosamino)-1-(3-pyridyl)-1-butanone induced tumorigenesis in A/J mice by green tea and black tea, *Cancer Res.,* 52: 1943–1947, 1992.

Weber, J.M., Ruzindana-Umunyana, A., Imbeault, L., and Sircar, S., Inhibition of adenovirus infection and adenain by green tea catechins, *Antiviral Res.,* 58:167–173, 2003.

Guava   Guava (*Psidium guajava* L.) is an evergreen native to Mexico and Cenral American countries. Guava leaves, roots, and fruits have been used to prevent and treat diarrhea (Lutterodt, 1989) and diabetes (Cheng and Yang, 1983). Studies have also reported that guava has antimutagenic activity, including the identification of (+)-gallocatechin, an antimutagenic compound in guava leaves (Grover and Bala, 1993; Matsuo et al., 1993). Popular Mexican medicine recommends the use of guava leaf water decoction to treat acute diarrhea, colic, flatulence, and gastric pain (Aguilar et al., 1994). Arima and Danno (2002) recently isolated four antibacterial compounds in guava leaves. In addition to guajavarin and quercetin, two new flavonoid glycosides were characterized. The latter were identified as morin-3-*O*-α-L-lyxopyranoside and morin-3-*O*-α-L-arabopyranoside, both of which were effective against *Salmonella enteritidis* and *Bacillus cereus*. Flavonoids, such as quercetin, are also associated with spasmolytic effect and antidiarrheic capacity of guava-leaf products. Lozoya and coworkers (2002) conducted a randomized, double-blinded clinical study that established the safety and efficacy of a phytodrug made from guava leaves standardized in its quercetin content. Decreased abdominal pain was experienced by adult patients suffering from acute diarrheic disease after taking a capsule containing 500 mg of the product every eight hours for three days. The research-ers suggested it could be a useful alternative as an antispasmodic product.

References

Aguilar, A., Argueta, A., and Cano, L., Flora medicinal indigena de Mexico, Treinta y cinco monografias del Atlas de las Plantas de la Medicina Tradicional Mexicana, *INI*, Mexico, 245, 1994.

Arima, H. and Danno, G., Isolation of antimicrobial compounds from guava (*Psidium guajava* L.) and their structural elucidation, *Biosci. Biotechnol. Biochem.* 66:1727–1730, 2002.

Cheng, J.T. and Yang, R.S., Hypoglycemic effect of guava juice in mice and human subjects, *Am. J. Chin. Med.,* 11:74–76, 1983.

Grover, I.S. and Bala, S., Studies on antimutagenic effects of guava (*Psidium guajava*) in *Salmonella typhimurium,* 300:1–4, 1993.

Lozoya, X., Reyes-Morales, H., Chavez-Soto, M.A., Martinez-Garcia, M del C., Soto-Conzalez, Y., and Doubova, S.V., Intestinal anti-spasmodic effect of a phytodrug of *Psidium guajava folia* in the treatment of acute diarrheic disease, *J. Ethnopharmacol.,* 83: 19–24, 2002.

Lutterodt, G.D., Inhibition of gastrointestinal release of acetylcholine by quercetin as a possible mode of action of *Psidium guajava* leaf extracts in the treatment of acute diarrhea disease, *J. Ethnopharmacol.,* 25:235–247, 1989.

Matsuo, T., Hanamura, N., Shimoi, K., Nakamura, Y., and Tomita, I., Identification of (+)-gallocatechin as a bio-antimutagenic compound in *Psidium guajava* leaves, *Phytochemistry,* 36:1027–1029, 1993.

Gum acacia *see* **Acacia gum**

Guar gum   Guar gum, a soluble fiber extracted from the endosperm of the Indian cluster bean (*Cyanopsis tetragonoloba* L.), is a summer legume grown mainly in Western India and Eastern Pakistan. It is a nongelling gum similar to locust-bean gum used extensively in the food industry. Guar gum is a galactomannan in which the molar ratio of galactose to mannose is approximately 1:2. Viscous fibers are very effective for glycemic control (Jenkins et al., 1979; Wolever et al., 1979; Wursch and Pi-Sunyer, 1997). Thus, guar gum, a viscous fiber, is considered to be effective as long as it is not hydrolyzed (Cabre, 2004). A partially hydrolyzed guar gum was shown by Slavin and Greenberg (2003) to have a number of clinical uses, including reducing the incidence of diarrhea in septic patients maintained on enteral nutrition, reducing symptoms of irritable-bowel syndrome, and increasing bifidobacterium in the gut.

Early studies by Jenkins et al. (1979) suggested guar gum could lower total plasma total cholesterol and LDL cholesterol. Castro and coworkers (2003), however, were unable to find any changes in serum lipids of hypocholesterolemic rats maintained on a diet containing 1.5 percent of several hydrocolloids, including guar gum.

The suggestion that guar gum may be beneficial for reducing weight is attributed to increasing viscosity of the bowel contents and the feeling of postprandial satiety (Blackburn et al., 1984; Van de Ven et al., 1994). Based on a number of clinical trials, guar gum is recommended for treating obese patients. Pittler and Ernst (2001) conducted a meta-analysis of randomized trials in which dietary guar gum was used for reducing body weight. Based on their findings they could not recommend guar gum as a treatment for reducing body weight.

References

Blackburn, N.A., Holgate, A.M., and Read, N.W., 1984. Does guar gum improve post-prandial hyperglycaemia in human by reducing small intestine area, *Br. J. Nutr.,* 52:197–204, 1984.

Cabre, E., Fibre supplementation of enetral formula-diets: a look to the evidence, *Clin. Nutr. Suppl.,* 1: 63–74, 2003

Castro, I.A., Tirapegui, J., and Benedicto, M.L., Effect of diet supplementation with three soluble polysaccharides on serum lipid levels of hypercholesterolemic rats, *Food Chem.,* 80:323–330, 2003.

Jenkins, D.J, Wolever, T.M.S., Leeds, A.R., Gassull, M.A., Haisman, P., Dilawari, J., Goff, D.K., Metz, G.L., and Alberti, K.G.M.M., Dietary fibres, fibre analogues, and glucose tolerance: Importance of viscosity, *Br. Med. J.,* 1:1392–1394, 1978.

Jenkins, D.J.A., Leeds, A.R., Slavin, B., Mann, J., and Jepson, E.M., Dietary fiber and blood lipids: Reduction in serum cholesterol in type II hyperlipidemia by guar gum, *Am. J. Clin. Nutr.,* 32:16–18, 1979.

Pittler, M.H. and Ernst, E., Guar gum for body weight reduction: Meta-analysis of randomized trials, *Am. J. Med.,* 110:724–730, 2001.

Slavin, J.L. and Greenberg, N.A., Partially hydrolyzed guar gum: Clinical nutrition uses, *Nutrition,* 19:549–552, 2003.

Van de Ven, M.L.H.M., Westerterp-Plantenga, M.S., Wouters, L., and Saris, W.H.M., Effects of liquid preloads with different fructose/fibre concentrations on subsequent food intake and ratings of hunger in women, *Appet.,* 23:129–146, 1994.

Wolever, T.M.S., Jenkins, D.J., Nineham, R., and Alberti, K.G., Guar gum and reduction of postprandial glycaemia: Effect of incorporation into solid food, liquid food and both, *Br. J. Nutr.,* 41:505–510, 1979.

Wursch, P. and Pi-Sunyer, F.X., The role of viscous soluble fiber in metabolic control of diabetes: A review with special emphasis on cereals rich in beta glucan, *Diabet. Care,* 20:1774–1780, 1997.

G

H

Halichondrin B Halichondrin B, a polyether macrolide isolated from marine sponges and tunicates, was shown to have potent cytotoxicity properties *in vitro* and anticancer properties *in vivo* (Hirata and Uemura, 1986; Litaudon et al., 1994; Fodstad et al., 1996). The sponge *Lissodendoryx* n. sp. 1 was the most promising

1: Halichondrin B

Halichondrin B. (From Seletsky et al., *Bioorg. Med. Chem. Lett.*, 14:5547–5550, 2004. With permission.)

source of halichondrin B components, although it is found in four other sponges. The potential of halichondrin B as an anticancer drug (Pettit et al., 1993a) is limited by its relative scarcity. Halichondrin B disrupts mitotic spindle formation and induces mitotic arrest by inhibiting tubulin assembly and microtubule assembly (Pettit et al., 1993b). A synthetic C(1)-C(38) halichondrin subunit was reported to exhibit anticancer properties similar to that of halichondrin B (Stamos et al., 1997; Towle et al., 2001). Wang et al. (2000) synthesized simplified analogues of halichondrin B that still retained cell growth inhibitory potency *in vitro*. Austad and coworkers (2002) synthesized C(37)-C(54) halichondrin subunits. The National Cancer Institute selected halichondrin B for drug development.

References

Austad, B.C., Hart, A.C., and Burke, S.D., Halichondrin B: Synthesis of the C(37)-C(54) subunit, *Tetrahedron*, 58:2011–2026, 2002.

Fodstad, O., Breistoel, K., Pettit, G.R., Shoemaker, R.H., and Boyd, M.P., Comparative antitumor activities of halichondrins and vineblastine against human tumor xenografts, *J. Exp. Therap. Oncol.*, 1:119–125, 1996.

Hirata, Y. and Uemura, D., Halichondrins — antitumor macrolides from marine sponge, *Pure. Appl. Chem.*, 58:701–710, 1986.

Litaudon, M., Hart, J.B., Blunt, J.W., Lake, R.J., and Munro, M.H.G., Isohomohalichondrin B: A new antitumor polyether macrolide from the New Zealand deep-water sponge *Lissodendoryx* sp., *Tetrahedron Lett.*, 35:9435–9438, 1994.

Pettit, G.R., Tan, R., Gao, F., Williams, M.D., Doubek, D.L., Boyd, M.R., Schmidt, J.M., Chapius, J.-C., Hamel, E., Bai, R., Hooper, J.N.A., and Tackett, L.P., Isolation and structure of halistan 1 from Eastern Indian Ocean marine sponge *Phakellia carteri*, *J. Org. Chem.*, 58:2538–2541, 1993a.

Pettit, G.R., Gao, F., Doubek, D.L., Boyd, M.R., Hamel, E., Bai, R.L., Schmidt, J.M., Tackett, L.P., and Rutzler, K., Antineoplastic agents, 252, Isolation and structure of halistatin-2 from the Comoros marine sponge *Axinella-carteri*, *Gazz. Chim. Ital.*, 123:371–377, 1993b.

Seletsky, B.M., Wang, Y., Hawkins, L.D., Palme, M.H., Habgood, G.J., DiPietro, L.V., Towle, M.J., Salvato, K.A., Wells, B.F., Alafs, K.K., Kishi, Y., Littlefield. B.A., and Yu, M.J., Structurally simplified macrolactone analogues of halichondrin B, *Bioorg. Med. Chem. Lett.*, 14:5547–5550, 2004.

Stamos, D.P., Sean, S.C., and Kishi, Y., New synthetic route to the C14-C.38 segment of halichondrins, *J. Org. Chem.*, 62:7552–7553, 1997.

Towle, M.J., Solvato, K.A., Budrow, J., Wels, B.F., Kutznetsov, G., Aalfs, K.K., Welsh, S., Zheng, W., Seletsky, B.M., Palme, M.N., Habgood, G.J., Singer, L.A., DiPietro, L.V., Wang, Y., Chen, J.J., Quincy, D.A., Davis, A., Yoshimatsu, K., Kishi, Y., Yu, M.J., and Littlefield, B.A., *In vitro* and *in vivo* anticancer activities of synthetic macrocyclic ketone analogues of halichondrin B, *Cancer Res.*, 61:1013–1021, 2001.

Wang, Y., Habgood, G.J., Christ, W.J., Kishi, Y., Littlefield, B.A., and Yu, M.J., Structure-activity relationships of halichondrin B analogues: Modifications of C.30-C.38, *Bioorg. Med. Chem. Lett.,* 10:1029–1032, 2000.

Hawthorn Hawthorn (*Crataegus*) grows in the northern temperate regions of the world, mainly in East Asia, Europe, and North America. The bright-red berries of hawthorn fruit contain fructose, flavonoids, proanthocyanidins, triterpenes, organic acids, vitamins, and minerals (Huang, 1993). Zhang et al. (2001) reported hawthorn fruit was rich in phenolic antioxidants, particularly hyperoside, isoquercitrin, epicatechin, chlorogenic acid, quercetin, rutin, and protocatechuic acid. The ability of hawthorn fruit to lower total serum cholesterol, LDL cholesterol, and triglycerides in hyperlipidemic individuals was reported by Chen and coworkers (1995). More recent studies by Zhang et al. (2002a) showed inclusion of a 0.5 percent aqueous ethanolic extract from hawthorn-fruit powder in a semisynthetic diet containing 0.1 percent cholesterol diet to rabbits lowered serum total cholesterol and triacylglycerols by 10 percent and 13 percent, respectively (Figure H.48). A possible mechanism involved greater bile-acid excretion mediated by upregulation of hepatic cholesterol 7α-hydroxylase and inhibition of cholesterol adsorption mediated by downregulation of intestinal acyl CoA: cholesterol acyltransferase activity.

Pittler et al. (2003) examined the efficacy of hawthorn extract in treating chronic heart failure by meta-analysis of randomized trials. Their results suggested a significant benefit was derived from hawthorn extract as an adjunctive treatment for chronic heart failure. A pilot study conducted by Walker and coworkers (2002) using 36 mildly hypertensive subjects found hawthorn extract reduced the diastolic blood pressure in 10 out of the 19 subjects, with a trend in the reduction of anxiety. The small number of subjects and the low levels of hawthorn extract used in this study, however, warrants further investigation.

References

Chen, J.D., Wu, Y.Z., Tao, Z.L., Chen, Z.M., and Liu, X.P., Hawthorn (Shan Zha) drink and its lowering effect on blood lipid levels in humans and rats, *World Rev. Nutr. Diet,* 77:147–154, 1995.

Huang, K.C., Shan Zha: *Crataegus pinnatifida,* in *The Pharmacology of Chinese Herbs*, CRC Press, Boca Raton, Florida, 1993.

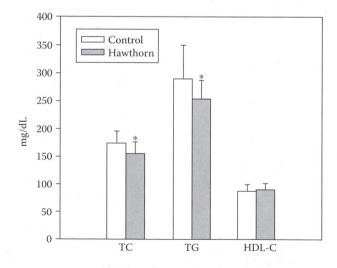

FIGURE H.48 Effects of supplementation of 0.5 percent hawthorn fruit ethanolic extract (equal to 2 percent dried-fruit powder) in diet on serum total cholesterol (TC), triacylglycerols (TG), and high-density lipoprotein cholesterol (HDL-C) in hamsters. Values are means ± S.D., n = 15. *Differs significantly at $p < 0.05$ (From Zhang et al., *Food Res. Inter.,* 35:885–891, 2002a. With permission.)

Pittler, M.H., Schmidt, K., and Ernst, E., Hawthorn extract for treating chronic heart failure: Meta-analysis of randomized trials, *Am. J. Med.,* 114:665–674, 2003.

Walker, A.F., Marakis, G., Morris, A.P., and Robinson, P.A., Promising hypotensive effect of hawthorn extract: A randomized double-blind pilot study of mild, essential hypertension, *Phytother. Res.,* 16:48–54, 2002.

Zhang, Z., Chang, Qi, Zhu, Min., Huang, Y., Ho, W.K.K., and Chen, Z.-Y., Characterization of antioxidants present in hawthorn fruits, *J. Nutr. Biochem.,* 12:144–152, 2001.

Zhang, Z., Ho, W.K.K., Huang, Y., and Chen, Z.-Y., Hypocholesterolemic activity of hawthorn fruit is mediated by regulation of cholesterol-7-α-hydroxylase and acyl CoA: Cholesterol acyltransferase, *Food Res. Inter.,* 35:885–891, 2002a.

Zhang, Z., Ho, W.K.K., Huang, Y., James, A.E., Lam, L.W., and Chen, Z.Y., Hawthorn fruit is hypolipidemic in rabbits fed a high cholesterol diet, *J. Nutr.,* 132:5–10, 2002b.

Hemp   The annual herbaceous plant hemp (*Cannabis sativa* L.) has been traditionally grown for its fiber and oil. Its seeds were reported to have a number of health benefits, including lowering cholesterol and high blood pressure (Jones, 1995). Hemp-seed oil is perfectly balanced with respect to the ratio (3:1) of the two essential polyunsaturated fatty acids, linoleic to linolenic acid. The presence of γ-linolenic acid in hemp oil makes it an excellent ingredient in light body oils and lipid-enriched creams (Rausch, 1995).

References

Jones, K., *Nutritional and Medicinal Guide to Hemp Seed,* Rainforest Botanical Laboratory, Gibsons, B.C., Canada, 1995.

Rausch, P., Verwendung von hanfsamenol in der kosmetik, in *Bioresource Hemp,* 2nd ed., Nova-Institute, Cologne, Germany, 1995, pp. 556–561, 1995.

Herbs *see also* **Individual herbs**   Herbs are used extensively and with increasing interest in North America in complimentary and alternative medicines (Eisenberg et al., 1998). Women (particularly white, middle-aged women) appear to be the major users of these nontraditional therapies (Astin, 1998; Druss and Rosenheck, 1999). Like pharmaceutical drugs, herbal medicines can be therapeutic at one dose and toxic at another (Fugh-Berman, 2001). Of particular concern, however, are the possible adverse effects of herbal–drug interactions. In a review of herbs commonly used by women, Tesch (2001) noted that some herbs, such as *Ginkgo biloba,* were more effective than the placebo for dementia. However, when taken with aspirin or warfarin, it inhibited the platelet-activating factor and was associated with serious bleeding. St. John's Wort, shown to be effective for treating mild to moderate depression in the short term, suffers from many drug interactions. Ginseng may attenuate postprandial glycemia and improve psychological symptoms in perimenopausal women. A decrease in certain cancers associated with ginseng, however, is offset by its impurity and possible side effects. A review of herbal medicines and epilepsy by Spinella (2001) noted that certain herbal sedatives (kava kava, valerian, chamomile, passion flower) may potentiate the effects of antiepileptic medications, increasing their sedative and cognitive effects. However, limited evidence suggests that many of these herbal medicines, particularly those containing ephedrine and caffeine, can exacerbate seizures. A list of the clinical reports for some herb–drug interactions is summarized in Table H.37. A review of alternative medicines for treating glaucoma by Rhee et al. (2001) indicated that while *Ginkgo biloba* and other Chinese herbal medicines do not affect intraocular pressure, they may have a beneficial effect by improving blood flow to the optic nerve. These researchers cautioned that using some herbal medicines could have possible toxicities and side effects.

Zou et al. (2002) examined the *in vitro* effects of 25 purified components from commonly used herbal products on the catalytic activity of cDNA-expressed cytochrome P450 isoforms. Herbal products containing kava kava, *Ginkgo biloba,* garlic, or St. John's Wort were capable of inhibiting the metabolism of coadministered medications in which the primary elimination route was via cytochrome

TABLE H.37
Clinical Reports of Selected Herb–Drug Interactions

Herb and Drug(s)	Results of Interaction
Ginkgo (*Ginkgo biloba*)	
Apirin	Serious hyphema
Warfarin	Intracerebral hemorrhage
Thiazide diuretic	Hypertension
Ginseng (*Panax* spp.)	
Warfarin	Decreased INR
Phenelzine	Headache and tremor
Alcohol	Increased alcohol clearance
St. John's Wort (*Hypericum perforatum*)	
Paroxetine	Lethargy/incoherence
Setraline	Mild serotonin syndrome
Combined oral contraceptive (ethyloestradiol and desogestrel)	Breakthrough bleeding
Valerian (*Valeriana officinalis*)	
Alcohol	A mixture of valepotriates reduces adverse effect of alcohol on concentration

Source: Adapted from Fugh-Berman, *Lancet*, 355:134–138, 2001.

P450. Constituents in these herbal products inhibited one or more of the cytochrome P450 isoforms at concentrations less than 10 µM. Of the three main isoforms (CYP2C9, CYP2C19, and CYP3A4) affected, CYP2C19 proved to be the most sensitive. These herbal components were capable of eliciting clinically significant drug interactions.

For a more detailed discussion of the risks associated with herbal medicines, the review articles by Izzo et al. (2004) and Zhou et al. (2004) are strongly recommended.

References

Astin, J.A., Why patients use alternative medicine: Results of a national study, *JAMA*, 279:1548–1553, 1998.

Druss, B.G. and Rosenheck, R.A., Association between use of unconventional therapies and conventional medical services, *JAMA*, 282:651–656, 1999.

Eisenberg, D.M., Davis, R.B., Ettner, S.L., Appel, S., Wilkey, S., Van Rompay, M., and Kessler, R.C., Trends in alternative medicine use in the United States, 1990–1997: Results of a follow-up national survey, *JAMA*, 280:1569–1575, 1998.

Fugh-Berman, A., Herb-drug interactions, *Lancet*, 355:134–138, 2001.

Izzo, A.A., Di Carlo, G., Borrielli, F., and Ernst, E., 2004. Cardiovascular pharmacotherapy and herbal medicines: The risk of drug interaction, *Inter. J. Cardiol.*, 98:1–14, 2004.

Rhee, D.J., Katz, L.J., Spaeth, G.L., and Myers, J.S., Complementary and alternative medicine for glaucoma, *Surv. Ophthamol.*, 46:43–55, 2001.

Spinelli, M., Herbal medicines and epilepsy: The potential for benefit and adverse effects, *Epilepsy Behav.*, 2:524–532, 2001.

Tesch, B.J., Herbs commonly used by women: An evidence-based review, *Clin. J. Women's Health*, 1: 89–102, 2001.

Zhou, S., Koh, H.-L., Gao, Y., Gong, Z., and Lee, E.J.D., Herbal bioactivation: The good, the bad and the ugly, *Life Sci.*, 74:935–968, 2004.

Zou, L., Harkey, M.R., and Henderson, G.L., Effects of herbal components on cDNA-expressed cytochrome P450 enzyme catalytic activity, *Life Sci.*, 71: 1579–1589, 2002.

Hesperidin   Hesperidin (3′,5,7-trihydroxy-4′-methoxyflavonone-7-rhamnoglucoside), is a naturally occurring bioflavonoid present in fruits and vegetables. As a component of citrus-fruit peel, it was shown to lower cholesterol in rats (Bok et al., 1999; Galati et al., 1994), as well as exhibit antioxidant activity *in vitro* (Van Acker et al., 1996; Chan et al., 1999).

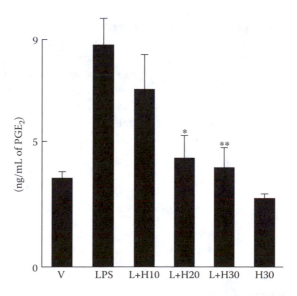

Hesperidin

(Adapted from Kanaze et al., *J. Pharm. Biomed. Anal.,* 36:175–181, 2004.)

A number of studies have shown dietary hesperidin, alone or in combination with diosmon, exerted anticarcinogenic effects in tongue, colon, esophageal, and urinary-bladder carcinogenic rat models (Tanaka et al., 1997a, b, 2000;

Yang et al., 1997). In addition, hesperidin was also shown to have anti-inflammatory activity in mouse skin exposed to a tumor promoter (Koyuncu et al., 1999). Using the rat model for testing arthritis, Guardia and coworkers (2001) showed hesperidin inhibited both acute and chronic phases of inflammation. Sakata et al. (2003) examined the modulating effects of hesperidin on the expression and activity of COX-2 and iNOS enzymes induced by the endotoxin lipopolysaccharide (LPS). COX-2 and iNOS are inducible enzymes, which, in association with inflammatory responses, play a key role in carcinogenesis. Using mouse macrophage cells, hesperidin dramatically suppressed prostaglandin E_2, nitric dioxide, and expression of iNOS protein, which could explain its anti-inflammatory and antimutagenic properties (Figure H.49).

Hesperidin and 6-methylapigenin were reported by Marder et al. (2003) as new *Valeriana* flavonoids with activity on the central nervous system. $2S$-(−)-hesperidin was found to have sedative and sleep-enhancing properties potentiated by 6-methylapigenin. The chemistry and pharmacology of the citrus bioflavonoid hesperidin were reviewed by Garg et al. (2001).

FIGURE H.49 PGE_2 production in RAW 264.7 cells. PGE_2 over production was induced by LPS (0.2 µg/mL medium, *L*) and suppressed by hesperidin (H), with various concentrations. v, cells treated with vehicle. *L + H10-L + H30*, cells treated with LPS and 10, 20, and 30 µM of hesperidin. *H30* cells treated with hesperidin 30 µM. Mean PGE_2 concentration ± SD of three separate experiments. *$p < 0.005$ and **$p < 0.003$ compared with *L* by Student's t-test. (From Sakata et al., *Cancer Lett.,* 199:139–145, 2003. With permission.)

References

Bok, S.H., Lee, S.H., Park, Y.B., Bae, K.H., Son, K.H., Jeong, T.S., and Choi, M.S., Plasma and hepatic cholesterol and hepatic activities of 3-hydroxy-3-methyl-glutaryl coenzyme A reductase and acyl coenzyme A: Cholesterol transferase are lower in rats fed citrus peel extract or a mixture of citrus biflavonoids, *J. Nutr.*, 128:1182–1185, 1999.

Chan, T., Galati, G., and O'Brien, P.J., Oxygen activation during peroxidase catalysed metabolism of flavones and flavonones, *Chem. Biol. Interact.*, 122:15–25, 1999.

Galati, E.M., Monforte, M.T., Kirjainen, S., Forestieri, A.M., Trovato, A., and Tripodo, M.M., Biological effect of hesperidin, a citrus flavonoid (note 1): Anti-inflammatory and analgesic activity, *Il Farmaco*, 49:709–712, 1994.

Garg, A., Garg, S., Zaneveld, L.J.D., and Singla, A.K., Chemistry and pharmacology of the citrus bioflavonoid hesperidin, *Phytother. Res.*, 15:655–669, 2001.

Guardia, T., Rotelli, A.E., Juarez, A.O., and Pelzer, L.E., Anti-inflammatory properties of plant flavonoids, effects of rutin, quercetin and hesperidin on adjuvant arthritis in rat, *Il Formaco.*, 56:683–687, 2001.

Kakumoto, M., Satoh, K., Horo, A., Sumida, T., Tanaka, T., and Ogawa, H., Chemoprevention of azoxymethane-induced rat colon carcinogenesis by the naturally occurring flavonoids diosmin and hesperidin, *Carcinogenesis*, 18:957–965, 1997b.

Kanaze, F.I., Kokkalou, E., Georgarakis, M., and Niopas, I., A validated solid-phase extraction HPLC method for the simultaneous determination of the citrus flavonone aglycones hesperitin and naringenin in urine, *J. Pharm. Biomed. Anal.*, 36:175–181, 2004.

Koyuncu, H., Berkada, B., Baykut, F., Soybir, G., Alati, C., Gul, H., and Altun, M., Preventive effect of hesperidin against inflammation in CD-1 mouse skin caused by tumor promoter, *Anticancer Res.*, 19:3237–3241, 1999.

Marder, M., Viola, H., Wasowski, C., Fernandez, S., Medina, J.H., and Paladini, A.C., 6-Methylapigenin and hesperidin: New valeriana flavonoids with activity on the CNS, *Pharmacol. Biochem. Behav.*, 75:537–545, 2003.

Sakata, K., Hirose, Y., Qiao, Z., Tanaka, T., and Mori, H., Inhibition of inducible isoforms of cyclooxygase and nitric oxide synthase by flavonoid hesperidin in

mouse macrophage cell line, *Cancer Lett.*, 199:139–145, 2003.

Tanaka, T., Kohno, H., Murakami, M., Shimada, R., Kagami, S., Sumida, T., Azuma, Y., and Ogawa, H., Suppression of azoxymethane-induced colon carcinogenesis in male F344 rats by mandarin juices in β-cryptoxanthin and hesperidin, *Int. J. Cancer*, 88:146–150, 2000.

Tanaka, T., Makita, H., Ohnishi, M., Mori, H., Satoh, K., Hara, A., Sumida, T., Fukutani, K., Tanaka, T., and Ogawa, H., Chemoprevention of 4-mitroquinoline 1-oxide induced oral carcinogenesis in rats by flavonoids diosmin and hesperidin, each alone and in combination, *Cancer Res.*, 57:246–252, 1997a.

Van Acker, S.A.B.E., Van Den Berg, D.J., Tromp, M.N.J.L., Griffioen, D.H., Van Bennekom, W.P., Van Der Vijgh, W.J.F., and Bast, A., Structural aspects of antioxidant activity of flavones or flavonones, *Free Rad. Biol. Med.*, 20:331–342, 1996.

Yang, M., Tanaka, T., Hirose, Y., Deguchi, T., Mori, H., and Kawada, Y., Chemoprotective effects of diosmin and hesperidin on *N*-butyl-*N*-(4-hydroxybutyl)-induced urinary bladder carcinogenesis in male 1CR mice, *Int. J. Cancer*, 73:719–724, 1997.

High-density lipoproteins *see* Lipoproteins

Honey   Honey, a complex mixture of carbohydrates, has been studied extensively (Horvath and Molnarl-Perl, 1998; Gomez Barez et al., 2000). In addition, some cyclitols or polyalcohols, such as myo-inositol and mannitol, have also been reported in edible honeys (Horvath and Molnarl-Perl, 1998). Sanz and coworkers

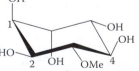

Myo-inositol and D-pinitol. (From Hart et al., *Carbohydr. Res.*, 339:1857–1871, 2004. With permission.)

TABLE H.38
Anti-inflammatory Effect of (+)-Pinitol on Carrageenan-Induced Paw Edema in Rats[1]

Treatment	Dose (mg/kg, i.p.)	Edema Volume (mL)	Inhibition (percent)
Control (saline, 3.0 mL/kg, i.p.)		0.90 ± 0.02	—
Phenylbutazone	100	0.23 ± 0.01*	74.44
(+)-Pinitol	2.5	0.53 ± 0.04*	41.11
	5	0.44 ± 0.02*	51.11
	10	0.31 ± 0.02*	65.55

[1] Values are mean ± S.E. (n = 6).
* $p < 0.001$ versus control; Student's t-test.

From Singh et al., *Fitoterapia*, 72:168–170, 2001. With permission.

H

(2004) identified quercitol, pinitol, 1-*O*-methyl-muco-inositol, and muco-inositol for the first time in edible honey. Of 28 honeys examined, most had myo-inositol and pinitol, while only in some samples were the other cyclitols detected. The anti-inflammatory nature of (+)-pinitol, isolated from *Abies pindrow* leaves, was demonstrated by Singh and coworkers (2001) using the carrageenan-induced paw edema in rats. A significant reduction in edema volume was evident in the presence of pinitol with a dose of 10 mg/kg comparable to that of phenylbutazone (Table H.38).

Certain honeys derived from such floral sources as *Leptospermum scoparium* (Manuka) and *L. polygalifolium* (Meadhoney) provide additional antioxidants, antibacterial agents, and other unidentified compounds and are referred to as therapeutic honeys (Lusby et al., 2002). The ability of these honeys to prevent microbial growth in the moist-wound environment accounts, in part, for their beneficial effects in wound healing. Tonks et al. (2003) examined the wound-healing ability of three honeys (manuka, pasture, and jelly bush) on the activation state of immunoincompetent cells, using the human monocytic cell-line model MonoMac-6. All of the honeys significantly increased the release of important inflammatory cytokines TNF-α, IL-1β, and IL-6 (Figure H.50). These cytokines are both proinflammatory and anti-inflammatory. While all three honeys showed significant increases in cytokines compared to the sugar-solution control, the

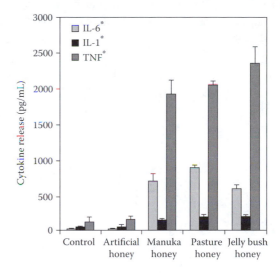

FIGURE H.50 Effect of 1 percent (w/v) honeys on TNF-α, IL-1β, and IL-6 release from isolated human peripheral-blood monocytes. Results are expressed as mean ± SD. *$p < 0.001$ analyzed by ANOVA and Tukey's pair-wise comparisons. (From Tonks et al., *Cytokine*, 21:242–247, 2003. With permission.)

Australian jelly-bush honey had the greatest effect. The ability of these honeys to regulate the production of cytokines is probably due to the presence of components other than sugar. These components have yet to be identified but could involve cyclitols.

References

Gomez Barez, J.A., Garcia Villanova, R.J., Elvira Garcia, S., Rivas Pala, T., Gonzalez Paramas, A.M., and Sanchez Sanchez, J., Geographical distribution of honeys through the employment of sugar patterns and common chemical quality parameters, *Eur. Food Res. Technol.*, 210:437–444, 2000.

Hart, J.B., Kroger, L., Falshaw, A., Falshaw, R., Farkas, E., Thiem, J., and Win, A.L., Enzyme-catalysed synthesis of galactosylated 1D- and 1L-*chiro*-inositol, 1D-pinitol, *myo*-inositol and selected derivatives using the β–galactosidase from the thermophile *Thermoanaerobacter sp.* strain TP6-B1, *Carbohydr. Res.*, 339:1857–1871, 2004.

Horvath, K. and Molnarl-Perl, I., Simultaneous GC-MS quantitation of *o*-phosphoric, aliphatic and aromatic carboxylic acids, proline, hydroxymethylfurfural and sugars as their TMS derivatives: In honeys, *Chromatographia*, 48:120–126, 1998.

Lusby, P.E., Coombes, A., and Wilkinson, J.M., Honey: A potent agent for wound healing? *JWOCN*, 29:295–300, 2002.

Sanz, M.L., Sanz, S.J., and Martinez-Castro, I., Presence of some cyclitols in honey, *Food Chem.*, 84:133–135, 2004.

Singh, R.K., Pandey, B.L., Tripathi, M., and Pandey, V.B., Anti-inflammatory effect of (+)-pinitol, *Fitoterapia*, 72:168–170, 2001.

Tonks, A.J., Cooper, R.A., Jones, K.P., Blair, S., Parton, J., and Tonks, A., Honey stimulates inflammatory cytokine production from monocytes, *Cytokine*, 21:242–247, 2003.

Hops (*Humulus lupulus* L.)   The bitter taste and aroma of beers is due to the bitter acids extracted from hops added to the sweet wort during brewing. These are composed of α- and β-acids, humulone, cohumulone, adhumulone, lupulone, colupulone, and adlupulone and their oxidation products (Scheme H.30) (Verzele and Potter, 1978). The potential of bitter acids, such as humulone, as chemotherapeutic or chemopreventive agents was evident by their ability to inhibit angiogenesis (Shimamura et al., 2001), suppress cyclooxygenase-2 transcription (Yamamoto et al., 2000), induce differentiation of

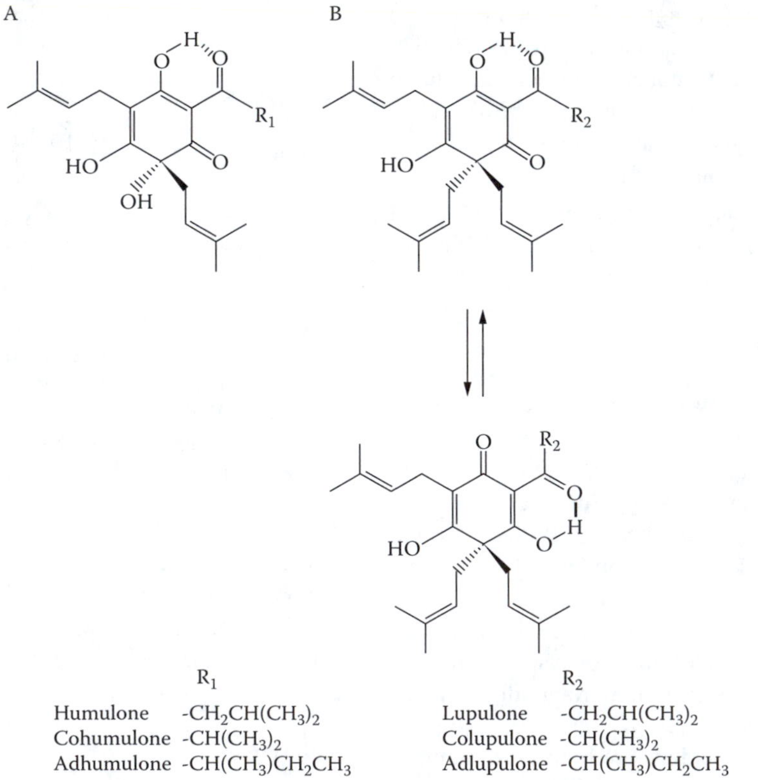

	R_1
Humulone	-CH$_2$CH(CH$_3$)$_2$
Cohumulone	-CH(CH$_3$)$_2$
Adhumulone	-CH(CH$_3$)CH$_2$CH$_3$

	R_2
Lupulone	-CH$_2$CH(CH$_3$)$_2$
Colupulone	-CH(CH$_3$)$_2$
Adlupulone	-CH(CH$_3$)CH$_2$CH$_3$

SCHEME H.30 Chemical structures of hop bitter acids: (A) α-acids; (B) β-acids. (From Chen and Lin, *J. Agric. Food Chem.*, 52:55–64, 2004. With permission.)

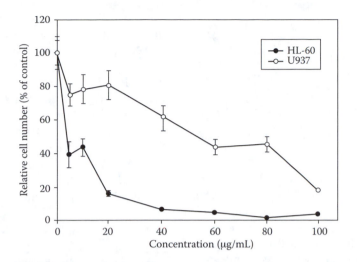

FIGURE H.51 Effect of hop bitter acids on cell viability, HL-60 and U937 cells when treated with either 5 µL/mL of DMSO as vehicle control or various concentrations of hop bitter acids for 24 h. Cell viability was determined by luminescent ATP detection assay kit, with data representing the means ± of three determinations. (From Chen and Lin, *J. Agric. Food Chem.*, 52:55–64, 2004. With permission.)

myelogenous leukemia cells (Honma et al., 1998), inhibit tumor promotion by 12-*O*-tetradecanoyl-phorbol-13-acetate (Yasukawa et al., 1995), and induce apoptosis in human leukemia HL-60 cells (Tobe et al., 1997). Chen and Lin (2004) attempted to delineate the mechanism whereby hop bitter acids triggered apoptosis in human leukemia-cell lines HL-60 and U937. The hop bitter acids inhibited HL-60 cell viability in a dose-dependent manner, with an IC$_{50}$ of 8.67 µg/mL (Figure H.51). The U937 cells proved much more resistant to the action of the hop bitter acids with an IC$_{50}$ value of around 58.87 µg/mL. Several mechanisms were proposed for triggering apoptosis involving Fas activation and mitochondrial dysfunction.

References

Chen, W.-J. and Lin, J.-K., Mechanisms of cancer chemoprevention by hop bitter acids (beer aroma) through induction of apoptosis mediated by Fas and caspase cascades, *J. Agric. Food Chem.*, 52:55–64, 2004.

Honma, Y., Tobe, H., Makishima, M., Yokoyama, A., and Okabe-Kado, J., Induction of differentiation of mycelogenous leukemia cells by humulone, a bitter in the hop, *Leuk. Res.*, 22:605–610, 1998.

Shimamura, M., Hazato, T., Ashino, H., Yamamoto, Y., Iwasaki, E., Tobe, H., Yamamoto, K., and Yamamoto, S., Inhibition of angiogenesis by humulone, a

bitter acid from beer hop, *Biochem. Biophys. Res. Commun.*, 289:220–224, 2001.

Tobe, H., Kubota, M., Yamaguchi, M., Kocha, T., and Aoyagi, T., Apoptosis to HL-60 by humulone, *Biosci. Biotechnol. Biochem.*, 61:1027–1029, 1997.

Verzele, M. and Potter, M.De, High-performance liquid chromatography of hop bitter substances, *J. Chromatogr. A.*, 166:320–326, 1978.

Yamamoto, K., Wang, J., Yamamoto, S., and Tobe, H., Suppression of cyclooxygenase-2 gene transcription by humulon of beer hop extract studied with reference to glucocorticoid, *FEBS Lett.*, 465:103–106, 2000.

Yasukawa, K., Takeuchi, M., and Takido, M., Humulon, a bitter in the hop, inhibits tumor promotion by 12-*O*-tetradecanoylphorbol-13-acetate in two-stage carcinogenesis in mouse skin, *Oncology*, 52:156–158, 1995.

Huperzine A and B   Huperzine A (HupA), a sesquiterpene alkaloid obtained from Chinese club moss (*Huperzia serrata*) or *Lycopodium serrata*, has been used as the folk medicine *Quian Ceng Ta* for centuries (Liu et al., 1986). It is a potent, highly specific, and reversible inhibitor of acetylcholinesterase, equivalent or superior to physostigmine, galanthamine, donepezil, and tacrine, approved drugs for treating

Huperzine A (1)   Huperzine B (2)

(From Lee et al., *Tetrahedron Lett.*, 45:285–287, 2004. With permission.)

Alzheimer's disease that are capable of crossing the blood–brain barrier (Wang et al., 1986; Wang and Tang, 1998). As a promising therapeutic agent for treating Alzheimer's disease, Wang et al. (2000) showed that huperzine A decreased the incidence rate of vascular dementia via multiple mechanisms involving the cholinergic system, oxygen free radicals, and energy metabolism. This was evident by its ability to significantly restore choline acetyl tranferase activity in the hippocampus of rats, as well as reducing superoxide dismutase, lipid peroxide, lactate, and glucose to normal levels (Table H.39). Zhao and Tang (2002) showed huperzine A preferentially inhibited the tetrameric molecular form of acetylcholinesterase in the cerebral cortex, hippocampus, and striatum of the rat brain, while tacrine and rivastigime preferentially inhibited the monomeric form. Physostigmine showed no form selectivity in any brain region. Donepezil varied from region to region with respect to its preferential inhibition of either the G4- and G1

selectivity. The different inhibitory preferences among acetylcholinesterase inhibitors require further study in relation to their effect on Alzheimer's disease. To understand the molecular events leading to Alzheimer's disease, Zhang and Tang (2003) examined the effect of huperzine A on staurosporine neuronal apoptosis in primary cultured rat cortical neurons. They demonstrated for the first time that huperzine A attenuated neurotoxin staurosporine-induced apoptosis, possibly via upregulation of bcl-2, downregulation of bax, and reduction in immunoreactive caspase-3 proenzyme.

The potential of huperzine A as a therapeutic agent for Alzheimer's disease was demonstrated by Zhang et al. (2004), who showed it increased the downregulation of secretory amyloid proteins by upregulating protein kinase C on infused rats and human embryonic kidney 293 Swedish mutant cells.

Tonduli and coworkers (2002) found huperzine A was extremely effective in preventing epileptic activity induced in rats by soman. Its ability to prevent toxicity was due to its protection of the enzyme acetylcholinesterase and reduction of hypercholinergy by soman at the electrophysiological level.

Huperzine B, a cogener of huperzine A in club moss, was reported to have a lower acetylcholinesterase inhibitory potency (Hu and Tang, 1987). Pretreatment of a rat pheochromocytoma cell line PC12 with huperzine B by

TABLE H.39

Effects of Huperzine A (HupA) on Superoxide Dismutase Activities and Lipid Peroxides in Rats Hypoperfused After Bilateral Ligation of the Common Carotoid Arteries[1]

Group	Superoxide Dismutase (nU/mg protein)			Lipid Peroxidase (nmol/mg protein)		
	Cortex	Hippocampus	Striatum	Cortex	Hippocampus	Striatum
Sham-operated	$40.1 \pm 1.5^{**}$	$46.3 \pm 1.9^{**}$	$46.2 \pm 2.6^{**}$	$2.69 \pm 0.07^{**}$	$2.88 \pm 0.10^{**}$	$3.55 \pm 0.17^{**}$
Saline-operated	69.0 ± 2.9	74.8 ± 6.0	97.3 ± 5.7	3.70 ± 0.14	4.11 ± 0.17	5.38 ± 0.27
HupA-treated[5] (0.1 mg/kg)	$36.3 \pm 1.7^{**}$	$43.0 \pm 2.0^{**}$	$42.1 \pm 1.8^{**}$	$2.80 \pm 0.07^{**}$	$3.08 \pm 0.13^{**}$	$3.36 \pm 0.07^{**}$

[1] Rats were killed 40 min. after the last administration of huperzine A on day 33 following bilateral ligation of the common carotoid arteries. From day 15 to day 33, huperzine A was administered orally twice per day.
** $p < 0.01$ versus saline-treated group.

Source: From Wang et al., *Bioorg. Med. Chem. Lett.*, 10:1029–1032, 2000. With permission.

Zhang and Tang (2000) showed it had similar neuroprotective effects to huperzine A against H_2O_2-induced injury. This neuroprotective effect could have application in the treatment of Alzheimer's disease.

Three new *Lycopodium* alkaloids were recently identified by Tan et al. (2003) in *Huperzia serrata* as huperzine S (2β,13β-epoxyalopecuridine), huperzine T (5α-hydroxy-6-oxodihydro-phlegmariu- rine A), and huperzine U (2,3-dihydro-12-hydroxyhuperzine B). The potential health benefits of these alkaloids still remain to be established.

References

Hu, H. and Tang, X.C., Cholinesterase inhibition by huperzine B, *Acta Pharmacol. Sin.*, 8:18–22, 1987.

Lee, I.Y.C., Hong, J.Y., Jung, M.H., and Lee, H.W., Synthesis of huerzine B through ring closing metathesis, *Tetrahedron Lett.*, 45:285–287, 2004.

Liu, J.S., Zhu, Y.L., Yu, C.M., Zhou, Y.-Z., Han, Y.-Y., F.-W., and Qui, B.-F., The structure of huperzine A and B, two new alkaloids exhibiting anticholinesterase activity, *Can. J. Chem.*, 64:837–839, 1986.

Tan, C.-H., Ma, X.-Q., Chen, G.-F., and Zhu, D.-Y., Huperzines S.T., and U: New *Lycopodium* alkaloids from *Huperzia serrata*, *Can. J. Chem.*, 81:315–318, 2003.

Tonduli, L.S., Testylier, G., Masqueliez, C., Lallement, T., and Monmaur, P., Effects of huperzine used as pre-treatment against soman-induced seizures, *Neurotoxicology*, 22:29–37, 2001.

Wang, L.M., Han, Y.F., and Tang, X.C., Huperzine A improves cognitive deficits caused by chronic cerebral hypoperfusion in rats, *Eur. J. Pharmacol.*, 398:65–72, 2000.

Wang, Y.E. and Tang, X.C., Anticholesterase effects of huperzine A, E2020 and tacrine, *Eur. J. Pharmacol.*, 349:137–142, 1998.

Wang, Y.E., Yue, D.X., and Tang, X.C., Anticholesterolase activity of huperzine A, *Acta Pharmacol. Sin.*, 7:110–113, 1986.

Zhang, H.Y. and Tang, X.C., Huperzine B, a novel acetylcholinesterase inhibitor, attenuates hydrogen peroxide induced injury in PC12 cells, *Neurosci. Lett.*, 292:41–44, 2000.

Zhang, H.Y. and Tang, X.C., Huperzine A attenuates the neurotoxic effect of staurosporine in primary rat cortical neurons, *Neurosci. Lett.*, 340:91–94, 2003.

Zhang, H.Y., Yan, H., and Tang, X.C., Huperzine A enhances the level of secretory amyloid precursor protein and protein kinase C-α in intracerebroventricular β-amyloid-(1-40) infused rats and human embryonic kidney 293 Swedish mutant rats, *Neurosci. Lett.*, 360:21–24, 2004.

Zhao, Q. and Tang, X.C., Effects of huperzine A on acetylcholinesterase isoforms *in vitro:* Comparison with tacrine, donepezil, rivastigimine and physostigmine, *Eur. J. Pharmacol.*, 455:101–107, 2002.

Hydratis canadensis see **Golden seal**

Hydroxymatairesinol Hydroxymatairesinol (HMR) found in Norway spruce (Ekman, 1976), is related to matairesinol, an abundant

Hydroxymatairesinol. (From Taskinen et al., *J. Mol. Struct.*, (Theochem), 677:113–124, 2004. With permission.)

lignan found in rye bran. Its structure shown below consists of two guaiacol (2-methoxyphenol) units bonded to α and β positions of a γ-butyrolactone (2-oxacyclopentanone) ring via carbon atoms (Taskinen et al., 2004). Using Apc[min] (adenomatous polyposis coli) mice, a genetically manipulated animal colon-cancer model, Oikarinen et al. (2000) found significantly lower numbers of adenomas in the small intestine of animals fed HMR compared to the other diets, including rye bran.

References

Ekman, R., Analysis of lignans in Norway spruce by combined gas chromatography-mass spectrometry. *Holzforschung*, 30:79–85, 1976.

Oikarinen, S.I., Pajari, A.-M., and Mutanen, M., Chemoprotective activity of crude hydroxymataires-inol (HMR) extract on Apc[min] mice, *Cancer Lett.*, 161:253–258, 2000.

Taskinen, A., Eklund, P., Sjoholm, R., and Hotokka, The molecular structure and some properties of hydroxymatairesinol, an *ab initio* study, *J. Mol. Struct.*, (Theochem), 677:113–124, 2004.

Hydroxytyrosol *see also* **Olive oil**   Hydroxytyrosol (2-(3,4-dihydroxyphenyl)ethanol, a naturally occurring phenolic compound in olive oil, is a potent antioxidant that prevents low-density lipoprotein from oxidation *in vivo* (Grignaffini et al., 1994) as well scavenges free radicals (Visioli et al., 1998). Studies showed

Hydroxytyrosol. (From Vogna et al., *Tetrahedron Lett.*, 44:8289–8292, 2003. With permission.)

hydroxytyrosol inhibited platelet aggregation and protected against damage by reactive-oxygen species (Petroni et al., 1995; Manna et al., 1997, 1999a, b). The ability of hydroxytyrosol to act *in vivo* was suggested, as it is rapidly taken up by intestinal cell lines by passive diffusion (Manna et al., 2000). Della Ragione and coworkers (2000) found hydroxytyrosol arrested cell proliferation and apoptosis in HL60 cells.

They attributed hydroxytyrosol's anti-inflammatory and chemopreventive effects to its ability to downregulate lymphocyte proliferation, which could prove beneficial in the treatment of chronic bowel pathologies, such as Chrone's disease.

References

Grignaffini, P., Roma, P., Galli, C., and Catapano, A.L., Protection of low-density lipoprotein from oxidation by 3,4-dihydroxyphenylethanol, *Lancet,* 343: 1296–1297, 1994.

Manna, C., Galleti, P., Cucciolla, V., Moltedo, O., Leone, A., and Zappia, V., The protective effect of the olive oil polyphenol (3,4-dihydroxyphenyl)-ethanol counteracts reactive oxygen metabolite-induced cytotoxicity in Caco-2 cells, *J. Nutr.,* 127:286–292, 1997.

Manna, C., Galleti, P., Cucciolla, V., Montedoro, G., and Zappia, V., Olive oil hydroxytyrosol protects human erythrocytes against oxidative damage, *J. Nutr. Biochem.,* 10:159–165, 1999a.

Manna, C., Ragione, F.D., Cucciolla, V., Borriella, A., D'Angelo, S., Galletti, P., and Zappia, V., Biological effects of hydroxytyrosol, a polyphenol from olive oil endowed with antioxidant activity, *Adv. Exp. Med. Biol.,* 472:115–130, 1999b.

Manna, C., Galletti, P., Maisto, G., Cucciolla, V., D'Angelo, S., and Zappia, V., Transport mechanism and metabolism of olive oil hydroxytyrosol in Caco-2 cells, *FEBS Lett.,* 470:341–344, 2000.

Petroni, A., Blasevich, M., Salami, M., Papini, N., Montedoro, G.F., and Galli, C., Inhibition of platelet aggregation and eicoisanoid production by phenolic components of olive oil, *Thromb. Res.,* 178:151–160, 1995.

Ragione, F.D., Cucciolla, V., Borriello, A., Della Petra, V., Pontoni, G., Racioppi, L., Manna, C., Galleti, P., and Zappia, V., Hydroxytyrosol, a natural molecule occurring in olive oil induces cytochrome *c*-dependent apoptosis, *Biochem. Biophys. Res. Commun.,* 278:733–739, 2000.

Visioli, F., Bellomo, G., and Galli, C., Free radical scavenging properties of olive oil polyphenols, *Biochem. Biophys. Res. Commun.,* 247:60–64, 1998.

Vogna, D., Pezzella, A., Panzella, L., Napolitano, A., and d'Ischia, M., Oxidative chemistry of hydroxytyrosol: Isolation and characterization of novel methanooxocinobenzodioxinone derivatives, *Tetrahedron Lett.,* 44:8289–8292, 2003.

Hyperforin *see also* **St. John's Wort**   The major lipophilic constituent in the herb St. John's Wort (*Hypericum perforatum*) is the acylphloroglucinol derivative, hyperforin (Laak-mann et al., 1998; Singer et al., 1999). In addition to its antibacterial activity (Gurevich et al.,

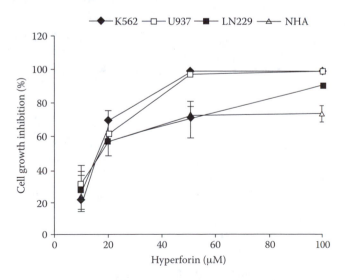

(From Hostanka, K. et al., *Eur. J. Pharmaceutics Biopharmaceutics*, 56:121–132, 2003. With permission.)

1971), hyperforin was also shown to inhibit the growth of autologous MT-450 breast carcinoma in immunocompetent Wistar rats in a similar manner to that of the cytotoxic drug paclitaxel (Schempp et al., 2002). The antiproliferative and apoptosis-inducing properties of hyperforin were recently demonstrated by Hostanka et al. (2003) in several leukemia cell lines (Figure H.52). Hyperforin treatment of leukemic cells resulted in inhibition of their growth in a dose-dependent manner. Apoptosis was induced by hyperforin in leukemia U937 and K562 cells by enhancement of caspase-9 and caspase-3, and caspase-8 and caspase-3, respectively. They also reported synergism between hyperforin and hypericin, a naphthodianthrone in St. John's Wort, on tumor-growth inhibition.

St. John's Wort (*Hypericum perforatum*) extracts have traditionally been used to treat mild depression, although not all clinical trials have confirmed this property (Whiskey et al., 2001; Kasper, 2001; Bilia et al., 2002). The antidepressant properties of hyperforin were attributed to its ability to inhibit monoamine reuptake (Muller et al., 1997; Chatterjee et al., 1998). These workers showed that in contrast to other antidepressants, hyperforin potently inhibited synaptosomal uptake of the amino-acid transmitters GABA and L-glutamate. Roz and coworkers (2002) reported hyperforin inhibited the uptake of monoamines by the rat-brain synaptic vesicles in a dose-dependent manner. To explain this phenomenon, Roz and Rehavi (2003) found hyperforin acted like a protonophore, reducing the pH across the synaptic-vesicle membrane, which interfered with monoamine storage.

H

FIGURE H.52 Effect of exposure to hyperforin on cell growth of leukemia K562, U937, LN229, and NHA cells. Cells (5×10^3/well) were grown for 48 h in the presence of various concentrations of hyperforin and cell growth assessed by the tatrazolium salt, WST-1. (From Hostanka et al., *Eur. J. Pharmaceutics Biopharmaceutics.*, 56:121–132, 2003. With permission.)

References

Bilia, A.R., Gallori, S., and Vincieri, F.F., St. John's wort and depression: Efficacy, safety and tolerability — an update, *Life Sci.,* 70:3077–3096, 2002.

Chatterjee, S.S., Bhattacharya, S.K., Wounemann, M., Singer, A., and Muller, W.E., Hyperforin as a possible antidepressant component of hypericum extracts, *Life Sci.,* 63:499–510, 1998.

Gurevich, A.I., Dobrynin, V.N., Kolosov, M.N., Popravko, S.A., Riabova, I.D., Chernov, B.K., Derbentseva, N.A., Aisenman, B.E., and Gargulya, A.D., Hyperforin an antibiotic from *Hypericum perforatum, Antibiotiki,* 16:510–513, 1971.

Hostanska, K., Reichling, J., Bommer, S., Weber, M., and Saller, R., Hyperforin a constituent of St. John's wort (*Hypericum perforatum* L.) extract induces apoptosis by triggering activation of caspases and with hypericin synergistically exerts cytotoxicity towards human malignant cells lines, *Eur. J. Pharmaceutics Biopharmaceutics.,* 56:121–132, 2003.

Kasper, S., *Hypericum perforatum* — a review of clinical studies, *Pharmacopsychiatry,* 34(Suppl. 1): 51–55, 2001.

Laakmann, G., Schule, C., Baghai, T., and Kieser, M., St. John's wort in mild to moderate depression: The relevance of hyperforin for the clinical efficacy, *Pharmacopsychiatry,* 31:54–59, 1998.

Muller, W.E., Rolli, M., Schafer, C., and Hafner, U., Effects of hypericum extract (LI 160) in the biochemical models of antidepressant activity, *Pharmacopsychiatry,* 30 (Suppl. 2):102–107, 1997.

Roz, N., Mazur, Y., Hirshfeld, A., and Rehavi, M., Inhibition of vesicular uptake of monoamines by hyperforin, *Life Sci.,* 71:2227–2237, 2002.

Roz, N. and Rehavi, M., Hyperforin inhibits vesicular uptake of monoamines by dissipating pH gradient across synaptic vesicle membrane, *Life Sci.,* 73:461–470, 2003.

Schempp, C.M., Kirkin, V., Simon-Haarhaus, B., Kersten, A., Kiss, J., Termeer, C.C., Gilb, B., Kaufman, T., Borner, C., Sleeman, J.P., and Simon, J.C., Inhibition of tumor cell growth by hyperforin, a novel anticancer drug from St. John's wort that acts by induction of apoptosis, *Oncogene.,* 21:1242–1250, 2002.

Singer, A., Wonnemann, M., and Muller, W.E., Hyperforin, a major antidepressant constituent of St. John's wort, inhibits serotonin uptake by elevating free intracellular Na[11], *J. Pharmacol. Exp. Ther.,* 290: 1363–1368, 1999.

Whiskey, E., Wernecke, U., and Taylor, D., A systematic review of meta-analysis of *Hypericum perforatum* in depression: A comprehensive clinical review, *Int. Clin. Psychopharmacol.,* 16(5):239–252, 2001.

Hypericin *see also* **St. John's Wort**   Hypericin, a naphthodianthrone present in St. John's wort (*Hypericum perforatum* L.), has received increasing attention because of its antiviral, antiretroviral, and photodynamic properties (Gulick et al., 1999; Kamuhabwa et al., 2000; Lavie et al., 1995). In the presence of oxygen and light stimulation, hypericin is one of the most powerful photosensitizers in nature by generating reactive-oxygen species (ROS) capable of destroying tumors (Agostinis et al., 2002). The phototherapeutic properties of hypericin are important in the new therapeutic approach to the treatment of superficial neoplastic lesion, known as photodynamic therapy (PDT). Chen and de Witte (2000) found hypericin was a potent and effective tumor photosensitizer as a PDT tool using a mouse P388 lymphoma-tumor model. Treatment with hypericin (2, 5, and 20 mg/kg, i.p.) 2 h prior to light irradiation significantly ($p < 0.01$) prolonged the life span of the mice (Figure H.53). The efficacy of PDT treatment with hypericin was highest after 2 h compared to 24- and 48-h intervals. Ali and coworkers (2001) showed that photoactivated hypericin induced apoptosis in

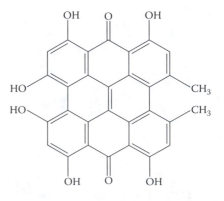

Hypericin. (From Hostanska et al., *Eur. J. Pharmaceutics Biopharmaceutics.,* 56:121–132, 2003. With permission.)

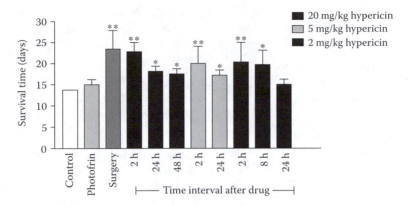

FIGURE H.53 Survival time of DBA/2 mice bearing subcutaneously transplanted P388 lymphoma cells after PDT and surgical excision. Tumor was exposed to 595 nm light 2–48 h after a 2, 5, or 20 mg/kg dose (i.p.) of hypericin and to 630 nm light 24 h after a 5 mg/kg dose (i.p.) of photofrin. For both cases, the light dose was 120 J/cm^2, delivered at the intensity of 1 mW/cm^2. The control group shown was the data of tumor-bearing mice without treatment. Each column represents the mean ± SD (bars) for at least four animals. **$p < 0.01$, *$p < 0.05$, compared with the control. (From Chen and de Witte, *Cancer Lett.*, 150:111–117, 2000. With permission.)

human mucosal carcinoma cells by activating caspase proteases, particularly caspase-3.

As an exogenous fluorophore, hypericin showed excellent sensitivity of above 90 percent in the fluorescent diagnosis of bladder cancer, suggesting its use in the early detection of this disease *in situ* (D'Hallewin et al., 2002). Using isolated crayfish neuron, Uzdensky et al. (2003) showed the potential of hypericin and its water-soluble derivative, developed using polyvinylpyrrolidone as carrier, for the visualization and selective photodynamic treatment of malignant gliomas.

The efficacy of St. John's wort for the treatment of mild and moderate depression still remains controversial. Nevertheless, more than 30 clinical trials have found similar efficacy between St. John's wort and low doses of tricyclic antidepressants, without their attendant side effects (Greeson et al., 2001; Schultz, 2002). Simmen and coworkers (2003) examined the effect of three St. John's wort constituents, hyperforin, hypericin, and pseudohypericin. The latter is the hydroxylated derivative of hypericin found in substantially larger amounts compared to hypericin, although no pharmacological effects have yet been ascribed to it. For the first time, these researchers showed the functional antagonism of corticotrophin-releasing factor (CRF$_1$) receptor by all three compounds, providing evidence for their role in the antidepressant efficacy of St. John's wort. This is because selective CRF$_1$ receptor agonists represent a new class of anxiolytics/antidepressants. Hypericin and hyperforin affected both CRF and calcitonin, while pseudohypericin selectively antagonized CRF and was considered the only real CRF$_1$ antagonist.

References

Agostinis, P., Vantieghem, A., Merlevede, W., and de Witte, P.A.M., Hypericin in cancer treatment: More light on the way, *Inter. J. Biochem. Cell Biol.*, 34: 221–241, 2002.

Ali, S.M., Chee, S.K., Yuen, G.K., and Olivo, M., Hypericin and hypercrellin induced apoptosis in human mucosal carcinoma cells, *J. Photochem. Photobiol.*, 65:59–73, 2001.

Chen, B. and de Witte, P.A., Photodynamic therapy efficacy and tissue distribution of hypericin in a mouse P388 lymphoma tumor model, *Cancer Lett.*, 150:111–117, 2000.

D'Hallewin, M.-A., Bezdetnaya, L., and Guillemin, F., Fluorescence detection of bladder cancer: A review, *Eur. Urol.*, 42:417–425, 2002.

Greeson, J.M., Sanford, B., and Monti, D.A., St. John's wort (*Hypercum perforatum*): A review of the current pharmacological, toxicological, and classical literature, *Psychophramacology*, 153:402–414, 2001.

Gulick, R.M., McAuliffe, V., Holden-Wiltse, J., Crumpacker, C., Liebes, L., Stein, D.S., Meehan, P., Hussey, J., and Forscht, F.T., Phase 1 studies of hypericin, the active compound in St. John's wort, as an antiretroviral agent in HIV-infected adults, AIDS Clinical Trials Group Protocols 150 and 258, *Ann. Intern. Med.,* 130:510–514, 1999.

Hostanska, K., Reichling, J., Bommer, S., Weber, M., and Saller, R., Hyperforin a constituent of St. John's wort (*Hypericum perforatum* L.) extract induces apoptosis by triggering activation of caspases and with hypericin synergistically exerts cytotoxicity towards human malignant cells lines, *Eur. J. Pharmaceutics Biopharmaceutics.,* 56:121–132, 2003.

Kamuhabwa, A.R., Agostinis, P.A., D'Hallewin, M.A., Kasran, A., and de Witte, P.A.M., Photodynamic activity of hypericin in human urinary bladder carcinoma cells, *Anticancer Res.,* 20:2579–2584, 2000.

Lavie, G., Mazur, D., Lavie, D., and Meruelo, D., The chemical and biological properties of hypericin: A compound with a broad spectrum of biological activities, *Med. Res. Rev.,* 15:111–119, 1995.

Schultz, V., Clinical trials with Hypericum extracts in patients with depression — results, comparisons, conclusions for therapy with antidepressant drugs, *Phytomedicine,* 9:468–474, 2002.

Simmen, U., Bobirnac, I., Ullmer, C., Lubbert, H., Buter, K.B., Schaffner, W., and Schoeffter, P., Antagonist effect of pseudohyerick at CRF, receptor, *Eur. J. Pharmacol.,* 458:251–256, 2003.

Uzdensky, A.B., Bragin, D.E., Kolosov, M.S., Kubin, A., Loew, H.G., and Moan, J., Photodynamic effect of hypericin and a water-soluble derivative on isolated crayfish neuron and surrounding glial cells. *J. Phtochem. Photobiol.,* 72:27–33, 2003.

H

Indole-3-acetic acid (IAA) Indole-3-acetic acid (IAA) is the major form of the plant hormone, auxin, a key regulator of cell division, elongation, and differentiation in higher plants (Goldsmith, 1993). Recent studies showed that

Indole-3-acetic acid. (Wu et al., *Sens. Actuat.*, B96: 658–662, 2003. With permission.)

a combination of IAA and horseradish peroxide (HRP) was cytotoxic to cancer cells and could be used as a novel cancer therapy (Folkes et al., 1998; Greco and Dachs, 2001; Wardman, 2002). IAA must undergo oxidative decarboxylation by HRP before it becomes cytotoxic (Folkes and Wardman, 2001). Since the activated form of IAA produced free radicals, including peroxy radicals, the combination of IAA and horseradish peroxidase could be used to enhance cellular oxidative stress and bring about apoptosis (Candeias et al., 1995). Kim

and coworkers (2004) showed that the combination of IAA and horseradish produced free radicals in a dose-dependent manner and induced apoptosis in G361 human melanoma cells. The presence of 1.2 µg/mL of HRP, 100 and 500 µM IAA, caused 50 percent and 100 percent of the cells to die, respectively (Figure I.54). The mechanism involved activation of caspase-8 and caspase-9, which in turn led to activation of caspase-3 and cleavage of poly(ADP-ribose)polymerase. Another examination of the mechanism of IAA cytotoxicity by de Melo et al. (2004) suggested induction of cell death by IAA involved the production of reactive-oxygen species by HRP.

References

Candeias, L.P., Folkes, L.K., Porssa, M., Parrick, J., and Wardman, P., Enhancement of lipid peroxidation by indole-3-acetic acid derivatives: Substituent effects, *Free Rad. Res.*, 23:403–418, 1995.

de Melo, M.P., de Lima, T.M., Pithon-Curi, T.C., and Curi, R., The mechanism of indole acetic acid cytotoxicity, *Toxicol. Lett.*, 148: 103–111, 2004.

Folkes, L.K., Candeias, L.P., and Wardman, P., Toward targeted "oxidation therapy" of cancer; peroxidase-catalysed cytotoxicity of indole-3-acetic acid, *Int. J. Radiat. Oncol. Biol. Phys.*, 42:917–920, 1998.

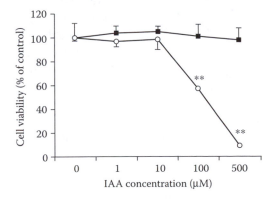

FIGURE I.54 Cytotoxic effect of IAA/HRP in G361 human melanoma cells. After serum-starvation cells were treated with varying concentrations (1–500 µM) of IAA in the absence (■) and presence (○) of HRP (1.2 µg/mL). Each experiment was repeated at least twice, independently and representative results shown. ** $p < 0.01$ compared to the untreated control. (From Kim et al., *Cell Signal*, 16:81–88, 2004. With permission.)

Folkes, L.K. and Wardman, P., Oxidative activation of indole-3-acetic acids to cytotoxic species—a potential new role for plant auxins in cancer therapy, *Biochem. Pharmacol.*, 61:129–136, 2001.

Goldsmith, M.H.M., Cellular signaling: New insights into the action of the plant growth hormone auxin, *Proc. Natl. Acad. Sci.*, 90:11442–11445, 1993.

Greco, O. and Dachs, G.U., Gene directed enzyme/prodrug therapy of cancer; Historical appraisal and future prospectives, *J. Cell Physiol.*, 187:22–36, 2001.

Kim, D.-S., Jeon, S.-E., and Park, K.-C., Oxidation of indole-3-acteic acid by horseradish peroxidase induces apoptosis in G361 human melanoma cells, *Cell Signal*, 16:81–88, 2004.

Wardman, P., *Curr. Pharm. Des.*, 8:1376–1374, 2002.

Wu, K., Sun, Y., and Hu, S., Development of an amperometric indole-3-acetic acid sensor based on carbon nanotubes film coated glassy carbon electrode, *Sens. Actuat.*, B96:658–662, 2003.

Indole-3-carbinol *see* **Diindoylmethane**

Inulin   Inulin, a naturally occurring, complex polysaccharide present in many plants, is obtained primarily from the roots of chicory (*Cicorium intybus* L.) (De Bruyn et al., 1992) or the tubers of Jerusalem artichoke (Baldini et al., 2003). Chicory inulin is composed of mixtures of linear β 2-1 fructans varying in length from 2 to approximately 65 fructose residues. In comparison, Jerusalem artichoke inulin has a much shorter chain length. The linear 1,2-β-linked D-frutofuranoside chains of inulin are attached via an α1-β2 type sucrose linkage to a terminal glucose molecule. The inability of digestive enzymes to digest these 1,2-β-link-ages ensures inulin reaches the gut intact, where it is fermented by the gut flora. In fact, inulin is a prebiotic, stimulating the growth of bifido-bacteria and inhibiting colon carcinogenesis in animal models (Reddy et al., 1997; Roberfroid et al., 1998; Reddy, 1999). Causey and cowork-ers (2000) showed inulin significantly lowered serum triglycerides in hypercholesterolemic men, as well as improved the gut flora. Koo et

Inulin   n = approx. 35

al. (2003) found inulin-stimulated NO synthesis *via* activation of protein kinase C (PKC)- α and protein tyrosinase kinase, which activated NF-κB in RAW 264.7 cells. The release of NO is important for its tumoricidal effects and may explain the anticarcinogenic effects associated with inulin. These results point to inulin having considerable promise as a functional ingredient in the diet.

Videla and coworkers (2001) showed dietary inulin reduced the severity of dextran sodium sulfate colitis in rats. Oral inulin prevented colonic mucosal inflammation by dextran sodium sulfate (DSS) that histologically resem-bles human ulcerative colitis (Okayasu et al., 1990). In addition to improving histological scores and decreasing the release of inflamma-tory mediators, it also lowered tissue myelo-peroxidase accumulation in DSS colitis in rats. These results suggested inulin may be a useful dietary or pharmacological intervention in patients suffering from ulcerative colitis.

References

Baldini, M., Danuso, F., Turi, M., and Vannozzi, G.P., Evaluation of new clones of Jerusalem artichoke (*Helianthus tuberosum* L.) for inulin and sugar yield from stalk and tuber, *Ind. Crops Prod.*, 19:25–40, 2003.

Causey, J.L., Feirtag, J.M., Gallaher, D.D., Tungland, B.C., and Slavin, J.L., Effects of dietary inulin on serum lipid, blood glucose and gastrointestinal environment in hypercholesterolemic men, *Nutr. Res.*, 20:191–201, 2000.

De Bruyn, A., Alvarez, A.P., Sandra, P., and DeLeenheer, L., Isolation and identification of O-β$_D$-fructofuranosyl-(2-1)-O-β$_D$-O-β$_D$-fructofuranosyl-(2-1)-$_D$ fructose: A product of the enzymatic hydrolysis of the inulin from *Cicorium intybus*, *Carbohydr. Res.*, 235:303–308, 1992.

Koo, H.-N., Hong, S.-H., Seo, H.-G., Yoo, T.-S., Lee, K.-N., Kim, N.-S., Kim, C.-H., and Kim, H.-M., Inulin stimulates NO synthesis via activation of PKC-α and protein tyrosine kinase, resulting in the activation of NF-κB by IFN-γ-primed RAW 264.7 cells, *J. Nutr. Biochem.*, 14:598–605, 2003.

Okayasu, I., Hatakeyama, S., and Yamada, M., A novel method in the induction of reliable experimental acute and chronic ulcerative colitis in mice, *Gastroenterology*, 98:694–702, 1990.

Reddy, B.S., Possible mechanisms by which pro- and prebiotics influence colon carcinogenesis and tumor growth, *J. Nutr.*, 129:1478S–1482S, 1999.

Reddy, B.S., Hamid, R., and Rao, C.V., Effect of dietary oligofructose and inulin on colonic preneoplastic aberrant crypt foci inhibition, *Carcinogenesis*, 18:1371–1374, 1997.

Roberfroid, M.B., Van Loo, J.A.E., and Gibson, G.R., The bifidogenic nature of chicory inulin and its hydrolysis products, *J. Nutr.*, 128:11–19, 1998.

Videla, S., Vilaseca, J., Antolin, M., Garcia-Lafuente, A., Guarner, F., Crespo, E., Casalots, J., Salas, A., and Malagelada, J.R., Dietary inulin improves distal colitis induced by dextran sodium sulfate in the rat, *Am. J. Gastroenterol.*, 96:1486–1493, 2001.

Isoflavones *see also* Daidzein and Genistein

Isoflavones represent a group of phytoestrogens that are chemically strikingly similar to mammalian estrogens. Phytoestrogens mainly bind to the second subtype of the estrogen receptor (ERβ), while mammalian estradiol has a higher binding affinity for the "classic" estrogen receptor ERα (Kuiper et al., 1998; Casanova et al., 1999). They can thus act as either estrogen agonists or antagonists (Setchell, 1998; Setchell and Cassidy, 1999). Legumes are good sources of isoflavones, with soybeans and soy products being the most abundant, containing approximately 0.2–1.6 mg/g dry weight (Kurzer and Xu, 1997). Fitpatrick (2003) recently reviewed the literature on the effects of soy isoflavones on lipid metabolism, osteoblasts and osteoclasts, bone markers, bone-mineral density, and cognition. Based on very limited human clinical data, it was hard to make definitive recommendations to clinicians other than moderate use for postmenopausal women. The low incidence of breast cancer, cardiovascular disease, and climacteric symptoms in Japanese women compared to Caucasians has been attributed to higher soybean intake. Watanabe et al. (2002) showed a slight improvement in elongation of the menstrual cycle in young women taking an isoflavone-rich tablet. Climacteric women also showed improvement in bone density, hypertension, and climacteric symptoms when maintained on these tablets.

References

Casanova, M., You, L., Gaido, K.W., Archibeque-Engle, S., Janszen, D.B., and Heck, H.A., Developmental effects of dietary phytoestrogens in Sprague–Dawley rats and interactions of genistein and daidzein with rat estrogen receptors alpha and beta *in vitro*, *Toxicol. Sci.*, 51:236–244, 1999.

Fitzpatrick, L.A., Soy isoflavones: Hope or hype? *Maturitas*, 44(1):S21–S29, 2003.

Kuiper, G.G.J.M., Lemmen, J.G., Carlsson, B., Corton, J.C., Safe, S.H., van der Saag, P.T., Van der Burg, B., and Gustafsson, J.A., Interaction of estrogenic chemicals and phytoestrogens with estrogen receptor β, *Endocrinology*, 139:4252–4263, 1998.

Kurzer, M.S. and Xu, X., Dietary phytoestrogens, *Ann. Rev. Nutr.*, 17:353–381, 1997.

Setchell, K.D., Phytoestrogens: The biochemistry, physiology, and implications for human health of soy isoflavones, *Am. J. Clin. Nutr.*, 68:1333S–1346S, 1998.

Setchell, K.D. and Cassidy, A. Dietary isoflavones: Biological effects and relevance to human health, *J. Nutr.*, 129:758S–767S, 1999.

Watanabe, S., Uesugi, S., and Kikuchi, Y., Isoflavones for prevention of cancer, cardiovascular diseases, gynecological problems and possible immune potentiation, *Biomed. Pharmacother.*, 56:302–312, 2002.

Isohomohalichondrin B (From Litaudon et al., *Tetrahedron Lett.*, 35:9435–9438, 1994. With permission.)

Isohomohalichondrin B   Isohomohalichon-drin B (IHB), a member of the halichondrin group, was isolated in New Zealand from the deep-water sponge *Lissodendoryx* sp. It was shown by Litaudon et al. (1994) to be highly toxic towards P388 (murine leukemia) cells. Bergamaschi and coworkers (1999) found IHB to be a potent, antitumor agent delaying cell cycle S-phase progress, mitotic block, tetrap-loidy, and inducing apoptosis in a human can-cer-cell line.

References

Bergamaschi, D., Ronzoni, S., Taverna, S., Faretta, M., De Feudis, P., Faircloth, G., Jimeno, J., Erba, E., and D'Incalci, M., Cell cycle perturbations and apo-ptosis induced by isohomohalichondrin B (IHB), a nairal marine compound., *Br. J. Cancer,* 79:267–277, 1999.

Litaudon, M., Hart, J.B., Blunt, J.W., Lake, R.J., and Munro, M., Isohomohalichondrin B, a new antitumor polyethermacrolide from New Zealand deep-water sponge *Lissodendoryx* sp., *Tetrahedron Lett.,* 35: 9435–9438, 1994.

Isoliquiritigenin   The chalcone isoliquiritige-nin (ISL), isolated from licorice and shallots, was shown by Yamamoto et al. (1991) to inhibit the formation of skin papilloma induced by 7,12-dimethylbenz[α]-anthracene (DMBA) and TP (phorbol acetate). Maggliolini et al. (2002) reported ISL exhibited both estrogenic and antiproliferative effects on MCF7 breast-cancer cells. High concentrations of this phy-toestrogen inhibited proliferation of MCF7 cells, while low concentrations stimulated

Isoliquiritigenin. (From Cao et al., *J. Chromatogr.,* A. 1042:203–209, 2004. With permission.)

progression of estrogen-dependent breast tumors. Based on these results, they cautioned that the level of ISL taken by menopausal women be carefully monitored.

The ability of ISL to suppress metastasis of mouse renal-cell carcinoma was reported by Yamazaki and coworkers (2002). The number of metastatic lung nodules was significantly reduced in the presence of ISL. Kanzawa and coworkers (2003) recently reported ISL effec-tively inhibited prostate cancer. They found that the cell growth of prostate-cancer cell line DU145 was significantly reduced by ISL in a dose- and time-dependent manner (Figure I.55). The mechanism of action appeared to involve induction of S- and G2/M-phase arrest and was associated with enhanced expression of GADD153. These results suggested ISL was a potential candidate for treating prostate cancer.

The potential of ISL in the treatment of lung cancer was recently demonstrated by Ii et al. (2004). They found ISL inhibited cell prolifer-ation of a human lung-cancer cell line in a dose- and time-dependent manner. Cell cycle progres-sion was arrested at the G2/M phase, which was associated with enhanced expression of p21[CIP1/WAF1], a universal inhibitor of cyclic-dependent kinases.

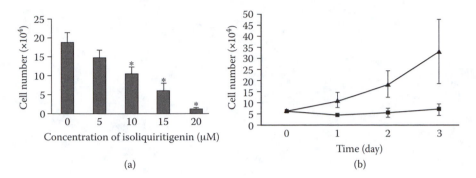

(a)   (b)

FIGURE I.55 Effect of ISL on the growth of the prostate cancer DU145 cell lines. (a) Dose-dependent effect: cells were exposed for 48 h to various concentrations of ISL or DMSO alone (control). $p < 0.05$ versus control. (b) Time-kinetics study: cells were exposed to 15 μM of ISL for 24, 48, and 72 h. ((▲) DMSO alone (control) (■)) (From Kanzawa et al., *Eur. Urol.*, 43:580–586, 2003. With permission.)

References

Cao, Y., Wang, Y., Ji, C., and Ye, J., Determination of liquiritigenin and isoliquiritigenin in *Glycyrrhiza uralensis* and its medicinal preparations by capillary electrophoresis with electrochemical detection, *J. Chromatogr.*, A. 1042:203–209, 2004.

Ii, T., Satomi, Y., Katoh, D., Shimada, J., Baba, M., Okuyama, T., Nishimo, H., and Kitamura, N., Induction of cell cycle arrest and p21[CIPI/WAFI] expression in human lung cancer cells by isoliquiritigenin, *Cancer Lett.*, 207:27–35, 2004.

Kanzawa, M., Satomi, Y., Mitzutani, Y., Ukimura, O., Kawauchi, A., Sakai, T., Baba, M., Okuyama, T., Nishino, H., and Miki, T., Isoliquiritigenin inhibits the growth of prostate cancer, *Eur. Urol.*, 43:580–586, 2003.

Maggliolini, M., Statti, G., Vivacqua, A., Gabriele, S., Rago, V., Loizzo, M., Menichini, F., and Amdo, S., Estrogenic and antiproliferative activities of isoliquiritigenin in MCF7 breast cancer cells, *J. Steroid Biochem. Mol. Biol.*, 82:315–322, 2002.

Yamamoto, S., Aizu, E., Jiang, H., Nakadate, T., Kiyoto, I., Wang, J.C., and Kato, R., The potent antitumor-promoting agent isoliquiritigenin, *Carcinogenesis*, 12:317–323, 1991.

Yamazaki, S., Morita, T., Endo, H., Hamamoto, T., Baba, M., Joichi, S., Kaneko, S., Okada, Y., Okuyama, T., Nishino, H., and Tokue, A., Isoliquiritigenin suppresses pulmonary mertastasis of mouse renal cell carcinoma, *Cancer. Lett.*, 183:23–30, 2002.

I

J

Jasmine (*Jasminum grandiflorum* L.) While jasmine grows in many parts of the world, jasmine absolute is produced mainly in Egypt by solvent extraction of the essential oil from its delicate flowers. In addition to odorant volatiles, the oil contains fats, pigments, and fat-soluble vitamins. It is used in aromatherapy as a holistic remedy for apathy, fear, hypersensitivity, panic, hysteria, uterine disorders, childbirth pain, skincare, frigidity, coughs, hoarseness, and muscular spasms (Tisserand, 1985; Lawless, 1995).

Konig et al. (1992) developed a GC column using a chiral stationary phase for measuring linalool and jasmine lactone in jasmine oil. Tamogami and coworkers (2001) compared the enantiometric ratios of chiral components in jasmine absolute obtained from Egypt, India, and France. Except for methyl epijasmonate, the other chiral components were not enantiometrically pure. Sensory evaluation indicated that the key flavoring odorants in jasmine were (R)-δ-jasmine lactone and $(1R, 2S)$-methyl epijasmonate. The very low enantiometric purity of the $(1R, 2R)$-enantiomer of methyl jasmonate in Indian juniper probably accounted for the difference in flavor quality compared to those grown in France and Egypt.

Some evidence suggests that spasmolysis or relaxation of smooth muscle in the pig ilieum *in vitro* (Lis-Balchin et al., 1996) is correlated with the holistic relaxant effect in man (Lis-Balchin and Hart, 1997). Lis-Balchin and coworkers (2002) reported that jasmine appeared to mediate its spasmolytic action by increasing intracellular cAMP with the possibility of some calcium-channel blockage. They suggested that the pharmacological activity observed in isolated guinea pig ileum may explain the effect of inhaled jasmine vapor by its action on the central nervous system.

References

Konig, W.A., Gercke, B., Icheln, D., Evers, P., Donnecke, J., and Wang, W., New selectively substituted cyclodextrins as stationary phases for the analysis of chiral constituents of essential oils, *J. High Resol. Chromatogr.,* 15:367–372, 1992.

Lawless, J., *The Illustrated Encyclopedia of Essential Oils,* Element Books Ltd., Dorset, U.K., 1995.

Lis-Balchin, M., Hart, S., Deans, S.G., and Eaglesham, E., Comparison of the pharmacological and antimicrobial action of commercial plant essential oils, *J. Herb Species Med. Plants,* 4:69–85, 1996.

Lis-Balchin, M. and Hart, S., Correlation of the chemical profiles of essential oil mixes with their relaxant and stimulant properties in man and smooth muscle preparations *in vitro,* in *Proc. 27th Int. Symp. Ess. Oils,* Franz, Ch., Math, A., and Buchbauer, G., Eds., Allured Pub. Corp., Vienna, 1997, pp. 8–111, Carol Stream IL, pp. 24–28.

Lis-Balchin, M., Hart, S., and Wan Hang-Lo, B., Jasmine absolute (*Jasmonium grandiflora* L.) and its mode of action on guinea-pig ilieum *in vitro, Phytother. Res.,* 16:437–439, 2002.

Tamogami, S., Awano, K., and Kitahara, T., Analysis of the enantiomeric ratios of chiral components in absolute jasmine, *Flav. Fragr. J.,* 16:161–163, 2001.

Tisserand, R., *The Art of Aromatherapy,* C.W. Daniel Co. Lts., Saffron Walden, 1985.

Jerusalem artichoke (*Helianthus tuberosum* L) *see* Inulin Jerusalem artichoke, a native North American plant, is capable of enduring high temperatures and severe water-stress conditions. It is one of the richest sources of inulin, a linear polysaccharide of fructose units attached to a terminal sucrose. Baldini and coworkers (2004) evaluated new clones of Jerusalem artichoke, reporting maximum inulin yields up to 8.0 t/ha. Since it cannot be digested by digestive enzymes, inulin enters the intestine intact, where it is fermented by bifidobacteria in the intestine and is therefore considered a prebiotic.

References

Baldini, M., Danuro, F., Turi, M., And Vannazzi, G.P., Evaluation of new clones of Jerusalem artichoke (*Helianthus tuberosum* L.) for inulin and sugar yield from stalks and tubers, *Ind. Crops Prod.,* 19: 25–40, 2004.

Jojoba   Jojoba (*Simmondsia chinensis*) is an arid perennial evergreen shrub native to Arizona, California, and northwestern Mexico (Hogan, 1978). The seeds contain a light yellow, odorless wax ester composed of straight-chain esters of monounsaturated C_{18}, C_{20}, and C_{24} acids and alcohols, referred to as jojoba liquid wax. Tobares et al. (2003) found cold-pressed wax had the best oxidative stability due to the higher retention of tocopherols and phenolic antioxidants. Jojoba liquid wax has traditionally been used in folk medicine for treating renal colic, sunburn, chaffed skin, hair loss, headache, wounds, and sore throat (Yaron, 1987). Human studies showed that sulfurized jojoba liquid wax was effective in treating acne, while the unmodified wax was used for treating psoriasis (Mosovich, 1985). The anti-inflammatory properties of jojoba liquid wax were recently demonstrated in several animal models by Habashy et al. (2004). Using the carrageenan-induced rat paw oedema model, jojoba liquid wax significantly reduced edema, as well as decreased prostaglandin E_2 (PGE_2) in the inflammatory exudates in a dose-dependent manner (Figure J.56).

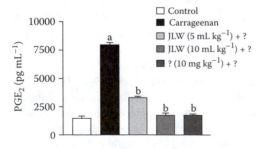

FIGURE J.56 Effect of jojoba liquid wax (JLW) on PGE_2 production in exudates from carrageenan-treated rats. [a]Statistically significant from the control group at $p < 0.05$; [b]Statistically significant from the carrageenan-induced group at $p < 0.05$. (Habashy et al., *Pharmacol. Res.,* 51:95–105, 2005. With permission.)

References

Habashy, R.R., Abdel-Naim, A.B., Khalifa, A.E., and Al-Azizi, M.M., Anti-inflammatory effects of jojoba liquid wax in experimental animals, *Pharmacol. Res.,* 51:95–105, 2005.

Hogan, L., Jojoba: A new crop for arid regions of the world? *Crops Soils Mag.,* 31(2):18–19, 1978.

Mosovich, B., Treatment of acne and psoriasis, in *Proceedings of the Sixth International Conference on Jojoba and its Uses*, Wisniak, J. and Zabicky, J., Eds., University of Negev, Beer Sheva, Israel, 1985, pp. 393–397.

Tobares, L., Guzman, C. and Maestri, D. Effect of extraction and bleaching processes on jojoba (Simmondsia chinensis) wax quality. *Eur. J. Lipid Sci. Technol.,* 105:749–753, 2003.

Yaron, A., Metabolism and physiological effects of jojoba oil, in *The Chemistry and Technology of Jojoba Oil*, Wisniak, J., Ed., American Oil Chemists' Society Press, Champaign, Illinois, 1987, pp. 251–265.

Juniper (*Juniperus communis* L.)   Juniper, an evergreen wind-pollinated shrub or small tree, grows extensively in the Northern Hemisphere. Its blue-black berries have a number of pharmacodynamic properties, including diuretic, nephrotoxic, and antioxidative (Sanchez de Medina et al., 1994; Schichter and Leuschner, 1997; Takacsova et al., 1995).

The berries contain an essential oil that is obtained by steam distillation (Newall et al., 1996). The oil is composed mainly of mono-terpenes (60 percent), which appear responsible for its biological properties. Filipowicz et al. (2003) recently attributed the antibacterial and antifungal activity of juniper-berry oil to the presence of (–)-α-pinene, *p*-cymene, and β-cymene in the oil. Muhlbauer and coworkers (2003) demonstrated for the first time that essential oils, such as sage, rosemary, pine, turpentine, eucalyptus, and juniper, and their monoterpenes effectively inhibited bone resorption in the rat. The latter has implications in preventing bone loss associated with osteoporosis.

Na and coworkers (2001) showed juniper oil inhibited heat shock-induced apoptosis of human astrocyte CCF-STTG1 cells. Astrocytes are the most abundant glial cell types in the brain, and their death, or apoptosis, has been implicated in the pathogenesis of a number of central-nervous diseases, including Alzheimer's disease. Thus, juniper oil may have therapeutic value in inhibiting astrocyte apoptosis by preventing activation of caspase-3, a key factor in the execution of apoptosis.

Juniper-berry oil is also rich in 5,11,14-eicosatrienoic acid, a polyunsaturated fatty acid similar to that found in fish oil. Jones et al. (1998) found juniper-berry oil was more effective than fish in protecting rat liver from reperfusion injury, a major cause of graft damage in liver transplants, as well as hepatic damage in alcohol-induced liver disease.

The Navajo tribe in northern Arizona and southern Utah have traditionally used ash from the branches and needles of the juniper tree as flavoring in their food products. In addition, a tea is also made from juniper ash to treat diarrhea, as well as injured muscles. Christensen et al. (1998) showed that, in addition to calcium, juniper ash also contributed significant amounts of magnesium and iron in the Navajo diet.

References

Christensen, N.K., Sorenson, A.W., Hendricks, D.G., and Munger, R., Juniper ash as a source of calcium in the Navajo diet, *J. Am. Diet. Assoc.*, 98:333–334, 1998.

Filipowicz, N., Kaminski, M., Kurlenda, J., Asztemborska, M., and Ochocka, J.R., Antibacterial and antifungal activity of juniper berry oil and its selected components, *Phytother. Res.*, 17:227–231, 2003.

Jones, S.M., Zhong, Z., Enomoto, N., Schemmer, P., and Thurman, R.G., Dietary juniper oil minimizes hepatic reperfusion injury in the rat, *Hepatol.*, 28: 1042–1050, 1998.

Muhlbauer, R.C., Lozano, A., Palacio, S., Reinli, A., and Felix, R., Common herbs, essential oils, and monoterpenes potently modulate bone metabolism, *Bone*, 32:372–380, 2003.

Na, H.-F., Koo, H.-N., Lee, G-G., Yoo, S.-J., Park, J.-H., Lyu, Y.-S., and Kim, H.-M., Juniper oil inhibits the heat shock-induced apoptosis via preventing the caspase-3 activation of human astrocytes CCF-STTG1 cells, *Clinica Chim. Acta*, 314:215–220, 2001.

Newall, C.A., Anderson, L.A., and Phillipson, J.D., *Herbal Medicine — A Guide for Healthcare Professionals*, The Pharmaceutical Press, London, U.K., 1996.

Sanchez de Medina, F., Gamez, M.J., Jimenez, I., Jimenez, J., Osuna, J.I., and Zarzuelo, A., Hypoglycemic activity of juniper "berries," *Planta Med.*, 60: 197–200, 1994.

Schichter, H. and Leuscher, F., The potential nephrotoxic effects of essential juniper oil, *Arzneimittelforschung*, 47:855–858, 1997.

Takacsova, M., Pribela, A., and Faktorova, M., Study of the antioxidative effects of thyme, sage, juniper and oregano, *Nahrung.* 39:241–243, 1995.

J

K

Kaempferol

Kaempferol Kaempferol (3,4′,5,7-tertahydroxyflavone) is a flavonol found in abundance in fruits, vegetables, and tea (Cao et al., 1997; Hertog et al., 1992). It has been shown to have

Kaempferol. (From Tian et al., *J. Mol. Struct.,* 691: 197–202, 2004. With permission.)

anti-inflammatory and antioxidant properties in macrophages and neurons. For example, kaempferol protected rat-cortical neurons from amyloid β protein toxicity by minimizing the production of reactive-oxygen species and inhibiting caspase activity (Wang et al., 2001). It was shown previously to reduce prostaglandin E_2 and nitrite production in mouse macrophages by suppressing inducible cyclooxygenase-2 and inducible nitric-oxide synthetase (Liang et al., 1999). Okamoto et al. (2002) examined the immunoregulating properties of kaempferol and found it useful for treating cell-mediated immune diseases, such as acute graft-versus-host disease (GVHD). *In vitro* studies with mice-spleen cells showed kaempferol acted directly on T cells by inhibiting Th1 cytokine production and suppressing expansion or generation of CD8+ CTLs. Subsequent treatment of C57BL/6-into-BDF 1 mice with kaempferol reduced GVHD-associated antihost CTL activity by activating Th2 cells and engraftment of the donor cells. The overall result was early recovery of body weight loss, increased survival, and reduced injury to the liver and large intestine.

Recent data suggest tea and vegetable consumption, such as onions, can provide protection against osteoporosis in older women (Hegarty et al., 2000; Muhlbauer and Li, 1999; New et al., 2000; Muhlbauer et al., 2002). This was attributed to the presence of flavonols, such as quercetin and kaempferol as rutin, a glycoside of quercetin. Rutin was shown previously by Horcajada-Molteni and coworkers (2000) to inhibit ovariectomy-induced osteopenia in rats. Using osteoclasts from 10-day-old rabbits, Wattel et al. (2003) showed kaempferol and quercetin both reduced bone resorption in a time- and dose-dependent manner (Figure K.57). Both flavonols induced apoptosis of mature osteoclasts in the same dose range that effectively inhibited bone resorption. Treatment of highly purified rabbit osteoclasts with 50 µM quercertin and kaempferol significantly reduced intracellular levels of reactive-oxygen species by 75 percent and 25 percent, respectively. Below this concentration, neither of these flavonols exhibited any antiradical activity, so that their antioxidant activity could not explain their inhibitory effect on bone resorption. However, they found that only kaempferol's inhibition of bone resorption was partially reduced by addition of a pure antiestrogen. This suggested that inhibition of bone resorption by kaempferol could be partly explained by its estrogenic effect. This study demonstrated the importance of dietary sources of flavonols, such as kaempferol, as inhibitors of osteoporosis.

References

Cao, G., Sofic, E., and Prior, L.P., Antioxidant and prooxidant behaviour of flavonoids: Structure-activity relationships, *Free Rad. Biol. Med.,* 22:749–760, 1997.

Hegarty, V.M., May, H.M., and Khaw, K.T., Tea drinking and bone mineral density in older women, *Am. J. Clin. Nutr.,* 71:1003–1007, 2000.

Hertog, M.G.L., Hollman, P.C.H., and Katan, M.B.J., Content of potentially anticarcinogenic flavonoids in 28 vegetables and 9 fruits commonly consumed in

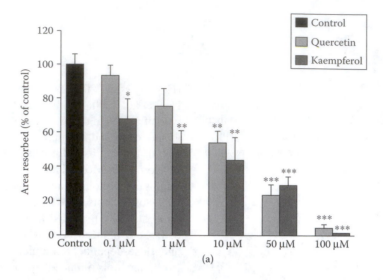

(a)

FIGURE K.57 Effect of different concentrations of quercetin and kaempferol on osteoclastic bone resorption. Osteoclasts were cultured on cortical bovine slices during 48 h in media containing either vehicle (0.1 percent DMSO = control) or flavonols, quercetin, and kaempferol (0.1–100 μM), and bone resorption assessed by measurement of total area of resorption pits. Results expressed as percent of control. Values are mean ± SEM of three independent experiments (N = 5 for pit-area measurement); (∗) $p < 0.05$, (∗∗) $p < 0.01$, and (∗∗∗) $p < 0.001$ compared with control group. (Wattel et al., *Biochem. Pharmacol.*, 65:35–42, 2003. With permission.)

the Netherlands, *J. Agric. Food Chem.*, 40:2379–2383, 1992.

Horcajada-Molteni, M.N., Crespy, V., Coxam, V., Davicco, M.J., Remesy, C., and Bartlet, J.P., Rutin inhibits ovariectomy-induced osteopenia in rats, *J. Bone Miner. Res.*, 15:2251–2258, 2000.

Liang, Y.-C., Huang, Y.-T., Tsai, S.-H., Lin-Shiau, Y.-J., Chen, C-F., and Lin, J.K., Suppression of inducible cyclooxygenase and inducible nitric oxide synthase by apigenin and related flavonoids in mouse macrophages, *Carcinogenesis*, 20:1945–1952, 1999.

Muhlbauer, R.C. and Li, F., Effect of vegetables on bone metabolism, *Nature*, 401:343–344, 1999.

Muhlbauer, R.C., Lozano, A., and Reinli, A., Onion and a mixture of vegetables, salads, and herbs affect bone resorption in the rat by a mechanism independent of their base excess, *J. Bone Miner. Res.*, 17:1230–1236, 2002.

New, S.A., Robins, S.P., Campbell, M.K., Martin, J.C., Garton, M.J., Bolton-Smith, C., Grubb, D.A., Lee, S.J., and Reid, D.M., Dietary influences on bone mass and bone metabolism: Further evidence of a positive link between fruit and vegetable consumption and bone health? *Am. J. Clin. Nutr.*, 71:142–151, 2000.

Okamoto, I., Iwaki, K., Koya-Miyata, S., Tanimoto, T., Kono, K., Ikeda, M., and Kurimoto, M., The flavonoid kaempferol suppresses the graft-versus-host

reaction by inhibiting type 1 cytokine production and CD8+ T cell engraftment, *Clin. Immunol.*, 103:132–144, 2002.

Tian, J., Liu, J., Tian, X., Hu, Z., and Chen, X., Study of the interaction of kaempferol with bovine serum albumin, *J. Mol. Struct.*, 691:197–202, 2004.

Wang, C.-N., Chi, C.-W., Lin, Y.-L., Chen, C.-F., and Shiao, Y.-J., The neuroprotective effects of phytoestrogens on amyloid β-protein-induced toxicity are mediated by abrogating the activation of caspase cascade in rat cortical neurons, *J. Biol. Chem.*, 276:5287–5295, 2001.

Wattel, A., Kamel, S., Mentaverri, R., Lorget, F., Prouillet, C., Petit, J.-P., Fardelonne, P., and Brazier, M., Potent inhibitory effect of naturally occurring flavonoids quercetin and kaempferol on *in vitro* osteoclastic bone resorption, *Biochem. Pharmacol.*, 65:35–42, 2003.

Kava-kava   Kava-kava (*Piper methysticum*), a plant native to the Pacific Islands, has been used for its soporific and narcotic effects (Bilia et al., 2002). Extracts were traditionally prepared from its macerated roots by mixing with water and coconut milk (Norton and Ruze,

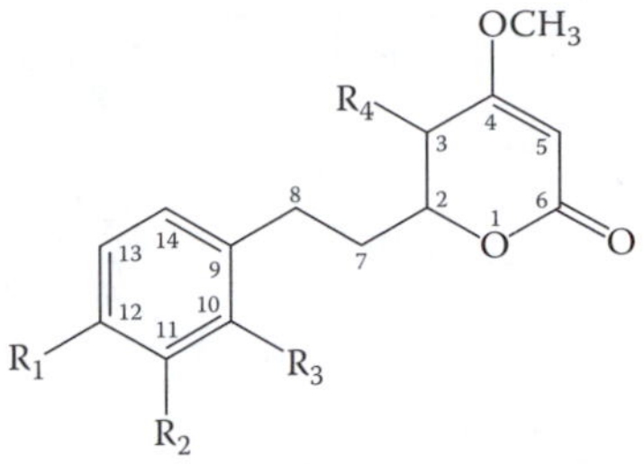

Kavalactones	R_1	R_2	C5–C6	C7–C8
Kacain				=
7,8-Dihydrokavain				
Methysticin		OCH_2O		=
Dihydromethysticin		OCH_2O		
Yangonin	OCH3		=	=
Desmethoxyyangonin			=	=
5,6,7,8-Tetrahydroyangonin				

SCHEME K.31 Kavalactone structures. (Adapted from Bilia et al., *J. Chromatogr. B.*, 812:203–214, 2004.)

1994). The active ingredients in kava-kava, known for their analgesic and anesthetic properties, are a group of lipophillic lactone derivatives with an arylethylene-α-pyrone skeleton. The major lactones are (+) kavain, (+)-methysticin, desmethoxyyangonin, yangonin, (+)-dihydrokavain, (+)-dihydromethysticin, and tetrahydroyangonin. Minor components include chalcones and essential oil. The kavalactone structures are shown in Scheme K.31.

In vitro studies showed isolated kavalactones directly affected the central nervous system and neurotransmitters by interacting with GABA-benzodiazepine receptors and by inhibiting noradrenaline uptake (Davies et al., 1992; Jussofie et al., 1994). Inhibition of noradrenaline uptake by kavalactones may explain some of their psychotropic properties (Seitz et al., 1997). The ability of kava-enriched extracts to inhibit human platelet MAO-B may also be an important mechanism for their psychotropic properties (Uebelhack et al., 1998).

Extensive clinical studies, using a number of rating scales (Hamilton Anxiety Scale and Clinical Global Impressions Scale), all showed the efficacy of kavalactones as an anxiolytic drug. For example, Lehmann et al. (1996) demonstrated the effectiveness of kava-kava extract for treating anxiety disorders, while Voltz and Kieser (1997) showed the same extract significantly

improved patients suffering from anxiety of nonpsychotic origin. Overall, studies showed good tolerance and low incidence of adverse effects associated with kava-kava treatment, including a systematic review and meta-analysis (Pittler and Ernst, 2000). Cagnacci and coworkers (2003) recently found an improvement in the mood of perimenopausal women, particular in anxiety, following administration of kava-kava. Lehrl (2004) reported that sleep disturbances associated with nonpsychotic disorders were effectively and safely treated with a kava extract WS®1490.

A number of adverse cases, however, were reported in Germany, where kava-kava was associated with dopamine antagonism (Schelosky et al., 1995), while seven cases of hepatitis were attributed directly to kava-kava intake (Strahl et al., 1998; Escher et al., 2001; Russmann et al., 2001). Stickel and coworkers (2003) pointed to the potential hepatoxicity of kava in Germany, which led to hepatic necrosis or cholestatic hepatitis in patients given alcoholic and acetonic kava extracts. High doses of kava lactones were recently shown by Gow et al. (2003) to have serious hepatoxic side effects. Such lactones are normally metabolized by the cytochrome P450 system in the liver (Schmidt et al., 1999) and by lactone hydrolases in the serum (Bargota et al., 2003). A recent study by

---

TABLE K.40
**Extraction of Kava Lactones from Roots of *P. Methysticum*
with Different Solvents[1]**

Extract	Percent Kava Lactones in Dried Extract
Acetone extract (standardized method)	100(0.001)
96 percent ethanol extract (standardized method)	100(0.001)
25 percent ethanol (traditional method)	15(0.02)
Water (traditional method)	2.97(0.03)

[1] Data presented as means (and standard deviation) for 10 samples in each solvent.

Source: Adapted from Whitton et al., *Phytochemistry,* 64:673–679, 2003. With permission.

Whitton et al. (2003) attributed the toxicity of kava-kava lactones to the particular extraction method, as they were 30 times higher in the standardized preparations compared to the traditional aqueous-extraction method. The various solvents used to extract kava lactones resulted in markedly different yields in the dried extract, ranging from 100 percent for the standardized methods involving acetone or 96 percent alcohol to 15 percent and 2.97 percent using the more traditional extractants of 25 percent ethanol or water, respectively (Table K.40). The higher levels in the more standardized extracts would saturate the detoxification pathways leading to hepato side effects. Since glutathione plays a crucial role in the phase II conversion of lactones to excretable waste products,

its depletion could explain the increased side effects observed for kavalactones. Schmidt and coworkers (2001) reported that sesquiterpene lactones bind to glutathione, allowing faster clearance by lactone hydrolases in the hepatocytes. Whitton and coworkers (2003) showed that supplementation with glutathione rendered the kava lactone nontoxic to eukaryotic cells by a similar mechanism in which the lactone ring was opened up via the Michael reaction (Scheme K.32), bypassing the cytochrome P50 pathway. The adverse hepatotoxic effects were found with the tablets and capsules made using standardized kava extracts in which glutathione was either absent or present at very low levels. Traditional preparations, on the other hand, contained high levels of glutathione, which probably

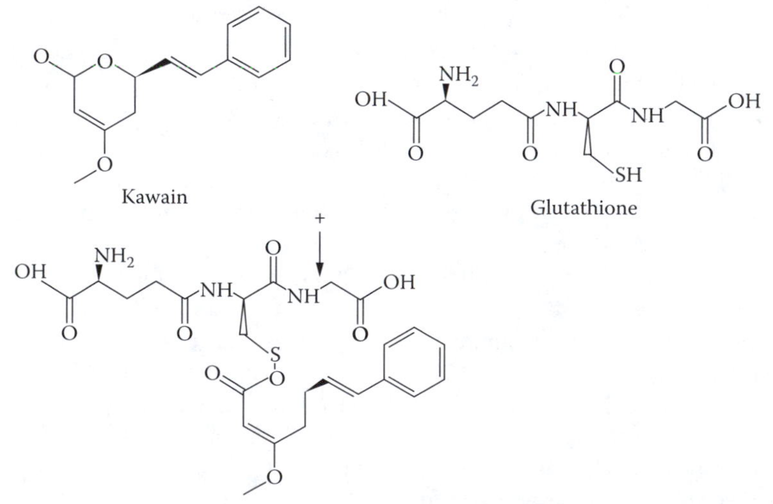

SCHEME K.32 The Michael reaction between kawain and glutathione. (From Whitton et al., *Phytochemistry,* 64:673–679, 2003. With permission.)

explains their safe use for many years. To avoid these adverse effects, supplementation with glutathione appears to be essential. The recent banning of kava in the U.K. and Europe is presently under review.

References

Bargota, R.S., Akhtar, M., Biggadike, K., Gani, D., and Allemann, R.K., Structure-activity relationship on human serum paraxonona (PONI) using substrate analogues and inhibitors, *Bioorg. Med. Chem. Lett.,* 13:1623–1626, 2003.

Bilia, A.R., Gallori, S., and Vincieri, F.F., Kava-kava and anxiety: Growing knowledge about the efficacy and safety, *Life Sci.,* 70:2581–2597, 2002.

Bilia, A.R., Scalise, L., Bergonzi, M.C., and Vincieri, F.F., Analysis of kava lactones from *Piper methyticum* (Kava-Kava), *J. Chromatogr.,* B., 812:203–214, 2004.

Cagnacci, A., Arangino, S., Renzi, A., Zanni, A.L., Malmusi, S., and Volpe, A., Kava-kava administration reduces anxiety in perimenopausal women, *Maturitas,* 44:103–109, 2003.

Davies, L., Drew, C.A., Duffield, P., Johnston, G.A.P., and Jamieson, D.D., Kava pyrones and resin studies on GABAA, GABAB and benzodiazepine binding sites in rodent brain, *Pharmacol. Toxicol.,* 71:120–126, 1992.

Escher, M., Desmeules, J., Giostra, E., and Mentha, G., Drug points: Hepatitis associated with kava, a herbal remedy for anxiety, *Br. Med. J.,* 322:139, 2001.

Gow, P.J., Connelly, N.J., Hill, R.L., Crowley, P., and Augus, P.W., Fatal fulminant hepatic failure induced by a natural therapy containing kava, *Med. J. Australia,* 178:442–443, 2003.

Jussofie, B., Schmiz, A., and Hiemke, C., Kavapyrone enriched extract from *Piper methysticum* as a modulator of GABA binding site in different regions of the rat brain, *Psychopharmacol.,* 116:469–474, 1994.

Lehmann, E., Kinzler, E., and Friedemann, J., Efficacy of a special Kava extract in patients with studies of anxiety, tension and restlessness of nonmental origin. A double-blind placebo-controlled study of four weeks treatment, *Phytomedicine,* 3:113–119, 1996.

Lehrl, S., Clinical efficacy of kawa extract WS® 1490 in sleep disturbances associated with anxiety disorders: Results of a multicenter, randomized, placebo-controlled double-blind clinical trial, *J. Affective Disorders,* 78:101–110, 2004.

Norton, S.A. and Ruze, P., Kava dermopathy, *J. Am. Acad. Dermatol.,* 31:89–97, 1994.

Pittler, M.H. and Ernst, E., Efficacy of kava for treating anxiety: Systematic and meta-analysis, *J. Clin. Psychopharmacol.,* 1:84–89, 2000.

Russman, S., Lauterburg, B.H., and Helbling, A., Kava hepatotoxicity, *Ann. Intern. Med.,* 135:68–69, 2001.

Schelosky, L., Raffauf, C., Jendroska, K., and Poewe, W., Kava and dopamine antagonism, *J. Neurol. Neurosurg. Psych.,* 58:639–640, 1995.

Schmidt, T.L. Ly-Pahl, H.L., and Merfort, I., Helananolide type sesquiterpene lactones, Part 5: The role of glutathione addition under physiological conditions, *Bioorg. Med. Chem.,* 7:2849–2855, 1999.

Schmidt, T.L., Lyss, G., Pahl, H.L., and Merfort, I., Helananolide type sesquiterpene lactones, Part 7: The role of glutathione addition under physiological conditions, *Biorg. Med. Chem.,* 9:2189–2194, 2001.

Seitz, U., Schule, A., and Gleitz, J., [^{3}H]-Monoamine uptake, inhibition properties of kavapyrones, *Planta Med.,* 63:548–549, 1997.

Stickel, F., Baumuller, H.-M., Seitz, K., Vasilakis, D., Seitz, G., Seitz, H.K., and Schuppan, D., Hepatitis induced by kava (*Piper methysticum rhizoma*), *J. Hepatol.,* 39:62–67, 2003.

Strahl, S., Ehret, V., Dahm, H.H., and Maier, K.P., Necrotizing hepatitis after taking herbal medication (extracts of kava or of a common or lesser celandine), *Dtsch. Med. Wochenschr.,* 123:1410–1414, 1998 (in German).

Uebelhack, R., Franke, L., and Schewe, H.-J., Inhibition of platelet MAO-B by kavapyrone-enriched extract from kava-kava, *Pharmacopsychiatry,* 31: 187–192, 1998.

Volz, H.P. and Kieser, M., Kava-kava extract WS1490 versus placebo in anxiety disorders — a randomized placebo-controlled 25-week outpatient trial, *Pharmacopsychiatry,* 30:1–5, 1997.

Whitton, P.A., Lau, A., Salisbury, A., Whitehouse, J., and Evans, C.S., Kava lactones and the kava-kava controversy, *Phytochemistry,* 64:673–679, 2003.

K

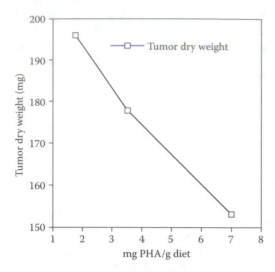

FIGURE K.58 Tumor growth expressed as dry tumor mass related to body dry weight in mice fed diets containing increasing amounts of phytohemagglutinins (PHA). (Pryme et al., *Cancer Lett.,* 146: 87–91, 1999. With permission.)

K

Kidney Bean *see also* **Beans and Lectins**

Kidney beans (*Phaseolus vulgaris*) are a variety of beans with a dark, red skin. Like most legumes, kidney beans contain a toxic lectin component that is normally inactivated by boiling to prevent gastric upset. Lectins or phytohemagglutinins, however, have been shown to exert beneficial health benefits. A number of studies reported that phytohemagglutinin in raw kidney bean diminished the growth of Krebs II non-Hodgkin lymphoma tumors in NMRI mice (Pryme et al., 1994a, b, 1996). Pryme and coworkers (1999) found that phytohemagglutinins curtailed the growth of established non-Hodgkin lymphoma tumors (five days after tumor development was initiated) by as much as 30–40 percent in female NMRI mice fed diets containing increasing levels of phytohemagglutinins in a dose-dependent manner, as shown in Figure K.58. These results further confirm the importance of red kidney bean as a functional food due, in part, to the presence of bioactive lectins.

References

Pryme, I.F., Bardocz, S., Grant, G., Duguid, T.J., Brown, D.S., and Pusztai, A., The plant lectin PHA as a tool for reducing the progression of tumor growth, in, *COST 98, Effects of Antinutients on the Nutritional Value of Legume Diets,* Vol. 5, Bardocz, S. and Pusztai, A., Eds., EC Publications, Luxembourg, 1996, pp. 24–29.

Pryme, I.F., Bardocz, S., and Pusztai, A., A diet containing the lectin phytohaemagglutinin (PHA) slows down the proliferation of Krebs II cell tumors in mice, *Cancer Lett.,* 76:133–137, 1994a.

Pryme, I.F., Bardocz, S., Pusztai, A., and Ewen, S.W.B., The growth of an established murine non-Hodgkin lymphoma tumor is limited by switching to a phytohaemagglutinin-containing diet, *Cancer Lett.,* 146:87–91, 1999.

Pryme, I.F., Pusztai, A., and Bardocz, S., The initial growth of Krebs II tumor cells, effect of phytohemagglutinin in the diet, *Int. J. Oncol.,* 5:1105–1107, 1994b.

Kiwifruit   Kiwifruit has become extremely popular over the past decade. Two varieties are grown, one with green flesh and the other with yellow flesh. In addition to being a rich source of vitamin C, those grown in Asia have been used in Chinese traditional medicine for the treatment of different cancers (Zhi, 1980). Sheng (1984) reported a 30–40 percent inhibition of sarcoma in mice fed kiwifruit, while Song (1984a, b) showed kiwifruit juice inhibited cancer-cell growth. Using the Ames' test, Liu and Peng (1994) found that some kiwi-fruit extracts exhibited a 95 percent inhibition of cancer. Motohashi and coworkers (2002) recently reported valuable bioactive compounds in kiwi gold fruit extracts. For example, hexane and acetone extracts proved selectively cytotoxic against human oral cell lines, while the more hydrophyllic 70 percent methanol fractions had higher anti-HIV, radical-generating, and O_2^--scavenging activities.

An antifungal, thaumatin-like protein composed of a single-chain 21 kDa was isolated by Wang and Ng (2002) from the green-flesh kiwifruit variety. The N-terminal sequences of thaumatin-like proteins (TLP) from mono- and dicotyledons exhibited 65–80 percent identity with TLP from kiwifruit (Table K.41). Of particular note was the presence of the fifth residue (F) not present in any of the other TLPs. The

TABLE K.41
Comparison of N-Terminal Sequences of Kiwifruit TLP with Other TLPSs[1]

Amino Acid	Residue Number	Identity	Percent
Kiwi TLP	1	ATFNFI·NNCPFTVWAAAVP·G	100
French Bean TLP	1	ANFN·IVNNCPYTVWAAASP·G	80
Wheat TLP	26	ATFN·IKNNCPYTVWPAATPIG	80
Barley TLP	1	ATFTVI·NKCQYTVWAAAVPAG	75
Maize TLP	1	AVFTVV·NQCPFTVWAASVP·G	65
Rice TLP	32	ATF·AITNRCQYTVWPAAVPSG	70
Chickpea TLP	22	ANFE·IVNNCPYTVWAAASP·G	75
Flaxseed TLP	1	ARFD·IQNKCPYTVWAASVP·G	70
Grape TLP	25	ATFD·ILNKCTYTVWAAASP·G	70

[1] Above sequences were obtained from a BLAST search and are aligned for maximal similarity. Amino-acid residues identical to the corresponding residues in kiwifruit TLP are underlined. Amino-acid residue number 26 for wheat TLP refers to A being the 26th amino-acid residue in the TLP.

Source: From Wang and Ng, *Phytochemistry,* 61:1–6, 2002. With permission.

kiwi protein exerted antifungal activity against *Botyris cinerea* and suppressed *Mycosphaerella arachidicola* and *Coprinus comatus*. Wang and Ng (2002) also found that kiwi TLP inhibited HIV-1 reverse transcriptase, similar to that reported for French bean TLP (Ye et al., 1999).

References

Liu, C. and Peng, M., *Big Dictionary of Anticancer Plants*, Hubei Science and Technology Publisher, Hubei, 1994, pp. 959–961.

Motohashi, N., Shirataki, Y., Kawase, M., Tani, S., Sakagami, H., Satoh, K., Kurihara, T., Nakashima, H., Mucsi, I., Varga, A., and Molnar, J., Cancer prevention and therapy with kiwifruit in Chinese folklore medicine: A study of kiwifruit extracts, *J. Ethnopharmacol.*, 81:357–364, 2002.

Sheng, Z., *Handbook of Chinese Cancer Treatment*, Chongqing Publishers, Chongqing, Sichuan Province, 1994, pp. 661–662.

Song, P., Healthy application by kiwifruit juice, *Nutr. Res.*, 6:35–40, 1984a.

Song, P., Anticancer activity of Chinese kiwifruit, *Nutr. Res.*, 6:109–114, 1984b.

Wang, H. and Ng, T.B., Isolation of an antifungal thaumatin-like protein from kiwi fruits, *Phytochemistry*, 61:1–6, 2002.

Ye, X.Y., Wang, H.X., and Ng, T.B., First chromatographic isolation of an antifungal thaumatin-like protein from French bean legumes and demonstration of its antifungal activity, *Biophys. Res. Commun.*, 263:1002–1013, 1999.

Zhi, C.-J., *Chinese Anti-Cancer Agents*, Hua-lian Publishers, Taipei, 1980, pp. 1, 74—75.

Kurosu   Kurosu is one of the traditional vinegars in Japan produced from unpolished rice by fermentation. It has been reported to have medicinal properties, such as improving blood fluidity and preventing hypertension (Nishikawa et al., 2001). Studies by Nishidai and coworkers (2000) showed an ethyl-acetate extract from Kurosu exhibited both antioxidant activity, as well as antitumor properties in mice. Shimoji et al. (2002) first identified dihydroferulic acid and dihydrosinapic acid as the major phenolics in Kurosu responsible for its radical-scavenging activity. These compounds were present at much higher levels in Kurosu compared to common rice vinegar (polished-rice vinegar), as shown in Table K.42. The higher content of antioxidant compounds in Kurosu, particularly dihydroferulic and dihydrosinapic acids, probably explains the almost twofold greater scavenging activity by Kurosu compared to rice vinegar.

K

TABLE K.42

Content of Antioxidative Compounds and Dihydroferulic Acid and Dihydrosinapic Acid in Kurosu and Rice Vinegar and Their I_{50} in DPPH Radical-Scavenging Activity

	Content (mg/L) in Kurosu	Content (mg/L) in Rice Vinegar	IC_{50} (μg/mL)
Kurosu Concentrate	29400		1710
Rice Vinegar Concentrate		23800	3340
Dihydroferulic Acid	24.8	0.09	15.1
Dihydrosinapic Acid	4.68	n.d.[a]	10.1

[a] Not detected.

Source: From Shimoji et al., *J. Agric. Food Chem.*, 50:6501–6503, 2002.

References

Nishidai, S., Nakamura, Y., Torikai, K., Yamamoto, M., Ishihara, N., Mori, H., and Ohigashi, H., Kurosu, a traditional vinegar produced from unpolished rice, suppresses lipid peroxidation *in vitro* and in mouse skin, *Biosci. Biotechnol. Biochem.*, 64:1909–1914, 2000.

Nishikawa, Y., Takata, Y., Nagai, Y., ori, T., Kawada, T., and Ishihara, N., Antihypertensive effect of Kurosu extract, a traditional vinegar produced from unpolished rice, in the SHR rats, *Nippon Syokuhin Kagaku Kogaku Kaishi*, 48:73–75, 2001 (in Japanese).

Shimoji, Y., Tamura, Y., Nakamura, Y., and Nanda, K., Shoho, N., Nishakawa, Y., Ishihara, N., Uenakai, K., and Ohigashi, H., Isolation and identification of DPPH radical scavenging activity compounds in Kurosu (Japanese unpolished rice vinegar), *J. Agric. Food Chem.*, 50:6501–6503, 2002.

K

α-Lactalbumin α-Lactalbumin, the major protein regulator of lactose synthase in milk, has the highest content of tryptophan (Trp) and the highest Trp/ΣLarge neutral amino-acids (LNAAs) ratio among food-protein sources (Heine et al., 1996). Tryptophan is the precursor of brain serotonin (5-hydroxy-tryptamine, 5-HT), which is involved in mood disorders, such as anxiety and depression (Berk, 2000). Consequently, tryptophan was proposed as a possible treatment for depression (Meyers, 2000; Young, 2000). Because of its high level of tryptophan, Markus et al. (2000) showed that ingestion of α-lactalbumin reduced depressive feelings in stress-vulnerable human subjects compared to a casein-enriched diet. Using male Wistar rats, Orosco and coworkers (2004a) also found that ingestion of an α-lactalbumin-enriched diet induced anxiolytic and rewarding effects compared to an enriched casein diet. These effects may be related to the enhanced release of serotonin in the medial hypothalamus in rats fed 30 min meals (acutely) but disappeared after 3–6 days of diet (chronic). Based on their research findings, together with the study by Markus et al. (2003), diets enriched with α-lactalbumin appeared to be beneficial in treating stress and anxiety in the short term.

Pelligrini et al. (1999) identified antimicrobial peptides in bovine α-lactalbumin by isolating and characterizing three bacteriocidal domains. Oevermann and coworkers (2003) showed that chemical modification of the lysine residues with 3-hydroxyphthalic anhydride (3-HP) in several bovine milk protein fractions, including α-lactalbumin, yielded compounds with antiviral activity against human herpes simplex virus type 1 (HSV-1). Digestion of these modified proteins produced short peptides that had considerable potential for the treatment of herpes, as they were economical, as well as

exhibited reduced antigenicity. Supplementation of an infant formula with α-lactalbumin and glycomacropeptide by Bruk et al. (2002) also benefited the human microflora by significantly reducing the presence of pathogenic bacteria.

Opioid active peptides are released from milk proteins, such as α-lactalbumin, by enzymatic hydrolysis. For example, α-lactorphin, a tetrapeptide (Tyr-Gly-Leu-Phe) released by peptic or tryptic hydrolysis of α-lactalbumin, had an amino-acid sequence corresponding to residues 50–53 in the original intact protein (Antila et al., 1991). The opioid properties associated with α-lactorphin reflected the similarity between its amino acid sequence and the N-terminal amino-acid residues of opioid peptides, such as β-endorphin, enkephalins, and dynorphin (Tyr-Gly-Gly-Phe) (Teschemacher et al., 1997). α-Lactorphin was found by Nurminen et al. (2000) to lower blood pressure in spontaneously hypertensive rats with established hypertension. Sipola and coworkers (2002) showed α-lactorphin improved vascular relaxation in the spontaneously hypertensive rats and involved nitric oxide but not vasodilatory prostanoids.

References

Antila, P., Paakkari, I., Jarvinen, A., Mattila, M.J., Laukkanen, M., Pihlanto-Leppala, A., Mantsala, P., and Hellman, J., Opioid peptides derived from *in vitro* proteolysis of bovine whey protein, *Int. Dairy J.,* 1:215–229, 1991.

Berk, M., Selective serotonin reuptake inhibitors in mixed anxiety-depression, *Int. Clin. Psychopharmacol.,* 15(Suppl. 2): S41–45, 2000.

Bruck, W.M., Graverholt, G., and Gibson, G.R., Use of batch culture and a two-stage continuous culture system to study the effect of supplemental α-lactalbumin and glycomacropeptide on mixed populations of human gut bacteria, *FEMS Microbiol. Ecol.,* 41: 231–237, 2002.

Heine, W., Radke, M., Wutzke, K.D., Peters, E., and Kundt, G., Alpha-lactalbumin-enriched low-protein infant formulas: A comparison to breast milk feeding, *Acta Paediatr.*, 85:1024–1028, 1996.

Markus, C.R., Olivier, B., Panhuysen, G.E.M., Van der Gusten, J., Alles, M.S., Tuiten, A., Wastenberg, H.G.M., Fekkes, D., Koppeschaar, H.F., and de Haan, E.E.H.F., The bovine protein α-plactalbumin increases the plasma ratio of tryptophan to other large neutral amino acids, and in vulnerable subjects raises brain serotonin activity, reduces cortisol concentration, and improves mood under stress, *Am. J. Clin. Nutr.*, 71:1536–1544, 2000.

Meyers, S., Use of neurotransmitter precursors for treatment of depression, *Altern. Med. Rev.*, 5:64–71, 2000.

Nurminen, M.-L., Sipola, M., Kaarto, H., Pihlanto-Leppala, A., Piilota, K., Korpela, R., Tossavainen, O., Korhonen, H., and Vapaatalo, H., α-Lactorphin lowers blood pressure measured by radiotelemetry in normotensive and in spontaneously hypertensive rats, *Life Sci.*, 66:1535–1543, 2000.

Oevermann, A., Engels, M., Thomas, U., and Pellegrini, A., The antiviral activity of naturally occurring proteins and their peptide fragments after chemical modification, *Antiviral Res.*, 59:23–33, 2003.

Orosco, M., Rouch, C., Beslot, F., Feurte, S., Regnault, A., and Dauge, V., Alpha-lactalbumin-enriched diets enhance serotonin release and induce anxiolytic and rewarding effects in the rat, *Behav. Brain Res.*, 148:1–10, 2004a.

Pellegrini, A., Thomas, U., Bramaz, N., Hunziker, P., and von Fellenberg, R., Isolation and identification of three bacteriocidal domains in the bovine α-lactalbumin molecule, *Biochem. Biophys. Acta*, 1426: 439–448, 1999.

Sipola, M., Finckenberg, P., Vapaatalo, H., Pihlanto-Leppala, A., Korhonen, H., Korpela, R., and Nurminen, M.-L., α-Lactorpin and β-lactorphin improve arterial function in spontaneously hypertensive rats, *Life Sci.*, 71:1245–1253, 2002.

Teschemacher, H., Koch, G., and Brantl, V., Milk protein-derived opioid receptor ligands, *Peptide Sci.*, 43:99–117, 1997.

Young, S.N., Behavioral effects of dietary neurotransmitter precursors: Basic and clinical aspects, *Neurosci. Biobehav. Rev.*, 20:313–323, 1996.

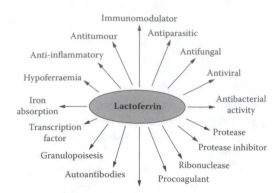

SCHEME L.33 Proposed roles for lactoferrin. (From Brock, *Biochem. Cell. Biol.*, 80:1–6, 2002. With permission.)

Lactoferrin and Lactoferricin *see also* **Bovine lactoferrin** Lactoferrin, an iron-binding glycoprotein present in milk, is a multifunctional protein with immunomodulation and antimicrobial activity (Vorland, 1999; Weinberg, 2001; Farnaud and Evans, 2003). These many roles for lactoferrin are summarized in Scheme L.33. In contrast, lactoferricin is a peptide released from the N-terminal part of lactoferrin by peptic digestion (Tomita et al., 1991). Compared to lactoferrin, a bilobal glycoprotein with a mass of 80 kDa, the lactoferricin-peptide structure is a loop with a cationic charge, containing 25 amino acids in the case of bovine lactoferricin (Lfcin B) and 47 amino-acid residues for human lactoferricin (Lfcin H) (Scheme L.34).

Lactoferrin is a potent inhibitor of different enveloped viruses, including herpes simplex virus (HSV) 1 and 2 (Marchetti et al., 1998), human immunodeficiency virus (HIV) (Puddu et al., 1998), human cytomegalovirus (Portelli et al., 1998), and human hepatitis C virus (Ikeda et al., 1998), as well as two naked viruses, SA-11 rotavirus and poliovirus type 1 (Marchetti et al., 1999; Superti et al., 1997). Arnold and coworkers (2002) found lactoferrin was the only milk protein that inhibited adenovirus replication in a dose-dependent manner by preventing replication at an early phase of viral replication.

Bovine and human lactoferricin (Lfcin B and Lfcin H) were both shown to exhibit antiviral activity against human cytomegalovirus

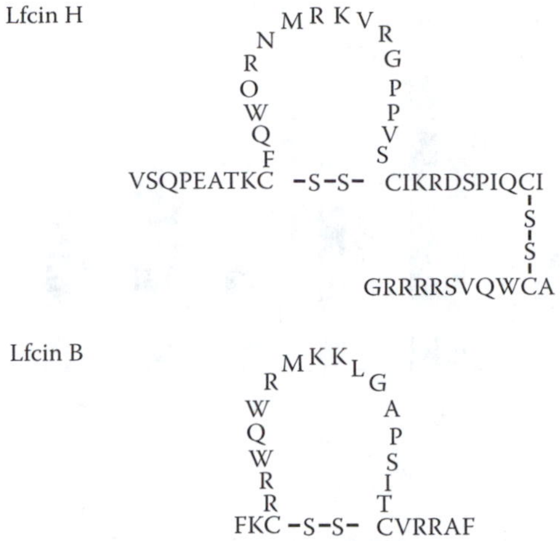

Lfcin H

```
            M R K V
         N           R
      R                 G
      O                 P
      W                 P
      Q                 V
      F                 S
VSQPEATKC  -S-S-  CIKRDSPIQCI
                               |
                               S
                               |
                               S
                               |
              GRRRRSVQWCA
```

Lfcin B

```
         M K K L
      R           G
    W                 A
    Q                 P
    W                 S
    R                 T
    R
  FKC -S-S- CVRRAF
```

SCHEME L.34 Loop structure of human (Lfcin H) and bovine (Lfcin B) lactoferricin. Single-letter code is used to indicate the amino-acid sequence of each peptide. (From Jenssen et al., *Antiviral Res.*, 61:101–109, 2004. With permission.)

(HCMV) by preventing its entry into human fibroplasts (Andersen et al., 2001). A synergy between Lfcin B and the drug acyclovir (ACV) in inhibiting HSV was observed by Andersen and coworkers (2003) by a sevenfold drop in EC_{50} for both ACV and Lfcin B. The potency of Lfcin B increased substantially in the presence of ACV, which could reduce the amount of the drug administered, as well as the incidence of drug-resistant strains. A similar synergy was observed between bovine lactoferrin and ACV. Jenssen et al. (2003) recently concluded that hydrophobicity, molecular size, special distribution of charged lipophilic amino acids, and cylic structure were features that affected the antiviral activity of Lfcin B against HSV.

References

Andersen, J.H., Jenssen, H., and Gutteberg, T.J., Lactoferrin and lactoferricin inhibit Herpes simplex 1 and 2 infection and exhibit synergy when combined with acyclovir, *Antiviral Res.*, 58:209–215, 2003.

Andersen, J.H., Osbakk, S.A., Vorland, L.H., Traavik, T., and Guttenberg, Lactoferrin and cyclic lactoferricin inhibit the entry of human cytomegalovirus into human fibroblasts, *Antiviral Res.*, 51:141–149, 2001.

Arnold, D., Di Biase, A.M., Marchetti, M., Pietrantoni, A., Valenti, P., Seganti, L., and Superti, F., Antiadenovirus activity of milk proteins: Lactoferrin prevents viral infection, *Antivira Res.*, 53:153–158, 2002.

Brock, J.H., The physiology of lactoferrin, *Biochem. Cell. Biol.*, 80:1–6, 2002.

Farnaud, S. and Evans, R.W., Lactoferrin — a multifunctional protein with antimicrobial properties, *Mol. Immunol.*, 40:395–405, 2003.

Ikeda, M., Sugiyama, K., Tanaka, T., Tanaka, K., Sekihara, H., Shimotohno, K., and Kato, N., Lactoferrin markedly inhibits hepatitis C virus infection in cultured human hepatocytes, *Biochem. Biophys. Res. Commun.*, 245:549–553, 1998.

Jenssen, H., Andersen, J.H., Uhlin-Hansen, L., Gutteberg, T.J., and Rekdal, O., Anti-HSV activity of lactoferricin analogues is only partly related to their affinity for heparin sulfate, *Antiviral Res.*, 61:101–109, 2004.

Marchetti, M., Pisani, S., Antonini, G., Valenti, P., Seganti, L., and Orsi, S., Metal complexes of bovine lactoferrin inhibit *in vitro* replication of herpes simplex virus type 1 and 2, *Biometals*, 11:89–94, 1998.

Marchetti, N.M., Superti, F., Ammendolia, M.G., Rossi, O., Valenti, P., and Seganti, L., Inhibition of poliovirus type 1 infection by iron-, manganese- and zinc-saturated lactoferrin, *Med. Microbiol. Immunol.*, 187:199–204, 1999.

Portelli, J., Gordon, A., and May, J.T., Effect of compounds with antibacterial activities in human milk on respiratory syncytial virus and cytomegalovirus *in vitro*, *J. Med. Microbiol.*, 47:1015–1018, 1998.

Puddu, P., Borghi, P., Gessani, S., Valenti, P., Belardelli, F., and Saganti, L., Antiviral effect of bovine lactoferrin saturated with metal ions on early steps of human immunodeficiency virus type 1 infection, *Int. J. Biochem. Cell Biol.*, 30:1055–1062, 1998.

Superti, F., Ammendolia, M.G., Valenti, P., and Seganti, L., Antirotaviral activity in milk proteins: Lactoferrin prevents rotavirus infection in the eneterocyte-like cell line HT-29, *Med. Microbiol. Immunol.*, 186:83–91, 1997.

Tomita, M., Bellamy, W., Takase, M., Yamauchi, K., Wakabayashi, H., and Kawase, K., Potent antibacterial peptides generated by pepsin digestion of bovine lactoferrin, *J. Dairy Sci.*, 74:4137–4142, 1991.

L

Vorland, L.H., Lactoferrin: A multifunctional glyco-protein, *APMIS*, 107:971–981, 1999.

Weinberg, E.D., Human lactoferrin: A novel thera-peutic with broad spectrum potential, *J. Pharm. Pharmacol.*, 53:1303–1310, 2001.

Lactokinin   Lactokinin is a short, biologically active peptide released by tryptic digestion of the whey milk protein β-lactoglobulin (Ala-Leu-Pro-His-Ile-Arg) (Mullally et al., 1997). It inhibits angiotensin-1-converting enzyme (ACE), an enzyme associated with the rennin–angiotensin system that regulates peripheral blood pressure, reducing blood pressure in hypertensive individuals. Fitzgerald and Meisel (1999) suggested that while ACE inhibitors derived from whey protein were not as potent as synthetic antihypertensive drugs, they were sufficiently active to exert an antihypertensive effect. Vermeirssen and coworkers (2002) reported that lactokinin was partly transported through a caco-2 cell monomer. Maes and coworkers (2004) showed for the first time that lactokinin modulated the release of endothelin-1 (ET-1) by porcine aortic endothelial cells (Figure L.59). ET-1 is a vasoconstrictive pep-tide that acts via a specific receptor. Compared to 0.1 mM of the drug captopril, which decreased ET-1 release by 42 percent, lactoki-nin produced a 29 percent decrease under the same conditions. Thrombrin significantly stim-ulated the basal release of ET-1 by 66 percent.

While incubation with 1 µM and 0.1 nM of captopril inhibited the stimulated ET-1 release by 45 percent and 62 percent compared to 32 percent and 43 percent when thrombrin was coincubated with 1 µM and 0.1 mM of lacto-kinin. While lactokinin was not quite as effec-tive as captopril, nevertheless, this milk-protein-derived peptide could still be a useful treat-ment of hypertension. Recent data by Maes et al. (2004) showed lactokinin modulated ET-1 release by endothelial cells, which explained the antihypertensive effect of milk-protein peptides.

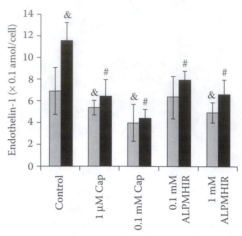

FIGURE L.59   Effect of captopril and lactokinin on basal and 10 µ/mL thrombrin-stimulated endothelial-1 release by porcine aortic endothelial cells. Drugs and peptide were solubilized in medium 199 supple-mented with 190 porcine serum. Cells were exposed to medium 199 with 1 percent serum, 1 µM and 0.1 mM captopril (cap), 0.1 and 1.0 mM lactokinin (ALPMHIR), with or without the addition of 10 µ/mL thrombrin (throm). & Different from ET-1 release without stimulation, $p < 0.01$. ᵍ Different from 10 µ/mL thrombrin-stimulated ET-1 release, $p < 0.01$. Values are means ± 2 SD., n = 10–15. (Maes et al., *Reg. Pept.*, 118(1–2):105–109, 2004. With per-mission).

References

Fitzgerald, R.J. and Meisel, H., Lactokinins: Whey protein ACE inhibitory peptides, *Nahrung*, 43:165–167, 1999.

Maes, W., Van Camp, J., Vermeirssen, V., Hemeryck, M., Ketelsleghers, J.M., Schrezenmeir, J., Oostveldt, P.V., and Huyghebaert, A., Influence of the lactokinin Ala-Leu-Pro-Met-His-Ile-Arg (ALPMHIR) on the release of endothelin-1 by enodothelial cells, *Reg. Pept.*, 118(1–2):105–109, 2004.

Mullally, M.M., Meisel, H., and Fitzgerald, R.J., Identification of a novel angiotensin-1-converting enzyme inhibitory peptide corresponding to a tryptic fraction of bovine β-lactoglobulin, *FEBS Lett.*, 402:99–101, 1997.

Vermeirssen, V., Deplancke, B., Tappenden, K.A., Van Camp, J., Gaskins, H.R., and Verstraete, W., Intestinal transport of the lactokinin Ala-Leu-Pro-Met-Ile-Arg through Caco-2 Bbe monolayer, *J. Pept. Sci.*, 8:95–100, 2002.

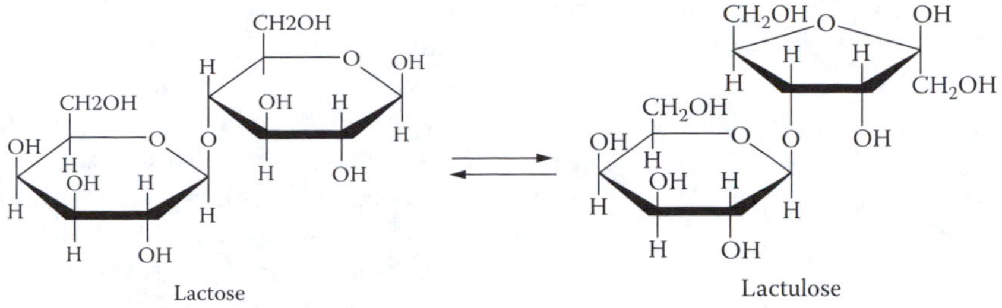

SCHEME L.35 Alkaline isomerization of lactose to lactulose. (From Montilla et al., *Food Chem.*, 90:883–890, 2005. With permission.)

Lactulose   Lactulose (4-*O*-β-D-galactopyra-nosyl-D-fructose), an isomerized product of lactose (Scheme L.35), is a registered medicinal drug in more than 100 countries (Schumann, 2002). While it does not occur naturally in milk, it is present in very small amounts in heated milk and in UHT milk. Unlike the α 1-4 glycosidic bond in lactose, the β 1-4 glycosidic bond in lactulose cannot be broken down by the digestive enzymes, so it passes through to the intestine, where it is metabolized by the colonic bacteria. Lactulose is a prebiotic, as it is the preferred food for lactic-acid bacteria compared to the proteolytic activity of various pathogenic bacteria in the colon. It is effective in the treatment of chronic constipation and is the standard, worldwide treatment for hepatic encephalopathy (Blei and Cordoba, 2001).

Lactulose also prevents tumors by protecting DNA in human-flora associated rats exposed to dimethylhydrazine (DMH) (Rowland et al., 1996). Although very little lactulose is absorbed (0.25–2 percent), it appears to have specific beneficial immunological effects when given intravenously or *in vitro* (Greve et al., 1980; Liehr and Heine, 1981). Lactulose has been found to reduce urinary tract infection (UTI) and pneumonia (McCutcheon and Fulton, 1989) and stimulate calcium absorption in postmenopausal women (Van de Heuvel and Weidauer, 1999). A preparation containing lactulose was reported by Bianchi and coworkers (1994) to lower blood glucose. Lhoste et al. (2001) reported Fischer male rats innoculated with *Clostridium paraputrificum* fed lactulose-enriched diets increased butyrate in the caesum.

The formation of butyrate has a number of beneficial effects, including preventing carcinogenesis (see butyric acid).

References

Bianchi, G.P., De Mitri, M.S., Bugianesi, E., Abbiati, R., Fabbri, A., and Marchesini, G., Lowering effects of a preparation containing fibres and lactulose on glucose and insulin levels in obesity, *Ital. J. Gastroenteol.* 26:174–178, 1994.

Blei, A.T. and Cordoba, J., Hepatic encephalopathy, *Am. J. Gastroenterol.*, 96:1968–1974, 2001.

Greve, J.W., Gouma, D.J., von Leeuwen, P.A.M., and Buurman, W.A., Lactulose inhibits endotoxins induced tumor necrosis factor production by monocytes. An *in vitro* study, *Gut*, 31:198–203, 1990.

Lhoste, E.F., Nugon-Baudon, L., Lory, S., Meslin, J.-C., and Andrieux, C., The fermentation of lactulose in rats inoculated with *Clostridium paraputrificum* influences the activities of liver and intestinal xenobiotic metabolizing enzymes, *J. Sci. Food Agric.*, 81:1397–1404, 2001.

Liehr, H. and Heine, W.D., Treatment of endotoxemia in galactosamine hepatitis by lactulose administered intravenously, *Hepato-Gastroenterol.*, 28: 296–298, 1981.

McCutcheon, J. and Fulton, J.D., Lowered prevalence of infection with lactulose therapy in patients in long term hospital care, *J. Hosp. Infect.*, 13:81–86, 1989.

Montilla, A., del Castillo, M.D., Sanz, M.L., and Olano, A., Egg shell as catalyst of lactose to lactulose, *Food Chem.*, 90:883–890, 2005.

Rowland, I.R., Bearne, C.A., Fischer, R., and Pool-Zobel, B.L., The effect of lactulose on DNA damage induced by DMH in the colon of human flora-associated rats, *Nutr. Can.*, 26:37–47, 1996.

Schumann, C., Medicinal, nutritional and technological properties of lactulose. An update, *Eur. J. Nutr.,* 41(Suppl. 1):17–25, 2002.

Van de Heuvel, E.G. and Weidauer, T., Role of non-digestible carbohydrate lactulose in the absorption of calcium, *Med. Sci. Monit.,* 5:1231–1237, 1999.

Lavender (*Lavandula angustifolia*) Lavender oil, used in aromatherapy, is obtained from the flowering tips of the plant *Lavandula angustifolia.* Shellie and coworkers (2002) identified 85 components in lavender essential oil, which accounted for more than 95 percent of the oil. Of nine samples analyzed, three were closest to the ISO Standard 3515, which included acceptable ranges for linalool, 25–38 percent; linalyl acetate, 25–45 percent; lavandulyl acetate minimum, 2 percent; terpinen-4-ol, 2–6 percent; lavandulol minimum, 0.3 percent; 1,8-cineole, 0–15 percent; limonene, 0–0.5 percent; trans-β-ocimene, 2–6 percent; *cis*-β-ocimene, 4–10 percent; 3-octanone, 0–2 percent; camphor, 0–0.5 percent; and α-terpineol, 0–1 percent. Lavender oil is a holistic relaxant thought to have carminative, antiflatulence, and anticolic properties (Tisserand, 1985). The oil was found to have a spasmolytic effect on guinea-pig ileum *in vitro* (Lis-Balchin et al., 1996), which is correlated with the holistic relaxant effect in man (Lis-Balchin and Hart, 1997). The spasmolytic effect of lavender and linalool were shown by Lis-Balchin and Hart (1999) to be mediated via cAMP.

The impact of aromatherapy on positive mood shifts by Knasko (1992) led to a study on the effect of lavender baths on psychological well-being by Morris (2002). Forty female university students and staff, with a mean age of 28.2 years, were randomly allocated either grapeseed oil or 80 percent grapeseed oil and 20 percent lavender oil to use in their daily bath for 14 days. Using the University of Wales Institute of Science and Technology (UWIST) Mood Adjective Checklist (Matthews et al., 1990), lavender oil was found to have a selective effect on anger–frustration in the first trial, while reducing negative responses about the future in the second trial. These results suggested lavender-oil baths may have a positive effect on psychological well-being. A recent study by Fernandez and coworkers (2004) showed differences in response to odors between newborn infants of depressed and non-depressed mothers. Only newborn infants of depressed mothers increased relative left frontal electroencephalographic (EEG) asymmetry following exposure to lavender or rosemary aroma, with no response by newborns of non-depressed mothers. The shift in right frontal EEG asymmetry is a pattern associated with a positive effect and response to positive stimuli and was related to significantly greater head turning and lip licking. A recent review of the scientific and clinical evidence for the psychological effects of lavender was prepared by Kirk-Smith (2003).

References

Fernandez, M., Hernandez-Reif, M., Field, T., Sanders, C., Diego, M., Sanders, C., and Roca, A., EEG during lavender and rosemary exposure in infants of depressed and non-depressed mothers, *Infant Behav. Develop.,* 27:91–100, 2004.

Kirk-Smith, M., The psychological effects of lavender II: Scientific and clinical evidence, *Intern. J. Aromather.,* 13(23):82–88, 2003.

Knasko, S.C., Ambient odour's effect creativity, mood, and perceived health, *Chem. Senses.,* 17:27–35, 1992.

Lis-Balchin, M. and Hart, S., Correlation of the chemical profiles of essential oil mixes with their relaxant and stimulant properties in man and smooth muscle preparations *in vitro*, in *Proc. 27th International Symposium on Essential Oils,* Franz, C.H., Mathe, A., and Buchbaer, G., Eds., Allured Pub. Corp., Carol Stream, IL, 1997, pp. 24–28.

Lis-Balchin, M. and Hart, S., Studies on the mode of action of the essential oil of lavender (*Lavandula angustifolia* P. Miller), *Phytother. Res.,* 13:540–542, 1999.

Lis-Balchin, M., Hart, S., Deans, S.G., and Eaglesham, E., Comparison of the pharmacological and antimicrobial action of commercial plant essential oils, *J. Herbs Spices Med. Plants,* 4:69–88, 1996.

Matthews, G., Jones, D., and Chamberlain, G., Refining measurement of mood: The UWIST Mood-Adjective Checklist, *Br. J. Psychol.,* 81:17–42, 1990.

Morris, N., The effects of lavender (*Lavandula angustifolium*) baths on psychological well-being: Two exploratory randomised control trials, *Complement. Ther. Med.*, 10:223–228, 2002.

Shellie, R., Mondello, L., Marriott, P., and Dugo, G., Characterisation of lavender essential oils by using gas chromatography-mass spectrometry with correlation of linear retention and comparison with comprehensive two-dimensional gas chromatography, *J. Chromatogr. A.*, 970:225–234, 2002.

Tisserand, R., *The Art of Aromatherapy*, C.W. Daniel Co. Ltd., Saffron Walden, U.K., 1985.

Lectins   Lectins are glycoproteins that combine reversibly with sugars and glycoconjugates. They cause agglutination of erythrocytes, as well as interfere with nutrient absorption by binding with glycoproteins on the epithelial surface of the small intestine (Lajolo and Genovese, 2002). They are found as phytohemagglutinins in a wide variety of plants, particularly legumes. Lectins may have possible medical uses by their ability to provoke hyperplasia of the small intestine, alter the bacterial flora, and interfere with hormone secretion, as well as enter systematic circulation (Pusztai, 1993; Pusztai and Bardocz, 1996). For example, mice fed a purified bean phytohemagglutinins had reduced tumor growth, indicating competition between the gut epithelium undergoing hyperplasia and the growing tumor (Pusztai et al., 1998). Gastman et al. (2004) reported wheat-germ agglutinin induced apoptosis by binding to surface carbohydrates (*N*-acetylmeuraminic or *N*-acetylglucosamine) of normal and malignant cells. The lectin-induced apoptosis was extremely fast and mediated via a mitochondrial pathway.

The possible use of lectins for treating obesity was shown by Pusztai and coworkers (1998) by the reduction in lipid accumulation in obese rats fed a diet containing raw kidney beans. This was attributed to a reduction in insulin levels by the bean lectins with no loss in body or muscle proteins observed.

Nishimura and coworkers (2004) recently found that bone-marrow mesenchymal stem cells, chondrocytes, and osteoblasts exposed to a lectin from the bean (*Phaseolus vulgaris*) increased their adhesion on plastic culture dishes or plates of hydroxyapatite, titanium, and poly-DL-lactic-co-glycolic acid (PLGA). The bean lectin, erythroagglutinin, enhanced resistance of these cells to proteases and mechanical stimuli, suggesting their potential in tissue engineering and cell therapy.

References

Gastman, B., Wang, K., Han, J., Zhu, Z., Huang, X., Wang, G.-Q., Rabinowich, H., and Gorelik, E., A novel apoptotic pathway as defined by lectin cellular initiation, *Biochem. Biolphys. Res. Commun.*, 316: 263–271, 2004.

Lajolo, F.M. and Genovese, M.I., Nutritional significance of lectins and enzyme inhibitors from legumes, *J. Agric. Food Chem.*, 50:6592–6598, 2002.

Nishimura, H., Nishimura, M., Oda, R., Yamanaka, K., Matsubara, T., Ozaki, Y., Sekiya, K., Hamada, T., and Kato, Y., Lectins induce resistance to proteases and/or mechanical stimulus in all examined cells — including bone marrow mesenchymal stem cells — on various scaffolds, *Exp. Cell Res.*, 295:119–127, 2004.

Pryme, I.F., Pusztai, A. Bardocz, S., and Ewen, S.W.B., The induction of gut hyperplasia by phyto-haemagglutinins in the diet and limitation of tumor growth, *Histol. Histopathol.*, 13:575–583, 1998.

Pusztai, A., Dietary lectins are metabolic signals for the gut and modulate immune and hormone functions, *Eur. J. Clin. Nutr.*, 47:691–699, 1993.

Pusztai, A. and Bardocz, S., Biological effects of plant lectins on the gastrointestinal tract: Metabolic consequences and applications, *Trends Glycosci. Glycotechnol.*, 8:149–165, 1996.

Pusztai, A., Grant, G., Buchan, W.C., Bardocz, S., de Carvalho, A.F.F.U., and Ewen, S.W.B., Lipid accumulation in obese Zucker rats is reduced by inclusion of raw kidney bean (*Phaseolus vulgaris*) in the diet, *Br. J. Nutr.*, 79:213–221, 1998.

Legumes *see also* **Beans, Bowman-Birk protease inhibitors, Chickpea, Kidney bean, Lectins, Lentils, Peas, Resistant starch, and Soybeans**   Legumes play an important role in human nutrition, as they are excellent sources of proteins and complex carbohydrates. In addition to being good sources of vitamins and minerals, legumes are considered low glycemic foods, as they elicit a low blood-glucose response (Tharanathan and Mahadevamma, 2003). Legumes have long been recognized as beneficial for controlling and treating metabolic diseases, such as diabetes mellitus, coronary heart disease, and colon cancer (Simpson et al., 1981). They are consumed as whole or grains, dehusked, or as split legumes and include peas, lentils, and a variety of beans, such as red gram, black gram, cowpea, broad bean, field bean, horse bean, and kidney bean.

A number of dietary components in legumes appear to be responsible for their beneficial physiological effects, including protein and starch. Chau and coworkers (1998) incorporated 12 percent protein concentrates from three Chinese legume seeds, *Phaeolus angularis, Phaseolus calcaratus,* and *Dolichos lablab* in the diets of male Golden Syrian hamsters and found a pronounced hypocholesterolemic effect. The three legume-protein concentrates significantly ($p < 0.05$) lowered serum triglyceride and total and LDL cholesterol levels and liver total lipids and cholesterol compared to casein. The more potent hypocholesterolemic effects were associated with *P. calacaratus* and *D. lablab*, while only the former significantly increased serum HDL cholesterol. During processing, the higher amylose content (30–40 percent) of legume starches compared to cereals (Madhusudhan and Tharanathan, 1995) results in the formation of large amounts of resistant starch. The latter is known to have important physiological benefits (Edwards, 1993).

Legumes are also rich in protease inhibitors and lectins, considered antinutritional factors (Lajolo and Genovese, 2002). However, the Bowman–Birk inhibitor was shown to have therapeutic properties that included anticarcinogenic and antiinflammatory, as well the ability to reduce ulcerative colitis in mice (Kennedy, 1998; Wan et al., 1999; Ware et al., 1999; Armstrong et al., 2000).

Lectins are also recognized for their beneficial properties, including preventing gastrointestinal atrophy during total parenteral nutrition and reducing tumor growth in mice, as well as treating obesity (Pryme et al., 1998; Pusztai et al., 1998; Jordinson et al., 1999).

References

Armstrong, W.B., Kennedy, A.R., Wan, X.S., Atiba, J., McLaren, G.E., and Meyskens, F.L., Jr., Single-dose administration of Bowman-Birk inhibitor concentrate in patients with oral leukoplakia, *Cancer Epidemiol. Biomarkers,* 9:43–47, 2000.

Chau, C.-F., Cheung, P.C.K., and Wong, Y.-S., Hypocholesterolemic effects of protein concentrates from three Chinese indigenous legume seeds, *J. Agric. Food Chem.,* 46:3698–3701, 1998.

Edwards, C.A., Interactions between nutrition and intestinal microflora, *Proc. Nutr.,* 52:375–382, 1993.

Jordinson, M., Goodlad, R.A., Brynes, A., Bliss, P., Ghatewi, M.A., Bloom, S.R., Fitzgerald, A., Grant, G., Bardocz, S., Pustzai, A., Pagnatelli, M., and Calam, J., Gastrointestinal responses to a panel of lectins in rats maintained on total parenteral nutrition, *Am. J. Physiol.-Gastr. Liver Physiol.,* 39:G1235–G1242, 1999.

Kenndey, A.R., The Bowman-Birk inhibitor from soybeans as anticarcinogenic agent, *Am. J. Clin. Nutr.,* 68: 1406S–1412S, 1998.

Lajolo, F.M. and Genovese, M.I., Nutritional significance of lectins and enzyme inhibitors from legumes, *J. Agric. Food Chem.,* 50:6592–6958, 2002.

Madhushan, B. and Tharanathan, R.N., Legume and cereal starch — why differences in digestibility? Part 1, Isolation and composition of legume (green gram and Bengal gram) starches, *Staerke,* 47:165–171, 1995.

Pryme, I.F., Pustzai, A., Bardocz, S., and Ewen, S.W.B., The induction of gut hyperplasia by phytohemagglutinin in the diet and limitation of tumor growth, *Histol. Histopathol.,* 13:575–583, 1998.

Pusztai, A., Grant, G., Buchan, W.C., Bardocz, S., de Carvalho, A.F.F.U., and Erwen, S.W.B., Lipid accumulation in obese Zucker rats is reduced by inclusion of raw kidney bean (*Phaseolus vulgaris*) in the diet, *Br. J. Nutr.,* 79:213–221, 1998.

Simpson, H.C., Lousley, R.S., Greekie, M., Hockaday, T.D.R., Carter, R.D., and Mann, J.I., A high carbohydrate leguminous fibre diet improves all aspects of diabetes control, *Lancet,* 1:1–4, 1981.

Tharanathan, R.N. and Mahadevamma, S., Grain legumes — a boon to human nutrition, *Trends Food Sci. Technol.,* 14:507–518, 2003.

Wan, X.S., Meyskens, F.L., Jr., Armstrong, W.B., Taylor, T.H., and Kennedy, A.R., Relationship between protease activity and neu oncongene expression in patients with oral leukoplakia treated with the Bowman-Birk inhibitor, *Cancer Epidemiol. Biomarkers,* 8:601–608, 1999.

Ware, J.H., Wan, X.S., Newberne, P., and Kennedy, A.R., Bowman-Birk inhibitor concentrate reduces colon inflammation in mice with dextran sulfate sodium-induced ulcerative colitis, *Digest. Dis. Sci.,* 44: 986–990, 1999.

Eriocitrin, hesperidin, and diosmin. (From Del Rio et al., *Food Chem.*, 84:457–461, 2004. With permission.)

Lemon *see also* Flavonoids and Hesperidin

Lemon juice is a rich source of ascorbic acid and flavonoids. The antioxidant properties of these compounds have been suggested to inhibit heart disease and certain types of cancers (Salah et al., 1995). Marin and coworkers (2002) found these nutraceuticals were higher in Fino lemon juice compared to the Vern variety. In addition, they found that different industrial-extraction systems affected the levels of these components. Miyake et al. (1997) identified the flavonoid, eriocitrin, in lemon fruit, which had considerable antioxidant activity. Ogata and coworkers (2000) showed this flavonoid induced apoptosis in HL-60 cells and may have therapeutic applications. A recent study of *Citrus limon* flavonoids by Del Rio et al. (2004) found that immature fruit from Lisbon and Fino-9 cultivars were excellent sources of the flavonone hesperidin, while mature fruits from Fino-9 and leaves of Eureka were good sources of the flavone diosmin and the flavonone eriocitrin. Each of these flavonoids have been shown to have pharmaceutical properties.

References

Del Rio, J.A., Fuster, M.D., Gonez, P., Porras, I., Garcia-Lidon, A., and Ortuno, A., *Citrius limon*: A source of flavonoids of pharmaceutical interest, *Food Chem.*, 84:457–461, 2004.

Marin, F.R., Martinez, M., Uribesalgo, T., Casillo, S., and Frutos, M.J., Changes in nutraceutical composition of lemon juices according to different industrial extraction systems, *Food Chem.*, 78:319–324, 2002.

Miyake, Y., Yamamoto, K., and Osawa, T., Isolation of eriocytrin (eryodictiol-7-rutinoside) from lemon fruit (*Citrus limon* BURM.f.) and its antioxidative activity, *Food Sci. Tecnol. Int. Tokio.*, 3:84–89, 1997.

Ogata, S., Miyaje, Y., Yamomoto, K., Okumura, K., and Taguchi, H., Apoptosis induced by the flavonoid from lemon fruit (*Citrus limon* BURM. f.) and its metabolites in HL-60 cells, *Biosci. Biotechnol. Biochem.*, 64:1975–1978, 2000.

Salah, N., Miller, N.J., Paganga, G., Tijburg, L., Bolwell, G.P., and Rice-Evans, C., Polyphenolic flavonols as scavenger of aqueous phase radicals and as chain-breaking antioxidants, *Arch. Biochem. Biophys.*, 322:339–346, 1995.

L

Lemon balm (*Melissa officinalis*)   The leaves of lemon balm, a perennial, lemon-scented herb, are used extensively as an herbal tea in Europe for its aromatic, digestive, and antispasmodic properties in treating sleep disturbances and gastrointestinal disorders (Bisset and Wichtl, 1994). It is generally sold in combination with other herbs that elicit "calming" or sedative effects. Cerny and Schmid (1999) showed that a combination of valerian and lemon balm significantly improved the quality of sleep of healthy volunteers during 30 days of treatment with 360 mg/day and 240 mg/day of valerian and lemon balm, respectively. Acute administration of lemon balm was shown by Kennedy and coworkers (2002) to modulate the mood and cognitive performance of healthy volunteers in a dose- and time-dependent manner, as assessed using the Congitive Drug Research (CDR) computerized-test battery and two serial subtraction tasks. The calming effect and possible cholinergic modulation of lemon balm may have application in the treatment of Alzheimer's disease. A recent double-blind, placebo-controlled study using lemon balm essential aromatherapy on 71 patients suffering from severe dementia by Ballard et al. (2004) also showed they were less agitated and socially withdrawn compared to the placebo.

Carnat and coworkers (1998) reported the presence of 0.13 percent citral (neral + geranial) and 11.8 percent total polyphenolic compounds in the essential oil of dried lemon-balm leaves. Of the latter, hydroxycinnamic compounds accounted for 11.3 percent, with rosmarinic acid 4.1 percent, and total flavonoids 0.5 percent. Herbal tea from lemon balm contained 10 mg/L essential oil, of which 74 percent was citral plus large amounts of polyphenolic compounds.

References

Ballard, C., O'Brien, J., Reichelt, K., and Perry, E., Aromatherapy as a safe and effective treatment for the management of agitation in severe dimentia: The results of a double-blind, placebo controlled trial with Melissa, *J. Clin. Psychiatry,* 63:553–558, 2002.

Bisset, N.G. and Wichtl, M., *Herbal Drugs*, Medpharm, Stuttgart, 1994.

Carnat, A.P., Carnat, A., Fraisse, D., and Lamaison, J.L., The aromatic and polyphenolic composition of lemon balm (*Melissa officinalis* L. subsp. *Officinalis*) tea, *Pharmaceutica Acta Helv.,* 72:301–305, 1998.

Cerny, A. and Schmid, K., Tolerability and efficacy of valerian/lemon balm in healthy volunteers: A double-blind, placebo-controlled, multicentre study, *Fitoterapia,* 70:221–228, 1999.

Kennedy, D.O., Scholey, A.B., Tildesley, N.T.J., Perry, E.K., and Wesnes, K.A., Modulation of mood and cognitive performance following acute administration of *Melissa officinalis* (lemon balm), *Pharmacol. Biochem. Behav.,* 72:953–964, 2002.

Lemon Grass (*Cymbopogon citratus*)   Lemon grass, native to India, is used in Thai and Vietnamese cooking. Most commercial crops for the United States are grown in California and Florida. Using the Salmonella mutation assay, Vinitketkumnuen and coworkers (1994) showed an ethanol extract from lemon grass exhibited antimutagenic activity against a number of different mutagens. Anticancer components in lemon grass extract were found by Suaeyun et al. (1997) to inhibit azoxymethane (AOM)-initiated colon carcinogenesis in the rat. Puatanachokchai et al. (2002) showed a similar lemon-grass extract inhibited the early stages of hepatocarcinogenesis in diethyl-nitrosamine (DEN)-treated male Fischer 344 rats by reducing the number of putatively preneoplastic, glutathione *S*-transferase placental form-positive lesions, as well as the level of oxidative hepatocyte nuclear DNA injury, assessed by 8-hydroxyguanosine production.

References

Puatanachokchai, R., Kishida, H., Denda, A., Murata, N., Konishi, Y., Vinitketkumnuen, U., and Nakae, D., Inhibitory effects of lemon grass (*cymbopogon citratus*) extract on the early phase of hepatocarcinogenesis after initiation with diethylnitrosamine in 344 male Fischer rats. *Cancer Lett.*, 183:9–15, 2002.

Suaeyun, R., Kinouchi, T., Arimochi, H., Vinitketkumnuen, U., and Ohnishi, Y., Inhibitory effects of lemon grass (*Cymbopogon citratus*, Stapf) on formation of azoxymethane-induced DNA adducts and aberrant crypt foci in the rat colon, *Carcinogenesis*, 18:949–955, 1997.

Vinitketkumnuen, U., Puatanachokchai, R., Kongtawelert, P., Lertprasertsuke, N., and Matsushima, T., Antimutagenicity of lemon grass (*Cymbopogon citrates*, Stapf) to various known mutagens in Salmonella mutation assay, *Mutat. Res.*, 341:71–75, 1994.

Lentils (*Lens culinaris* L.) Legume seeds such as lentils provide an inexpensive source of protein for a large part of the world's population. Like other legumes, lentils contain phytohemagglutinins and protease inhibitors, which must be destroyed by cooking before they can be utilized in the diet. Duenas and coworkers (2003) identified proanthocyanidins in the seed coat of lentils. The major monomeric flavan-3-ol identified was (+) catechin-3-glucose followed by smaller amounts of (+)-catechin and (–)-epicatechin. The latter compounds were reported to exhibit potent antioxidant and free-radical-scavenging activities and to inhibit platelet aggregation and antiulcer activity against stomach-mucosa injury (Vinson et al., 1995; Cook and Samman, 1996; Duenas et al., 2003). The large amounts of these bioactive compounds in lentil seed coats represent a potential source of nutraceuticals

References

Cook, N.C. and Samman, S., Flavonoids — chemistry, metabolism, cardiopreventive effects, and dietary source, *J. Nutr. Biochem.*, 7:66–76, 1996.

Duenas, M., Sun, B., Hernandez, T., Estrella, I., and Spranger, M.I., Proanthocyanidin composition in the seed coat of lentils (*Lens culinaris* L.), *J. Agric. Food Chem.*, 51:7999–8004, 2003.

Vinson, J.A., Dabbagh, Y.A., Serry, M.M., and Jang, J., Plant flavonoids, especially tea flavonols, are powerful antioxidants using an *in vitro* oxidation model for heart disease, *J. Agric. Food Chem.*, 43:2800–2802, 1995.

Lettuce (*Lactuca sativa*) Lettuce leaves are quite low in phenolics, but Kang and Saltveit (2002) reported a fourfold increase in iceberg and romaine lettuce following heat-shock (45°C for 2.5 min. in water) treatment or wounding. This increase in phenolics was accompanied by a corresponding increase in antioxidant power (FRAP). Serafini and coworkers (2002) showed that ingestion of 260 g fresh lettuce raised the plasma-antioxidant levels in 11 healthy volunteers compared to the same lettuce stored at 5°C under modified atmosphere-packaging conditions (MAP: O_2-N_2, 5:95 v/v). Ingestion of the fresh lettuce resulted in significantly higher plasma total radical-trapping potential (TRAP) compared to the MAP stored lettuce. In addition, there was a significant increase in plasma quercetin, *p*-coumaric, caffeic acid, β-carotene, and vitamin C following consumption of fresh lettuce, which was not observed following ingestion of MAP lettuce. Thus, optimized MAP storage conditions were needed to better preserve the bioactive components of fresh-cut produce.

Nicolle and coworkers (2004) recently found male Wistar rats fed a diet containing 20 percent freeze-dried lettuce over a three-week period had increased excretion of cholesterol end products, as well as enhanced antioxidant status (Figure L.60). A slight but significant ($p < 0.05$) decrease in cholesterol was observed in rats on the lettuce-fed diet, while triacylglycerol levels were unaffected. A decrease of –23 percent in cholesterol levels in the plasma triacylglycerol-rich lipoprotein (with a minor contribution of LDL) fraction was accompanied by an increase of +18 percent in the HDL fraction and a slight decrease of –7 percent in triacylglycerol levels in the lettuce-fed rats compared to the control. Nicolle and coworkers (2004) attributed these

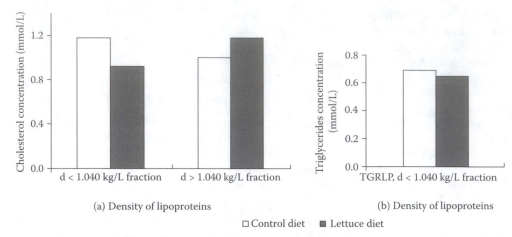

(a) Density of lipoproteins   (b) Density of lipoproteins

□ Control diet   ■ Lettuce diet

FIGURE L.60 (a) Changes in the distribution of cholesterol in the various lipoprotein fractions in rats fed control or lettuce diets. The fractions with $d < 1.040$ kg/L correspond chiefly to triacyclyglycerol-rich lipoproteins (TGRLP), with a lower contribution of LDL. The fractions with $d < 1.040$ kg/L correspond essentially to HDL; (b) differences in the repartition of triacylglycerols in plasma-lipoprotein fractions of rats fed control or lettuce diets. Each value is the mean of triplicate analyses of a pool of eight plasma. (Nicolle et al., *Clinical Nutr.,* 23:605–614, 2004. With permission.)

TABLE L.43
Fiber and Antioxidant Content of Lettuce[1]

	Lettuce
Energy (kJ/g)	9.4
Fiber (mg/g.d.w.)	260
Vitamin C (µg/g.d.w.)	840 ± 11
Vitamin E (µg/g.d.w.)	577 ± 14
Lutein (µg/g.d.w)	176 ± 13
Nonidentified xanthophyll (µg/g.d.w.) as lutein equivalent	114 ± 8
β-carotene (µg/d.w.w.)	66 ± 2.3
Total phenolic compounds (mg/g.d.w.) as gallic-acid equivalent	28.5 ± 11

[1] On a dry-weight basis. Values expressed as means of triplicate analysis ± SEM.

Source: Nicolle et al., *Clinical Nutr.,* 23:605–614, 2004. With permission.

beneficial effects to the fiber and antioxidant content of lettuce (Table L.43).

References

Kang, H.-M. and Saltveit, M.E., Antioxidant capacity of lettuce leaf tissue increases after wounding, *J. Agric. Food Chem.,* 50:7536–7541, 2002.

Nicolle, C., Cardinault, N., Gueux, E., Jaffrelo, L., Rock, E., Mazur, A., Amourex, P., and Remesy, C., Health effect of vegetable-based diet: Lettuce consumption improves cholesterol metabolism and antioxidant status in the rat, *Clin. Nutr.,* 23:605–614, 2004.

Serafini, M., Bugianesi, R., Salucci, M., Azzinni, E., Ragguzzini, A., and Maiani, G., Effect of acute ingestion of fresh and stored lettuce (*Lactuca sativa*) on plasma total antioxidant levels in human subjects, *Br. J. Nutr.,* 88:615–623, 2002.

Licochalcone A   Licochalcone A is an oxygenated chalcone first isolated from Chinese licorice roots, which has considerable biological activity (Nadelmann et al., 1997). Barfod and coworkers (2002) found licochalcone A and

Licochalcone A. (From Fukai et al., *Fitoterapia,* 74: 720–724, 2003. With permission.)

four synthetic analogues inhibited proliferation of lymphocytes, as well as the production of proinflammatory and anti-inflammatory cytokines. These results suggested that these compounds exert immunomodulatory effects, which may be useful for treating some diseases. Oral administration of licochalcone A (30 mg/kg/day) to mice with glomerular disease (Masugi-nephritis) was found by Fukai et al. (2003) to reduce the urinary-protein excretion compared to nephritic mice. Licochalcone A also exhibited weak scavenging activity against superoxide radicals.

References

Barfod, L., Kemp, K., Hansen, M., and Kharazmi, A., Chalcones from Chinese licorice inhibit proliferation of T cells and production of cytokines, *Inter. Immunopharmacol.,* 2:545–555, 2002.

Fukai, T., Satoh, K., Nomura, T., and Sakagami, H., Antinephritis and radical scavenging activity of prenylflavonoids, *Fitoterapia,* 74:720–724, 2003.

Nadelmann, L. Tjørnelund, J., Christensen, E., and Hansen, H., High-performance liquid chromatographic determination of licochalcone A and its metabolites in biological fluids, *J. Chromatogr. B.,* 695:389–3900, 1997.

Licorice *see also* **Glabridin, Glycyrrhin, and Glycyrrhizic acid**   Licorice root, one of the oldest and most commonly used botanicals in Chinese medicine, has been used worldwide for medicinal purposes since ancient times (Liu et al., 2000). The key components associated with its medicinal properties are triterpenes, polyphenols, polysaccharides, flavonoids, alkaloids, polyamines, and essential oils. Licorice triterpenes are nonsteroidal agents exhibiting both antioxidant and anti-inflammatory properties (Wang and Nixon, 2001). The most important triterpene in licorice, glycyrrhizin (GL), is hydrolyzed to its major metabolite, glycyrrhetinic acid (GA) (Wang et al., 1998). GA exists in two different forms, 18α-glycyrrhetinic acid (α-GA) and 18β-glycyrrhetinic acid (β-GA), both of which are antimutagens capable of inhibiting monooxygenase activity (Wang et al., 1991). Tamir and coworkers (2000) showed glabridin, an isoflavan in licorice root, acted as a phytoestrogen by inhibiting the proliferation of estrogen responsive (ER+) and estrogen nonresponsive (ER-) human breast cells at concentrations greater than 15 μm.

Rafi et al. (2001) found a novel polyphenol in licorice root, 1-(2,4-dihydroxyphenyl)-3-(4′-hydroxyphenyl) 1-propanone (β-hydroxy DHP), that was more inhibitory against Bcl-2 phosphorylation in tumor cells compared to its stereoisomer α-hydroxy DHP. Bcl-2, a protein that prevents cell death, inhibits cytochrome c

L

Glycyrrhetinic acid (glycyrrhizic acid). (From Wang et al., *J. Chromatogr. A.,* 811:219–224, 1998. With permission.)

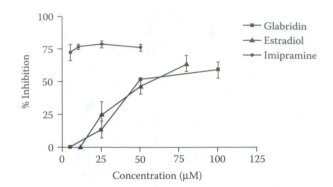

FIGURE L.61 The effect of increasing concentration of glabridin (■), estradiol (▲), and imipramine (●) on the inhibition of hSERT reuptake. 293-hSERT cells were incubated for 20 min with estradiol or ipramine at various concentrations (0–100 μM). Cells were harvested, and the incorporated radioactivity was measured with a scintillation liquid. Data are presented as percent inhibition of controls. Values are means ± SD of three experiments. (Ofir et al., *J. Mol. Nurosci.,* 20:135–140, 2003. With permission.)

from being released from mitochondria, which is essential for cell apoptosis to occur. Thus, licorice components appear to act as chemopreventive agents with potential as new pharmaceuticals for treating cancers.

Ofir and coworkers (2003) recently showed that licorice isoflavans and isoflavene were capable of inhibiting serotinin re-up, a known pharmacological treatment for major depression, as well as anxiety, appetite, and obsessive-compulsive disorders (Barker and Blakely, 1995). Glabridin, for example, mimicked estradiol by

Glabridin. (Adapted from Tamir et al., *J. Steroid Biochem. Mol. Biol.,* 78:291–298, 2001.)

inhibiting serotonin reuptake in a dose-dependent manner (Figure L.61). The ability to inhibit serotonin reuptake was facilitated by the lipophilic part of the isoflavans, as well as the hydroxyl at position 2′ in the B ring. These licorice constituents appear to have considerable potential for the therapeutic treatment of

mild to moderate depression in premenopausal and postmenopausal women.

References

Barker, E.L. and Blakely, R.D., Norepinephrine and serotonin transporter: Molecular targets of antidepressant drugs, in *Psychopharmacology: The Fourth Generation of Progress,* Bloom, F.E. and Kupfer, D.J., Eds., Raven Press, New York, 1995, pp. 321–333.

Liu, H.-M., Naoki, S., Takimi, A., and Tamio, M., Constituents and their sweetness of food additive enzymatically modified licorice extract, *J. Agric. Food Chem.,* 48:6044–6047, 2000.

Ofir, R., Tamir, S., Khatib, S., and Vaya, J., Inhibition of serotonin re-uptake by licorice constituents, *J. Mol. Neurosci.,* 20:135–140, 2003.

Rafi, M.M., Vastano, B.C., Zhu, N., Ho, C-T., Ghai, G., Rosen, R.T., Gallo, M., and Di Paola, R.S., Novel polyphenol molecule isolated from licorice root (*Glycyrrhiza glabra*) induces apoptosis, G2/M cycle arrest, and Bcl-2 phosphorylation in tumor cell lines, *J. Agric. Food Chem.,* 50:677–684, 2002.

Tamir, S., Eizenberg, M., Somjen, D., Israel, S., and Vaya, J., Estrogen-like activity of glabrene and other constituents isolated from licorice root, *J. Steroid Biochem. Mol. Biol.,* 78:291–298, 2001.

Tamir, S., Eizenberg, M., Somjen, D., Stern, N., Shelach, R., Kaye, A., and Vaya, J., Estrogenic and antiproliferative properties of glabridin from licorice in human breast cancer cells, *Cancer Res.,* 60:5704–5709, 2000.

Wang, Z., Argarwal, R., Zhou, Z.C., Bickers, D.R., and Mukhtar, H., Inhibition of mutagenicity in *Salmonella typhymurium* and skin tumor initiating and tumor promoting activities in SENCAR mice by glycyrrhetinic acid: Comparison of 18α- and 18β-stereoisomers, *Carcinogenesis,* 12:187–192, 1991.

Wang, P., Li, S.F.Y., and Lee, H.K., Determination of glycyrrhizic acid and 18-β-glycyrrhetinic acid in biological fluids by micellar electrokinetic chromatography, *J. Chromatogr. A.,* 811:219–224, 1998.

Wang, Z. and Nixon, D., Licorice and cancer, *Nutr. Cancer,* 39:1–11, 2001.

Lignans *see also* **Flaxseed, Matairesinol, and Secoisolariciresinol** Lignans are a complex group of phenolic compounds widely distributed in the plant kingdom, composed of phenylpropane dimers linked by β–β bonds with a 1,4-diarylbutane structure (Smeds and Hakala, 2003). Flaxseed is the richest source of lignans compared to other food sources, such as soybean, oat bran, and lentils, as summarized in Table L.44. The main lignan precursors in flaxseed are secoisolariciresinol (SEC) and matairesinol (MAT) (Scheme L.36). SEC is normally present in the form of secoisolariciresinol diglucoside (SDG), which is converted by bacteria in the gastrointestinal tract to enterodiol and enterolactone. Both enterodiol and enterolactone were shown to inhibit the growth of human colon-cancer cells at a concentration of 100 μmM (Sung et al., 1998). Supplementation of flaxseed in the diets of rats decreased the number of aberrant crypts and foci in AOM-treated rats (Serraino and Thompson, 1992). A dose-dependent reduction in

TABLE L.44
Level of Lignans in Some Plant Food Sources

Food	Lignans (total) (ugg^{-1})
Flaxseed meal	675
Flaxseed flour	527
Lentils	17
Soy bean	8.6
Oat bran	6.5
Wheat bran	5.6
Kidney bean	5.6

Source: Adapted from Reinli and Block, *Nutr.Cancer,* 26: 123–148, 1996.

metastasis and the growth of secondary tumors observed in mice fed flaxseed by Yan et al. (1998) indicated its potential for preventing metastasis.

Niemeyer and Metzler (2002) examined the oxidative metabolism of lignans SEC and MAT and showed they were both excellent substrates for cytochrome P450 hydroxylation at the aliphatic and aromatic positions in the molecule. The different pathways involved are outlined in Scheme L.37. However, the genotoxic potential of these hydroxylated products, including isolariciresinol (ISL) and lariciresinol (LAR), have yet to be determined.

Owen and coworkers (2000) showed for the first time that lignans (+)-1-acetoxypinoresinol and (+)-pinoresinol were major components of the phenolic fractions in extra-virgin olive oils. They were virtually absent in the corresponding refined oils. Nurmi and coworkers (2003) reported that lignans in red wine ranged from 0.812 to 1.406 mg/L, with isolariciresinol being the main one.

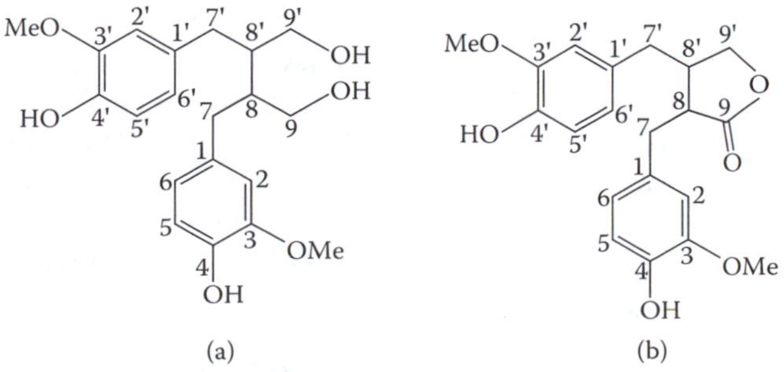

(a)   (b)

SCHEME L.36 Structure and numbering of secoisolariciresinol (a) and matairesinol (b). (From Saarinen et al., *J. Chromatogr. B.,* 777:311–319, 2002. With permission.)

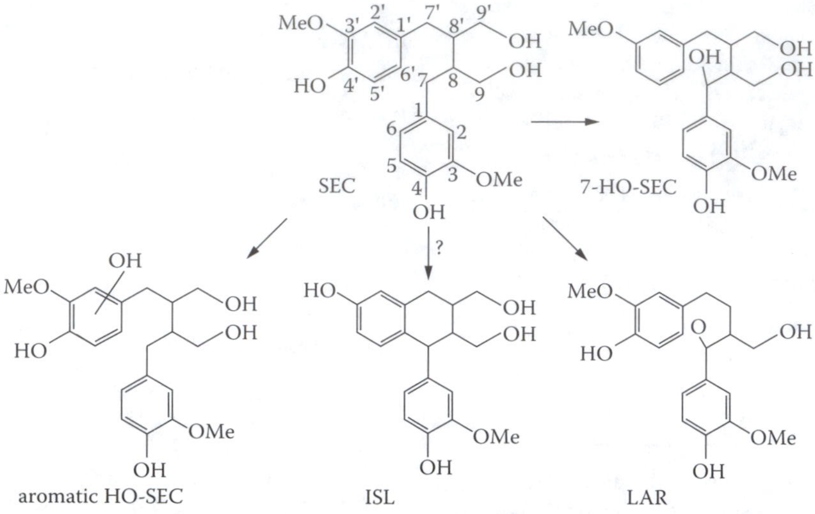

SCHEME L.37 Oxidative pathways in the metabolism of SEC. (Niemeyer and Metzler, *J. Chromatogr. B.*, 777:321–327, 2002. With permission.)

References

Niemeyer, H.B. and Metzler, M., Oxidative metabolites and genotoxic potential of mammalian and plant lignans *in vitro*, *J. Chromatogr. B.*, 777:321–327, 2002.

Nurmi, T., Haeinonen, S., Mazur, W., Deyama, T., Nishibe, S., and Adlercreutz, H., Lignans in selected wines, *Food Chem.*, 83:303–309, 2003.

Owen, R.W., Mier, W., Giacosa, A., Hull, W.E., Spiegelhalder, B., and Bartsch, H., Identification of lignans as major components in the phenolic fraction of olive oil, *Clin. Chem.*, 46:976–988, 2000.

Reinli, K. and Block, G., Phytoestrogen content of foods — a codium of literature values, *Nutr. Cancer*, 26:123–148, 1996.

Saarinen, N.M., Smeds, A., Makela, S.I, Ammala, J., Hakala, K., Pihlava, J.-M., Ryhanen, E.-L., Sjoholm, R., and Santti, H., Structural determinants of plant lignans for the formation of enterolactone *in vivo*, *J. Chromatogr.*, 777:311–319, 2002.

Serraino, M. and Thompson, L.U., The effect of flaxseed supplementation on the imitation and promotional stages of mammary tumorigenesis, *Nutr. Cancer*, 17:153–159, 1992.

Setchell, K.D.R. and Adlercreutz, H.A., Mammalian lignans and phytoestrogens. Recent studies on their formation, metabolism and biological role in health and disease, in *Role of Gut Flora in Toxicity and Cancer*, Rowland, I.R., Ed., Academic Press, New York, 1988, pp. 315–345.

Smeds, A. and Hakala, K., Liquid chromatographic-tandem mass spectrometric method for the plant lignan 7-hydroxymatairesinol and its potential metabolites in human plasma, *J. Chromatogr. B.*, 793:297–308, 2003.

Sung, M.-K., Lautens, M., and Thompson, L.U., Mammalian hormones inhibit the growth of estrogen-independent human colon cells, *Anti. Cancer Res.*, 18:1405–1408, 1998.

Taskinen, A., Eklund, P., Syoholm, R., and Hotokha, M., The molecular structure and properties of hydroxymatairesinol, an *ab initio* study, *J. Mol. Struct.*, (Theochem), 677:113–124, 2004.

Yan, L., Yee, J.A., Li, D., McGuire, M.H., and Thompson, L.U., Dietary flaxseed supplementation and experiential metastasis of melanoma in mice, *Cancer Lett.*, 124:181–186, 1998.

Limes (*Citrus aurantifolia*) Limes, members of the Rutaceae family, only grow in a tropical climate. Many different varieties are cultivated in the Middle East, tropical Asia, and in Florida in the United States. Kawaii and coworkers (1999) examined the antiproliferative effects of the readily extractable fraction from 34 important citrus juices on four different human cancer cells. Of these extracts, sweet lime inhibited the proliferation of three of these lines but was much less toxic towards normal human cell

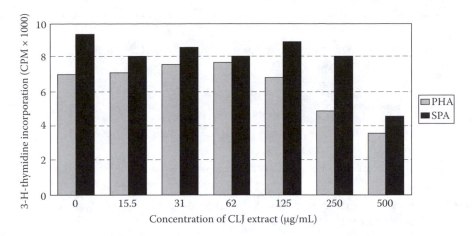

FIGURE L.62 Inhibitory effect of concentrated lime juice (CLJ) on the proliferation of PHA- and SPA-activated mononuclear cells. Proliferation of PHA-activated mononuclear cells was significantly inhibited by 250 and 500 µg/mL of CLJ extract, whereas only 500 µg/mL of the extract could induce significant inhibition in proliferation of SPA-activated mononuclear cells. Each value represents the mean ± SD of at least three independent measurements. $p < 0.05$ was considered significant with regard to unstimulated control (0 µg/mL of CLJ extract). (From Gharagozloo and Ghaderi, *J. Ethnopharmacol.*, 77:85–90, 2001. With permission.)

lines. Gharagozloo and Ghaderi (2001) later reported a concentrated lime-juice extract exhibited immunomodulatory effects on activated cultured human mononuclear cells. The levels of extract needed to inhibit proliferation of phytohemagglutinin (PHA)-activated mononuclear cells were 250 and 500 µg/mL, while inhibition of staphyloccocal protein (SPA)-activated mononuclear cells required 500 µg/mL (Figure L.62). They suggested that it was the protein components in the lime-juice extract that appeared responsible for its immunomodulatory properties.

References

Gharagozloo, M. and Ghaderi, A., Immunomodulatory effect of concentrated lime juice extract on activated human mononuclear cells, *J. Ethnopharmacol.*, 77:85–90, 2001.

Kawaii, S., Tomono, Y., Katase, E., Ogawa, K., and Yano, M., Antiproliferative effects of the readily extractable fractions prepared from various citrus juices on several cancer cell lines, *J. Agric. Food Chem.*, 47:2509–2512, 1999.

Limonene *d*-Limonene is a monocyclic monoterpene in essential oils of citrus fruits, spices, and herbs. Orange peel is a particularly

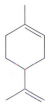

d-Limonene. (Adapted from Casuscelli et al., *Appl. Cat.*, A: General, 274:115–122, 2004.)

rich source, ranging from 90–95 percent (w/w). Limonene has been reported to exhibit chemoprotective activity against spontaneously and chemically induced tumors in the skin (Elegbede et al., 1988), liver (Dietrich and Swenberg, 1991), mammary gland (Elson et al., 1988; Maltzman et al., 1989), and lung and forestomach of rodents (Wattenberg et al., 1989; Watenberg and Coccia, 1991). Kawamori et al. (1996) showed *d*-limonene was effective against azoxymethane (AOM)-induced colon cancer in F344 rats. Those treated with 0.5 percent *d*-limonene in the drinking water had a significantly lower number of 2, 3, and 4 crypts compared to (AOM)-treated rats (Table L.45). These researchers confirmed the ability of *d*-limonene to inhibit formation of colonic ACF by blocking formation of (AOM)-induced ACF in the colon. Uedo and coworkers (1999) examined the mechanism involved in inhibiting gastric

TABLE L.45
Effect of *d*-Limonene on Aberrant Crypt/Focus Induced by AOM in Rat Colon[1]

Treatment	ACF/Focus				
	1 crypts	2 crypts	3 crypts	4 crypts	5 crypts
AOM alone	46.0 ± 6.6	48.5 ± 11.7	28.8 ± 5.4	6.6 ± 1.1	1.5 ± 1
AOM + *d*-limonene	40.5 ± 11.5	32.8 ± 6.0^b	14.2 ± 4.1^c	1.5 ± 0.5^c	0.5 ± 0.8

[1] Significantly different from AOM alone by Student's t test (b, $p < 0.05$; c, $p < 0.001$).
From Kawamori et al., *Carcinogenesis,* 17:369–372, 1996. With permission.

carcinogenesis in Wistar rats induced by *N*-methyl-*N'*-nitrosoguanidine. Feeding 2 percent limonene significantly inhibited the induced cancer through increased apoptosis and decreased DNA synthesis.

References

Casuscelli, S.G., Crivello, M.E., Perez, C.F., Ghione, G., Herrero, E.R., Pizzio, L.R., Vasquez, P.G., Caceres, C.V., and Blanco, M.N., Effect of reaction conditions on limonene epoxidation with H_2O_2 catalyzed by supported Keggin heteropolycompounds, *Appl. Cat.,* A: General, 274:115–122, 2004.

Dietrich, D.R. and Swenberg, J.A. The presence of α2u-globulin is necessary for *d*-limonene promotion of male rat kidney tumor, *Cancer Res.,* 51:3512–3521, 1991.

Elegbede, J.A., Maltzman, T.H., Verma, A.K., Tanner, M.A., Elson, C.E., and Gould, M.N., Mouse skin tumor promoting activity of orange peel and *d*-limonene: A re-evaluation, *Carcinogenesis,* 7:2047–2049, 1986.

Elson, C.E., Maltzman, T.H., Boston, J.L., Tanner, M.A., and Gould, M.N., Anticarcinogenic activity of *d*-limonene during the initiation and promotion/progression stages of DMBA-induced rat mammary carcinogenesis, *Carcinogenesis,* 9:331–332, 1988.

Kawamori, T., Tanaka, T., Hirose, Y., Ohnishi, M., and Mori, H., Inhibitory effect of *d*-limonene on the development of colonic aberrant crypt foci induced by azoxymethane in F344 rats, *Carcinogenesis,* 17:369–372, 1996.

Maltzman, T.H., Hurt, L.M., Elson, C.E., Tanner, M.A., and Gould, M.N., The prevention of nitrosomethylurea-induced mammary tumors by *d*-limonene and orange oil, *Carcinogenesis,* 10:781–783, 1989.

Uedo, N., Tatsuta, M., Iishi, H., Baba, M., Sakai, N., Yano, H., and Otani, T., Inhibition by *d*-limonene of gastric carcinogenesis induced by *N*-methyl-*N'*-nitrosoguanidine in Wistar rats, *Cancer Lett.,* 137: 131–136, 2002.

Wattenberg, L.W., Sparnins, V.L., and Barany, G., Inhibition of *N*-nitrosodiethylamine carcinogenesis in mice by naturally occurring organosulfur and monoterpenes, *Cancer Res.,* 49:2689–2692, 1989.

Wattenberg, L.W. and Coccia, J.B., Inhibition of 4-(methylnitrosoamino)-1-(3-pyridyl)-1-butanone carcinogenesis in mice by *d*-limonene and citrus fruit oils, *Carcinogenesis,* 12:115–117, 1991.

Limonin *see also* **Limonoids**   Limonin glucoside, one of the most abundant limonoids in citrus fruit, is readily available in orange-juice and citrus-juice processing byproducts (Schoch et al., 2001; Ifuku et al., 1998). Together with nomilin, they both inhibited forestomach, buccal pouch, lung, and skin carcinogenesis in rodents (Lam et al., 1989; Wada, 1996). Tanaka and coworkers (2000) clearly demonstrated inhibition of AOM-induced colonic ACF by dietary limonin or obacunone with suppression of preneoplasia to malignancy. This was evident by significantly lower incidences of multiplicities in the treated groups compared to the AOM control (Table L.46).

References

Ifuku, Y., Maseda, H., Miyake, M., Inaba, N., Ayano, S., Ozaki, Y., Maruyama, K., and Hasegawa, S., Method for manufacturing limonoid glucosides, U.S.Patent 5734046, 1998.

Kelly, C., Jewell, C., and O'Brien, N.M., The effect of dietary supplementation with the citrus limonoids, limonin and nobilin on xenobiotic-metabolizing enzymes in the liver and small intestine of the rat, *Nutr. Res.,* 23:681–690, 2003.

Citrus limonoids, limonin (a) and nomilin (b). (From Kelly et al., *Nutr. Res.,* 23:681–690, 2003. With permission.)

TABLE L.46
Incidence and Multiplicity of Large-Intestinal Neoplasm of Rats Fed Obacunone or Limonin (During or After Exposure to AOM)

Group No.	Treatment	No. of Rats Examined	Incidence of Rats with Neoplasm			Multiplicity (No. or Tumors/rat, Mean ± SD)		
			Total	AD[1]	ADC	Total	AD[1]	ADC
1	AOM only	25	10(75%)	2(8%)	18(72%)	0.84 ± 0.61	0.08 ± 0.27	0.76 ± 0.51
2	AOM + 500 ppm obacunone	16	5[a](31%)	1(6%)	4[b](25%)	0.38 ± 0.60[c]	0.04 ± 0.24	0.31 ± 0.58[d]
3	AOM + 500 ppm limonin	16	3[e](19%)	2(13%)	1[f](6%)	0.19 ± 0.39[g]	0.13 ± 0.33	0.06 ± 0.24[g]
4	AOM⇄500 ppm obacunone	16	2[h](13%)	0(0%)	2[h](13%)	0.13 ± 0.33[g]	0	0.13 ± 0.33[g]
5	AOM⇄500 ppm limonin	16	3[e](19%)	1(6%)	2[e](13%)	0.19 ± 0.39[g]	0.06 ± 0.24	0.13 ± 0.33[g]
6	500 ppm obacunone	8	0(0%)	0(0%)	0(0%)	0	0	0
7	500 ppm limonin	8	0(0%)	0(0%)	0(0%)	0	0	0
8	No treatment	8	0(0%)	0(0%)	0(0%)	0	0	0

[1] AD, adenoma; ADC, adenocarcinoma.

[2] O, obacunone; L, limonin.

[a–h] Statistically significant from group 1: [a]$p = 0.012$; [b]$p = 0.004$; [c]$p < 0.05$; [d]$p < 0.02$; [e]$p = 0.001$; [f]$p = 0.00003$; [g]$p < 0.001$; [h]$p = 0.0002$.

Source: Tanaka et al., *Carcinogenesis,* 22:193–198, 2001. With permission.

Lam, L.K.T., Li, Y., and Hasegawa, S., Effects of citrus limonoids on glutathione *S*-transferase activity in mice, *J. Agric. Food Chem.,* 37:878–880, 1989.

Schoch, T.K., Manners, G.D., and Hasegawa, S., Analysis of limonoid glucosides from citrus by electrospray ionization liquid chromatography-mass spectrometry, *J. Agric. Food Chem.,* 49:1102–1108, 2001.

Tanaka, T., Maeda, M., Kohno, H., Murakami, M., Kagami, S., Miyake, M., and Wada, K., Inhibition of azoxymethane-induced colon carcinogenesis in male F344 rats by the citrus limonoids obacunone and limonin, *Carcinogenesis,* 22:193–198, 2001.

Wada, K., 1996. Studies on the constituents of edible and medicinal plants to affect metabolizing system in mammals, *Natural Med.,* 50:195–203, 1996 (in Japanese).

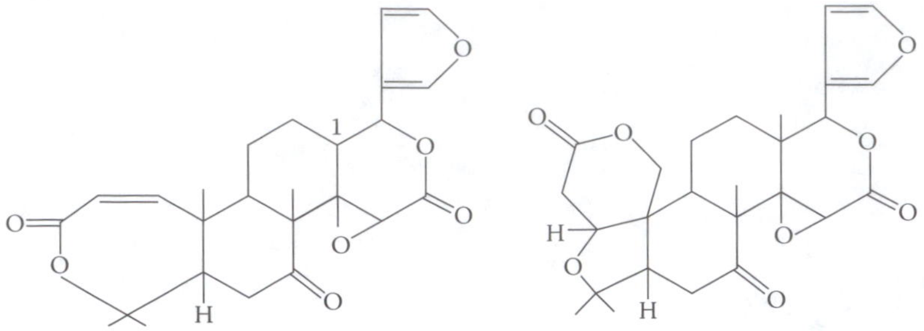

SCHEME L.38 Chemical structures of (a) obacunone and (b) limonin. (Tanaka et al., *Carcinogenesis*, 22: 193–198, 2000. With permission.)

Limonoids *see also* **Limonin**   Limonoids are a group of highly oxygenated triterpenoids found in members of the Rutaceae (citrus fruits) and Maliaceae (neem) families. Citrus fruits are particularly rich sources of limonoids, with the most prevalent being obacunone and limonin (Scheme L.38). They impart bitterness to citrus juices, but as the fruit matures, they form glycosides, which are tasteless and water soluble. The anticancer properties of limonoids are attributed to their induction of the phase II enzyme, glutathione *S*-transferase (Lam et al., 1989; Kelly et al., 2003). Administration of high doses of citrus limonoids to four groups of healthy male and female subjects were shown by Manners and coworkers (2003) to be readily bioavailable and nontoxic.

References

Kelly, C., Jewell, C., and O'Brien, N.M., The effect dietary supplementation with the citrus limonoids, limonin and nomilin on xenobiotic-metabolizing enzymes in the liver and small intestine of the rat, *Nutr. Res.,* 23:681–690, 2003.

Lam, L.K.Y., Li, Y., and Hasegawa, S., Effect of citrus limonoids on glutathione *S*-transferase in mice, *J. Agric. Food Chem.,* 37:878–880, 1989.

Manners, G.D., Jacob, R.A., Breksa, A.P., III, Schoch, T.K., and Hasegawa, S., Bioavailability of citrus limonoids in humans, *J. Agric. Food Chem.,* 51:4156–4161, 2003.

α-Lipoic acid   α-Lipoic acid (thioctic acid), a short-chain fatty acid with two sulfur atoms, is a naturally occurring coenzyme of pyruvate and α-ketoglutarate dehydrogenases. It can be reduced to dihydrolipoic acid, with the two sulfur atoms converted to sulfhydryl groups. Lipoic acid is found mainly in meat and liver and could not be detected in vegetables (Hiroyuki, 1998). It appears to be a useful, therapeutic agent for neurological and liver disorders (Packer et al., 1995; Bustamante et al.,

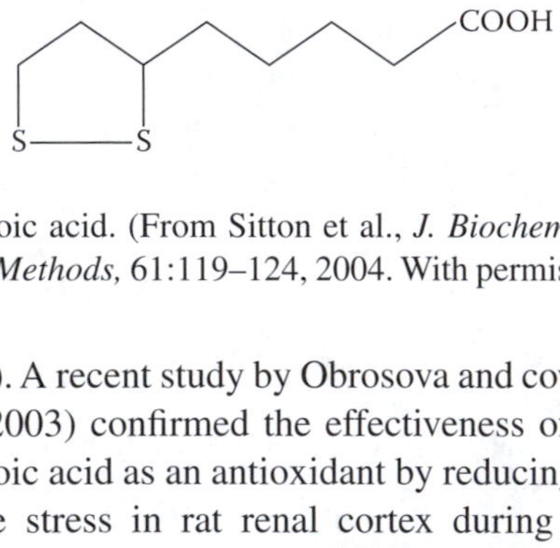

α-Lipoic acid. (From Sitton et al., *J. Biochem. Biophys. Methods,* 61:119–124, 2004. With permission.)

1998). A recent study by Obrosova and coworkers (2003) confirmed the effectiveness of DL-α-lipoic acid as an antioxidant by reducing oxidative stress in rat renal cortex during early diabetes. Preclinical trials were recommended to assess the efficacy of lipoic acid for treating diabetic complications, such as diabetic nephropathy. Gibson et al. (2003) also confirmed the major role of oxidative stress in diabetic autonomic and somatic neuropathy, by the ability of α-lipoic acid to protect autonomic nerves of gastric fundus and the vascular supply of these nerves and neuronal-cell bodies from damage by reactive-oxygen species (ROS). As seen in Figure L.63, α-lipoic acid corrected the defective,

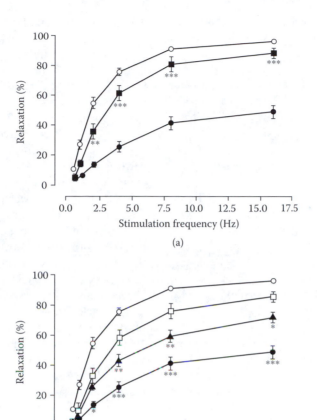

FIGURE L.63 (a,b) Effect of diabetes and chronic α-lipoic-acid treatment on NANC-mediated frequency–response curves in 5-hydroxytryptamine (5-HT) precontracted rat gastric fundus longtitudinal muscle strips. (a) Prevention study: nondiabetic control group, n = 18. Eight-week diabetic control group, n = 20;, α-lipoic-acid prevention treatment diabetic group, n = 9. Data are mean ± SEM. **$p < 0.01$, ***$p < 0.001$ compared to eight-week diabetic control group. (b) Intervention study: nondiabetic ( ) and 8 week diabetic ( ) control groups as in (a), plotted for comparison; 4 week diabetic control group, n = 17; α-lipoic acid intervention group treated for 4 weeks following 4 weeks of untreated diabetes, n = 8. Data are mean ±. *$p < 0.05$, **$p < 0.01$, ***$p < 0.001$ vs. α-lipoic acid intervention treatment group (Gibson et al., *Free Rad. Biol. Med.*, 35:160–168, 2003. With permission.)

relaxation-impaired gastric fundus nonadrenergic, noncholinergic (NANC) nerves caused by diabetes by providing 82.8 percent protection for maximum relaxation (16 Hz, $p < 0.001$).

Lapenna et al. (2003) recently showed that it was the reduced form of lipoic acid, dihydrolipoic acid, not lipoic acid, that inhibited 15-lipoxygenase-dependent lipid peroxidation, suggesting possible antioxidant and antiathrogenic properties.

References

Bustamante, J., Lodge, J.K., Marcocci, L., Trischler, H.J., Packer, L., and Rihn, B.H., Alpha-lipoic acid in liver metabolism and disease, *Free Rad. Biol. Med.*, 24:1023–1039, 1998.

Gibson, T.M., Cotter, M.A., and Cameron, N.E., Effects of alpha-lipoic acid on impaired gastric fundus innervation in diabetic rats, *Free Rad. Biol. Med.*, 35:160–168, 2003.

Hiroyuki, K., Chromatographic analysis of lipoic acid and related compounds, *J. Chromatogr.*, B717: 247–262, 1998.

Lapenna, D., Ciofani, G., Pierdomenico, S.D., Giamberardino, M.A., and Cuccurullo, F., Dihydrolic acid inhibits 15-lipoxygenase-dependent lipid peroxidation, *Free Rad. Biol. Med.*, 35:1203–1209, 2003.

Obrosova, I.G., Fathallah, L., Liu, E., and Nourooz-Zadeh, J., Early oxidative stress in the diabetic kidney: Effect of DL-α-lipoic acid, *Free Rad. Biol. Med.*, 34:186–195, 2003.

Packer, L., Witt, E.H., and Tritschler, H.J., Alpha-lipoic acid as a biological antioxidant, *Free Rad. Biol. Med.*, 19:227–250, 1995.

Sitton, A., Schmid, M.G., Gubitz, G., and Aboul-Enein, H.Y., Determination of lipoic acid in dietary supplement preparations by capillary electrophoresis, *Biochem. Biophys. Methods*, 61:119–124, 2004.

Lipoproteins Lipoproteins are conjugated proteins in which simple proteins are combined with lipid components, such as cholesterol or triacylglycerols. They are classified according to their density as low-density (LDL) or high-density (HDL) lipoproteins. LDL and HDL both transport lipids in the watery fluids of the body; however, HDL transports cholesterol from the peripheral tissues to the liver for oxidation. High LDL and low HDL levels are associated with a high risk of ischemic heart disease (Gordon and Rifkind, 1989). However, a high level of HDL cholesterol appears to protect the arterial wall from the formation of atherosclerotic lesions by removing lipids (Yancey et al., 2003).

The protective effect afforded by HDL against ischemic heart disease appears to be mediated via a reduced cardiac tumor necrosis factor-α (TNF-α) content and enhanced cardiac prostaglandin release (Calabresi et al., 2003). Apoliprotein-specific synthetic HDLs made by combining phosphatidylcholine and apolipoprotein A-1 were proposed by Sirtori et al. (1999) as novel, therapeutic tools for treating cardiovascular diseases. They reported that it was possible to produce synthetic HDLs on a large scale and to safely administer high doses to humans. Subsequent research showed the effectiveness of these synthetic HDLs in animal models of atherosclerosis, arterial thrombosis, and hemorrhagic and septic shock (Sha et al., 2001; Cockerill et al., 2001; Chiesa et al., 2002). Rossoni et al. (2004) demonstrated the cardioprotective effects of administering synthetic HDLs to isolated rat hearts 10 min prior to ischemia by the rapid and dose-dependent improvement in postischemic cardiac function. The left ventricular developed pressure recovered to 71 ± 3.2 compared to 40.5 ± 3.8 mm Hg for the saline-treated hearts, while cardiac perfusion pressure increased to 100.3 ± 6.2 compared to 132.0 ± 9.0 mm Hg.

LDL cholesterol, because of its detrimental relationship to cardiovascular disease, cannot be considered a nutraceutical. Nevertheless, the oxidized form of this low-density lipoprotein (OxLDLs) appears to function as a specific delivery system for photosensitizers to the scavenger receptors expressed on the macrophages in atherosclerotic lesions, enhancing the benefits of photodynamic therapy (De Vries et al., 1999). Photodynamic therapy, a promising new therapy for cardiovascular pathologies, such as atherosclerosis and retetenosis, involves the specific delivery of a photosensitizer, such as aluminum phthalcyanine chloride (AIPc), to the atherosclerotic plaque, where it is activated by light of a specific wavelength, reducing the narrowing of the artery (Nyamekye et al., 1996).

References

Calabresi, L., Rossoni, G., Gomaraschi, M., Sisto, F., Berti, F., and Franceschini, G., High-density lipoprotein protect isolated rat hearts from ischemia-reperfusion injury by reducing cardiac tumor necrosis factor-α content and enhancing prostoglandin release, *Circ. Res.*, 92:330–337, 2003.

Chiesa, G., Monteggia, E., Marchesi, M., Lorenzon, P., Laurello, M., Lorusso, V., Di Mario, C., Karvouni, E., Newton, R.S., and Bisgaier, C.L., Franceshini, G., and Sirtoni, C.R., Recombinant apolipoprotein A-1$_{Milano}$ infusion into rabbit carotid artery rapidly removes lipid from fatty streaks, *Circ. Res.*, 90:974–980, 2002.

Cockerill, G.W., McDonald, M.C., Mota-Filipe, H., Cuzzocrea, S., Miller. N.E., and Thiemermann, C., High density lipoproteins reduce organ injury and organ dysfunction in a rat model of hemorrhagic shock, *FASEB J.*, 15:1941–1952, 2001.

De Vries, H.E., Moor, A.C.E., Dubbelman, T.M.A.R., Van Berkel, T.J.C., and Kuiper, J., Oxidized low-density lipoprotein delivery system for photosensitizers: Implications for photodynamic therapy of atherosclerosis, *J. Pharmacol. Exp. Ther.,* 289:528–534, 1999.

Gordon, D.J. and Rifkind, B.M., High density lipoprotein: The clinical implications of recent studies, *N. Engl. J. Med.,* 321:1311–1316, 1989.

Nyamekye, I., Buonaccorsi, G., McEwan, J., MacRobert, A., Bown, S., and Bishop, C., Inhibition of intimal hyperplasia in balloon injured arteries with adjunctive phthalocyanine sensitized photodynamic therapy, *Eur. J. Endovasc. Surg.,* 11:19–28, 1996.

Rossoni, G., Gomaraschi, M., Berti, F., Sirtori, C.R., Franceschini, G., and Calabresi, L., Synthetic high-density lipoprotein exert cardioprotective effects in myocardial ischemia/reperfusion injury, *J. Pharmacol. Exp. Ther.,* 308:79–84, 2004.

Sha, P.K., Yano, J., Reyes, O., Chyu, R.Y., Kaul, S., Bisgaier, C.L., Drake, S., and Cercek, B., High-dose recombinant apolipoprotein A-1$_{Milano}$ mobilizes tissue cholesterol and rapidly reduces plaque lipid and macrophage content in apolipoprotein E-deficient mice: Potential implications for acute plaque stabilization, *Circulation,* 103:3047–3050, 2001.

Sirtori, C.R., Calabresi, L., and Franceschini, G., Recombinant apolipoproteins for the treatment of vascular diseases, *Atherosclerosis,* 142:29–40, 1999.

Yancey, P.G., Bortnick, A.E., Kellner-Weibel, G., Llera-Moya, M., Phillips, M.C., and Rothblat, G.H., Importance of different pathways of cellular cholesterol efflux, *Arterioscler. Thromb. Vasc. Biol.,* 23: 712–719, 2003.

Lobeline   Lobeline, an alkaloid constituent of Indian tobacco (*Lobelia inflata*), is a nicotine antagonist and may be useful as a smoking cessation agent. A clinical trial by Schneider and Olsson (1996) found that treatment with 7.5 mg lobeline resulted in a sustained abstinence from tobacco over the last four weeks of the study in 10 out of 34 treated subjects compared to 8 out of 47 subjects on the placebo. A multicenter study of sublingual lobeline tablet use and cessation of smoking with 750 subjects by Glover

Lobeline. (From Dwoskin and Crooks, *Biochem. Pharmacol.,* 63:89–98, 2002. With permission.)

and coworkers (1998) found no statistical differences between lobeline and the placebo. In one of three sites, however, there was significant efficacy so that lobeline as a smoking-cessation agent still remains controversial. The ability of lobeline to inhibit amphetamine-induced release of dopamine *in vitro* and amphetamine-induced hyperactivity suggested to Dwoskin and Crooks (2002) that lobeline and its analogues could act as therapeutic agents for treating methamphetamine abuse. The potential of lobeline as a novel pharmacotherapy for treating psychostimulant abuse was further confirmed by Miller and coworkers (2003), who showed lobeline attenuated locomotor stimulation in rats induced by the repeated nicotine administration.

References

Dwoskin, L.P. and Crooks, P.A., A novel mechanism of action and potential use of lobeline as a treatment for psychostimulant abuse, *Biochem. Pharmacol.,* 63:89–98, 2002.

Glover, E.D., Leischow, S.J., Rennard, S.I., Glover, P.N., Daughton, D., Quirin, J.N., Schneider, F.H., and Mione, P.J., A smoking cessation trial with lobeline sulfate: A pilot study, *Am. J. Health Behav.,* 22:62–74, 1998.

Miller, D.K., Harrod, S.B., Green, T.A., Wong, M.-Y., Bardo, M.T., and Dwoskin, L.P., Lobeline attenuates locomotor stimulation induced by repeated nicotine administration in rats, *Pharmacol. Biochem. Behav.,* 74:279–286, 2003.

Schneider, F.H. and Olsson, T.A., Clinical-experience with lobeline as a smoking cessation agent, *Med. Chem. Res.,* 6:562–570, 1996.

Lovage (*Levisticum officinale* Koch.)   Lovage, a member of the *Apiaceae* family, is an aromatic and perennial medicinal herb grown extensively in Europe. The name is derived from its reputation as a love charm or aphrodisiac (Stuart, 1989). The essential oil from its leaves, seeds, and roots is used in food, beverages, and perfumery (Cu et al., 1990). Of 191 compounds identified in the oil, Toulemonde and Noleau (1988) showed that β-phellandrene accounted for 63 percent of the seed oil, while *n*-butyl-idene-4,5-dihydrophthalide was the major constituent in root oil (67 percent). Bylaite and coworkers (1998) showed that lovage seeds and flowers were the richest sources of oil with α-terpinyl acetate, the major constituent in the leaves and stems (up to 70 percent), while β-phellandrene accounted for 61.5 percent and 40.8 percent of the seed and flower oils, respectively. They also identified Z-ligustilide as a major phthalide in lovage leaves and stem oils, ranging from 4.4 percent–11.7 percent and 4.8–13.8 percent, respectively, depending on the harvesting time. Later work by Bylaite and coworkers (2000), using dynamic headspace-gas chromatography and olfactometry analysis, showed that while β-phellandrene was the dominant constituent in lovage oil, its impact on aroma was not the most significant.

The medicinal properties of lovage can be traced back to the Benedictine monks who recommended chewing the seed to aid digestion and relieve flatulence (Stuart, 1989). Lovage roots were also known for centuries to possess carminative and spasmolytic activity (Segebrecht and Schilcher, 1989). Its use as a folk medicine in Europe is related to its calming effect on the stomach, as well as in the treatment of congestion, rheumatism, and migraine headaches. It was approved in Germany for inflamed urinary tract and preventing kidney stones (Hogg et al., 2001). Excessive dosages of lovage should be avoided by pregnant women, as it promotes the onset of menstruation, while its irritant action can cause kidney damage (Maybe et al., 1988; Stuart, 1989)

References

Bylaite, E., Roozen, J.P., Legger, A., Venskutonis, R.P., and Posthumus, M.A., Dynamic headspace-gas chromatography-olfactometry analysis of different anatomical parts of lovage (*Levisticum officinale* Koch.) at eight growing stages, *J. Agric. Food Chem.*, 48:6183–6190, 2000.

Bylaite, E., Venskutonis, R.P., and Roozen, J.P., Influence of harvesting time on the composition of volatile components in different anatomical parts of lovage (*Levisticum officinale* Koch.), *J. Agric. Food Chem.*, 46:3735–3740, 1998.

Cu, J.-Q., Pu, F., Shi, Y., Perineu, F., Delmas, M., and Gaset, A., The chemical composition of lovage headspace and essential oil produced by solvent extraction with various solvents, *J. Essent. Oil Res.*, 2:53–59, 1990.

Hogg, C.L., Svoboda, K.P., Hampson, J.B., and Brocklehurst, S., Investigation into the composition and bioactivity of essential oil from lovage (*Levisticum officinale* W.D.J. Koch), *Inter. J. Aromather.*, 11:144–151, 2001.

Matbe, R., McIntyre, M., Michael, P., Duff, G., and Stevens, J., *The Complete New Herbal*, Hamilton, London, 1988.

Segebrecht, S. and Schilcher, H., Ligustilide: Guiding component for preparation of *Levisticum officinale* roots, *Planta Med.*, 55:572–573, 1989.

Stuart, M., *The Encyclopedia of Herbs and Herbalism*, Macdonald and Co. Ltd., 1989

Toulemonde, B. and Noleau, I., Volatile constituents of lovage (*Levisticum officinale* Koch.), in *Flavors and Fragrances, A World Perspective*, Lawrence, B.M., Mookherjee, B.D., and Willis, B.J., Eds., Elsevier Science Publishers, Netherlands, 1988, pp. 641–657.

Low-density lipoprotein *see* **Lipoproteins**

Lunasin Lunasin, a soybean peptide consisting of 43 amino acids, contains at the carboxyl end none Asp(D) residues, an Arg-Gly-Arg (RGD) cell adhesion motif, and a predicted helix with structural homology to a conserved region of chromatin-binding proteins. Galvez and de Lumen (1999) reported that transfection of mammalian cells with the lunasin gene arrested mitosis, resulting in cell death. Galvez et al. (2001) further confirmed the chemopreventive properties of soybean lunasin by its ability to induce apoptosis in the SENCAR mouse-skin cancer model. Application of lunasin (250 μg/week) reduced skin-tumor incidence/mouse by 70 percent, as well as delayed the appearance of tumors by two weeks compared to the control. The antitumor activity of lunasin action resulted from its ability to prevent histone acetylation by binding preferentially to deacylated histone H4 *in vitro*. Jeong and coworkers (2003) showed the feasibility of large-scale production of soybean lunasin capable of suppressing the formation of mammalian cells by an oncongene.

Using Western blot analysis, Jeong et al. (2002) isolated and purified a lunasin peptide from barley. Different barley lunasin fractions

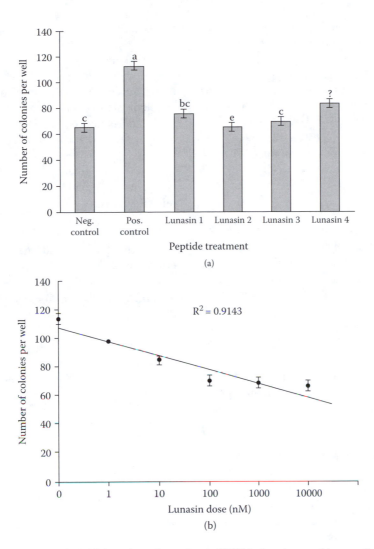

FIGURE L.64 Purified lunasin inhibits colony formation in IPTG-induced *ras* stably transformed 2-12 cells. (a) At a concentration of 10 μM, barley lunasin purified using different methods was as effective in inhibiting colony formation as synthetic lunasin. Negative control was not treated with IPTG, while positive control was treated with IPTG without lunasin. Lunasin 1 is the crude extract of barley lunasin; lunasin 2 is lunasin 1 purified by ion-exchange chromatography by elution at 0.7 M NaCl and not dialyzed before bioassay; lunasin 3 is lunasin 2 purified by immunoaffinity chromatography; and lunasin 4 is synthetic lunasin. Treatment means (± standard errors) with similar letters are not significantly different from each other, as analyzed by a One-Way ANOVA followed by Duncan's Multiple Range Test. (b) Dose response of immuno-purified barley lunasin fraction in suppression of colony formation. Each lunasin dose represents the means (± standard error) of triplicate experiments. (Jeong et al., *J. Agric. Food Chem.*, 50:5903–5908, 2002. With permission)

were shown to inhibit colony formation in iso-propyl-β-D-thiogalactoside (IPTG)-induced, *ras*-stably infected mouse-fibroblast cells as effectively as a chemically synthesized lunasin at a concentration of 10 μM (Figure L.64). These fractions also inhibited histone acetylation, attributed previously to the antitumor properties of soybean lunasin. Identification of

lunasin in barley suggests it could be present in other plant seeds.

References

Galvez, A.F., Chen, N., Macbieh, J., and de Lumen, B.O., Chemopreventive property of a soybean peptide (lunasin) that binds to deacylated histones and inhibits acetylation, *Cancer Res.*, 61:7473–7478, 2001.

L

Galvez, A.F. and de Lumen, B.O., A soybean cDNA encoding a chromatin-binding peptide inhibits mitosis of mammalian cells, *Nat. Biotech.,* 17:495–500, 1999.

Jeong, H.J., Lam, Y., and de Lumen, B.O., Barley lunasin suppresses *ras*-induced colony formation and inhibits core histone acetylation in mammalian cells, *J. Agric. Food Chem.,* 50:5903–5908, 2002.

Jeong, H.J., Park, J.H., Lam, Y., and de Lumen, B.O., Characterization of lunasin isolated from soybean, *J. Agric. Food Chem.,* 51:7901–7906, 2003.

Lutein   Lutein is a 40-carbon hydroxylated carotenoid or xanthophyll yellow pigment in dark-green vegetables, as well as in egg yolk, corn, orange juice, melon, and orange peppers masked by chlorophyll (Pfander, 1992; Sommerburg et al., 1998). It is found, together with zeaxanthin, in large concentrations in the area of the human retina involved in central vision, known as macula lutea.

Both of these pigments are implicated in the pathogenesis of macular degeneration, a condition leading to loss of vision in the elderly (Seddon et al., 1994).

Epidemiological evidence pointed to an association between macular degeneration and carotenoid intake. The concentration of lutein and zeaxanthin were significantly lower in eyes suffering from macular degeneration compared to healthy controls (Beatty et al., 2001). Researchers at the University of Pennsylvania showed that supplementation of lutein by patients suffering from choroideremia, a genetically linked retinal disease, significantly increased the macular optical density (Duncan et al., 2002). A 50 percent increase in macular pigment optical density was also reported by Richer and coworkers (2002), which further established the role of lutein in improving visual function in patients suffering from age-related macular degeneration. Semba and Dagnelie (2003) concluded that lutein and zeaxan-

thin acted as antioxidants reducing photo-oxidative stress in the retina by deactivating highly reactive singlet oxygen $^1O_2$. A two-year, double-blind, placebo-controlled study by Olmedilla and coworkers (2003) showed that only supplementation with lutein improved visual acuity of patients with age-related cataracts compared to α-tocopherol and the placebo (Figure L.65). These results suggested that long-term supplementation with lutein could be beneficial to individuals suffering from age-related cataracts.

References

Alves, Rodrigues, A., and Shao, A., The science behind lutein, *Toxicol. Lett.,* 150:57–83, 2004.

Beatty, S., Murray, I.J., Henson, D.B., Carden, D., Koh, H.H., and Boulton, M.E., Macular pigment and risk for age-related macular degeneration in subjects from a northern European population, *Invest. Ophthamol. Vis. Sci.,* 40:439–446, 2001.

Duncan, J.L., Aleman, T.S., Gardner, L.M., De Castro, E., Marks, Bennett, J.D.A., Emmons, J.M., Bieber, M.L., Steinberg, J.D., Stone, E.M., MacDonald, I.M., Cideciyan, A.V., Maguire, M.G., and Jacobson, S.G., Macular pigment and lutein supplementation in choroideremia, *Exp. Eye Res.,* 74:371–381, 2002.

Olmedilla, B., Pharm, D., Granado, F., Blanco, I., and Vaquero, M., Lutein, but not α-tocopherol, supplementation improves visual function in patients with age-related cataracts: A 2 year double-blind, placebo-controlled pilot study, *Nutrition,* 19:21–24, 2003.

Pfander, H., Carotenoids: An overview, *Methods Enzymol.,* 213:3–13, 1992.

Richer, S., Stiles, W., Statkute, L., Pei, K.Y., Frankowski, J., Nyland, J., Pulido, J., and Rudy, Y., The lutein antioxidant trial (LAST)(Abstract), *ARVO,* B539, 2002.

Seddon, J., Ajani, U.A., Sperduto, R.D., Hiller, R., Blair, N., Burton, T.C., Farber, M.D., Grogouda, E.S., Haller, J., and Miller, D.T., Dietary carotenoids, vitamins A, C, and E and advanced age-related macular degeneration, Eye disease case-control study group, *J. Am. Med. Assoc.,* 272:1413–1420, 1994.

Lutein. (Adapted from Alves-Rodrigues and Shao, *Toxicol. Lett.,* 150:57–83, 2004.)

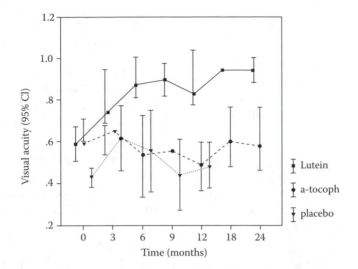

FIGURE L.65 Changes in visual acuity of patients with cataracts during supplementation study (eyes were assessed individually). Lutein group (n = 9), α-tocopherol (n = 10), and placebo group (n = 7), CI, confidence interval. (Olmedilla et al., *Nutrition,* 19:21–24, 2003. With permission.)

Semba, R.D. and Dagnelie, G., Are lutein and zeax-anthin conditionally essential nutrients for eye health? *Med. Hypoth.,* 61:465–472, 2003.

Sommerburg, O., Kuenen, J.E.E., Bird, A.C., and van Kiujik, F.J.G.M., Fruits and vegetables that are sources of lutein and zeaxanthin: Macular pigments in human eyes, *Br. J. Ophthamol.,* 82:907–910, 1998.

Luteolin Luteolin, a 3′, 4′, 5,7-tetrahydroxy-flavone, is found in the glycosylated form in celery, green pepper, perilla leaf, and chamomile tea (Shimoi et al., 1998). It has been shown to exhibit antimutagenic, antitumorigenic, anti-oxidant, and anti-inflammatory properties (Samejima et al., 1995; Kim et al., 1999; Casagrande and Darbon, 2001; Xagorari et al., 2001). Casagrande and Darbon (2003) found luteolin was a potent inhibitor of lipopolysac-charide (LPS)-stimulated nuclear factor-kappa B (NF-κB) transcriptional activity in Rat-1

Luteolin. (From Li et al., *J. Pharm. Biomed. Anal.,* 37:615–620, 2005. With permission.)

fibroplasts by modulating the transcription complex assembly in the fibroplasts. Miagkov et al. (1998) showed NF-κB played a critical role in chronic inflammation.

References

Casagrande, F. and Darbon, J-M., Effects of structurally related flavonoids on cell cycle progression of human melanoma cells: Regulation of cyclin-dependent kinases CDK2 and CDK1, *Biochem. Pharmacol.,* 61:1205–1215, 2001.

Kim, H.K., Cheon, B.S., Kim, Y.-H., Kim, S.Y., and Kim, H.P., Effects of naturally occurring flavonoids on nitric oxide production in the macrophage cell line RAW 264.7 and their structure-activity relationships, *Biochem. Pharmacol.,* 58:759–765, 1999.

Kim, S.-H., Shin, K.-J., Kim, Y.-H., Han, M.S., Lee, T.G., Kim, E., Ryu, S.H., and Suh, P.-G., Luteolin inhibits the nuclear factor κB transcriptional activity of rat-1 fibroblasts, *Biochem. Pharmacol.,* 66:955–963, 2003.

Li, L., Jiang, H., Wu, H., and Zeng, S., Simultaneous determination of luteolin and apigenin in dog plasma by RP-HPLC, *J. Pharm. Biomed. Anal.,* 37:615–620, 2005.

Miagkov, A.V., Kovalenko, D.V., Brown, C.E., Didsbury, J.R., Cogswell, J.P., Stimpson, S.A., Baldwin, A.S., and Makarov, S.S., NF-κB activation provides the potential link between inflammation and hyperplasia in the arthritic joint, *Proc. Natl. Acad. Sci.,* 95:13859–13864, 1998.

Samejima. K., Kanazawa, K., Ashida, H., and Danno, G., Luteolin: A strong antimutagen against dietary carcinogen, Tr-P-2, in peppermint, sage, and thyme, *J. Agric. Food Chem.*, 43:410–414, 1995.

Shimoi, K., Okada, H., Furugori, M., Goda, T., Takase, S., Suzuki, M., Hara, Y., and Kinae, N., Intestinal absorption of luteolin and luteolin 7-*O*-beta-glucoside in rats and humans, *FEBS Lett.*, 438:220–224, 1998.

Xagorari, A., Papapetropolous, A., Mauromatis, A., Economou, M., Fotsis, T., and Roussos, C., Luteolin inhibits an endotoxin-stimulated phosphorylation cascade and proinflammatory cytokine production in macrophages, *J. Pharmacol. Exp. Ther.*, 296:181–187, 2001.

Lycopene Lycopene is an acyclic isomer of the carotenoid β-carotene without any vitamin A activity (Stahl and Sies, 1996). It is found in abundance in fresh, ripe tomatoes and to a lesser extent in watermelon, papaya, guava, and grapefruit. Structurally, lycopene is a highly unsaturated, straight-chain hydrocarbon in which 11 of its 13 double bonds are conjugated (Argawal and Rao, 2000). It occurs predominantly in the *trans* isomer but undergoes isomerization to the *cis* isomer during heat processing. In fact, the increased levels of the *cis* isomer accounts for the much greater absorption of lycopene in processed tomato products (Stahl and Sies, 1992). Lycopene is a potent antioxidant with singlet oxygen-quenching ability twice that of β-carotene and 10 times that of α-tocopherol and is also able to inactivate hydrogen peroxide and nitrogen dioxide (Bohm et al., 2001; Heber and Lu, 2002).

Epidemiological studies showed that diets supplemented with lycopene reduced the risk of many chronic diseases, such as cancer and heart disease (Edward, 1999). The benefits associated with lycopene are related to its potent antioxidant properties through its ability to scavenge free radicals (Mortensen et al., 1997). Porrini and Riso (2000) showed that a daily consumption of 25 grams of tomato paste by healthy young women significantly increased plasma and lymphocyte lycopene concentrations after 14 days. Exposure of collected blood lymphocyte samples to free radicals using the Comet Test showed a significant reduction of 50 percent DNA damage compared to the control samples. A further study by Chen and associates (2001) showed that dietary lycopene fed to men with prostate cancer significantly reduced hydroxylated guanosine (8-OHdG), a by-product and useful biomarker of oxidative DNA damage in cell nuclei, by 21.3 percent. This indicated that lycopene exerted a protective effect on white blood cells by reducing oxidative damage in cancerous prostate tissue. Bowen and coworkers (2002) showed that consumption of tomato-sauce dishes containing 30 mg of lycopene per day for three weeks by 22 patients with localized prostate adenocarcinoma significantly reduced serum-prostate-specific antigen (PSA) levels and DNA oxidation. A recent examination of patients undergoing colonoscopy for colorectal adenomas by Erhardt et al. (2003) showed plasma lycopene concentrations were inversely related to adenoma risk, further supporting the protective role of lycopene against colorectal cancer.

Nara and coworkers (2001) reported that only when HL-60 human promyelocytic leukemia cells were exposed to an autoxidized mixture of lycopene (6 µM) for five days did they undergo apoptosis. Zhang et al. (2003) subsequently identified an oxidized cleavage product of lycopene, (*E,E,E*)-4-methyl-8-oxo-2,4,6-nonatrienal (MON), which they found induced

(*E,E,E*)-4-methyl-8-oxo-2,4,6-nonatrienal (MON). (From Zhang et al., *Free Rad. Biol. Med.*, 35:1653–1663, 2003. With permission.)

Lycopene. (Adapted from Alves-Rodrigues, A. and Shao, A., *Toxicol. Lett.*, 150:57–83, 2004.)

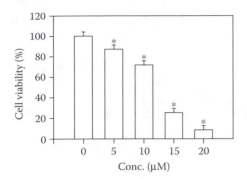

FIGURE L.66 Effect of (*E,E,E*)-4-methyl-8-oxo-2,4,6-nonatrienal on the viability of HL-60 cells. The cell viability was evaluated by the MTT method and is expressed as the percentage of the value of the control culture treated with the vehicle (THF) alone. Values represent means ± SD of eight wells. The asterisk indicates a value significantly different from the vehicle value ($p < 0.01$). Statistical comparisons were made by the Scheff's F-test. (Zhang et al., *Free Rad. Biol. Med.,* 35:1653–1663, 2003.)

DNA fragmentation and apoptosis in a time- and dose-dependent manner. Cell viability was reduced to 71.6 percent of the control in the presence of 10 μM MON (Figure L.66).

Lycopene can also prevent cardiovascular disease. Supplementing the diet of six healthy human subjects with 60 mg/day of lycopene for three months significantly reduced their plasma LDL cholesterol levels by 14 percent (Furhman et al., 1997). Treatment of hypertensive patients with 15 mg per day of lycopene in the form of a capsule was found by Paran and Engelhard (2001) to reduce systolic blood pressure by almost 100 mm Hg over an eight-week period. Mohanty et al. (2002) also found that lycopene protected the human lens from oxidative damage and had potential as an anticataract agent.

Lycopene's potent antioxidant property could provide a treatment for neurodegenerative diseases. A recent study by Suganuma and coworkers (2003) found dietary lycopene attenuated the age-related learning in senescence-accelerated mice (SAMPS) by ameliorating the memory deficits in these animals. A recent review of lycopene and human health by Rao and Rao (2003) is recommended.

References

Alves, Rodrigues, A. and Shao, A., The science behind lutein, *Toxicol. Lett.,* 150:57–83, 2004.

Argawal, S. and Rao, A.V., Carotenoids and chronic diseases, *Drug Metab. Drug Interact.,* 17:189–210, 2000.

Bohm, F., Edge, R., Burke, M., and Truscott, T.G., Dietary uptake of lycopene protects human cells from singlet oxygen and nitrogen dioxide-ROS components from cigarette smoke, *J. Photochem. Photobiol. B. Biol.,* 64:176–178, 2001.

Bowen, P., Chen, L., Stacewicz-Sapuntzakis, M., Duncan, C., Sharifi, R., Ghosh, L., Kim, H.S., Christov-Tzelkov, K., and van Breemen, R., Tomato sauce supplementation and prostate cancer: Lycopene accumulation and modulation of biomarkers of carcinogenesis, *Exp. Biol. Med.,* 227:886–893, 2002.

Chen, L., Stacewicz-Sapuntzakis, M., Duncan, C., Sharafi, R., Ghosh, L., Van Breeman, R., Ashton, D., and Bowen, P.E., Oxidative damage in prostate cancer patients consuming tomato sauce-based entrees as a whole food intervention, *J. Natl. Cancer Inst.,* 93:1872–1879, 2001.

Erhardt, J.G., Meisner, C., Bode, J.C., and Bode, C., Lycopene, β-carotene and colorectal adenomas, *Am. J. Clin. Nutr.,* 78:1219–1224, 2003.

Furhman, B., Elis, A., and Aviram, M., Hypocholesterolemic effect of lycopene and β-carotene is related to suppression of cholesterol synthesis and augmentation of LDL receptor activity in macrophage, *Biochem. Biophys. Res. Commun.,* 233:58–662, 1997.

Edward, G., Tomato, tomato-based products, lycopene, and cancer: Review of epidemiological literature, *J. Natl. Cancer Inst.,* 91:317–331, 1999.

Giovannucci, E., Tomatoes, tomato-based products, lycopene, and cancer: Review of the epidemiologic literature, *J. Natl. Cancer Inst.,* 91:317–331, 1999.

Giovannucci, E., Ascherio, A., Rimm, E.B., Stampfer, M.J., Colditz, G.A., and Willett, W.C., Intake of carotenoids and retinol in relation to risk of prostate cancer, *J. Natl. Cancer Inst.,* 87:1767–1776, 1995.

Heber, D. and Lu, Q.-Y., Overview of mechanisms of action of lycopene, *Exp. Biol. Med.,* 227:920–923, 2002.

Hurham, B., Elis, A., and Aviram, M., Hypocholesterolemic effect of lycopene and β-carotene is related to suppression of cholesterol synthesis and augmentation of LDL receptor activity in macrophage, *Biochem. Biophys. Res. Commun.,* 233:658–662, 1997.

L

Mohanty, I., Joshi, S., Trivedi, D., Srivastava, S., and Gupta, S.K., Lycopene prevents sugar-induced morphological changes and modulates antioxidant status of human lens epithelial cells, *Br. J. Nutr.,* 88:347–354, 2002.

Mortensen, A., Skibsted, L.H., Sampson, J., Rice-Evans, C., and Everett, S.A., Comparative mechanisms and rates of free scavenging by carotenoid antioxidants, *FEBS Lett.,* 418(1–2):91–97, 1997.

Nara, E., Hayashi, H., Kotake, M., Miyashita, K., and Nagao, A., Acyclic carotenoids and their oxidation mixtures inhibit the growth of HL-60 human promyelocytic leucemia cells, *Nutr. Cancer,* 39:273–283, 2001.

Paran, E. and Engelhard, Y., Effect of Lyc-O-Mato, standardized tomato extract on blood pressure, serum lipoproteins, plasma homocysteine and oxidative stress markers in grade 1 hypertensive patients, *Proceedings of the 16th Annual Scientific Meeting of the Society of Hypertension,* San Francisco, 2001.

Porrini, M. and Riso, P., Lymphocyte lycopene concentration and DNA protection from oxidative damage is increased in women after a short period of tomato consumption, *J. Nutr.,* 130:189–192, 2000.

Rao, A.V. and Rao, L.G., Lycopene and human health, *Nutr. Genom. Funct. Foods,* 1:35–44, 2003.

Stahl, W. and Sies, H., Uptake of lycopene and its geometrical isomers is greater from heat-processed than from unprocessed tomato juice in humans, *J. Nutr.,* 122:2161–2166, 1992.

Stahl, W. and Sies, H., Lycopene: A biologically important carotenoid in humans? *Arch. Biochem. Biophys.,* 336:1–9, 1996.

Suganuma, H., Hiran, T., Kaburagi, S., Hayakawa, K., and Inakuma, T., Ameliorative effects of dietary carotenoids on memory deficits in senescence-accelerated mice (SAMPS), *Int. Congress Series,* 1260:129–135, 2003.

Zhang, H., Kotake-Nara, E., Ono, H., and Nagao, A., A novel cleavage product formed by autoxidation of lycopene induces apoptosis in HL-60 cells, *Free Rad. Biol. Med.,* 35:1653–1663, 2003.

Lysine The essential amino acid, L-lysine, has been used for many years as its monohydrochloride salt (LMH) to improve the diets of many Third World countries (Flodin, 1993). Research in the 1970s suggested that oral supplements of lysine monohydrochloride

suppressed recurrent herpes simplex infections (Griffith et al., 1978). As a result, pharmaceutical-grade LMH supplements are readily available in 500-mg tablets. An excellent review of the pharmacology and toxicology of lysine was published by Flodin (1997). Sarubin (2003) suggested that daily supplements of up to 3 grams of lysine appear to be safe. However, Marcason (2003) cautioned that diets high in lysine or with high lysine:arginine ratios were found to be hypercholesterolemic in some animal studies.

Poly-L-lysine has also been shown to inhibit the herpes simplex virus type 1 (HSV) by possibly preventing its adsorption (Langeland et al., 1988; WuDunn and Spear, 1989). Egal and coworkers (1999) found that magainins, a class of cationic peptides rich in lysine and octanoyl groups originally isolated from the skin of the African clawed frog (*Xeenopus laevis*), had a direct antiviral effect on HSV.

References

Egal, M., Conrad, M., MacDonald, D.L., Maloy, W.L., Motley, M., and Genco, C.A., Antiviral effects of synthetic membrane-active peptides on herpes simplex virus type 1, *Int. J. Antimicrob. Agents,* 13:57–60, 1999.

Flodin, N.W., Lysine supplementation of cereal foods: A retrospective, *J. Am. Coll. Nutr.,* 12:486–500, 1993.

Flodin, N.W., The metabolic roles, pharmacology, and toxicology of lysine, *J. Am. Coll. Nutr.,* 16:7–21, 1997.

Griffith, R.S., Norins, A.L., and Kagan, C., A multicentered study of lysine therapy in herpes simplex infection, *Dermatologica,* 156:257–267, 1978.

Langeland, N., Moore, L.J., Holmsen, H., and Haar, L., Interaction of polylysine with the cellular receptor for herpes simplex virus type 1, *J. Gen. Virol.,* 69:1137–1145, 1988.

Marcason, W., Will taking the amino acid supplement lysine prevent or treat herpes simplex virus? *J. Am. Diet. Assoc.,* 103:351, 2003.

Sarubin, F., Lysine, *The Health Professional's Guide to Popular Dietary Supplements,* 2nd ed., American Dietetic Association, Chicago, 2003, pp. 269–273.

WuDunn, D. and Spear, P.G., Initial interaction of herpes simplex virus with cells is binding to heparan sulfate, *J. Virol.,* 63:52–58, 1989.

M

Maca Maca (*Lepidium meyenii*) Walp is a cruciferous vegetable native to the Andes of Peru. The tuber is consumed because of its nutritional value and phytochemical content (Dini et al., 1994). Its ethnomedicinal properties are connected to fertility and vitality. A recent study by Sandoval et al. (2002) showed Maca had strong antioxidant activity by its ability to inhibit peroxynitrite, DPPH, peroxyls, and deoxyribose degradation. The concentration of catechins is much lower in Maca compared to green tea; nevertheless it still has the capacity to scavenge free radicals and protect cells against oxidative stress.

References

Dini, F., Migliuolo, G., Rastrelli, L., Saturnino, P., and Schettino, O., Chemical composition of *Lepidium meyenii, Food Chem.,* 49:347–349, 1994.

Sandoval, M., Okuhama, N.N., Angeles, F.M., Melchor, V.V., Condezo, L.A., Lao, J., and Miller, M.J.S., Antioxidant activity of the cruciferous vegetable Maca (*Lepidium meyenii*), *Food Chem.,* 79: 207–213, 2002.

Macrolactin A Macrolactin A, a 24-member polyene macrolide containing three sets of conjugated dienes and four stereogenic centers, was first isolated from deep-sea bacterium in 1989 (Gustafson et al., 1989). It was shown to exhibit significant antiviral and anticancer properties, including inhibition of B16-F10 murine melanoma cells (Rychonovsky et al., 1992). The lack of an adequate supply of macrolactin for therapeutic purposes has resulted in attempts to synthesize macrolactin A and analogues (Marino et al., 2002; Kobayashi et al., 2004).

References

Barmann, H., Prahlad, V., Tao, C., Yun, Y.K., Wang, Z., and Donaldson, W.A., Development of organoiron methodology for preparation of the polyene natural product monolactin A, *Tetrahedron,* 56: 2283–2295, 2000.

Gustafson, K., Roman, M., and Fenical, W.J., The macrolactins, a novel class of antiviral and cytotoxic macrolides from deep-sea marine bacterium, *J. Am. Chem. Soc.,* 111:7519–7524, 1989.

Kobayashi, Y., Fukuda, A., Kimachi, T., Ju-ichi, M., and Takemoto, Y., Asymmetric synthesis of macrolactin A analogue, *Tetrahedron Lett.,* 45:677–680, 2004.

Marino, J.P., McClure, M.S., Holub, D.P., Comasseto, J.V., and Tucci, F.C., Stereocontrolled synthesis of (–)-macrolactin A, *J. Am. Chem. Soc.,* 124:1664–1668, 2003.

Rychnovsky, S.D., Skalitzky, D.J., Pathirana, C., Jensen, P.R., and Fenical, W.J., Stereochemistry of macrolactins, *J. Am. Chem. Soc.,* 114:671–677, 1992.

Microlactin A. (From Barmann et al., *Tetrahedron,* 56:2283–2295, 2000. With permission.)

Madonna lily (*Lilium candidum*) Madonna lily, known by the botanical name *Lilium candidum*, belongs to the N.O. *Lililaceae* family, which grows throughout Europe. In the early days of Christianity, it was dedicated by the church to the Madonna (hence, its popular name), probably because its delicate whiteness was considered a symbol of purity. It produces stiff, erect stems, 3–5 feet high, clothed with lance-shaped leaves. The white, bowl-shaped flowers appear in June, flowering into July, and have a strong, sweet, penetrating perfume. The bulbs were long known for their therapeutic effects. They have highly demulcent and also somewhat astringent properties. They were reported as effective medicinal materials for the external treatment of burns and swellings and as emollient cataplasms for tumors, ulcers, and external inflammation. The fresh bulb, bruised and applied to hard tumors, can often ripen them in quite a short time. Antiyeast activity was observed by Mucaji et al. (2002), while the use of *Lilium candidum* bulbs as an antiviral agent to treat shingles (*Herpes zoster*) was reported by Pieroni (2000). Spirostanol saponins and jatropham isolated from the ethanolic extract of *Lilium candidum* proved potent inhibitors (> 60 percent) of 12-*O*-tetradecanoyl-phorbol-13-acetate, a specific tumor promoter for an epidermal carcinogenesis, and in the presence of a polyaromatic carcinogenic substance 7,12-dimethylbenz(*a*)-anthracene (Vachalkova et al., 2000). Phytochemical studies on *Lilium candidum* demonstrated the existence of dimeric pyrroline derivatives, 3-methylsuccinoyl-flavone, pyrrilidineylflavone, steroidal saponins (Eisenreichova et al., 2000; Mimaki et al., 1993, 1998), and sterols (Mucaji et al., 2000). Spirostanol and furostanol saponins had inhibitory effects on Na+/K+ ATPase (Mimaki et al., 1999) and etioline, a steroidal alkaloid (Erdogan et al., 2001).

References

Eisenrichova, E., Haladova, M., Mucaji, P., Budensky, M., and Ubik, K., A new steroidal saponin from the bulbs of *Lilium candidum* L., *Pharmazie,* 55: 549–550, 2000.

Erdogan, I., Sener, B., and Attar-u-Rahman, Etioline, steroidal alkaloid from *Lilium candidum* L, *Biochem. Syst. Ecol.,* 29:535–536, 2001.

Mimaki, Y., Satou, T., Kuroda, M., Sashida, Y., and Hatakeyama, Y., New steroidal constituents from the bulbs of *Lilium candidum, Chem. Pharm. Bull.,* 46: 1829–1832, 1998.

Mimaki, Y., Satou, T., Kuroda, M., Sashida, Y., and Hatakeyama, Y., Steroidal saponins from the bulbs of *Lilium candidum* L., *Ceska Slov. Farm.,* 51:567–573, 1999.

Mucaji, P., Haladova, M., Eisenrichova, E., Budensky, M., and Ubik, K., Sterols in *Lilium candidum* L., *Ceska Slov. Farm.,* 49:29–31, 2000.

Mucaji, P., Hedecova, D., Haladova, M., and Eisenrichova, E., Anti-yeast activity of ethanol extracts of *Lilium candidum* L., *Ceska Slov. Farm.,* 51:297–300, 2002.

Pieroni, A., Medicinal plants and food medicines in the folk traditions of the upper Lucca Province, Italy, *J. Ethnopharmacol.,* 70:235–273, 2000.

Resnikova, S.A., Bugara, A.M., and Erokhina, A.I., Cytochemical study of the DNA and istone? In the tissues of the lily anther in the course of microsporo- and gametogenesis, *Onogenez,* 10:276–284, 1979 (Russian).

Vachalkova, A., Eisenrichova, E., Haladova, M., Mucaji, P., Jozova, B., and Novotny, L., Potential carcinogenic and inhibitory activity of compounds isolated from *Lilium candidum* L., potential carcinogenic and inhibitory activity of compounds isolated from *Lilium candidum* L., *Neoplasma,* 47:313–318, 2000.

Mangiferin Mangiferin, 1,3,6,7-tetrahydroxyxanthone-C2-β-D-glucoside, found in higher plants, such as the stem bark of *Manginfera indica* L., is a constituent of folk medicines. It has attracted considerable attention because it is pharmacologically active, exhibiting antitumor and antiviral (Guha et al., 1996; Yoosook et al., 2000), antidiabetic (Ichiki et al., 1998; Miura et al., 2001), antibone resorption (Li et al., 1998), and antioxidant properties (Sanches et al., 2000). Yoshimi et al. (2001) showed 0.1 percent mangiferin significantly inhibited the development of aberrant crypt foci (ACF) in azoxymethane-induced tumorigenesis in F344 rats. Leiro and coworkers (2003) reported

Structure of mangiferin. (From Yoshimi et al., *Cancer Lett.,* 163:163–170, 2001. With permission.)

TABLE M.47
Effect of Mangiferin Given Intraperitoneally Daily for 28 Days on Erythrocyte MDA, CAT, and SOD in STZ-Induced Diabetic Rats

Treatment	Erythrocyte		
	nM of MDA/mL Packed RBC	CAT ($\times 10^3$)[a]U	SOD (U)
Normal rats	5.86 ± 0.06	6.06 ± 1.15	81.00 ± 7.15
Negative results	0.43 ± 0.76	3.46 ± 0.49	52.10 ± 13.59
Insulin (6 UI/kg)	5.93 ± 0.51*	4.90 ± 1.22	73.51 ± 16.57
Mangiferin (10 mg/kg)	5.43 ± 1.06*	4.28 ± 1.32	65.86 ± 8.97
Mangiferin (20 mg/kg)	5.74 ± 0.86*	3.92 ± 0.38	82.54 ± 10.46

U-one unit of SOD is the amount (in :g) of protein required to inhibit MTT reduction by 50%.

Values are means ± SE of six animals.

* $p < 0.05$ as compared to negative control.

[a] U-velocity constant/s

Source: From Muruganandan et al., *Toxicology,* 176:165–173, 2002. With permission.

mangiferin was a potent antioxidant that scavenged superoxide ions. Mangiferin also modulated gene expression of iNOS and cytokines, which regulate macrophage activity and participate in the regulation of NOS production, such as TNF-α and TNF-β. Thus, mangiferin may be useful for the treatment of inflammatory diseases, atherosclerosis, or septic shock. Stimulation of TNF-β, a cytokine inhibitor of angiogenesis (Mandriota et al., 1996), could also provide a useful treatment for blocking tumor growth or protect against autoimmune diseases. Garrido et al. (2004) reported, for the first time, inhibition of TNF-α and NO production by an aqueous extract of *Mangiferin indica* L. against endotoxic septic shock and microglia in rats.

A protective effect was also exerted by mangiferin in streptozotocin-induced oxidative damage to cardiac and renal tissues in rats (Muruganandan et al., 2002). This was evident by a decrease in renal and erythrocyte malondialdehyde (MDA) and catalase (CAT) and an increase in superoxide dismutase (SOD) in rats fed mangiferin intraperitoneally daily for 28 days (Table M.47).

References

Garrido, G., Delgado, R., Lemus, Y., Rodriguez, J., Garcia, D., and Nunex-Selles, A.J., Protection against septic shock and suppression of tumor necrosis factor alpha and nitric oxide production on macrophages and microglia by a standard aqueous extract *Mangifera indica* L. (VIMANG®): Role of mangiferin isolated from the extract, *Pharmacol. Res.,* 50:165–172, 2004.

Guha, S., Ghosal, S., and Chattopadhyay, U., Anti-tumor, immunodilatory and anti-HIV effect of mangiferin, a naturally occurring glucosylxanthone, *Chemother.,* 42:4432–4451, 1996.

Ichiki, H., Miura, T., Kubo, M., Ishihara, E., Komastu, Y., Tanigawa, K., and Okada, M., New antidiabetic compounds, mangiferin and its glucoside, *Biol. Pharm. Bull.,* 21:1389–1390, 1998.

Leiro, J.M., Alvarez, E., Arranz, J.A., Siso, I.G., and Orallo, F., *In vitro* effects of mangiferin on superoxide concentrations and expression of the inducible nitric oxide synthase, tumor necrosis factor-α and transforming growth factor-β genes, *Biochem. Pharmacol.,* 65:1361–1371, 2003.

Li, H., Miyahara, T., Tezuka, Y., Namba, T., Nemoto, N., Tonami, S., Seto, H., Tada, T., and Kadota, S., The effect of Kampo formulae on bone resorption *in vitro* and *in vivo*, 1, Active constituents of Tsu-Kan-yan, *Biol. Pharm. Bull.,* 21:1322–1326, 1998.

Mandriota, S.J., Menoud, P.-A., and Peppers, M.S., Transforming growth factor β1 down-regulators vascular endothelial growth receptor 2/flk-1 expression in vascular endothelial cells, *J. Biol. Chem.,* 271:11500–11505, 1996.

Miura, T., Ichiki, H., Hashimoto, L., Iwamoto, N., Kato, M., Kubo, M., Ishihara, E., Komatsu, Y., Okada, M., Ishida, T., and Tanigawa, K., Antidiabetic activity of a xanthone compound, mangiferin, *Phytomedicine,* 8:85–87, 2001.

M

Muruganandan, S., Gupta, S., Kataria, M., Lal, J., and Gupta, P.K., Mangiferin protects the streptozotocin-induced oxidative damage to cardiac and renal tissues in rats, *Toxicology,* 176:165–173, 2002.

Sanchez, G.M., Re, L., Giuliani, A., Nunez-Selles, A.J., Davison, G.P., and Leon-Fernandez, O.S., Protective effects of *Mangifera indica* L. extract, mangiferin and selected antioxidants against TPA-induced biomolecules oxidation and peritoneal macrophage activation in mice, *Pharmacol. Res.,* 42: 565–573, 2000.

Yoosook, C., Bunyapraphatsara, N., Boonakiat, Y., and Katasuk, Y., Anti-herpes simplex virus activities of crude water extracts of Thai medicinal plants, *Phytomedicine*, 6:411–419, 2000.

Yoshimi, N., Matsunaga, K., Katayama, M., Yamada, Y., Kuno, T., Qiao, Z., Hara, A., Yamahara, J., and Mori, H., The inhibitory effects of mangiferin, a naturally occuring glucosylxanthone, in bowel carcinogenesis of male F344 rats, *Cancer Lett.,* 163: 163–170, 2001.

M

Mangoes *see also* Maginiferin Mangoes (*Mangifera indica* L.) belong to the family *Anacardiaceae*, order *Rutales*. They grow naturally or are cultivated mainly in tropical and subtropical regions and are deeply entrenched in Indian history. Mangoes were mentioned in early Arialkrit literature, with Alexander the Great seeing his first in 326 BC when he traveled with his army to India. Every part of the mango is used in India. The dry twigs are used in sacrificial fires for religious ceremonies, while oil is extracted from the leaves and mixed with lime juice to treat skin ailments. Smoke from burning mango leaves are used as a cure for hiccups and sore throats; kernels are dried, ground, and used as a cure for asthma, while mango pulp is used to nurse cholera patients back to health. Dried mango flowers, containing 15 percent tannin, serve as an astringent in cases of diarrhea, chronic dysentery, catarrh of the bladder, and chronic urethritis resulting from gonorrhea. The bark contains mangiferin, polyphenols, terpenoids, steroids, fatty acids, and microelements and is astringent and employed against rheumatism and diphtheria. The resinous gum from the trunk is applied on cracks in the skin of the feet and on scabs, and is believed to be helpful in cases of syphilis.

Mangoes are an ideal summer food, as they are high in carotenoids, especially β-carotene, as well as other organic acids, such as citric acid, together with smaller amounts of shikimic, malic, and quinic acids. The sugar content varies, particularly among treatments during the storage period, although sucrose is the major sugar present in mangoes, followed by fructose and glucose (Gonzalez-Aguilar et al., 2000). Terpenes accounted for the majority of the volatile aroma components in mangoes (Macleod, 1984), while the main antioxidants are vitamins C, E, and selenium. Clinical studies showed the benefits of the high carotenoid levels in mangoes to eye health by their ability to prevent sties, corneal ulcers, and night blindness (Carlier et al., 1992; Christian et al., 1998). Extremely wide, seasonal variations in plasma ascorbic-acid levels associated with the consumption of mangoes is well known. For example, one of the first studies observed pregnant and lactating women in Keneba and Manduar, two neighboring, rural Gambian villages, showed ascorbic-acid levels peaked during the mango season in May and June, attaining a mean level of 1.4 mg/dL. The lowest levels, average 0.2 mg/dL, were observed during the rainy season in September and October (Bates et al., 1982).

The average mango (±350 g) contains 13,615 IU β-carotene (Puerto Rican analyses of 30 cultivars showed β-carotene ranged from a low of 4,171 IU/100 g in > Stringless Peach = to a high of 7,900 IU in > Carrie), 95 mg vitamin C (ascorbic acid ranged from 3.43 mg/100 g in > Keitt = to 62.96 in > Julie), and about 3.5 mg vitamin E. The mango fruit also contains B complex vitamins and minerals, such as iron, calcium (14 mg/100 g), magnesium, potassium, phosphorus, selenium, and zinc. The carotenoid composition of mango is affected by ripening, cultivar differences, and processing. Ripening affects the major carotenoids, violaxanthin and β-carotene. All *trans*-β-carotene, all *trans*-violaxanthin, and 9-*cis*-violaxanthin increased in the ripe fruit in comparison to the mature green fruits. Geographic effects also appeared to be substantial. In commercially processed mango juice, violaxanthin was not detected, while auroxanthin was present at appreciable levels, with β-carotene the main carotenoid (Mercadante and Rodriguez-Amaya, 1998). Mango seed kernel is a good source of fat (5–10 percent) (Lakshminarayana et al., 1983; Asad and Bukhari, 1996), protein (7 percent), and macronutrients, Ca (15–45 mg/100 g), Na (237–239 mg/100 g), and P (31–92 mg/100 g). It was reported to enhance the oxidative stability of clarified butter, ghee (Parmar and Sharma, 1986). Recently, antimicrobial activity of the ethanol extract of mango seed kernel against foodborne, pathogenic bacteria was demonstrated (Kabuki et al., 1997). The antioxidant activity of a high-dietary-fiber mango-peel product was also recently reported (Larrauri et al., 1997).

Mango dermatitis is a common term given to allergic contact dermatitis associated with the sap or skin of the fruit *Mangifera indica*. Patch testing with diluted sap (known to contain mangiferin, resinous acid, mangiferic acid, and the resinol, mangiferol), crushed leaf, crushed stem, and fruit skin is usually positive in these cases (Calvert et al., 1996).

References

Asad, Q. and Bukhari, S.M.Z., Study of macro and micronutrients in mango seed kernels, *Sci. Int.,* 8: 37–38, 1996.

Bates, C.J., Prentice, A.M., Prentice, A., Paul, A.A., and Whitehead, R.G., Seasonal variations in ascorbic acid status and breast milk ascorbic acid levels in rural Gambian women in relation to dietary intake, *Trans. R. Soc. Trop. Med. Hyg.,* 76:341–347, 1982.

Calvert, M.L., Robertson, I., and Samaratunga, H., Mango dermatitis: Allergic contact dermatitis to *Mangifera indica, Austrlas. J. Dermatol.,* 37:59–60, 1996.

Carlier, C., Etchepare, M., Ceccon, J.F., Mourey, M.S., and Amedee-Manesme, O., Efficacy of massive oral doses of retinyl palmitate and mango (*Mangifera indica* L.) consumption to correct existing vitamin A deficiency in Sengalese children, *Br. J. Nutr.,* 68:529–540, 1992.

Christian, P., West, K.P., Jr., Khatry, S.K., Katz, J., Shrestha, S.R., Pradhan, E.K., LeClerq, S.C., and Pokhrel, R.P., Night blindness of pregnancy in rural Nepal — nutritional health risks, *Int. J. Epidemiol.,* 27:231–237, 1998.

Gonzalez-Aguilar, G.A., Wang, C.Y., and Buta, J.G., Maintaining quality of fresh-cut mangoes using anti-browning agents and modified atmosphere packaging, *J. Agric. Food Chem.,* 48:4204–4208, 2000.

Kabuki, T., Nakajima, H., Arai, M., Ueda, S., Kuwabara, Y., and Dosako, S., Characterization of novel antimicrobial compounds from mango (*Mangifera indica* L.) kernel seeds, *Food Chem.,* 71:61–66, 2000.

Lakshminarayana, G., Chandrasekhara Rao, T., and Ramalingaswamy, P.A., Varietal variations in content, characteristic and composition of mango seeds and fat, *J. Am. Oil Chem. Soc.,* 60:88–89, 1983.

Larrauri, J.A., Ruperz, P., and Saura-Calixto, F., Mango peel fibers with antioxidant activity, Zeitschrift fuer Lebensmittel-Unterschung und Forschung A, *Food Res. Tech.,* 205:39–42, 1997.

Macleod, A.J. and Pieris, N.M., Comparison of the volatile components of some mango cultivars, *Phytochemistry,* 23:361–366, 1984.

Mercandante, A.Z. and Rodriguez-Amaya, D.B., Effect of ripening, cultivar differences, and processing on the carotenoid composition of mango, *J. Agric. Food Chem.,* 46:128–130, 1998.

Parmar, S.S. and Sharma, R.S., Use of mango seed kernels in enhancing the oxidative stability of ghee, *Asian J. Dairy Res.,* 5:91–99, 1986.

M

Manoalide   Manoalide(1), a sesquiterpenoid metabolite from the Pacific sponge *Luffariella variablis*, is a potent analgesic and anti-inflammatory agent isolated in 1980 (De Silva and Scheuer, 1980; de Freitas et al., 1984). The anti-inflammatory activity of manoalide is due to

Structure of manoalide. (From De Rosa et al., *Tetrahedron,* 56:2095–2102, 2000. With permission.)

inhibition of phospholipase A_2 (PLA_2) a hydro-lytic enzyme catalysing the release of arachidonic acid from membrane-bound phospholipids. This reaction initiates a complex cascade of biochemical reactions, leading to the formation of proinflammatory mediators, such as leukotrienes and prostaglandins. Thus, it is a key therapeutic target for the suppression of inflammation and pain (Mayer et al., 1988). Manoalide has long been known as a potent and irreversible inhibitor of PLA_2 from the venoms of different species, such as cobra, bee, and rattlesnake (Lombardo and Dennis, 1985; Reynolds et al., 1991). Structure–activity relationship studies suggest that the closed-ring form of manoalide is the predominant molecular species that accounts for the selective and potent inhibition of PLA_2 (Glaser et al., 1988). The sterioselective synthesis of manoalide was carried out for the first time by Soriente et al. (1999a). Pretreatment with manoalide was found to significantly inhibit PLA_2 activity in the synovial fluid, prevent loss of proteoglycan from the condylar cartilage, and reduce proteoglycan levels in the lavage fluids, which suggested manoalide may be an effective antiarthritic agent (Schrier et al., 1996). Manoalide was also reported to inhibit superoxide release in the pathogenesis of LPS hepatoxicity (Mayer and Spitzer, 1993). As an inhibitor of the major enzyme phospholipase A, known to be involved in different inflammatory mechanisms, manoalide was broadly studied as an anti-inflammatory agent (Mayer et al., 1988; Soriente et al., 1999b). The synthesis of potentially anti-inflammatory manoalide hybrid was recently reported by Izzo et al. (2004).

References

De Freitas, J.C., Blankmeier, L.A., and Jacobs, R.S., *In vitro* inactivation of the neurotoxin action of b-bungarotoxin by the marine product, manoalide, *Experentia,* 40:864–865, 1984.

De Rosa, M., Soriente, A., Sodano, G., and Scettri, A., Enantioselective synthesis of pyranofuranone moieties of manoalide and cacospongioinolide B by enzymatic and chemical approach, *Tetrahedron,* 56: 2095–2102, 2000.

De Silva, E.D. and Scheuer, P.J., Manoalide, an antibiotic sesquiterpenoid from marine sponge *Luffariella*

variabilis (polejaeff), *Tetrahedron Lett.,* 21:1611–1614, 1980.

Glaser, K.B., de Carvalho, M.S., Jacobs, R.S., Kerman, M.R., and Faulkner, D.J., Manoalide: structure-activity studies and definition of the pharmacophire for phospholipase A_2 inactivation, *Mol. Pharmacol.,* 36:782–786, 1989.

Glaser, K.B., Vedvick, T.S., and Jacobs, R.S., Inactivation of phospholipase A_2 by manoalide, localization of the manoalide binding site on bee venom phospholipase A_2 *Biochem. Pharmacol.,* 37:3639–3646, 1988.

Izzo, I., Avallone, E., Della Monica, C., Casapullo, A., Amigo, M., and De Riccardis, F., Synthesis of potentially anti-inflammatory IPL,576,092-contignasterol and IPL576,092-manoalide hybrids, *Tetrahedron,* 60:5587–5593, 2004.

Lombardo, D. and Dennis, E.A., Cobra venom phospholipase A_2, inhibition by manoalide, a novel type phospholipase inhibitor, *J. Biol. Chem.,* 260:7234–7240, 1985.

Mayer, A.M., Glaser, K.B., and Jacobs, R.S., Regulation of eicosanoid biosynthesis *in vitro* and *in vivo* by the marine natural product manoalide: A potent inactivator of venom phospholipases, *J. Pharmacol. Exp. Ther.,* 244:871–878, 1988.

Mayer, A.M. and Spitzer, J.A., Modulation of superoxide anion generation by manoalide, arachidonic acid and staurosporine in liver infiltrated neutrophils in a rat model of endotoxemia, *J. Pharmacol. Exp. Ther.,* 267:400–409, 1993.

Reynolds, L.J., Mihelich, E.D., and Dennis, E.A., Inhibition of venom phospholipase A_2 by manoalide and manolalogue. Stoichioretry of incorporation, *J. Biol. Chem.,* 266:16512–16517, 1991.

Schrier, D.J., Flory, C.M., Finkel, M., Kuchera, S.L., Lesch, M.E., and Jacobson, P.B., The effects of the phospholipase A_2 inhibitor, manoalide, on cartilage degradation, stromelysin expression, and synovial fluid cell count induced by intraarticular injection of human recombinant interleukin-1 alpha in the rabbit, *Arthritis Rheum.,* 39:1292–1299, 1996.

Soriente, A., De Rosa, M., Apicella, A., Scettri, A., and Sodano, G., First enantioselective synthesis of manoalide: Application of aldehyde-dioxinone enantioselective condensation, *Tetrahedron Assymm.,* 10: 4481–4484, 1999.

Soriente, A., De Rosa, M.M., Scettri, A., Sodano, G., Terencio, M.C., Paya, M., and Alcaraz, M.J., Manoalide, *Curr. Med. Chem.,* 6:415–431, 1999.

Manzamine A   Manzamine A is an alkaloid isolated from the Okinawan marine sponge, genus *Haliclona* (Sakai et al., 1986). It consists of a complex pentacyclic-ring system with a pendant β-carboline moiety.

Many related alkaloids of the manzamine family have since been isolated from different sponge genera (Edrada et al., 1996; Tsuda et al., 1997; Magnier et al., 1998; Watanabe et al., 1998; Urban et al., 2000; Sayed et al., 2001). Manzamine A was initially described as an anti-tumor agent against mouse leukemia cells (Sakai et al., 1986), and recently was shown to be an antimalarial agent against rodent malaria parasite *Plasmodium berghei* and an antituber-culosis agent (Ang et al., 2000; Higa et al.,

Manzamine A. (From Kasanah et al., *Tetrahedron Lett.*, 44:1291–1293, 2003. With permission.)

2001). Its potent biological activities and its unusual chemical structure led researchers to synthesize and study this compound (Magnier, 1998; Winkler, 1998; Coldham, 2002; Herde-mann, 2002; Humphrey, 2002). A synthetic analogue of manzamine, Mana-Hox, was shown by Tu and coworkers (2004) to be cyto-toxic against tumor cells with an IC_{50} ranging from 1 to 5 μM. Apoptosis was induced as a result of chromosome missaggregation.

References

Ang, K.K.H., Holmes, M.J., Higa, T., Hamann, M.T., and Kara, U.A.K., *In vivo* antimalarial activity of the beta-carboline alkaloid manzamine A, *Antimicrob. Agents Chemother.*, 44:1645–1649, 2000.

Ang, K.K., Holmes, M., and Kara, U., Immune-mediated parasite clearance in mice infected with *Plasmodium berghei* following treatment with man-zamine A, *Parasitol. Res.*, 87:715–721, 2001.

Coldham, I., Crapnell, K.M., Fernandez, J.C., Mose-ley, J.D., and Rabot, R., Synthesis of the ABC ring system of manzamine A, *J. Org. Chem.*, 67:6181–6187, 2002.

Edrada, R.A., Proksch, P., Wray, V., Witte, L., Muller, W.E.G., and Van Soest, R.W.M., Four new bioactive manzamine-type alkaloids from the Phillipine marine sponge *Xestospongia ashmorica*, *J. Nat. Prod.*, 59:1056–1060, 1996.

El-Sayed, K.A., Kelly, M., Kara, U.A., Ang, K.K., Katsuyama, I., Dunbar, D.C., Khan, A.A., and Hamann, M.T., New manzamine alkaloids with potent activity against infectious diseases, *J. Am. Chem. Soc.*, 123:1804–1809, 2001.

Herdemann, M., Al-Mourabit, A., Martin, M.T., and Marazano, C., From a biogenetic scenario to a syn-thesis of the ABC ring of manzamine A, *J. Org. Chem.*, 67:1890–1897, 2002.

Higa, T., Tanaka, J., Ikuko, I., Nusman, M., Roy, M.C., and Kuvoola, I., Bioactive compounds from coral reef invertebrates, *Pure Appl. Chem.*, 73:589–593, 2001.

Humphrey, J.M., Liao, Y., Ali, A., Rein, T., Wong, Y.L., Chen, H.J., Courtney, A.K., and Martin, S.F., Enantioselective total syntheses of manzamine A and related alkaloids, *J. Am. Chem. Soc.*, 124:8584–8592, 2002.

Kasanah, N., Yousaf, M., Rao, K.V., Wedge, D.E., and Hamann, M.T., The biocatalytic conversion of 8-hydroxymanzamine A to manzamine A using Fusarium solari, *Tetrahedron Lett.*, 44:1291–1293, 2003.

Lynch, V.M., Liao, Y., Martin, S.F., and Davis, B.E., Structure of a tricyclic subunit of manzamine A, *Acta Crystallogr.*, 48(Pt. 9):1703–1705, 1992.

Magnier, E. and Langlois, Y., Manzamine alkaloids, syntheses and synthetic approaches, *Tetrahedron*, 54:6201–6258, 1998.

Martin, S.F., Humphrey, J.M., Ali, A., and Hillier, M.C., Enantioselective total synthesis of ircinal A and related manzamine alkaloids, *J. Am. Chem. Soc.*, 121:866–867, 1999.

Matzanke, N., Gregg, R., and Weinreb, S., Biomi-metic and synthetic approaches to marine sponge alkaloids derived from bis-pyridine macrocyles, a review, *Org. Prep. Proc. Int.*, 30:1–51, 1998.

Sakai, R., Higa, T., Jefford, C.W., and Bernardinelli, G., Manzamine A, a novel antitumor alkaloid from a sponge, *J. Am. Chem. Soc.*, 108:6404–6405, 1986.

Tsuda, M. and Kobayashi, J., Structures and biogen-esis of manzamines and related alkaloids, *Heterocy-cles*, 46:765–794, 1997.

M

Tu, L.C., Chou, C.-K., Chen, C.-Y., Chang, Y.-T., Shen, Y.-C., and Yeh, S.-F., Characterization of the cytotoxic mechanism of Mana-Hox, an analog of manzamine alkaloids, *Biochem. Biophys. Acta,* 1672: 148–156, 2004.

Watanabe, D., Tsuda, M., and Kobayashi, J., Three new manzamine congeners from amphimedon sponge, *J. Nat. Prod.,* 61:689–692, 1998.

Winkler, J.D. and Axten, J.M., The first total synthesis of ircinol A, ircinal A, and manzamine A and D, *J. Am. Chem. Soc.,* 120:6425–6426, 1998.

Marine products, *see also* **Bryostatin, Glucosamine/Chondroitin sulfate, Halichondrin B, Manoalide, and Manzamine A**   Over the past several decades, scientists have identified a core group of bioactive marine products with potential therapeutic properties. In a review by Faulkner (2000), a number of pharmacologically active products were reviewed, including bryostatins, curacin A, debromohymenialdisine, didemnin, discodermolide, dolastatin, ecteinascidin, eleutherobin, halichondrin B manoalides, pseudopterosins, topsetins, scytonemin, and debromohymenialdisine. One of the limitations is the lack of availability of some of these compounds, although chemical synthesis of manzamine analogues has provided an alternative source (Tu et al., 2004). In addition, aquaculture of marine invertebrates provides an alternative technology for their production, as well as tissue culture of invertebrate cells.

References

Faulkner, D.J., Marine pharmacology, *Antonie van Leeuwenhock,* 77:135–145, 2000.

Tu, L.C., Chou, C.-K., Chen, C.-Y., Chang, Y.-T., Shen, Y.-C., and Yeh, S.-F., Characterization of Mana-Hox, an analog of manzamine alkaloids, *Biochem. Biophys. Acta,* 1672:148–156, 2004.

Marine sponges *see also* **Manzamine A** Marine sponges found in Korean waters included genus *Petrosia*, which contains a number of polyacetylenes that are cytotoxic against several human tumor-cell lines. Kim et al. (1998) first isolated four new polyacetylenes from marine sponge, *Petrosia* sp., with cytotoxicity toward human tumor-cell lines. Several structures were identified, including duryne (1) and petrosynol (2). Kim and coworkers (2002) later showed these polyacetylenes inhibited DNA replication and predominantly inhibited the initiation stage of DNA replication.

References

Kim, J.S., Im, K.S., Jung, J.H. Kim, Y-L., Kim, J., Shim, C-J., and Lee, C-O., New bioactive polyacetylenes from the marine sponge *Petrosia* sp, *Tetrahedron,* 54:3151–3158, 1998.

Kim, D.-K., Lee, M.-Y., Lee, H.S., Lee, D.S., Lee, J.-R., Lee, B.-J., and Jung, J.H., Polyacetylenes from a marine sponge *Petrosia* sp. inhibit DNA replication at the level of initiation, *Cancer Lett.,* 185:95–101, 2002.

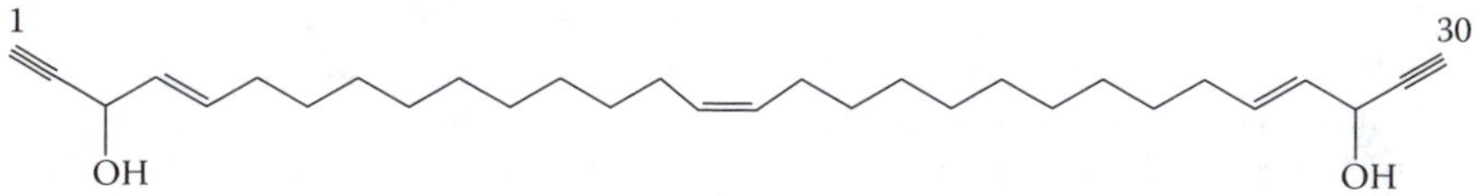

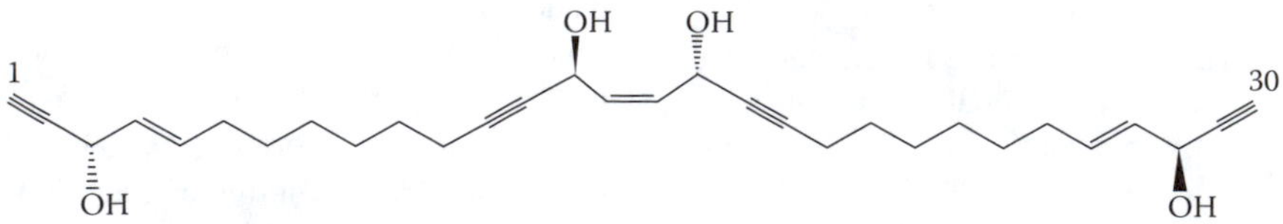

Structures of duryne (1) and petrosynol (2). (From Kim et al., *Tetrahedron,* 54:3151–3158, 1998. With permission.)

Meadowfoam (*Limnanthes alba*) Meadowfoam is an emerging specialty oilseed crop grown in the Northwestern United States. Its seeds contain 28 percent oil (on a dry basis) and are rich in C20 and C22 monounsaturated fatty acids (Holser, 2003). The low skin irritability and high stability of meadowfoam oil makes it suitable for use in cosmetic formulations and as lubricants (Burg and Kleiman, 1991; Emken et al., 1991; Ricks, 1991).

As mentioned earlier, meadowfoam pressed seed oil is extremely stable, although refining reduces its oxidative stability. Isbell et al. (1999) reported that meadowfoam oil enhanced the oxidative stability of other vegetable oils, suggesting the presence of antioxidants in this oil. Meadowfoam is rich in glucosinolates, such as glucolimnanthin, but these have little or no antioxidant activity (Plumb et al., 1996). However, Abbott and coworkers (2002) isolated a number of compounds in meadowfoam oil capable of forming 1,3-di(3-methoxybenzyl)thiourea (3MBTU) or its oxidation products. Several degradation products from glucolimnanthin, 3-methoxybenzyl isothiocyanate, and 3-methoxybenzylamine, were identified as both capable of forming 3MBTU. The latter compound proved to be an effective antioxidant by enhancing the oxidative stability of a number of vegetable oils, including rapeseed, jojoba, and sunflower oils at a level of 0.1 percent. The potential nutraceutical benefits from meadowfoam remain to be established, although the presence of glucosinolates and their corresponding isothiocyanates are known for their health benefits.

References

Abbott, T.P., Wohlman, A., Isbell, T., Momany, F.A., Cantrell, C., Garlotta, D.V., and Wiesleder, D., 1,3-di(Methoxybenzyl) thiourea and related lipid antioxidants, *Ind. Crops Prod.*, 16:43–57, 2002.

Burg, D.A. and Kleiman, R., Preparation of meadowfoam dimer acids and dimer esters, and their use as lubricants, *J. Am. Oil Chem. Soc.*, 68:600–603, 1991.

Emken, E.A., Adlof, R.O., and Abraham, S., Metabolism of meadowfoam oil fatty acids in mice, *Lipids*, 26:736–742, 1991.

Hosler, R.A., Seed conditioning and meadowfoam press oil quality, *Ind. Crops Prod.*, 17:23–26, 2003.

Isbell, T.A., Abbott, T.P., and Carlson, K.D., Oxidative stability index of vegetable oils in binary mixtures with meadowfoam oil, *Ind. Crops Prod.*, 9:115–123, 1999.

Plumb, G.W., Lambert, N., Chambers, S.J., Wanigatunga, S., Heany, R.K., Plumb, J.A., Arouma, O.L., Haliwell, B., and Miller, N.J., Are whole extracts and purified glucosinolates from cruciferous vegetables antioxidants, *Free Rad. Res.*, 25:75–86.

Ricks, D.J., Functional natural oils, *Cosm. Toiletries*, 106:77–79, 1991.

M

Meadowsweet (*Filipendula ulmaria*) Meadowsweet, a fragrant herb with small, white flowers that appear like umbels at the top of the stalks, blossoms from June to September. It can be found by river banks and in moist meadows. Historically, meadowsweet was used by herbalists for a wide variety of conditions, such as rheumatic complaints, muscle aches, headaches, colds and flu, digestive upsets, menstrual cramps, congestive heart failure, and as a diuretic agent (Gruenwald et al., 1998; Duke, 2000; Skidmore-Rose, 2001).

The primary constituents in meadowsweet are salicylates, including salicin, salicaldehyde, and methyl salicylate, which are thought to contribute to its antiplatelet activity. In the digestive

Salicin   Salicylaldehyde   Methyl salicylate

Adapted from Brenna, et al., *J. Agric. Food Chem.*, 52:7747–7751, 2004.

tract these compounds are oxidized to salicylic acid, a substance closely related to aspirin (acetyl-salicylic acid), which may give it a mild anti-inflammatory effect (Bernaulov and Denisenko, 1980) and an ability to reduce fevers during a cold or flu. The complimentary inhibitory activities reported by Halkes et al. (1997) are in line with its therapeutic value in inflammatory diseases.

Other constituents include flavonoids, mainly in the flowers, which exhibit considerable antioxidant and antimicrobial activity (Rauha et al., 2000), phenol glycosides (Horhammer, 1956; Thieme, 1966), tannins (Novikova, 1969), and essential oil. Kudriashov et al. (1990) reported that the flowers also contained a heparin-like anticoagulant factor, which demonstrated fibrinolytic properties *in vivo* activities (Peresun'ko, 1993).

References

Barnaulov, O.D. and Denisenko, P.P., Anti-ulcer action of a decoction of the flowers of the dropwort, *Filipendula ulmaria* (L), *Maxim Farmakol. Toksikol.*, 43:700–705, 1980.

Brenna, G., Fronza, G., Fuganti, C., Gatti, F.G., Pinciroli, M., and Serra, S., Differentiation of extractive and synthetic salicin. The ^{2}H aromatic pattern of natural 2-hydroxybenzl alcohol. *J. Agric. Food Chem.*, 52:7477–7717, 2004.

Duke, J.A., *The Green Pharmacy Herbal Handbook*, Rodale Press, Emmaus, Pennsylvania, 2000.

Gruenwald, J., Brendler, T., and Jaenicke, C., *The PDR for Herbal Medicines*, Medical Economics Co., Montvale, New Jersey, 1998.

Halkes, S.B.A., Beukelman, C.J., Kroes, B.H., Van den Berg, A.J.J., Van Dijk, H., and Labadie, R.P., Strong complement inhibitor from the flowers of *Filipendula ulmaria*, *Pharmaceut. Pharmacol. Lett.*, 7(2/3):79–82, 1997.

Horhammer, L., Hansel, R., and Endres, W., The flavone-glycosides of the *Filipendula* and *Spirae* species, *Arch. Pharm.*, 289:133–140, 1956.

Kudriashov, B.A., Liapina, L.A., and Zieva, L.D., The content of a heparin-like anticoagulant in the flowers of the meadowsweet *Filipendula ulmaria*, *Farmakol Toksikol.*, 53:39–41, 1990.

Novikova, N.N., Use of Filipendula ulmaria in medicine, *Permskogo Farmatsevticheskogo Instituta.*, 3:267–270, 1969.

Peresun=ko, A.P., Bespalov, V.G., Limarenko, A.I., and Aleksandrov, V.A., Clinoco-experimental study of using plant preparations from the flowers of *Filipendula ulmaria* (L.) Maxim for the treatment of precancerous changes and prevention of uterine cervical cancer, *Vopr. Onkol.*, 39:291–295.

Rauha, J.P., Remes, S., Heinonen, M., Hopia, A., Kahkonen, M., Kujala, T., Pihlaja, K., Vuorela, H., and Vuorela, P., Antimicrobial effects of Finnish plant extracts containing flavonoids and other phenolic compounds, *Int. J. Food Microbiol.*, 56:3–12, 2000.

Skidmore-Rose, L., *Mosby's Handbook of Herbs and Natural Supplements*, Mosby Inc., St. Louis, Missouri, 2001.

Thieme, H., Isolation of a new phenolic glycoside from the blossoms of *Filipendula ulmaria* (L.) Maxim, *Pharmazie*, 21:123, 1966.

Melatonin Melatonin (*N*-acetyl-5-methoxytryptamine), the main hormone of the pineal gland, is synthesized from the amino acid tryptophan via serotonin. It decreases with age so that supplementation may be beneficial in

Melatonin. (Adapted from Sun et al., *Bioorg. Med. Chem. Lett.*, 20:5157–5160, 2004.)

delaying age-related conditions. In addition to being a potent scavenger of free radicals (Reiter, 1997), melatonin may modulate the immune system and the growth of cancer cells (Maestroni et al., 1986; Blask et al., 1992). Hattori and coworkers (1995) identified melatonin in edible plants that would increase the amount of circulating levels in vertebrates. Medicinal plants, such as feverfew, was shown to be a good source of melatonin (Murch et al., 1997). A significant source of melatonin was found by Zielinski and coworkers (2001) in germinated legumes, which increased fourfold to eightfold in soybean, vetch, and lentil seeds, respectively, compared to the raw seeds. Of the three legumes examined, germinated vetch and soybean were almost twice as high in melatonin compared to germinated lentil seeds.

Melatonin was also found to prevent gastric ulceration in pigs (Ayles et al., 1996; Khan et al., 1990) and reduce the severity of colitis in mice (Pentney and Bubenik, 1995). Teplitzky et al. (2001) showed that a combination of melatonin and 9-*cis*-retinoic acid significantly inhibited tumor development in an *N*-nitroso-*N*-methylurea (NMU)-induced rat mammary-tumor model. Stavinsky et al. (2005) showed melatonin enhanced *in vivo* and *in vitro* plasmalemmal fusion (PEG-fusion) of severed rat sciatic axons. This may prove beneficial in repairing crush-type injuries to sciatic nerves and spinal chords in accidents involving humans.

References

Ayles, H.L., Ball, R.O., Friendship, R.M., and Bubenik, G.A., The effect of graded levels of melatonin on performance of gastric ulcers in pigs, *Can. J. Anim. Sci.,* 76:607–611, 1996.

Blask, D.E., Lemus-Wilson, A.M., Wilson, S.T., and Cos, T., Neurohormonal modulation of cancer growth by pineal melatonin, in *Melatonin and the Pineal Gland, From Basic Science to Clinical Application,* Touitou, Y., Arendt, J., and Pevet, P., Eds., 1992, pp. 303–310.

Hattori, A., Migitaka, H., Ligo, M., Itoh, M., Yamamoto, K., Ohtani-Kaneko, R., Hara, M., Suzuki, T., and Reiter, R.J., Identification of melatonin in plants and its effects on plasma melatonin levels and binding to melatonin receptors in vertebrates, *Biochem. Mol. Biol. Int.,* 35:627–634, 1995.

Maestroni, G.J.M., Conti, A., and Pierpaoli, W., Role of the pineal gland in immunity Circadian synthesis and release of melatonin modulates the antibody response and antagonizes the immunosuppressive effect of corticosterone, *J. Neuroimmunol.,* 13:19–30, 1986.

Murch, S.J., Simmons, C.B., and Saxena, P.K., Melatonin in feverfew and other medicinal plants, *Lancet,* 350:1598, 1997.

Pentney, P.T. and Bubenik, G.A., Melatonin reduces the severity of dextran-induced colitis in mice, *J. Pineal Res.,* 19:31–39, 1995.

Reiter, R.J., Antioxidant actions of melatonin, *Adv. Pharmacol.,* 38:103–117, 1997.

Stavinsky, R.C., Britt, J.M., Zuzek, A., Truong, E., and Bittner, G.D., Melatonin enhances the *in vitro* and *in vivo* repair of severed rat sciatic axons, *Neurosci. Lett.,* 376:98–101, 2005.

Sun, L.-Q., Takaki, K., Chen, J., Iben, L., Knipe, J.O., Pajor, L., Mahle, C.D., Ryan, E., and Xu, C., N-2[2-(4-Phenylbutyl)benzofuran-4-yl]cyclopropyl-methylacetamide: An orally bioavailable melatonin receptor agonist, *Bioorg. Med. Chem. Lett.,* 14:5157–5160, 2004.

Teplitzky, S.R., Kiefer, T.L., Cheng, Q., Dwivedi, P.D., Moroz, K., Myers, L., Anderson, M.B., Collins, A., Dai, J., Yuan, L., Spriggs, L.L., Blask, D.E, and Hill, S.M., Chemoprevention of NMU-induced rat mammary carcinoma with the combination of melatonin and 9-*cis*-retinoic acid, *Cancer Lett.,* 168:155–163, 2001.

Zielinski, H., Lewczuk, B., Przybylska-Gornowicz, B., and Kozlowska, H., Melatonin in germinated legume seeds as a potentially significant agent for health, *R. Soc. Chem.,* 269:110–117, 2001.

M

Mengkudu

Mengkudu Mengkudu (*Morinda citrifola* L.), or Indian mulberry, is found in tropical Asia or Polynesia. Its roots are reported to be good sources of anthroquinones (Thomson, 1971; Zenk et al., 1975). Studies by Zin and coworkers (2002) showed that a methanol extract of Mengkudu root had equivalent antioxidant activity to that of α-tocopherol and butylated hydroxyquinone (BHT). Some of the medicinal properties associated with this tree, such as the relief of rheumatic and other pains, may be due to its antioxidant capacity.

References

Thomson, R.H., *Naturally Occuring Quinones,* 2nd ed., Academic Press, London and New York, 1971.

Zenk, M.N., El-Shagi, H., and Schulte, U., Anthraquinone production by cell suspension cultures of *Morinda citrifolia, Planta Med., Suppl.* 79–101, 1975.

Zin, Z.M., Abdul-Hamid, A., and Osman, A., Antioxidative activity of extracts from Mengkudu (*Morinda citrifola* L.) root, fruit and leaf, *Food Chem.,* 78:227–231, 2002.

S-Methylmethane thiosulfonate   *S*-Methyl-methane thiosulfonate is found in cruciferous vegetables such as cabbage, onions, and cauliflower. It is formed from its precursor, *S*-methyl-L-cysteine sulfoxide. Coadministration of *S*-methylmethane thiosulfonate, isolated from cauliflower, with the nonsteroidal, antiinflammatory drug sulindac, was shown by Reddy et al. (1999) to inhibit chemically induced colon cancer in weanling male F344

$$H_3C-S-\overset{\displaystyle O}{\underset{\displaystyle O}{S}}-CH_3$$

S-Methylmethane thiosulfonate. (From Reddy et al., *Carcinogenesis*, 20:1645–1648, 1999. With permission.)

rats. A combination of 40 ppm *S*-methylmethane thiosulfonate and 160 ppm sulindac resulted in a far more significant ($p < 0.05$) inhibition of noninvasive adenomas (59 percent) during the promotion/progression stages, as well the multiplicity of noninvasive (71 percent inhibition), invasive (39 percent inhibition), and total colon adenomas (48 percent) compared to administration with either *S*-methylmethane thiosulfonate or sulindac, separately. This confirms earlier work by Kawamori and coworkers (1995) who showed that a diet containing *S*-methylmethane thiosulfonate inhibited azoxymethane-induced colon carcinogenesis in male F344 rats. The mechanism of action by *S*-methylmethane thiosulfonate was attributed to its ability to decrease mucosal ornithine decarboxylase, a rate-limiting enzyme in polyamine biosynthesis and cell proliferation.

References

Kawamori, T., Tanaka, T., Ohnishi, M., Hirose, Y., Nakamura, Y., Satoh, K., Hara, A., and Mori, H., Chemoprevention of azoxymethane-induced colon carcinogenesis by dietary feeding of *S*-methylmethane thiosulfonate in male F344 rats, *Cancer Res.*, 55:4053–4058, 1995.

Reddy, B.S., Kawamori, T., Lubet, R., Steele, V., Kelloff, G., and Rao, C.V., Chemopreventive effect of *S*-methylmethane thiosulfonate and sulindac administered together during the promotion/progression stages of colon carcinogenesis, *Carcinogenesis*, 20:1645–1648, 1999.

Methylxanthines *see also* **Caffeine**   Methylxanthines include any of the methylated derivatives of xanthine, such as caffeine, theobromine, and theophylline, and their derivatives. Caffeine is found in coffee, tea, cola nuts, mate, and guarana. Its major effects include stimulation of the central nervous system, cardiac muscle, respiratory system, and diuretic delays disease. Theophylline, a methylxanthine found in tea, is a cardiac stimulant, smooth-muscle relaxant, diuretic, and vasodilator. Theobromine, the main methylxanthine in cocoa beans (1.5–3 percent), cola nuts, and tea, is a diuretic agent, smooth-muscle relaxant, cardiac stimulant, and vasodilator (Shively and Tarka, 1984; Spiller, 1984; Youd et al., 1999; Vajner et al., 2002; Nawrot et al., 2003).

In humans, caffeine acts on the brain and skeletal muscles, while theophylline targets heart, bronchia, and kidneys. Recent interest in these alkaloids is centered on their potential reproductive toxicities.

CF: $R_1 = -CH_3$ $R_2 = -CH_3$
TB: $R_1 = -CH_3$ $R_2 = -H$
TP: $R_1 = -H$ $R_2 = -CH_3$

Methylxanthine structures: CF, caffeine; TB, theobromine; and TP, theophylline. (From Lopez-Martinez et al., *Analytica Chemica Acta*, 493:83–94, 2003. With permission.)

Caffeine and theobromine are known to cross the placental and blood–brain barriers, potentially capable of inducing fetal malformation by affecting expression of genes vital in development. The developing fetus may not have developed enzymes for detoxification of these methylxanthine alkaloids via demethylation. Evidence in favor of the toxicity of these compounds in experimental animals was presented by Eteng and coworkers (1997), who cautioned against the use of caffeine and theobromine pending further and more elaborate investigations. On the other hand, Slattery et al. (1999) showed that among men, low levels of coffee intake were associated with increased risk of colon cancer relative to nonconsumers of coffee, while at high levels of coffee consumption, caffeine and theobromine both inhibited the doxorubicin efflux from tumor cells, increased the doxorubicin concentration in a tumor, and thus enhanced the antitumor effect of doxorubicin, suggesting these xanthine derivatives may be useful for biochemical modulators.

Methylxanthines are used clinically as bronchodilators (Henderson-Smart and Steer, 2000, 2001). The precise mechanism whereby methylxanthines exert their beneficial effect in apnea, a problem of ventilatory control in the premature infant, defined as cessation of inspiratory gas flow for 20 sec or less if accompanied by bradycardia, cyanosis, or pallor, is not known. Proposed mechanisms include increased respiratory drive secondary to increased carbon-dioxide sensitivity and increased oxygen consumption. Other mechanisms postulated include adenosine antagonism, enhanced diaphragmatic contractility, and increased cyclic 3′,5′-cyclic AMP (Henderson-Smart and Steer, 2000, 2001). Johnson and coworkers (2003) demonstrated that the discrimination in the binding affinity of the methylxanthines, theophylline, theobromine, and caffeine with RNA molecule shows that strong, RNA-binding drugs, such as theophylline, can selectively be delivered to RNA targets of microbial pathogens having the mechanism of RNA catalysis. The controversies surrounding xanthine therapy for apnea in premature infants was reviewed by Millar and Schmidt (2003). They reported that an international trial was under way to examine the long-term efficacy and safety of methylxanthine therapy for very low-birth-weight babies.

References

Eteng, M.U., Eyong, E.U., Akpanyung, E.O., Agiang, M.A., and Aremu, C.Y., Recent advances in caffeine and theobromine toxicities: A review, *Plant Foods Hum. Nutr.,* 51:231–243, 1997.

Henderson-Smart, D.J. and Steer, P., Prophylactic methylxanthine for preventing of apnea in preterm infants, *Cochrane Database Syst. Rev.,* (2): CD000432, 2000.

Henderson-Smart, D.J. and Steer, P., Methylxanthine treatment of apnea in preterm infants, *Cochrane Database Syst. Rev.,* (3):CD000140, 2001.

Johnson, I.M., Kumar, S.G., and Malathi, R., RNA binding of theophylline, theobromine and caffeine, *J. Biomol. Struct. Dyn.,* 20:687–689, 2003.

Kakuyama, A. and Sadzuka, Y., Effect of methylxanthine derivatives on doxorubicin transport and antitumor activity, *Curr. Drug Metab.,* 2:379–395, 2001.

Lopez-Martinez, L., Lopez-de-Alba, P.L., Garcia-Campos, R., and De Leon-Rodriguez, L.M., Simultaneous determination of methylxanthines in coffees and teas by UV-Vis spectrophotometry and partial least squares, *Anal. Chem. Acta,* 493:83–94, 2003.

Millar, D. and Schmidt, B., Controversies surrounding xanthine therapy, *Sem. Neonatol.,* 9:239–244, 2003.

Nawrot, P., Jordan, S., Eastwood, J., Rostein, J., Hugenholtz, A., and Feeley, M., Effects of caffeine on human health, *Food Addit. Contam.,* 20:1–30, 2003.

Shively, C.A. and Tarka, S.M., Jr., Methylxanthine composition and consumption patterns of cocoa and chocolate products, *Prog. Clin. Biol. Res.,* 158:149–178, 1984.

Slattery, M.L., Caan, B.J., Anderson, K.E., and Potter, J.D., Intake of fluids and methylxanthine-containing beverages: Association with colon cancer, *Int. J. Cancer,* 81:199–204, 1999.

Spiller, G.A., Overview of the methylxanthine beverages and foods and their effect on health, *Prog. Clin. Biol. Res.,* 158:1–7, 1984.

Vajner, L., Konradova, V., Uhlik, J., and Zocova, J., The effects of intravenously administered methylxanthine preparations on the glycoconjugate composition of goblet cells in rabbit tracheal epithelium, *Acta Histochem.,* 104:107–112, 2002.

Youd, J.M., Newman, J.M., Clark, M.G., Appleby, G.J., Rattigan, S., Tong, A.C., and Vincent, M.A., Increased metabolism of infused 1-methylxanthine by working muscle, *Acta Physiol. Scand.,* 166:301–308, 1999.

M

Milk proteins *see also* **Casein and Whey Proteins Lactoglobulin**   Milk proteins, caseins, and whey proteins serve as important nutritional sources in the diet. The susceptibility of caseins to proteolysis, however, produces physiologically functional peptides, immunostimulating peptides (Parker et al., 1984), and angiotensin 1-converting enzyme inhibitors (ACEI). There have been many antihypertensive peptides produced by enzymic digestion of bovine and human caseins (Yamamoto and Takono, 1999). Those high in ACEI activity tend to be fairly short peptides with proline in the C-terminus. There is limited work on ACEI peptides from whey proteins due to the rigid structure and resistance to digestive enzymes of the major component, β-lactoglobulin. Nevertheless the enzymatic production of ACEI peptides from whey proteins was recently reported (Mullaly and coworkers, 1996, 1997). ACEI peptides were also found to be present in sour milk produced by starter cultures, *Lactobacillus helveticus* and *Saccharomyces cerevisiae* (Nakamura et al., 1995a, b). Balansky and coworkers (1999) showed that freeze-dried milk fermented by a *Lactobacillus bulgaricus* strain inhibited 1,2-dimethylhydrazine (DMH)-induced carcinogenesis. The effect varied with the particular *Lactobacillus bulgaricus* strain studied. For example, strain LBB.B144, whose product, FFM.B144, inhibited the intestinal carcinogenesis induced by DMH, as well as decreased tumor incidence and multiplicity in male and female rats in the large bowel, caecum, and duodenum. This contrasted with strain LBB.B5, whose product, FFM.B5, selectively inhibited DMH-induced carcinogenesis of the large bowel only. Both products significantly inhibited (26–33 percent) the induction of earduct tumors in rats, while only FFMB144 inhibited tracheal carcinogenesis induced by diethylnitrosamine (DEN) in Syrian hamsters. These results pointed to the potential of some fermented-milk products in the chemoprevention of cancer.

References

Balansky, R., Gyosheva, B., Ganchev, G., Mircheva, Z., Minkova, S., and Georgiev, G., Inhibitory effects of freeze-dried milk fermented by selected *Lactobacillus bulgaricus* strains on carcinogenesis induced by 1,2-dimethylhydrazine in rats and by diethylnitrosamine in hamsters, *Cancer Lett.,* 147:125–137, 1999.

Mullaly, M.M., Meisel, H., and FitzGerald, R.J., Synthetic peptides corresponding to α-lactalbumin and β-lactoglobulin sequences with angiotensin-1-converting enzyme inhibitory activity. *Biol. Chem. Hoppe-Seyler,* 377:259–260, 1996.

Mullaly, M.M., Meisel, H., and FitzGerald, R.J., Identification of novel angiotensin-1-converting enzyme inhibitory peptide corresponding to a tryptic fragment of bovine β-lactoglobulin, *FEBS Lett.,* 402: 99–101, 1997.

Nakamura, Y., Yamamoto, N., Sakai, K., Okuba, A., Yamazaki, S., and Takano, T., Purification and characterization of angiotensin-1-converting enzyme inhibitors from sour milk, *J. Dairy Sci.,* 78:777–783, 1995a.

Nakamura, Y., Yamamoto, N., Sakai, E., and Takano, T., Antihypertensive effect of sour milk and peptides isolated from it that are inhibitors to angiotensin — coinverting enzyme, *J. Dairy Sci.,* 78:1253–1257, 1995b.

Parker, F., Migliore-Amour, D.., Floch, F., Zerial, A., Werner, G.G., Jolles, J., Casaretto, M., Zahn, H., and Jolles, P., Immunostimulating hexapeptide from human casein: Amino acid sequence, synthesis and biological properties, *Eur. J. Biochem.,* 145:677–682, 1984.

Yamamoto, N. and Takano, T., Antihypertensive peptides derived from milk proteins, *Nahrung,* 43:159–164, 1999.

Milk thistle   Milk thistle, a medicinal herb native to the Mediterranean region, has been used for centuries as a remedy for liver ailments. The active ingredient in milk thistle is silymarin, a bioflavonoid mixture composed mainly of silybin with silydianin and silychristin (Scheme M.39). They are all liver protectants (antihepatotoxic agents), as studies showed they protect the liver from a wide range of toxins, including the deadly *Amanita phalloides* mushroom, or Death Cap mushroom. Silymarin has also been found to protect the liver from dangerous solvents, such as carbon tetrachloride and ethanol. Studies in Germany showed considerable improvement in patients suffering from chronic hepatitis after three months of treatment with silymarin. Daily doses of up to 420 mg of silymarin were shown to improve almost 50 percent of patients suffering

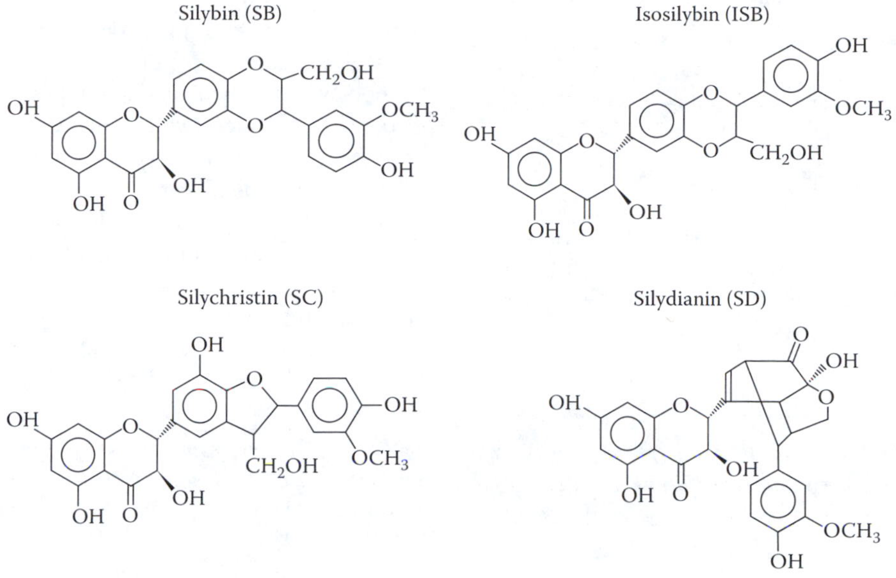

SCHEME M.39 Structures of the main silymarin components (From Kvasnicka et al., *J. Chromatogr. A.*, 990: 239–245, 2003. With permission.)

from cirrhosis of the liver. Silymarin appears to accelerate regeneration and production of liver cells. Because silymarin is insoluble in water, it is available in capsule form. In the United States, it is marketed as a food supplement in 200–250 mg capsules containing up to 80 percent silymarin. The beneficial effects are attributed to its antioxidant properties, as silymarin was reported to prevent lipid peroxidation (Velussi et al., 1997; Lahiri-Chaterjee et al., 1999), inhibit LDL oxidation (Skottova et al., 1999), and scavenge free radicals (Dehmlow et al., 1996a, b).

A systematic review and meta-analysis of milk thistle by Jacobs and coworkers (2002) concluded that milk thistle was safe and well-tolerated. However, the authors felt that the data were too limited to exclude a substantial benefit or harm from milk thistle on mortality or to recommend its efficacy for treating liver disease. Nevertheless, recent work by Gurley and coworkers (2004) using human subjects reported that botanical supplements, such as milk thistle, posed minimal risk for CYP-mediated herb–drug interactions in humans.

References

Dehmlow, C., Erhard, J., and de Groot, H., Inhibition of Kupffer cell functions as an explanation for the hepatoprotective properties of silibinin, *Hepatology*, 23:749–754, 1996a.

Dehmlow, C., Murawski, N., and de Groot, H., Scavenging of reactive oxygen species and inhibition of arachidonic acid metabolism by silibinin in human cells, *Life Sci.*, 58:1591–1600, 1996b.

Gurley, B.J., Gardner, S.F., Hubbard, M.A., Williams, K., Gentry, B., Carrier, J., Edwards, D., and Khan, I., Assessment of botanical supplementation on human cytochrome P450 phenotype: Citrus aurantium, echinacea, milk thistle, saw palmetto, *Clin. Pharmacol. Ther.*, 75:P35, 2004.

Jacobs, B.P., Dennehy, C., Ramirez, G., Sapp, J., and Lawrence, V.A., Milk thistle for the treatment of liver disease: A systematic review and meta-analysis, *Am. J. Med.*, 113:506–515, 2002.

Kvasnicka, F., Biba, B., Sevcik, R., Voldrich, M., and Kratka, J., Analysis of the active components of silyayarwalmarin, *J. Chromatogr. A.*, 990:239–245, 2003.

Lahiri-Chaterjee, M., Katiyar, S.K., Mohan, R.R., and Argawal, R.A., A flavonoid antioxidant, silymarin, affords exceptionally high protection against

M

tumor promotion in the SENCAR mouse skin tumorigenesis model, *Can. Res.*, 59:622–632, 1999.

Skottova, N., Kreeman, V., and Simaneck, V., Activities of silymarin and its flavonolignans upon low density lipoprotein oxidizability *in vitro*, *Phytotherapy Res.*, 13:535–537, 1999.

Velussi, M., Cernigoni, A.M., De Monte, A., Dapas, F., Caffau, C., and Zilli, M., Long-term (12 months) treatment with an anti-oxidant drug (silymarin) is effective on hyperinsulinemia, exogenous insulin need and malondialdehyde levels in cirrhotic diabetic patients, *J. Hepatol.*, 26:871–879, 1997.

Mistletoe (*Viscum album* L.)   Mistletoe is a half-parasitic plant that grows on deciduous trees all over the world (Barney et al., 1998). A traditionally valued medicinal plant, it has been used against high blood pressure, arthritis, cardiovascular illness, epilepsy, and as a narcotic. Extracts from mistletoe have been used in the treatment of cancers for decades. The anticancer activities are ascribed to the plant's viscotoxins (Konopa et al., 1980; Jung et al., 1990), lectins (Jung et al., 1990; Bussing, 1996), alkaloids (Khwaja et al., 1986), and polysaccharides (Jordan and Wagner, 1986), which vary, depending on the host tree, the subspecies of mistletoe, and the parts used and the time of harvest (Jaggy et al., 1995; Barberaki and Kintzios, 2002). Numerous preclinical and *in vitro* studies showed the mistletoe extracts standardized in terms of their lectin content have highly potent cytotoxic and immunostimulating effects, predominantly on the cellular immune system (Schink, 1997; Beuth, 1997; Elsaesser-Beile et al., 1998; Stauder, 2002). The immunostimulating effect is correlated with the apoptosis of immunologically active cells at low concentrations. Cytotoxic effects on tumor cells are likewise, but at high level, necrotic cell death predominates. Due to these properties, mistletoe extracts exhibited antitumoral activities in different animal models (Mengs et al., 2002). Pryme et al. (2002) showed that the growth of murine non-Hodgkin lymphoma (NHL) tumor was reduced by incorporating mistletoe lectin into the diet. The degree of lymphocyte infiltration was increased in tumors from mistletoe-lectin-fed mice, and this was accompanied by a high incidence of apoptotic bodies. Visual observation of NHL tumors from individual mice fed mistletoe-lectin-rich diets showed a reduction in tumor weight followed by poorly developed blood supply in contrast to control-fed mice, which suggested an anti-angiogenic response. Translation of these effects into a clinical response continues to pose a problem. While a number of clinical studies found improvement in the quality of life, data on the efficacy of mistletoe to prolong survival are conflicting and of variable quality (Mansky, 2002; Stauder and Kreuser, 2002).

References

Barberaki, M. and Kintzios, S., Accumulation of selected macronutrients in mistletoe tissue cultures: Effect of medium composition and explant source, *Sci. Hortic.*, 95:133–150, 2002.

Barney, C.W., Hawsworth, E.G., and Geils, B.W., Hosts of *Viscum album*, *Eur. J. For Path.*, 28:187–208, 1998.

Beuth, J., Clinical relevance of immunoactive mistletoe lectin-I, *Anticanc. Drugs,* 1:S53–55, 1997.

Bussing, A., Suzart, K., Bergmann, J., Pfuller, U., Schietzal, M., and Schweizer, K., Induction of apoptosis in human lymphocytes treated with *Viscum album* L. is mediated by mistletoe lectins, *Cancer Lett.,* 99:59–72, 1996.

Elsaesser-Beile, U., Lusebrink, S., Grussenmeyer, T., Wetterauer, U., and Schultze-Seeman, W., Comparison of the effects of various clinically applied mistletoe preparations on peripheral blood leukocytes, *Arzneimittel-Forschung,* 48:1185–1189, 1998.

Jaggy, C., Musielshi, H., Urech, K., and Schaller, G., Quantitative determination of lectins in mistletoe preparations, *Azneimittel-Forsch/Drug Res.,* 45:905–909, 1995.

Jordan, E. and Wagner, H., Structures and properties of polysaccharides from *Viscum album* (L). *Oncology,* 42:8–15, 1986.

Jung, M.L., Bandino, S., Ribereau-Gayon, G., and Beck, J.P., Characterization of cytotoxic proteins from mistletoe (*Viscum album* L.), *Cancer Lett.,* 51: 103–108, 1990.

Khwaja, T.A., Dias, C.B., and Pentecost, S., Recent studies on the antitumor activities of mistletoe (*Viscum album*) and its alkaloids, *Oncology,* 43:42–50, 1986.

M

Konopa, J., Woynarowski, J.M., and Lewandowska, M., Isolation of viscotoxin, cytotoxic basic polypeptides from mistletoe *Viscum album* L., *Hoppe Seyer's Z. Physiol. Chem.*, 361:1525–1533, 1980.

Mansky, P.J., Mistletoe and cancer: Controversies and perspectives, *Semin. Oncol.*, 29:589–594, 2002.

Mengs, U., Gothel, D., and Leng-Peschlow, E., Mistletoe extracts standardized to mistletoe lectins in oncology: Review on current status of preclinical research, *Anticancer Res.*, 22:1399–1407, 2002.

Pryme, I.F., Bardocz, S., Pusztai, A., and Ewen, S.W., Dietary mistletoe lectin supplementation and reduced growth of a murine non-Hodgkin lymphoma, *Histol. Histopathol.*, 17:261–271, 2002.

Schink, M., Mistletoe therapy for human cancer: The role of the natural killer cells, *Anticancer Drugs*, 8(Suppl. 1):S47–51, 1997.

Stauder, H. and Kreuser, E.D., Mistletoe extracts standardised in terms of mistletoe lectins (ML I) in oncology: Current state of clinical research, *Onkol.*, 25:374–380, 2002.

Monoterpenes *see also* **Geraniol, Limonene, Menthol, Perillyl alcohol, and Perrialdehyde** Monoterpenes are found in essential oils of citrus fruits, cherry, mints, and herbs. These 10-carbon isoprenoids are synthesized in plants via the mevalonate pathway but cannot be produced by fungi or mammals. Monoterpenes are largely responsible for the distinctive fragrance of many plants and function as chemoattractants or chemorepellents (McGarvey and Croteau, 1995). Limonene, one of the first monoterpenes produced from mevalonate, acts as precursor for a wide array of oxygenated, monocyclic monoterpenes, including carveol, carvone, menthol, perillyl alcohol, and perrillaldehyde.

Some monoterpenes have been shown to have antitumor activity capable of not only preventing the formation and progression of cancer but also to regress malignant tumors (Crowell, 1999). These include *d*-limonene (Kawamori et al., 1996), carveol (Crowell et al., 1992), menthol (Russin et al., 1989), geraniol (Yu et al., 1995), and perillyl alcohol (Mills et al., 1995). Chan (2001) reviewed the potential medicinal uses of monoterpenoid compounds, as well as assay methods.

The cancer-suppressing activity of monoterpenes during the promotion phase of mammary and liver carcinogenesis is thought to be due to inhibition of tumor-cell proliferation, acceleration of the rate of tumor death, and induction of tumor-cell differentiation (Morse and Stoner, 1993). Antitumor activity by limonene and other monoterpenes appears to be due to the induction of phase I and phase II carcinogen-metabolizing enzymes. Inhibition of protein isoprenylation prevents carcinogenesis, as prenylation of Ras enables it to associate with the plasma membrane, an essential step for its oncogenic activity (Clarke, 1992). Consequently, the antitumor activity of monoterpenes appears to be due to their effect on prenylation-independent mechanisms or prenylation of proteins other than Ras.

M

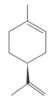 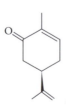 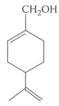

| Limonene | (−)-*trans*-Carveol | (−)-Carvone | Perillyl alcohol | Menthol |

Structures of monoterpenes. (Adapted from Chan, *J. Chromatogr. A.*, 936:47–57, 2001; Carter et al., *Phytochemistry*, 64:425–433, 2003; Tasarti et al., *J. Catal.*, 224:484–488, 2004.)

References

Carter, O.A., Peters, R.J., and Croteau, R., Mono-terpene biosynthesis pathway construction in *Escherichia coli*, *Phytochemistry,* 64:425–433, 2003.

Chan, K.K., Quantitation of monoterpenoid compounds with potential medicinal use in biological fluids, *J. Chromatogr. A.,* 936:47–57, 2001.

Clarke, S., Protein isoprenylation and methylation at carboxyl-terminal cysteine residues, *Annu. Rev. Biochem.,* 61:355–386, 1992.

Crowell, P.L., Prevention and therapy of cancer by dietary monoterpenes, *J. Nutr.,* 129:775–778, 1999.

Crowell, P.L., Kennan, W.S., Haag, J.D., Ahmad, S., Vedejs, E., and Gould, M.N., Chemoprevention of mammary carcinogenesis by hydroxylated derivatives of *d*-limonene, *Carcinogenesis,* 13:1261–1264, 1992.

Kawamori, T., Tanaka, T., Hirose, Y., Ohnishi, M., and Mori, H., Inhibitory effects of *d*-limonene on the development of colonic aberrant crypt foci induced by azoxymethane in F344 rats, *Carcinogenesis,* 17: 369–372, 1996.

McGarvey, D.J. and Croteau, R., Terpenoid metabolism, *Plant Cell,* 7:1015–1026, 1995.

Mills, J.J., Chari, R.S., Boyer, I.J., Gould, M.N., and Jirtle, R.L., Induction of apoptosis in liver tumors by the monoterpene perilly alcohol, *Cancer Res.,* 55: 979–983, 1995.

Morse, M.A. and Stoner, G.D., Cancer chemoprevention: Principles and prospects, *Carcinogenesis,* 14:1737–1746, 1993.

Russin, W.A., Hoesly, J.D., Elson, C.E., Tanner, M.A., and Gould, M.N., Inhibition of ubiquinone and cholesterol synthesis by monoterpenes does not involve Ras plasma membrane association, *Carcinogenesis,* 10:2161–2165, 1989.

Tasarti, A.F., Marchi, A.J., and Apesteguia, C.R., Highly selective synthesis of menthols from citral in a one-step process, *J. Catal.,* 224:484–488, 2004.

Yu, S.G., Hildebrandt, L.A., and Elson, C.E., Geranioo, an inhibitor of mevalonate biosynthesis, suppresses the growth of hepatomas and melanomas transplanted to rats and mice, *J. Nutr.,* 125:2763–2767, 1995.

Mushrooms *see also* **Oyster mushroom**
Yang and coworkers (2001) recently examined the nutritional values of a number of commercial mushrooms. Some of these mushrooms were found to have medicinal properties, including antitumor, antiviral, and immuno-modulating effects (Wasser and Weis, 1999). Of these mushrooms, shiitake and oyster mushrooms were shown by Yang et al. (2002) to exhibit antioxidant activity as assessed by the formation of TBA-active components and the scavenging of 1,1-diphenyl-2-picrylhydrazyl radicals. Oyster mushrooms exhibited to highest scavenging activity

Kim et al., (2004) recently reported that in addition to anti-angiogenic activity, a butyl alcoholic extract from the orange color mushroom, *Phillenus linteus,* exhibited anti-inflammatory and antinociceptive activities.

References

Kim, S.-H., Song, Y.-S., Kim, S.-K., Kim, B.-C., Lim, C.-J., and Park, E.-H., Anti-inflammatory and related pharmacological activities of the n-BuOH subfraction of mushroom *Phellinus linteus*, *J. Ethnopharmacol.,* 93:141–146, 2004.

Wasser, S.P. and Weis, A., Medicinal properties of substances occuring in higher *Basidiomycetes* mushrooms: Current perspectives, *Int. J. Med. Mushrooms,* 1:31–62, 1999.

Yang, J.H., Lin, H.C., and Mau, J.L., Antioxidant properties of several commercial mushrooms, *Food Chem.,* 77:229–235, 2002.

Yang, J.H., Lin, H.C., and Mau, J.L., Non-volatile taste components of several commercial mushrooms, *Food Chem.,* 72:465–471, 2001.

Mustard *see* **Yellow mustard**

Mycalolide A-C   Mycalolides A-C are cytotoxic macrolides isolated from a sponge of the genus Mycale. They are trisoxazole-containing natural products and include ulapualides, kabiramides, halichondramides, and jaspisamides. These natural products display a wide range of biological activities, such as antifungal,

Chemical structure of mycalolide-B. (From Hori et al., *FEBS Lett.*, 322:151–154, 1993. With permission.)

antileukemic, and ichthyotoxic properties. Mycolalide A exhibits potent antifungal activity against a diverse array of pathogenic fungi and cytotoxicity towards B-16 melanoma cells with IC_{50} values of 0.5–1.0 ng/mL (Fusetani et al., 1989). The ability of mycolalide-B to selectively inhibit actin polymerization and actin-activated myosin Mg(2+)-ATPase activity using purified actin and myosin from rabbit skeletal muscle or chicken gizzard was reported by Saito et al. (1994) and Hori et al. (1993), respectively. They suggested that these macrolides can act as actin-depolymerizing agents and may be involved in actin-mediated cell functions, such as muscle contraction, cell motility, and cell division. The relationship between the concentration of total actin and F-actin at different concentrations of mycalolide-B suggests it forms a 1:1 complex with platelet aggregation by interfering with actin polymerization (Sugidachi et al., 1998). Treatment of highly polarized MDCK cells with mycalolide B induced a decrease of transepithelial resistance, which demonstrates the involvement of actin in the paracellular gate, which seals the paracellular space of opposing cells (Takakuwa et al., 2000). Because actin filaments play a critical role in transporting nascent HIV-1 proteins in host cells, Sasaki et al. (2004) examined the effect of mycalolide-B in the process. Mycolalolide-B depolymerized actin, which appeared to prevent HIV- envelope proteins and core proteins from being transported toward the plasma membrane of the host cell. These researchers suggested that chemical modification of mycalolide-B, to reduce its toxicity, might lead to its application in treating AIDS by HIV-1 infection.

A number of novel, stereochemically complex macrolides having a large macrolactone (22- to 44-membered) ring that interact with the actin cytoskeleton have been isolated from different marine sources. Although the details of these interactions are still under investigation, these marine macrolides are important as novel molecular probes to help elucidate the cellular functions of actin (Yeung and Paterson, 1992). These macrolide properties led researchers to synthesize myocalolides as depolymerizing agents (Panek and Liu, 2000).

References

Fusetani, N., Yasumuro, K., Matsunaga, S., and Hashimoto, K., Mycalolides A-C, hybrid macrolides of ulapualides and halichondramide, from a sponge of the genus Mycale, *Tetrahedron. Lett.*, 30:2809–2812, 1989.

Hori, M., Saito, S., Shin, Y.Z., Ozaki, H., Fusetani, N., and Karaki, H., Mycalolide-B, a novel and specific inhibitor of actomyosin ATPase isolated from marine sponge, *FEBS Lett.*, 322:151–154, 1993.

Panek, J.S. and Liu, P., Total synthesis of the actin-depolymerizing agent (–)-mycalolide A: Application of chiral silane-based bond construction methology, *J. Am. Chem. Soc.*, 122:11090–11097, 2000.

Saito, S. and Karaki, H., A family of novel actin-inhibiting marine toxins, *Clin. Exp. Pharmacol. Physiol.*, 23:743–746, 1996.

Saito, S., Watabe, S., Ozaki, H., Fusetani, N., and Karaki, H., Mycalolide B, a novel actin depolymerizing agent, *J. Biol. Chem.*, 269:29710–29714, 1994.

Sasaki, H., Ozaki, H., Karaki, H., and Nonomura, Y., Actin filaments play an essential role for transport of nascent HIV-1 proteins in host cells, *Biochem. Biophys. Res. Commun.*, 316:588–593, 2004.

M

Sugidachi, A., Ogawa, T., Asai, F., Saito, H., Ozaki, H., Fusetani, B.N., Karaki, H., and Koike, H., Inhibition of rat platelet aggregation by mycalolide-B, a novel inhibitor of actin polymerization with a different mechanism of action from cytochalasin, *D. Thromb. Haemost.*, 79:614–619, 1998.

Takakuwa, R., Kokai, Y., Kojima, T., Akatsuka, T., Tobioka, H., Sawada, N., and Mori, M., Uncoupling of gate and fence functions of MDCK cells by the actin-depolymerizing reagent mycalolide B, *Exp. Cell Res.*, 257:238–244, 2000.

Yeung, K.S. and Paterson, I., Actin-binding marine macrolides: Total synthesis and biological importance, *Angew Chem. In. Ed. Engl.*, 41:4632–4653, 2002.

Mycalamide A, B   Mycalamides A, B, and D, isolated from the New Zealand marine sponge Mycale sp., showed close structural similarity to the insect toxin pederin, and exhibited potent cytoxicity and antitumor activity. All members of the pederin family are rare, difficult to isolate, and comparatively frail.

1 Mycalamide A (R=H)
2 Mycalamide B (R=Me)

Structures of mycalamide A and B. (Gardiner et al., *Tetrahedron lett.*, 45:1215–1217, 2004. With permission.)

Mycalamides A and B exhibited potent *in vitro* toxicity and *in vivo* efficacy against murine and human tumor cells. They were reported to inhibit HL-60, HT-29, and A549 human cell tumor lines. Mycalamide A was also active against BV16 melanoma, Lewis lung carcinoma, M5076 ovarian sarcoma, colon 26 carcinoma, and the human MX-1, CX-1, and Burkitt's lymphoma tumor xenografts. Mechanistic studies indicated mycalamides inhibited protein synthesis (Burres and Clement, 1989). Moreover, mycalamide A blocked T-cell activation in mice (Galvin et al., 1993) and induced apoptosis in several cell lines (Hood et al., 2001).

Mycalamides A and B were reported to convert the morphology of *ras*-transformed NRK-cells to normal morphology by preferentially inhibiting the biosynthesis of p21 protein (Ogawa, 1991). In addition to their biological activity, their unique framework and scarcity from natural sources make these molecules attractive synthetic targets (Jason et al., 2003). Trost and coworkers (2004) recently achieved an efficient formal synthesis of (–)-mycalamide A.

References

Burres, N.S. and Clement, J.J., Antitumor activity and mechanism of action of the novel marine natural products mycalamide-A and -B and onnamide, *Cancer Res.*, 49:2935–2940, 1989.

Galvin, F., Freeman, G.J., Razi-Wolf, Z., Benacerraf, B., Nadler, L., and Reiser, H., Effects of cyclosporin A, FK 506, and mycalamide A on the activation of murine CD4+ T cells by the murine B7 antigen, *Eur. J. Immunol.*, 23:283–286, 1993.

Gardiner, J.M., Mills, R., and Fessard, T., Synthesis of model ring systems related to C10-C18 analogues of the mycalamides/theopederins, *Tetrahedron Lett.*, 45:1215–1217, 2004.

Hood, K.A., West, L.M., Northcote, P.T., Berridge, M.V., and Miller, J.H., Induction of apoptosis by the marine sponge (*Mycale*) metabolites, Mycalamide A and patearnine. *Aptosis,* 6:207–219, 2001.

Ogawara, H., Higashi, K., Uchino, K., and Perry, N.B., Change of *ras*-transformed NRK-cells back to normal morphology by mycalamides A and B, antitumor agents from a marine sponge, *Chem. Pharm. Bull.*, 39:2152–2154, 1991.

Rech, J.C. and Floreancig, P.E., An oxidative entry into the amido trioxadecalin ring system, *Org. Lett.*, 5:1495–1498, 2003.

Trost, B.M., Yang, H., and Probst, G.D., A formal synthesis of (–)-mycalamide A, *J. Am. Chem. Soc.*, 126:48-49, 2004.

West, L.M., Northcote, P.T., Hood, K.A., Miller, J.H., and Page, M.J., Mycalamide D, a new cytotoxic amide from New Zealand marine sponge mycale species, *J. Nat. Prod.*, 63:707–709, 2000.

Myristic acid   This short-chain, saturated fatty acid (C14:0) is generally associated with increasing plasma total cholesterol, particularly

$$CH_3(CH_2)_{12}COOH$$

LDL cholesterol, in humans (Hays and Khosla, 1997; Hegsted et al., 1965). This was based on diets in which myristic acid accounted for 16 percent of the total dietary energy (Salter et al., 1998) or where cholesterol doses were too low or too high (Nicolosi et al., 1997). Recent research suggests myristic acid is an important cell component, as proteins need to be myristoylated for the transduction pathway, vesicular trafficking, and structural positioning (Boutin, 1997). Maternal milk, considered to be well balanced, contains 9 percent myristic acid, or about 3–4 percent of total energy. Most of it is located in the *sn*-2 position of the triacylglycerol molecule (Jensen et al., 1990). Using golden Syrian hamsters, because of their similarity with human cholesterol metabolism, Loison and coworkers (2002) tested the hypothesis that myristic-acid-containing diets ranging from 0.5–2.4 percent of the total dietary energy had no detrimental effect on plasma cholesterol. In fact, these researchers, for the first time, found that myristic acid actually increased HDL-cholesterol (HDL-C) via regulation of the hepatic expression of the scavenger receptor B1 (SR-B1). Because of the atheroprotective role of HDL-C, it appears that myristic acid exerted a beneficial effect under these conditions.

References

Boutin, J.A., Myristoylation, *Cell Sig.,* 9:15–35, 1997.

Hays, K.C. and Khosla, P., Dietary fatty acid thresholds and cholesterolemia, *FASEB J.,* 6:2600–2607, 1992.

Hegsted, D.M., McGrandy, R.B., Myers, M.L., and Stare, F., Quantitative effects of dietary fat on serum cholesterol in man, *Am. J. Clin. Nutr.,* 17:281–295, 1965.

Jensen, R.G., Ferris, A.M., Lammi-Keefe, C.J., and Henderson, R.A., Lipids of bovine and human milks: A comparison, *J. Dairy Sci.,* 73:223–240, 1990.

Loison, C., Mendy, F., Serougne, C., and Louton, C., Dietary myristic acid modifies the HDL-cholesterol concentration and liver scavenger receptor B1 in hamsters, *Br. J. Nutr.,* 87:199–210, 2002.

Nicolosi, R.J., Dietary saturation effects on low-density lipoprotein concentrations and metabolism in various animal models, *Am. J. Clin. Nutr.,* 65:1617S–1627S, 1997.

Salter, A.M., Mangiapane, E.H., Bennet, A.J., Bruce, J.S., Billet, M.A., Anderton, K.L., Marenah, C.B., Lawson, N., and White, D.A., The effect of different dietary fatty acids on lipoprotein metabolism: Concentration-dependent effects of diet enriched in oleic acid, myristic, palmitic and stearic acids, *Br. J. Nutr.,* 79:195–202, 1998.

M

N-Acetyl-L-cysteine (NAC)

N-Acetyl-L-cysteine (NAC), a powerful antioxidant and immune enhancer, is the acylated form of the amino acid cysteine found naturally in foods. NAC is a precursor of glutathione, which functions as a detoxicant and antioxidant in the body

N-Acetyl cysteine (NAC). (Adapted from Coleman et al., *Environ. Toxicol. Pharmacol.* 17:143–148, 2004.)

(Aruoma et al., 1989; De Flora et al., 1995). NAC supplements were reported to improve symptoms, as well as prevent recurrences of chronic bronchitis in patients (Grandjean et al., 2000). A short-term study of patients with adenomatous colonic polyps found NAC significantly decreased the proliferative index (PI) (Estensen et al., 1999). Several case reports with Unverricht-Lundborg disease, an inherited degenerative disorder, was dramatically improved by supplementation with NAC (Hurd et al., 1996; Selwa, 1999). NAC is used as a possible treatment for HIV because *in vitro* studies showed that glutathione-deficient cells are particularly sensitive to inflammatory cytokines, such as tumor necrosis alpha (TNF) (Staal et al., 1992). Using NAC therapy to increase intracellular glutathione levels should prevent stimulation by TNF of nuclear transcription factor kB (NF-κB) in HIV-infected cells, virus transcription, and replication. Certain medications, however, may interact with NAC and should be avoided.

The isomers of NAC, LNAC, and DNAC were recently found by Neal and coworkers (2003) to be effective antioxidants, protecting mice lung from increased malondialdehyde levels and mice liver from increased 8-hydroxy-deoxyguanosine, following 18 Gy whole-body radiation. These results were consistent with the radioprotection and repair processes associated with NAC. Serrano-Mollar et al. (2003) found NAC reduced primary inflammatory events, which prevented cellular damage and pulmonary-fibrosis development in bleomycin-induced lung damage in rats.

References

Aruoma, O.I., Halliwell, B., Hoey, B.M., and Butler, J. The antioxidant activity of *N*-acetylcysteine: Its reaction with hydrogen peroxide, hydroxyl radicals, superoxides and hypochlorous acid, *Free Rad. Biol. Med.,* 6:593–597, 1989.

Coleman, M.D., Khan, N., Welton, G., Lambert, P.A., Tims, K.J., and Rathbone, D.L., Effects of glutathione, N-acetyl-cysteine, α-lipoic acid and dihydrolipoic acid on the cytotoxicity of a 2-pyridylcarboxamidrazone antimycobacterial agent in human mononuclear leucocytes *in vitro, Environ. Toxicol. Pharmacol.,* 17:143–148, 2004.

De Flora, S., Cesarone, C.F., Balansky, R.M., Albini, R., D'Agostini, F., Bennicelli, C., Bagnasco, Camoirano, A.M., Scatolini, A., Rovida, A., and Izzotti, A., Chemoprevention properties and mechanisms of *N*-acetylcysteine: The experimental background, *J. Cell Biochem.,* 22:33–41, 1995.

Estensen, R.D., Levy, M., Klopp, S.J., Galbraith, A.R., Mandel, J.S., Bloomquist, J.A., and Wattenerg, L.W., *N*-Acetylcysteine suppression of the proliferative index in the colon of patients with previous adenomatous colonic polyps, *Cancer Lett.,* 147:109–114, 1999.

Grandjean, E.M., Berthet, P., Ruffman, R., and Leuenberger, P., Efficacy of oral long-term *N*-acetylcysteine in chronic bronchopulmonary disease: A meta-analysis of published double-blind, placebo-controlled clinical trials, *Clin. Ther.,* 22:209–221, 2000.

Hurd, R.W., Wilder, B.J., Helveston, W.R., and Utham, B.M., Treatment of four siblings with progressive myoclonus epilepsy of the Unverricht-Lundborg type with *N*-acetyl cysteine, *Neurology,* 47:1264–1268, 1996.

Neal, R., Matthews, R.H., Lutz, P., and Ercal, N., Antioxidant role of *N*-acetyl cysteine isomers following high dose irradiation, *Free Rad. Biol. Med.,* 34: 689–695, 2003.

Selwa, L.M., *N*-Acetylcysteine therapy for Unverricht-Lundberg disease, *Neurol.,* 52:426–427, 1999.

Serrano-Mollar, A., Closa, D., Prats, N., Blesa, S., Martinez-Losa, M., Cortijo, J., Estrela, J.M., Morcillo, E.J., and Bulbena, O., *In vivo* antioxidant treatment protects against bleomycin-induced lung damage in rats, *Br. J. Pharmacol.,* 138:1037–1048, 2003.

Staal, F.J., Ela, S.W., Roederer, M., Anderson, M.T., and Herzenberg, L.A., Glutathione deficiency and human immunodeficiency virus infection, *Lancet,* 339:909–912, 1992.

Nacystelyn

Nacystelyn Nacystelin (NAL), a newly developed lysine salt of *N*-acetyl-L-cytokine (NAC), has been shown to have mucolytic and antioxidant properties. Antonicelli and coworkers (2002) showed NAL had therapeutic potential in inflammatory-lung diseases by its ability to inhibit cytokine release.

References

Antonicelli, F., Parmentier, M., Drost, E.M., Hirani, N., Rahman, I., Donaldson, K., and MacNee, W., Nacystelyn inhibits oxidant-mediated interleukin-8 expression and NF-κB nuclear binding in alveolar epithelial cells, *Free Rad. Biol. Med.,* 32:492–502, 2002.

Naringin and Naringenin

Naringin and Naringenin Naringin (4′,5,7-trihydroxyflavonone-7-rhamnoglucoside), the major flavonone glycoside in grapefruit, was shown to have antiulcer, as well as superoxide, scavenging and antioxidant properties (Kroyer, 1986; Chen et al., 1990). When digested, naringin is hydrolyzed by the intestinal bacteria to its absorbable aglycone metabolite, naringenin (4′,5,7-trihydroxyflavonone) (Ameer et al., 1996). The properties associated with naringin are probably reflected by similar properties observed for naringenin (Parmar, 1983; Kroyer, 1986). In addition, naringenin was also found to have vasodilatory, as well as anticancer, properties (Rojas et al., 1996; So et al., 1996). The health benefits reported for naringin are probably due to the formation of its hydrolyzed metabolite, naringenin. For example, recent studies by Singh and Chopra (2004) attributed the radical-scavenging and antioxidant properties of naringin to its renoprotective effect against reactive-oxygen species, which play a major role in the pathogenesis of renal ischemia, a common cause of acute renal failure. Because of the absence of acute or chronic toxicity, they suggested naringin had clinical application in the prevention of ischemia-reperfusion. However, the antioxidant properties of naringin were also shown by Kanno and coworkers (2004) to interfere with the cytotoxicity and apoptosis-inducing oxidative stress exerted by the antimetabolite chemotherapeutic drug, cytosine arabinoside, in the treatment of acute leukemia.

The ability of naringin to inhibit HMG-CoA reductase, a key enzyme in cholesterol biosynthesis, pointed to its potential as a cholesterol-lowering and antiatherogenic agent (Bok et al., 2000; Shin et al., 1999). Using the rabbit as the animal model, Jeon et al. (2004) recently compared the hypocholesterolemic action of naringin and lovastatin, a drug used for lowering cholesterol. Male rabbits were maintained on a 0.5 percent high-cholesterol diet with either 0.05 percent naringin or 0.03 percent lovastatin

Structure of naringin and naringenin. (From Kanaze et al., *J. Chromatgr.* B., 801:363–367, 2004.)

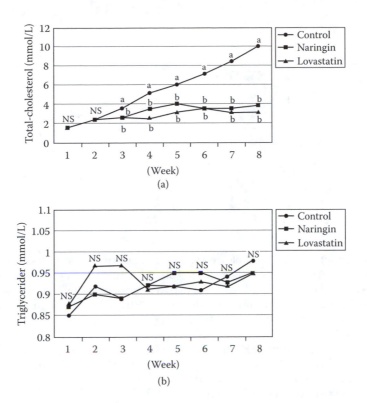

FIGURE N.67 Effects of naringin and lovastatin supplements for eight weeks on changes of plasma total cholesterol (a) and triglyceride (b) concentrations in high-cholesterol-fed rabbits. Values are mean ± SEM, n = 5. [a,b]Values not sharing a common letter are significantly different among groups at $p < 0.05$. [NS]Values are not significantly different among groups at $p < 0.05$. (Jeon et al., *Clin. Nutr.*, 23:1025–1035, 2004. With permission.)

over eight weeks. While the plasma triacylglycerols were unaffected by any of the treatments, there was a significant ($p < 0.05$) decrease in plasma total cholesterol, LDL cholesterol, and atherogenic index in animals treated with naringin or lovastatin. Naringin appeared to be as effective as lovastatin in lowering cholesterol, as shown in Figure N.67, for plasma total-cholesterol levels. Plasma HDL cholesterol was significantly higher in the naringin-fed group only. The cholesterol-lowering action of naringin was attributed to being mediated by a combination of acyl-CoA: cholesterol acyltransferase (ACAT) inhibition and increased sterol excretion.

The hypocholesterolemic properties of naringenin and several derivatives have also been demonstrated by Lee et al. (2003a). Two classes of naringenin derivatives, naringenin 7-*O*-oleic acid and naringenin 7-*O*-cetyl ether, both significantly reduced the formation of atherosclerotic lesions in rabbits fed a high-cholesterol (1 percent) diet, as shown in Figure N.68. However, the antiatherogenic effects could not be attributed to plasma-lipid levels so that another mechanism must be involved. Using rats, Lee and coworkers (2003b) showed naringenin 7-*O*-cetyl ether inhibited HMG-CoA reductase, as well as modulated plasma and hepatic lipids, when fed a high-cholesterol diet. Bernini and coworkers (2003) showed that naringenin lactone, formed from naringenin by the Baeyer–Villiger reaction, induced apoptosis in an E2 human lymphoma-cell line, normally resistant to apoptosis.

References

Ameer, B., Weintraub, R.A., Johnson, J.V., Yost, R.A., and Rouseff, R.L., Flavonone absorption after naringin, hesperidin, and citrus administration, *Clin. Pharmacol. Ther.*, 60:34–40, 1996.

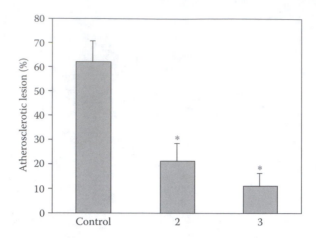

FIGURE N.68 Effects of naringenin 7-*O*-oleic ester (2) and naringenin 7-*O*-cetyl ether (3) on the aortic fatty-streak formations in rabbit model fed a high-cholesterol diet for eight weeks. A graph of atherosclerotic lesion size expressed as a percentage of the oil red-0 positive area/measured internal surface in each group. Bars represent standard deviations. * is significantly different ($p < 0.01$) from control group. (Lee et al., *Bioorg. Med. Chem. Lett.*, 13:3901–3903, 2003a. With permission.)

Bernini, R., Mincione, E., Cortese, M., Saladino, R., Gualandi, G., and Belfiore, M.C., Conversion of naringenin and hesperetin by heterogenous catalytic Baeyer-Villiger reaction into lactones exhibiting apoptotic activity, *Tetrahedron Lett.*, 44:4823–4825, 2003.

Bok, S.H., Shin, Y.W., Bae, K.H., Jeong, T.S., Kwon, Y.K., Park, Y.B., and Choi, M.S., Effects of narigin and lovastatin on plasma and hepatic lipids in high-fat and high-cholesterol fed rats. *Nutr. Res.*, 20:1007–1014, 2000.

Chen, Y., Zheng, R., Jia, Z., and Ju, Y., Flavonoids as superoxide scavengers and antioxidants, *Free Rad. Biol. Med.*, 9:19–21, 1990.

Galati, E.M., Trovato, A., Kirjavanein, S., Forestieri, A.M., Rossito, A., and Monforte, M.T., *Il Farmaco.*, 49:709–714, 1994.

Jeon, S.-M., Park, Y.B., and Choi, M.-S. Antihypercholesterolemic property of naringin alters plasma and tissue lipids, cholesterol-regulating enzymes, fecal sterol and tissue morphology in rabbits, *Clin. Nutr.*, 23:1025–1035, 2004.

Kanaze, F.I., Kokkalou, E., Georgarakis, M. and Niopas, I., Validated high-performance chromatographic method utilizing solid-phase extraction for the simultaneous determination of narigenin and hesperetin in human plasma, *J. Chromatogr.* B., 801:363–367, 2004.

Kanno, S., Shouji, A., Hirata, R., Asou, K., and Ishikawa, M., Effects of naringin on cytosine arabinoside (Ara-C)-induced cytotoxicity and apoptosis in P388 cells, *Life Sci.*, 75:353–365, 2004.

Kroyer, G., The antioxidant activity of citrus fruit peels, *Z. Ernahrungswiss.*, 25:63–69, 1986.

Lee, S., Lee, C.-H., Moon, S.-S., Kim, E., Kim, C.-T., Kim, B.H., Bok, S.-H., and Jeong, T.-S., Naringenin derivatives as anti-atherogenic agents, *Bioorg. Med. Chem. Lett.*, 13:3901–3903, 2003a.

Lee, M.K., Moon, S.S., Lee, S.E., Bok, S.H., Jeong, T.S., Park, Y.B., and Choi, M.S., Naringenin 7-*O*-cetyl ether as inhibitor of HMG-CoA reductase and modulator of plasma and hepatic lipids in high cholesterol-fed rats, *Bioorg. Med. Chem.*, 11:393–398, 2003b.

Parmar, N.S., The gastric antiulcer activity of naringenin, a specific histidine decarboxylase inhibitor, *Int. J. Tissue React.*, 5:415–420, 1983.

Rojas, D., Sanchez, V.R., Somoza, B., Ortega, T., and Villar, A., Vasodilatory effect of naringenin in rat aorta, *Phytother. Res.*, 10:S123–S125, 1996.

Ruh, M.F., Zacharewski, T., Connor, K., Howell, J., Chen, I., and Safe, S., Naringenin: A weakly estrogenic biflavoid that exhibits antiestrogenic activity, *Biochem. Pharmacol.*, 50:1485–1493, 1995.

Shin, Y.W., Bok, S.H., Jeuog, T.S., Bae, K.H., Jeoung, N.H., Choi, M.S. and Park, Y.B. Hypercholesterolemic effect of naringin associated with hepatic cholesterol regulating enzyme charges in rats, *Int. J. Vitamin Nutr.*, 69:27–31, 1994.

N

Singh, D. and Chopra, K., The effect of naringin, a bioflavonoid on ischemia-reperfusion induced renal injury in rats, *Pharmacol. Res.,* 50:187–193, 2004.

So, F.V., Guthrie, N., Chambers, A.F., Moussa, M., and Carroll, K.K., Inhibition of human breast cancer cell proliferation and delay of mammary tumorigenesis by flavonoids and citrus juices, *Nutr. Cancer*, 26: 167–181, 1996.

Nettle (*Urtica dioica* L.)   Nettles (*Urtica dioica* L.) are recognized for the stinging hairs on the leaves and stems, which release formic acid and histamine on the skin when touched. Nevertheless, many of these constituents (formic acid, acetylcholine, 5-hydroxytryptamine, and histamine) appear to have antiarthritic and antirheumatic properties. One of the best-known uses of nettles is for the treatment of gout and other rheumatic conditions by mobilizing uric acid from the joints and eliminating it through the kidney.

Aqueous extracts from nettles are used to treat a variety of ailments. In Morocco, for example, it is used as a hypotensive and antidiabetic agent (Bnouham et al., 2002). Significant antihyperglycemic effects observed with aqueous extracts from *Urtica dioica* were attributed, in part, to a reduction in intestinal glucose absorption (Bnouham et al., 2003). Farzami and coworkers (2003) also examined the blood-glucose-lowering effect of nettles and identified an active fraction, F_1, in extracts from nettles that enhanced insulin secretion from Islets of Langerhans.

The efficacy of nettle extracts as adjuvants in the treatment of rheumatism was attributed to their ability to inhibit expression of cytokines, as well as eicosanoid formation, in stimulated peripheral blood cells (Obetreis et al., 1996; Teucher et al., 1996). Subsequent work by Reihemann and coworkers (1999) showed that part of the anti-inflammatory action by nettle extracts involved inhibition of NF-κB activation. NF-κB, a family of transcription factors, is involved in the inducible expression of many genes involved in inflammatory responses (Baeuerle and Henkel, 1994; Barnes and Karin, 1997). These results are consistent with traditional antirheumatic drugs, which also exert part of their anti-inflammatory effects by interfering with the NF-κB pathway (Auphan et al., 1995; Sheinman et al., 1995; Wahl et al., 1998) A recent study by Gulcin et al. (2004) showed that a water extract from nettles exhibited antioxidant, antimicrobial, antiulcer, and analgesic properties.

References

Auphan, N., DiDonato, J.A., Rosette, C., Helmberg, A., and Karin, M., Immunosuppression by glucocorticoids: Inhibition of NF-κB activity through induction of IkB synthesis, *Science*, 270:286–290, 1995.

Barnes, P.J. and Karin, M., Mechanisms of disease: Nuclear Factor-κB-A pivotal transcription factor in chronic inflammatory diseases, *N. Engl. J. Med.,* 336:1066–1071, 1997.

Baeuerle, P.A. and Henkel, T., Function and activation of NF-κB in the immune system, *Annu. Rev. Immunol.,* 12:141–179, 1994.

Bnouhan, M., Mekhfi, H., Legssyer, A., and Ziyyat, A., Medicinal plants used in the treatment of diabetes in Morocco, *Int. J. Diab. Metab.,* 10:33–50, 2002.

Bnouhan, M., Merhfour, F.-Z., Ziyyat, A., Mekhfi, H., Aziz, M., and Legssyer, A., Antihyperglycemic activity of the aqueous extract of Urtica dioica, *Fitoterapia*, 74:677–681, 2003.

Farzami, B., Ahmadvand, D., Vardasbi, S., Majin, F.J., and Khagani, Sh., Induction of insulin secretion by a component of *Urtica dioica* leave extract in perifused Islets of Langerhans and its *in vivo* effects in normal and streptozotocin diabetic rats, *J. Ethnopharmacol.,* 89:47–53, 2003.

Gulcin, I., Kufrevioglu, O.I., Oktay, M., and Buyukokuroglu, M.E., Antioxidant, antimicrobial, antiulcer and analgesic activities of nettle (*Urtica dioica* L.), *J. Ethnopharmacol.,* 90:205–215, 2004.

Obertreis, B., Ruttkowski, T., Teucher, T., Behnke, B., and Shmitz, H., Anti-inflammatory effect of *Urtica folia* extract in comparison to caffeic malic acid, *Arzneim-Forsch Res.,* 46:389–394, 1996.

Reihemann, K., Behnke, B. and Schulze-Ostho, K., Plant extracts from stinging nettle (*Urtica dioica*), an antirheumatic remedy, inhibit the proinflammatory transcription factor-NF-κB. *FEBS Lett.,* 442:89–94, 1999.

Scheinman, R.I., Cogswell, P.C., Lofquist, A.K., and Baldwin, A.S., Jr., Role of transcriptional IkBa in mediation by immunosuppresion by glucocorticoids, *Science*, 270:283–286, 1995.

N

Teucher, T., Obertreis, B., Ruttkowski, T., and Shmitz, H., Cytokine secretion in whole blood of healthy volunteers after oral ingestion of an *Urtica dioica* L. leaf extract, *Arzneim-Forsch. Res.*, 46:906–910, 1996.

Wahl, C., Liptay, S., Adler, G., and Schmid, R.M., Sulfasalazine: A potent and specific inhibitor of nuclear factor κB, *J. Clin. Invest.*, 101:1163–1174, 1998.

Niacin and Nicotinamide   Niacin or nicotinic acid, β-pyridine carboxylic acid, is a water-soluble B vitamin that is readily converted into its physiologically active form, nicotinamide. Nicotinic acid was first reported a half a century ago by Altschul et al. (1955) to lower serum cholesterol in man. A subsequent study by Canner et al. (1986) used pharmacological doses of nicotinic acid as a hypolipidemic agent in the Coronary Drug Project to improve long-term survival after myocardial infarction. Niacin lowered plasma triglycerides and total and LDL cholesterol, while increasing HDL levels. The mechanism of action appeared to involve inhibition of peripheral lipolysis and VLDL synthesis and shunt of apolipoprotein B degradation, together with decreased apo A-I removal (Grundy et al., 1981; Jin et al., 1989). The reduced cellular cholesterol content and enhanced HDL-mediated cholesterol efflux appeared to result from the effects of niacin on the transcription of several key transporters and receptors involved in reverse cholesterol transport (Rubic et al., 2004). Signaling pathways transmitting niacin effects suggested a role for naicin-induced prostaglandin D_2 formation and activation of peroxisome proliferator-activated receptor gamma (PPARγ) in expression of the combined adhesion and scavenger receptor CD36.

A combination of statins, cholesterol-lowering drugs, and niacin were reported to produce clinical and angiographic benefits in patients suffering from coronary heart disease in an HDL-Atherosclerosis Treatment Study (HATS) (Brown et al., 2001). A three-year study by Zhao et al. (2004) on 160 patients with coronary heart disease found that a mean daily dose of simvastatin-niacin (13 mg and 4 mg, respectively) halted the progression of angiographic atherosclerosis. In addition, patients with low HDL had a reduction of 60 percent in the major clinical events associated with the disease compared to the placebos. A combination of simvastatin and niacin proved to be an effective and safe treatment that was well-tolerated by patients with or without diabetes mellitus. The therapeutic potential of niacin/statin combinations was also demonstrated by Bays and coworkers (2003) in a 16-week treatment of 315 patients (with elevated LDL cholesterol and low HDL cholesterol). A combination of extended-release niacin (niacin ER) and lovastatin proved far more effective in improving lipid profiles than either simvastatin or atorvastatin, as summarized in Table N.48.

In addition to the cholesterol-lowering effects of nicotinic acid, the cytoprotective and antiviral properties of nicotinamide is also receiving increasing attention. Maiese and Chong (2003) suggested nicotinamide may slow down degenerative diseases associated with the central nervous system. Another study implicated nicotinamide in the prevention of AIDS (Murray, 1999). Gaudineau and Auclair (2004) recently reported inhibition of human P450 enzymes by nicotinic acid and nicotinamide. The ability to inhibit P450 enzymes raises serious questions regarding the consumption of large, pharmacologically active doses of this vitamin in light of potential drug interactions when using multidrug therapies. Several recent reviews on the lipid-lowering properties of niacin are recommended (Ganji et al., 2003; Rosenson, 2003).

References

Altschul, R., Hoffer, A., and Stephen, J.D., Influence of nicotinic acid on serum cholesterol in man, *Arch. Biochem. Biophys.*, 54:558–559, 1955.

Bays, H.E., Dujovne, C.A., McGovern, M.E., White, E.T., Kashyap, M.L., Hutcheson, G.H., and Crouse, J.R., Comparison of once daily, niacin extended-release/lovastatin with standard simvastatin (The Advicor Versus Other Cholesterol-Modulating Agents Trial Evaluation [Advocate]), *Am. J. Cardiol.*, 91:667–672, 2003.

Brown, B.G., Zhao, X.-Q., Chait, A., Fisher, L.D., Mrse, J.S., Dowdy, A.A., Marino, E.K., Bolson, E.L., Alaupic, P., Frohlich, J., and Albers, J.J., Simvastatin

TABLE N.48
Percent Change from Baseline Following Niacin/Lovastatin, Atorvastatin, and Simvastatin Treatments

	Niacin ER/Lovastatin		Atorvastatin	Simvastatin
Week 8	1,000/40 mg	1,000/40 mg	10 mg	10 mg
LDL cholesterol	−38%[†]	−40%[†]	−38%[†]	−28%
HDL cholesterol	+20%[†‡]	+20%[†‡]	+3%	+7%[‡]
Triglycerides	−30%[†‡]	−35%[†‡]	−20%	−18%
Lipoprotein(a)	−16%[†‡]	−14%[‡]	+8%	0%[‡]
Week 12*	1,000/40 mg	1,500/40 mg	20 mg	20 mg
LDL cholesterol	−42%[†]	−42%[†]	−45%[†]	−35%
HDL cholesterol	+19%[†‡]	+24%[†‡]	+4%	+8%[‡]
Triglycerides	−36%[†‡]	−42%[†‡]	−30%[†]	−15%
Lipoprotein(a)	−20%[†‡]	−17%[†‡]	+2%	−1%
Week 16*	1,000/40 mg	2,000/40 mg	40 mg	40 mg
LDL cholesterol	−39%	−42%	−49%[†§]	−39%
HDL cholesterol	+17%[†‡]	+32%[†‡]	+6%	+7%
Triglycerides	−29%[†]	−49%[†]	−31%[†]	−19%
Lipoprotein(a)	−19%[†‡]	−21%[†‡]	0%	−2%

Note: LDL and HDL cholesterol are expressed as mean values, and triglycerides and Lp(a) are expressed as median values.

* Dosage is milligrams per day.

[†] $p \leq 0.05$ versus simvastatin.

[‡] $p \leq 0.05$ versus atorvastatin.

[§] $p \leq 0.05$ versus niacin ER/lovastatin 1,000/40 and 2,000/40 mg.

Source: From Bays et al., *Am. J. Cardiol.*, 91:667–672, 2003. With permission.

N

and niacin, antioxidant vitamins, or the combination for the prevention of coronary disease, *N. Engl. J. Med.*, 345:1583–1592, 2001.

Canner, P.L., Berge, K.G., Wenger, N.K., Stamler, J., Friedman, L., Prineas, R.J., and Friedewald, W., Fifteen years mortality in Coronary Drug Project patients: Long-term benefits with niacin, *J. Am. Coll. Cardiol.*, 8:1245–1255, 1986.

Ganji, S.H., Kamanna, V.S., and Kashyap, M.L., Niacin and cholesterol: Role in cardiovascular disease (Review), *J. Nutr. Biochem.*, 14:298–305, 2003.

Gaudineau, C. and Auclair, K., Inhibition of human P450 enzymes by nicotinic acid and nicotinamide, *Biochem. Biophys. Res. Commun.*, 317:950–956, 2004.

Grundy, S.M., Mok, H.Y., Zech, L., and Berman, M., Influence of nicotinic acid on metabolism of cholesterol and triglycerides in man, *J. Lipid Res.*, 22:24–36, 1981.

Jin, F.Y., Kamanna, V.S., and Kashyap, M.L., Niacin accelerates intracellular Apo B degradation by inhibiting triacylglycerol synthesis in human hepatoblastoma

(HepG2) cells, *Arterioscler. Thromb. Vasc. Biol.*, 19: 1051–1059, 1999.

Maiese, K. and Chong, Z.Z., Nicotinamide: Necessary nutrient emerges as a novel cytoprotectant for the brain, *Trends Pharmacol. Sci.*, 24:228–232, 2003.

Murray, M.F., Niacin as a potential AIDS preventive factor, *Med. Hypoth.*, 53:375–379, 1999.

Rosenson, R.S., Antiatherothrombotic effects of nicotinic acid, *Atherosclerosis*, 171:87–96, 2003.

Rubic, T., Trottmann, M., and Lorenz, R.L., Stimulation of the CD36 and the key effector of reverse cholesterol transport ATP-binding cassette A1 in monocytoid cells by niacin, *Biochem. Pharmacol.*, 67:411–419, 2004.`

Zhao, X.-Q., Morse, J.S., Dowdy, A.A., Heise, N., DeAngelis, D., Frohlich, J., Chait, A., Albers, J.J., and Brown, B.G., Safety and tolerability of simvastatin plus niacin in patients with coronary artery disease and low-high-density lipoprotein cholesterol (The HDL Atherosclerosis Treatment Study), *Am. J. Cardiol.*, 93:307–312, 2004.

Nicotinic Acid *see* Niacin

Nobiletin Nobiletin (5,6,7,8,3′,4′-hexa-methoxyflavone) is a polymethoxyflavonoid present in citrus fruit, including tangerines, sweet orange peel (*Citrus sinensis*), and in bitter orange (*Citrus aurantium*) (Horowitz and Gentilli, 1977). Kohno et al. (2001) reported that nobiletin suppressed the formation of azoxymethane (AOM)-induced colonic aberrant crypt foci (ACF) in rats. This was evident by the significant reduction in the frequency of

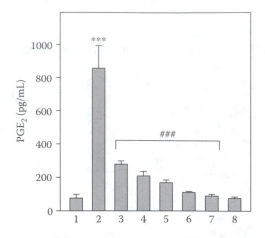

FIGURE N.69 Suppression of PGE_2 production by nobiletin in human synovial fibroblasts. Confluent synovial cells, at passage 10, were treated in 24-multiwell plates with recombinant human interleukin-1 a (rhIL-a) (1 ng/mL) and nobiletin in 1.0 mL of DMEM/0.2 percent LAH for 24 h. The amount of PGE_2 released in the culture medium was determined by enzyme immunoassay. Treatments: 1, control; 2, rhIL-1a; 3–7, rhIL-1a plus nobiletin (4, 8, 16, 32, and 64 mM, respectively); and 8, nobiletin (64 mM). Data are the means of ± SD for quadruplicate wells. Key: (***) and (###), significantly different from the control ($p < 0.001$) and the rhIL-1a-treated cells ($p < 0.001$), respectively, (Lin et al., *Biochem. Pharmacol.*, 65:2065–2071, 2003. With permission.)

Nobiletin. (From Iwase et al., *Cancer Lett.*, 163:7–9, 2001. With permission.)

ACF of 55 percent and 50 percent when nobiletin was fed over a five-week period at doses of 0.01 percent and 0.05 percent, respectively. The anti-inflammatory action of nobiletin was demonstrated by Ishiwa et al. (2000), who showed it suppressed the production of promatrix metalloproteinase (proMMP)-9/progelatinase B in rabbit synovial fibroblasts. High levels of the latter are found in the synovial tissues and fluid of patients with rheumatoid arthritis (Tetlow et al., 1993). Lin et al. (2003) further explored the anti-inflammatory properties of nobiletin and showed it interfered with the production of PGE_2 (Figure N.69). In contrast to interleukin-1a (IL-1α), which augmented PGE_2 production tenfold (treatment 2), nobiletin suppressed the IL-1-α mediated production of PGE_2 in a dose-dependent manner (4–64 mM; treatments 3–7). For example, a 65 percent reduction of IL-1α-induced PGE_2 production was evident by the presence of 4 mM nobiletin (treatment 3). Nobiletin interfered with PGE_2 production in human synovial fibroblasts by

down regulating of the COX-2 gene, while decreasing the expression of IL-1α, IL-1β, TNF-α, and IL-6 mRNAs in mouse macrophages. Based on these results, nobiletin appeared to have considerable potential as an immunomodulatory and anti-inflammatory drug.

The possible role of nobiletin in the prevention of atherosclerosis was reported by Whitman et al. (2005) because of its ability to reduce plasma cholesterol levels. Nobiletin inhibited acetylated LDL (acLDL)-mediated accumulaion of cholesterol esters in culture murine macrophages by 50–72 percent by an unknown mechanism, as it did not affect SR-A protein expression. In addition to reducing plasma cholesterol, it may also inhibit macrophage foam-cell formation.

Tanaka and coworkers (2004) proposed nobiletin as a new sunscreen reagent because of its ability to inhibit PGE_2 production by ultraviolet B (UVB) irradiation. Nobiletin suppressed COX-2 expression and decreased the activity of cytosolic phospholipase A (CPLA) in UVB-irradiated human keratinocytes. Its ability to prevent UVB-induced photoinflammation and photoaging of human keratinocytes makes nobiletin a potential sunscreen reagent.

References

Horowitz, R.M. and Gentilli, B., Flavonoid constituents of citrus, in *Citrus Science and Technology*, Nagy, S., Shaw, P.E., and Veldius, M.K., Eds., Avi Publishing Co., Westport, Connecticut, 1977, pp. 397–426.

Iwase, Y., Takemura, Y., Ju-ichi, M., Yano, M., Ito, C., Furukawa, H., Mukainaka, T., Kuchide, M., Tokuda, H., and Nishino, H., Cancer preventive activity of 3,5,6,7,8,3′,4′-heptamethoxyflavone from the peel of citrus plants, *Cancer Lett.,* 163:7–9, 2001.

Ishiwa, J., Sato, T., Mimaki, Y., Sushida, Y., Yano, M., and Ito, A., Citrus flavonoid nobiletin, suppresses the production and gene expression of matrix metalloproteinase 9/geratinase B in rabbit synovial fibroblasts, *J. Rheumatol.,* 271:20–25, 2000.

Kohno, H., Yoshitani, S., Tsukio, Y., Murakami, A., Koshimuzu, K., Yano, M., Tokuda, H., Nishino, H., Ohigashi, H., and Tanaka, T., Dietary administration of citrus nobiletin inhibits azoxymethane-induced colonic aberrant crypt foci in rats, *Life Sci.,* 69:901–913, 2001.

Lin, N., Sato, T., Takayama, Y., Mimaki, Y., Sashida, Y., Yano, M., and Itoh, A., Novel anti-inflammatory actions of nobiletin, a citrus polymethoxyflavonoid on human synovial fibroblasts and mouse macrophages, *Biochem. Pharmacol.,* 65:2065–2071, 2003.

Tanaka, S., Sato, T., Akimoto, N., Yano, M., and Ito, A., Prevention of UVB-induced photoinflammation and photoaging by the polymethoxyflavonoid, nobiletin, in human keratinocytes *in vivo* and *in vitro*, *Biochem. Pharmacol.,* 68:433–439, 2004.

Tetlow, L.C., Lees, M., Ogata, Y., Nagase, H., and Woolley, D.E., Differential expression of gelatinase B (MMP-9) and stromelysin-1 (MMP3) by rheumatoid synovial cells *in vitro* and *in vivo*. *Rheumatol. Int.,* 13:53–59, 1993.

Whitman, S.C., Kurowska, E.M., Manthey, J.A., and Duaghtery, A., Nobiletin, a citrus flavonoid isolated from tangarenes, selectively inhibits class A scavenger receptor-mediated metabolism of acetylated LDL by mouse macrophages, *Atherosclerosis,* 178:25–32, 2005.

Nordihydroguaiaretic acid   Nordihydroguaiaretic acid (NDGA) is also known as β, γ-dimethyl-α, delta-*bis*-(3,4-dihydroxyphenyl)butane; 4.4′-(2,3-dimethyltetramethylene)

Nordihyroguaiaretic acid. (From Lambert et al., *Toxicon.,* 40:1701–1708, 2002.)

dipyrocatechol. It is a constituent of the creosote bush *Larrea divaricata* and well known to be a selective inhibitor of lipoxygenases.

NDGA can also inhibit platelet-derived growth factor and the protein kinase C intracellular signaling family, which both play an important role in proliferation and survival of cancers. In fact, NDGA was shown to induce apoptosis in tumor xenografts (McDonald et al., 2001). NDGA is a lignan also found in large amounts (up to 10 percent by dry weight) in the leaves and twigs of *L. tridentata* capable of inducing cystic nephropathy in the rat, with intraperitoneal administration of NDGA being lethal in the mouse (LD$_{50}$ = 75 mg/kg) (Lambert et al., 2002). It can also block protein transport from the endoplasmic reticulum (ER) to the Golgi complex and induce the redistribution of Golgi proteins intro the ER (Fujiwara et al., 2003). Ono and coworkers (2002) showed NDGA inhibited fAbeta formation from Abeta and breaks down fAbeta *in vitro,* which suggests it could be a key molecule for the development of therapeutics for Alzheimer's disease. More recently Nakamura et al. (2003) reported NDGA protected microtubules in NRK cells from depolymerization caused by diverse drugs, suggesting NDGA belonged to a novel family of microtubule-stabilizing drugs.

NDGA has been used as an antioxidant in oils and foods. Specific inhibition of peroxidase, catalase, ethyl alcohol dehydrogenase, was shown to occur in the presence of 2×10^{-4} M of the antioxidant. Nonspecific inhibition of ascorbic-acid oxidase, D-amino-acid oxidase, the cyclophorase system, and urease have been reported in the presence of 2×10^{-4} M NDGA (Tappel and Marr, 1954). Acute toxicity studies indicated that the guinea pig is more sensitive than the rat (Griepentro, 1961). Published, long-term studies in the rat and mouse provided little detailed information and left some of the investigators in doubt regarding its safety (Cranston et al., 1947; Mannell, 1964).

References

Cranston, E.M., Jensen, M.J., Moren, A., Brey, T., Bell, E.T., and Bieter, R.N., The acute and chronic toxicity of nordihydroguaiaretic acid, *Fed. Proc.,* 6: 318–319, 1947.

Fujiwara, T., Misumi, Y., and Ikehara, Y., Direct interaction of the Golgi membrane with the endoplasmic membrane caused by nordihydroguaiaretic acid, *Biochem. Biophys. Res. Commun.,* 301:927–933, 2003.

Griepentrog, F., Allergy studies with simple compounds VII, Nordihydroguaiaretic acid, *Arzneimittel-Forsch,* 11:920–922, 1961.

Lambert, J.D., Zhao, D., Meyers, R.O., Kuester, R.K., Timmerman, B.N., and Dorr, R.T., Nordihydroguaiaretic acid: Hepatoxicity and detoxification in the mouse, *Toxicon.,* 40:1701–1708, 2002.

Lehman, A.J., Fitzhugh, O.G., Nelson, A.A., and Woodard, G., The pharmacological evaluation of antioxidants, *Adv. Food Res.,* 3:197–208, 1951.

Mannell, W.A., Canadian Food and Drug Directorate, Ottawa (letter, September 23), 1964.

McDonald, R.W., Bunjobpon, W., Liu, T., Fessler, S., Pardo, O.E., Glaser, M., Seckl, M.J., and Robins, D.J., Synthesis and anticancer activity of nordihydroguaiaretic acid (NDGA) and analogues, *Anticancer Drug Des.,* 16:261–270, 2001.

Nakamura, M., Nakazawa, J., Usui, T., Osada, H., Kono, Y., and Takatsuki, A., Nordihydroguaiaretic acid, of a new family of microtubule-stabilizing agents, shows effects differentiated from paclitaxel, *Biosci. Biotechnol. Biochem.,* 67:151–157, 2003.

Ono, K., Hasegawa, K., Yoshiike, Y., Takashima, A., Yamada, M., and Naiki, H., Nordihydroguaiaretic acid potently breaks down pre-formed Alzheimer's β-amyloid fibrils *in vitro,* J. *Neurochem.,* 81:434–440, 2002.

Tappel, A.L. and Marr, A.G., Antioxidants and enzymes, effect of α-tocopherol, propyl gallate, and nordihydroguaiaretic acid on enzymatic reactions, *J. Agric. Food Chem.,* 2:554–558, 1954.

Nuts *see* **Almonds and Walnuts** Albert et al. (2002) prospectively assessed whether increasing the frequency of nut consumption was associated with a lower risk of sudden cardiac death and related coronary heart disease points among 21,454 males enrolled in the U.S. Physicians' Health Study. Participants were monitored over an average of 17 years, and the results suggested an inverse association between nut consumption and the total coronary heart disease deaths.

References

Albert, C.M., Gaziano, M., Willett, W.C., and Manson, J.E., Nut consumption and decreased risk of sudden cardiac death in the Physicians' Health Study, *Arch. Intern. Med.,* 162:1382-1387, 2002.

N

O

Oatmeal Using a lauryl sulfate-irritation model, Boyer and coworkers (1998) demonstrated the anti-inflammatory and healing properties of several processed oatmeal extracts from *Avena Rheala* and *Avena Sativa*. Incorporating 20 percent of each oatmeal extract in a petrolatum ointment resulted in a similar 60 percent inhibition of perfusion blood flow, a measure of inflammation following application of 50 μl of 1 percent solution of lauryl sulfate to the forearm of 12 healthy volunteers, compared to the control. Oatmeal is recommended by veterinarians for treating skin allergies in pets.

References

Boyer, F., Dane, G.S., Borrel, M.T., Dupuy, P., and Gall, Y., Anti-inflammatory properties of oatmeal extracts using a lauryl-sulfate irritation model, *J. Dermatol. Sci.,* 16 (Suppl. 1):S217, 1998.

Oats The first health claim permitted by the Food and Drug Administration (FDA) in the U.S.A. under the Nutrition Labelling and Education Act (1990) for a specific food was made for diets high in oatmeal, oat bran, or oat flour. These diets were associated with a reduction in coronary heart disease. Food and feed oats belong to the species *Avena sativa*. Katz et al. (2001a) was the first to report the beneficial effects of daily supplementing the diet of 50 healthy subjects with whole-grain oats or wheat cereal by ameliorating the fat-induced impairment of vascular reactivity. The results observed were comparable to that of vitamin E. In fact, endothelial dysfunction following acute fat ingestion was shown by Katz et al. (2001b) to be concomitant with ingestion of vitamin E and oats, but not wheat.

The reduction in blood-cholesterol levels by oats was attributed to the presence of high levels of soluble fiber in the bran. This proved to be a linear, high-molecular-weight β-glucan, composed of β-1,4-linked glucose units separated by a single β-1,3-linked glucose every two or three units (Braaten et al., 1999).

Behall and coworkers (1997) examined the hypolipidemic effects of this soluble fiber by incorporating it into a typical diet of 7 men and 16 women. They found that β-glucan reduced total and LDL cholesterol, particularly in subjects maintained on a high β-glucan diet (Table O.49). No changes in triacylglycerol levels were observed.

Using a randomized, blind, placebo-controlled crossover design, Braaten et al. (1999) further established the relationship between oat-bran consumption and reduction in blood cholesterol in hypercholesterolemic individuals. Davy et al. (2002) showed that the addition of two large servings of oats also significantly reduced total and LDL cholesterol, thereby reducing the risk of cardiovascular disease.

Oat mixed-linkage β-glucan [(1→3)(1→4)-β-D-glucan. (From Colleoni-Sirghie et al., *Carbohydr. Polym.,* 54: 237–249, 2003. With permission.)

TABLE O.49
Mean Plasma Lipids in Subjects on Controlled Diets

	Maintenance diet mmol/L	Low β-glucan diet (1 percent)	High β-glucan diet (1 percent)
Total Cholesterol	5.47 ± 0.19	4.95 ± 0.19	4.67 ± 0.19
LDL Cholesterol	3.65 ± 0.16	3.11 ± 0.16	2.89 ± 0.16

Source: From Behall et al., *J. Am. Coll. Nutr.,* 16:46–51, 1997. With permission.

References

Behall, K., Schofield, D., and Hallfrisch, J., Effect of β-glucan in oat fiber extracts on blood lipids in men and women, *J. Am. Coll. Nutr.,* 16:46–51, 1997.

Braaten, J.T., Wood, P.J., Scott, F.W., Wolneytz, M.S., Lowe, M.K., Bradley-White, P. and Collins, M.W., Oats β-glucan reduces blood cholesterol concentration in hypercholesterlemic subjects, *Eur. J. Clin Nutr.,* 48:465–475, 1994.

Colleoni-Sirghie, M., Fulton, D.B., and White, P.J., Structural features of water soluble (1,3) (1,4)-b-D-glucans from high-b-glucan and traditional oat lines, *Carbohydr. Polym.,* 54:237–249, 2003.

Davy, B.M., Davin, K.P., Ho, R.C., Beske, S.D., Davrath, L.R., and Melby, C.L., High-fiber oat cereal compared with wheat cereal consumption favorably alters LDL-cholesterol subclass and particle numbers in middle-aged and older men, *Am. J. Clin. Nutr.,* 76: 351–358, 2002.

Katz, D.L., Nawaz, H., Boukhalil, J., Chan, W., Ahmadi, R., Giannamore, V., and Sarrel, P.M., Effects of oats and wheat cereals on endothelial responses, *Prev. Med.,* 33:476–484, 2001a.

Katz, D.L., Nawaz, H., Boukhalil, J., Giannamore, C.V.T., Chan, W., Ahmadi, R., and Sarrel, P.M., Acute effects of oats and vitamin E on endothelial responses to ingested fat, *Am. J. Prev. Med.,* 20:124–129, 2001b.

Oat avenanthramides   A group of novel alkaloids containing phenolic groups was identified by Collins (1989) in oat groats and hulls and identified as avenanthramides. They are substituted hydroxycinnamic-acid conjugates, with more than 25 types identified. The three most abundant avenanthramides, N-(4′-hydroxy-3′-cinnamoyl)-5-hydroxy-anthranilic acid (Bf), N-(4′-hydroxycinnamoyl)-5-hydroxy-anthranilic acid (Bp), and N-(3′,4′-dihydroxycinnamoyl)-5-hydroxyanthranilic acid (Bc), were shown to exhibit antioxidant activity using two *in vitro* systems (Scheme O.40) (Peterson et al., 2002). The levels of avenanthramides in oat groats were shown by Emmons and Peterson (2001) to be affected by genotype and growing conditions. Further breeding or growing in a particular environment could enhance the antioxidant capacity. Ji et al.

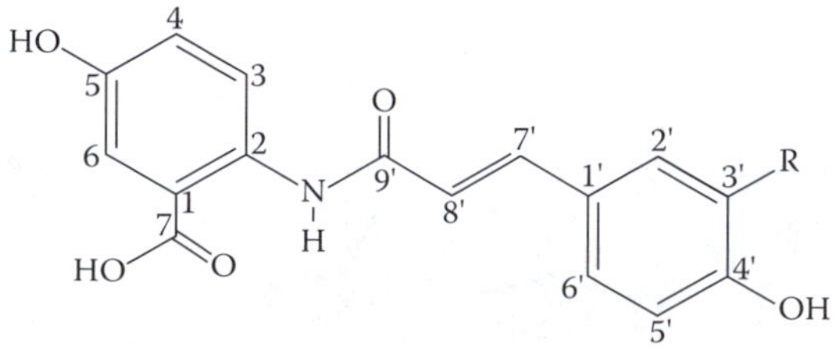

Avenanthramide	R
Bp	H
Bf	OCH$_3$
Bc	OH

SCHEME O.40 Oat aventhramides Bc, Bp, and Bf structures. (Peterson et al., *Food Chem.,* 79:473–478, 2002. With permission.)

(2003) showed for the first time that a diet supplemented with 0.1 percent synthetic Bc was tissue specific by only attenuating exercise-induced ROS in the soleus muscle and lipid peroxidation in the heart of female Sprague–Dawley rats compared to the control. A recent study by Liu and coworkers (2004) provided further evidence for the anti-inflammatory and antiatherogenic properties of oat avenanthramides.

References

Collins, F.W., Oat phenolics: Avenanthramides, novel substituted *N*-cinnamoylanthranilate alkaloids from oat groats and hulls, *J. Agric. Food Chem.*, 37:60–66, 1989.

Emmons, C.L. and Peterson, D.M., Antioxidant activity and phenolic contents of oat as affected by cultivar and location, *Crop Sci.*, 41:1676–1681, 1999.

Ji, L.L., Lay, D., Chung, E., Fu, Y., and Peterson, D.M., Effects of avenanthramides on oxidant generation and antioxidant enzyme activity in exercised rats, *Nutr. Res.*, 23:1579–1590, 2003.

Liu, L., Zubik, L., Collins, W.F., Marko, M.G., and Meydani, M., The antiatherogenic potential of oat phenolic compounds, *Atherosclerosis*, 175:39–49, 2004.

Peterson, D.M., Hahn, M.J., and Emmons, C.L., Oat avenanthamides exhibit antioxidant activities *in vitro*, *Food Chem.*, 79:473–478, 2002.

Ocimum sanctum   *Ocimum sanctum*, an annual herb grown throughout India, is considered sacred by the Hindus as *tulsi*, or "holy basil" in English. It has been reported to possess therapeutic properties, such as anticarcinogenic, antiseptic, antirheumatic, antistress, antihelmintic, and antibacterial activities (Bhargava and Singh 1981; Singh et al., 1996; Singh and Majumdar, 1999; Godhwani et al., 1987, 1988). Singh and Majumdar (1997) attributed the anti-inflammatory activity of *O. sanctum* to the ability of linolenic acid present in the fixed oil to block both the cyclooxygenase and lipoxygenase pathways of arachidonate metabolism. In addition to anti-inflammatory properties, Singh and Majumdar (1999) also reported *O. sanctum*-fixed oil had antiulcer activity. A recent study by

Dharmani et al. (2004) confirmed the antiulcer and ulcer-healing properties of *O. sanctum*. Using acetic acid-induced chronic gastric-ulcer animal models, they found the ulcers were completely healed within 20 days of treatment. They attributed this effect to the cytoprotective properties of *O. sanctum*, which has considerable potential for treating peptic ulcers.

Using an anaesthetized dog, Singh et al. (2001) showed the oil from *O. sanctum* exhibited hypotensive and anticoagulant activities comparable to that of aspirin. The ability of the oil to increase the pentobarbitone-induced sleeping time in rats was attributed to its possible inhibition of the cytochrome system involved in the hepatic metabolism of this drug.

The potential of *O. sanctum* for treating diabetes mellitus was examined by Vats and coworkers (2002), using an ethanolic extract from its leaves. They found a small but significant hypoglycemic effect in normal rats, as a single administration of 100, 200, and 400 mg/kg of the extract decreased glucose levels by 7.64 percent, 17.18 percent, and 19.78 percent, respectively. A significant reduction in plasma glucose levels was also observed in alloxanized rats. Recent work by Vats et al. (2004) showed *O. sanctum* significantly increased the activity of glucokinase, hexokinase, and phospho-fructokinase, the three key enzymes of carbohydrate metabolism, in streptozotocin-induced rats. The increase in these glycolytic enzymes observed in animals treated with *O. sanctum* could be secondary to the release of insulin. Since streptozotocin diabetes is an insulin-deficient model, it is likely that the component in *O. sanctum* exerts insulinomimetic activity. Further clinical studies are needed, however, to more conclusively establish *O. sanctum* as an antidiabetic herb. An earlier *in vitro* study by Halder et al. (2003) showed that the anticataract properties of an aqueous extract from *O. sanctum* was a significant inhibitor of aldose reductase in the rat lens. The latter enzyme plays a key role in sugar-induced cataract formation.

References

Bhargava, K.P. and Singh, N., Antistress activity of *Ocimum sanctum* Linn, *Ind. J. Med. Res.*, 73:443–451, 1981.

Dharmani, P., Kuchibhotla, V.K., Maurya, R., Srivastava, S., Sharma, S., and Palit, G., Evaluation of anti-ulcerogenic and ulcer-healing properties of *Ocimum sanctum* Linn, *J. Ethnopharmacol.*, 99:361–366, 2004.

Godhwani, S., Godhwani, J.L., and Was, D.S., *Ocimum sanctum* — an experimental study evaluating its anti-inflammatory, analgesic and antipyretic activity in animals, *J. Ethnopharmacol.*, 21:153–163, 1987.

Godhwani, S., Godhwani, J.L., and Vyas, D.S., *Ocimum sanctum* — a preliminary study evaluating its immunoregulatory profile in albino rats, *J. Ethnopharmacol.*, 24:193–198, 1998.

Halder, N., Joshi, S., and Gupta, S.K., Lens aldose reductase inhibiting potential of some indigenous plants, *J. Ethnopharmacol.*, 86:113–116, 2003.

Singh, S. and Majumdar, D.K., Evaluation of anti-inflammatory activity of fatty acids of *Ocimum sanctum* fixed oil, *Ind. J. Exp. Biol.*, 35:380–383, 1997.

Singh, S. and Majumdar, D.K., Evaluation of the gastric antiulcer activity of fixed oil of *Ocimum sanctum* (Holy Basil), *J. Ethnopharmacol.*, 65:13–19, 1999.

Singh, S., Majumdar, D.K., and Rehan, H.M.S., Evaluation of anti-inflammatory potential of fixed oil of *O. sanctum* and its possible mechanism of action, *J. Ethnopharmacol.*, 54:19–26, 1996.

Singh, S., Rehan, H.M.S., and Majumdar, D.K., Effect of *Ocimum sanctum* fixed oil on blood pressure, blood clotting time and pentobarbitone-induced sleeping time, *J. Ethnopharmacol.*, 78:139–143, 2001.

Vats, V., Grover, J.K., and Rathi, S.S., Evaluation of anti-hyperglycemic and hypoglycemic effect of *Trigonella foenum-graecum* Lnn, *Ocimum sanctum* Linn and *Pterocarpus marsupium* Linn in normal and alloxanized diabetic rats, *J. Ethnopharmacol.*, 79: 95–100, 2002.

Vats, V., Yadav, S.P., and Grover, J.K., Ethanolic extract of *Ocimum sanctum* leaves partially attenuates stroptozotocin-induced alterations in glycogen content and carbohydrate metabolism in rats. *J. Ethnopharmacol.*, 90:155–160, 2004.

Oleuropein Oleuropein is a polyphenolic glycoside constituent in the leaves, fruit, and oil of olives (*Olea europaea*) responsible for the bitter taste of olives (Panizzi et al., 1960). Its ability to inhibit platelet aggregation induced by arachidonic acid and adenosine diphosphate was first reported by Petroni et al. (1995). The effect of oleuropein on the platelet-activating factor (PAF), the third and most potent pathway

Oleuropein. (From Furneri et al., *Int. J. Antimicrob. Agents*, 20:293–296, 2002. With permission.)

causing platelet aggregation, was investigated by Andrikopoulos and coworkers (2002). Addition of 10 µM oleuropein, a level equivalent to the average intake of olive oil or olive pieces in the Mediterranean diet, reduced *in vitro* oxidation of LDL cholesterol by total polar compounds formed during oil frying by approximately 50 percent. Oleuropein also inhibited human-plasma aggregation irrespective of its induction by arachidonic acid, adenosine diphosphate, or PAF. These results suggested oleuropein could play a role in the prevention of atherogenic plaques and thus reduce the risk for cardiovascular disease. The first experimental evidence for the direct cardioprotective effect of oleuropein following coronary occlusion was reported recently by Manna and coworkers (2004). The antioxidant properties of oleuropein appeared to prevent postischemic oxidative burst by reducing the amount of oxidized glutathione, a sensitive marker of the heart's exposure to oxidative stress. The presence of oleuropein also reduced lipid-membrane peroxidation by reducing thiobarbituric-acid reactive substances in cardiac tissue after ischemia/reperfusion of isolated rat hearts (Figure O.70).

Oleuropein also inhibited or delayed the growth of a number of bacteria and microfungi (Tranter et al., 1993; Capasso et al., 1995;

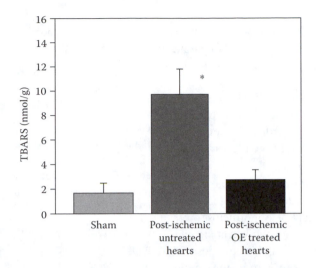

FIGURE O.70 Effect of oleuropein (OE) on thiobarbituric-reactive substance (TBARS) formation in the cardiac tissue after ischemia/reperfusion of isolated rat hearts. Isolated hearts were subjected to 30 min of global ischemia and then reperfused. After 1 h of reperfusion, hearts were removed from the perfusion apparatus and TBARS measured. Data (mean $\pm$ SD; n = 6) were analyzed by the Student t test. $^*p < 0.05$ compared to SHAM samples. (Manna et al., *J. Nutr. Biochem.*, 15:461–466, 2004. With permission.)

Tassou et al., 1995). Bisignano et al. (1999) reported oleuropein exhibited antimicrobial activity against the human pathogenic bacteria ATTC and clinically isolated Gram-positive and Gram-negative strains of *Salmonella* spp., *Vibrio* spp., and *Staphylococcus aureus*. Further work by Furneri et al. (2002) confirmed the *in vitro* antimycoplasmal activity of oleuropein by its inhibition of *Mycoplasma fermentans* and *Microplasma hominis* strains. The latter are normally resistant to erythromycin and very often to tetracyclines. However, further research is needed to determine whether oleuropein retains its antimycoplasmal properties *in vivo*.

References

Andrikopoulos, N.K., Antonopoulou, S., and Kaliora, A.C., Oleuropein inhibits LDL oxidation induced by cooking oil frying by-products and platelet aggregation induced by platelet-activating factor, *Lebensm-Wiss u-Technol.*, 35:479–484, 2002.

Bisignano, G., Tomaino, A., Lo Cascio, R., Crisafi, G., Uccella, N., and Saija, A., On the *in-vitro* antimicrobial activity of oleuropein and hydroxytyrosol, *J. Pharm. Pharmacol.*, 51:253–259, 1999.

Capasso, R., Evidente, A., Schivo, L., Orru, G., Marcialis, M.A., and Cristinzio, G., Antibacterial polyphenols from olive oil mill waste waters, *J. Appl. Bacteriol.*, 79:393–398, 1995.

Furneri, P.M., Marino, A., Saija, A., Uccella, N., and Bisignano, G., *In vitro* antimycoplasmal activity of oleuropein, *Int. J. Antimicrob. Agents*, 20:293–296, 2002.

Manna, C., Migliardi, V., Golino, P., Scognamiglio, A., Galletti, P., Chiariello, M., and Zappia, V., Oleuropein prevents oxidative myocardial injury induced by ischemia and reperfusion, *J. Nutr. Biochem.*, 15:461–466, 2004.

Panizzi, A., Scarpati, M.L., and Oriente, G., Chemical structure of oleuropein, bitter glycoside of olive with hypotensive activity, *Gaz. Chim. Ital.*, 90:1449–1485, 1960.

Petroni, A., Blasevich, M., Salami, M., Papini, N., Montedoro, G.F., and Galli, C., Inhibition of platelet aggregation and eicosanoid production by phenolic components of olive oil, *Thrombosis Res.*, 78:151–160, 1995.

Tassou, C.C. and Nychas, G.J.E., Inhibition of *Salmonella enteridis* by oleuropein in broth and in a model system, *Lett. Appl. Microbiol.*, 20:120–124, 1995.

Tranter, H.S., Tassou, C.C., and Nychas, G.J.E., The effect of the olive phenolic compound, oleuropin, on growth and enterotoxin B production by *Staphylococcus aureus*, *J. Appl. Bact.*, 74:253–259, 1995.

Oligofructose *see also* **Inulin, Prebiotics**
Oligofructose, a nondigestible carbohydrate composed of fructose units, including inulin, provide a number of benefits, such as constipation relief (Den Hond et al., 2000), prebiotics (Gibson et al., 1995), stimulation of calcium absorption from food (Van den Heuvel et al., 1999), and cancer prevention (Taper et al., 1998; Reddy et al., 1997).

The prebiotic nature of oligofructose was demonstrated by Rao (2001), who fed eight healthy subjects 5 g/day of oligofructose over three weeks compared to an equivalent amount of sucrose. Consumption of this low dose of oligosaccharides caused a one-log cycle increase in bifidobacterium after 11 days, indicative of an improved fecal-bacteria composition. A quantitative approach by Vulevic et al. (2004) derived an equation for measuring the prebiotic effect (MPE) of dietary fructooligosaccharides that included the production of lactic acid, as well as short-chain fatty acids (SCFA), acetic, proprionic, and butyric acids. The production of SCFA, such as the proprionate/acetate ratios, was reported to affect plasma glucose and lipid metabolism (Todesco et al., 1991; Boillot et al., 1995). Giacco and coworkers (2004) found that a moderate intake of short-chain fructooligosaccharides (10.6 g/day) by subjects with mild hypercholesterolemia, had no clinically relevant effect on either glucose or cholesterol levels, both at fasting or in the postprandial period. However, a small but significant increase was observed for Lp(a) levels, together with a reduction in postprandial insulin response.

Kelly-Quagliana and coworkers (2003) found that oligofructose and inulin both modulated immune function in mice by increasing the level of natural killer (NK) cell activity of splenocytes and phagocytic activity of peritoneal macrophages. Both upregulated the macrophage-dependent immune responses in a dose-dependent manner.

References

Boillot, J., Alamowitch, C., and Berger, A.M., Effects of dietary proprionate on hepatic glucose production, whole-body glucose utilization, carbohydrate and lipid metabolism in normal rats, *Br. J. Nutr.,* 73:241–251, 1995.

Den Hond, E., Geypens, B., and Ghoos, Y., Effects of long chain chicory inulin on constipation, *Nutr. Res.,* 20:731–736, 2000.

Giacco, R., Clemente, G., Luongo, D., Lasorella, G., Fiume, I., Brouns, F., Bornet, F., Patti, L., Cipriano, P., Rivellese, A.A., and Riccardi, G., Effects of short-chain fructo-oligosaccharides on glucose and lipid metabolism in mild hypercholesterolaemic individuals, *Clin. Nutr.,* 23:331–340, 2004.

Gibson, G.R., Beatty, E.R., Wang, X., and Cummings, J.H., Selective stimulation of bifidobacteria in the human colon by oligofructose and insulin, *Gasteroenterol.,* 108:975–982, 1995.

Kelly-Quagliana, K.A., Nelson, P.D., and Buddington, R.K., Dietary oligofructose and inulin modulate immune functions in mice, *Nutr. Res.,* 23:257–267, 2003.

Rao, V.A., The prebiotic properties of oligofructose at low intake levels, *Nutr. Res.,* 21:843–848, 2001.

Reddy, B.S., Hamid, R., and Rao, C.V., Effect of dietary oligofructose and inulin on colonic preneoplastic aberrant crypt foci inhibition, *Carcinogenesis,* 18:1371–1374, 1997.

Taper, H.S., Lemort, C., and Roberfroid, M.B., Inhibitory effect of dietary inulin and oligofructose on the growth of transplantable mouse tumor, *Anticancer Res.,* 18:4123–4126, 1998.

Todesco, T., Rao, A.V., Bosello, A., and Jenkins, D.J.A., Proprionate lowers blood glucose and alters lipid metabolism in healthy subjects, *Am. J. Clin. Nutr.,* 54:860–865, 1991.

van den Heuvel, E.G.H., Muys, Th., van Dokkum, W., and Schaafsma, G., Oligofructose stimulates calcium absorption in adolescents, *Am. J. Clin. Nutr.,* 69:544–548, 1999.

Vulevic, J., Rastall, R.A., and Gibson, G.R., Developing a quantitative approach for determining the *in vitro* prebiotic potential of dietary oligosaccharides, *FEMS Microbiol. Lett.,* 236:153–159, 2004.

Oligosaccharides *see* **Oligofructose and Inulin**

Olives *see also* **Hydroxytyrosol and Oleuropein** Olives are oval fruits composed of water, oil, sugar, protein, organic acids, and cellulose. The oil, which accounts for around 20 percent of the olive, is located mainly in the pulp. In addition to being a rich source of the monounsaturated fatty acid oleic acid, olives also contain large amounts of polyphenols, of which the secoiridoid glycoside oleuropein is the most abundant. The latter is composed of elenolic acid (oleoside-11-methylester) and hydroxytyrosol (3,4-dihydroxyphenyl ethanol) (Blekas et al., 2002). Oleuropein is responsible for the very bitter taste of unprocessed olives and is normally eliminated prior to human consumption by lye treatment or fermentation. Nevertheless, oleuropein has been shown to enhance nitric-oxide production in mouse macrophages, considered beneficial for the protection of the organism (Visioli et al. 1998). During ripening, oleuropein is hydrolyzed to smaller molecules, such as hydroxytyrosol, which gives extra-virgin oil its rich and complex flavor. Other phenolics reported in unprocessed olives include ligstroside (ester of elenolic acid with 4-hydroxyphenyl ethanol or tyrosol) and hydroxycinnamic acids, caffeic and ferulic.

The beneficial effects of olive oil are not only due the presence of monounsaturated fatty acids but also to the antioxidant properties of polyphenols in the oil. Hydroxytyrosol (3,4-dihydroxyphenyl) ethanol (DHPE), which accounts for 70–80 percent of total phenols in extra-virgin olive oil, was shown to be a very effective scavenger of peroxy radicals, protecting human erythrocytes from oxidative damage (Manna et al., 1998). In addition to tyrosol and hydroxytyrosol, Bonoli et al. (2003) identified a number of other phenolic compounds in olive oil by capillary-zone electrophoresis, including 2,3-dihydroxyphenylethanol. The lower incidence of cardiovascular disease was attributed to their contribution in the Mediterranean diet. Olive polyphenols have also been associated with a lower incidence of some cancers (Trichopoulou, 1995; Trichopoulou et al., 2000). Visioli and Galli (2003) recently reviewed the waste products of olives as sources of bioactive compounds for the treatment of chronic diseases.

References

Blekas, G., Vassilakis, C., Harizanis, C., Tsimidou, M., and Boskou, D.G., Biophenols in table olives, *J. Agric. Food Chem.,* 50:3688–3692, 2002.

Bonoli, M., Montanucci, M., Toschi, T.G., and Lerker, G., Fat separation and determination of tyrosol, hydroxytyrosol and other phenolic compounds in extra-virgin olive oil by capillary zone electrophoresis with ultraviolet-diode array detection, *J. Chromatogr. A,* 1011:163–172, 2003.

Manna, C., Galleti, P., Cucciolla, V., Montedoro, G., and Zappia, V., Olive oil hydroxytyrosol protects human erythrocytes against oxidative damages, *J. Nutr. Biochem.,* 10:159–169, 1999.

Trichopoulou, A., Olive oil and breast cancer, *Cancer Causes Contrl.,* 6:475–476, 1995.

Trichopoulou, A., Lagiou, P., Kuper, H., and Trichopoulos, D., Cancer and Mediterranean dietary traditions, *Cancer Epidemiol. Biomarkers Prev.,* 9:869–873, 2000.

Visioli, F., Bellosta, S., and Galli, C., Oleuropein, the bitter principle of olives, enhances nitric oxide production by mouse macrophages, *Life Sci.,* 62: 541–546, 1998.

Visioli, F. and Galli, C., Olives and their production waste products as sources of bioactive compounds, *Curr. Topics Nutraceutical Res.,* 1:85–88, 2003.

Omega-3 fatty acids *see also* **Eicosapentaenoic and Docosahexaenoic acids** Omega-3 fatty acids belong to the family of long-chain polyunsaturated fatty acids with the first double bond located at the third carbon from the terminal methyl end of the molecule between carbons three and four. They are the precursors of prostaglandins, thromboxanes, and leukotrienes, chemical messengers that control a number of important biochemical processes, including cell growth and division, blood pressure and clotting, immune reactions, and inflammation. The essential fatty acid, α-linolenic acid (C18:3ω3), is the precursor of eicosapentaenoic acid (EPA) (C20:5 ω-3) and docosahexaenoic acid (DHA) (C22:6 ω-3). It has been suggested that 1.5 percent of the daily total calories should be derived from omega-3 fatty acids (3 g for men and 2 g for women) or EPA and DHA (1.4 g for men and 1.2 g for women). The richest sources of omega-3 are fish oils, such as herring, mackerel, sardines, and salmon (Eskin, 2002). To meet these levels requires eating three (200–300 g) portions per week of these fatty fish. Increasing omega-3 intake is important for individuals with a family history of heart or circulatory problems. Omega-3 fatty acids reduce the risk of heart attacks by reestablishing a more normal lipid profile among people with hypertriglyceridemia. Eritsland et al. (1995) reported a 19 percent reduction in triglyceride levels when fed 4 g of fish. Epidemiological studies suggest that in societies where diets are high in fish, heart attacks, strokes, and circulatory problems are relatively rare. A 20-year study in the Netherlands by Simon (1994) showed that men who ate 30 g of fish daily were half as likely to die from coronary heart disease. Lau et al. (1993) also found that treating rheumatoid arthritis sufferers with supplements containing EPA (171 mg) and DHA (114 mg) reduced the amount of nonsteroidal, anti-inflammatory drugs (NSAIDs) needed. A marked improvement was observed after a year, in which there was a significant reduction in tender-joint counts and morning stiffness compared to the control group. This was confirmed in a later study by Kremer et al. (1995). The level of interleukin-1 β decreased significantly in patients consuming fish oils, suggesting omega-3 fatty acids reduced the underlying disease process. Other areas in which omega-3 fatty acids appear to play a beneficial role include possible protection to smokers against chronic obstructive pulmonary disease (COPD). Britton (1995) postulated that omega-3 fatty acids reduce prostaglandin and leukotriene synthesis, inhibit migration of proinflammatory neutrophils into the lung, and reduce the lung's response to allergens. The importance of omega-3 fatty acids in the synthesis of prostaglandins and other inflammatory mediators led to their role in other inflammatory disease. For example, fish oils have been shown to lessen itching and inflammation in psoriasis, while essential fatty acids exert anti-inflammatory action in infantile seborrheic dermatisis and diaper dermatitis. A recent application is the possible use of omega-3 fatty acids for reducing the relapse in the inflammatory disease of the GI tract, Crohn's disease.

Epidemiological and experimental evidence suggests that omega-3 fatty acids exert a protective effect against common cancers, most notably breast and colon (Rose and Connolly, 1999; Klein et al., 2000; Maillard et al., 2002). Animal studies provided convincing evidence that omega-3 fatty acids inhibited mammary-tumor growth and metastasis. Hardman (2002) reviewed the evidence for omega-3 fatty acids as an anticancer agent, suggesting it may augment cancer therapy. Kato and coworkers (2002) showed dietary omega-3 fatty acids exerted significant tumor-suppressing activities on the growth of human colon carcinoma xenograft in athymic nude mice. The primary tumor-suppressing acid was found to be docosahexaenoic acid.

References

Britton, J., Dietary fish oil and airways obstruction, *Thorax.,* 50 (Suppl. 1): s11–s15, 1995.

Eristland, I., Arnesen, H., Seljefolt, I. and Hostmark, A.T., Long-term metabolic effects of n-3 polyunsaturated fatty acids in patients with coronary heart disease, *Am. J. Clin. Nutr.,* 61:831–836, 1995.

Eskin, N.A.M., Authentication of borage, evening primrose and fish oils, in *Authentication of Fats and Oils,* Jee, T., Ed., CRC Press, U.S.A., and Blackman Pub., U.K., 2002, pp. 95–114.

Hardman, W.E., Omega-3 fatty acids to augment cancer therapy, *J. Nutr.,* 132:3508–3512, 2002.

Kato, T., Hancock, R.L., Mohammadpour, H., McGregor, B., Manalo, P., Khaiboullina, S., Hall, M.R., Pardini, L., and Pardini, R.S., Influence of omega-3 fatty acids on the growth of human colon carcinoma in nude mice, *Cancer Lett.,* 187:169–177, 2002.

Klein, V., Chajes, V., Germain, E., Schulgen, G., Pinault, M., Malvy, D., Lefrancq, T., Fignon, A., Le Floch, O., Lhuillery, C., and Bognoux, P., Low alpha linolenic acid content of adipose tissue is associated with an increased risk of breast cancer, *Eur. J. Cancer,* 36:335–340, 2000.

Kremer, J.M., Lawrence, D.A., Petrillo, G.F., Litts, L.L., Mullaly, P.M., Rynes, R.I., Stocker, R.P., Parhami, N., Greenstein, N.S., and Fuchs, B.R., Effects of high-dose fish oil on rheumatoid arthritis after stopping nonsteroidal anti-inflammatory drugs: Clinical and immune correlates, *Arthritis Rheum.,* 38: 1107–1114, 1995.

Lau, C.S., Morley, K.D., and Belch, J.J., Effects of fish oil supplementation on non-steroidal anti-inflammatory drug requirement in patients with mild rheumatoid arthritis — a double blind placebo controlled study, *Br. J. Rheumatol.,* 32:982–989, 1993.

Maillard, V., Bougnoux, P. Ferrari, P., Jourdan, M-L., Pinault, M., Lavillonniere, F., Body, G., Le Floch, O., and Chajes, V., N-3 and N-6 fatty acids in breast adipose tissue and relative risk of breast cancer in a case control study in Tours, France, *Int. J. Cancer,* 98:78–83, 2002.

Rose, D.P. and Connolly, J.M., Omega-3 fatty acids as cancer chemopreventative agents, *Pharmacol. Ther.,* 83:217–244, 1999.

Simon, H.B., Patient-directed, non-prescription approaches to cardiovascular disease, *Arch. Int. Med.,* 154:2283–2296, 1994.

Onions (*Allium cepa* Liliacae) Onions are one of the major sources of flavonoids in the Western diet (Knekt et al., 1996). They are particularly rich in quercetin, and its glycosides have been used in traditional medicine for their antiasthmatic, antithrombotic, antihypertensive, antihyperglycemic, antihyperlipidemic, and antitumor properties (Bordia et al., 1975, 1977; Belman, 1983; Dorsch et al., 1985; Kleijnen et al., 1990; Wagner et al., 1990). These health benefits are attributed to the presence of flavonoids and alk(en)yl cysteine sulphoxides in onions (Griffiths et al., 2002).

In vitro studies by Glasser et al. (2002) showed quercetin, a flavonoid in onion, inhibited hepatic cholesterol biosynthesis. Kumari and Augusti (2002) found (+)-S-methyl-L-cysteine sulfoxide in onion exhibited antidiabetic and antioxidant activities comparable to standard drugs. However, Ali and coworkers (2000) found onion extracts ineffective in lowering serum cholesterol in rabbits kept on a cholesterol-supplemented diet compared to garlic.

The presence of quercetin, alkyl sulfides, and diallyl disulfide in onions suggested it had strong anticancer properties. Seki et al. (2000) found that both onions and garlic equally suppressed the growth of leukemia HL-60 cells. Hu and coworkers (1999) reported an inverse relationship between onions in the diet and the risk of brain cancer. Shon and coworkers (2004) found the antioxidant and antimutagenic activities of ethyl-acetate extracts from red, yellow, and white onion extracts could be attributed to the presence of phenols and flavonoids.

References

Ali, M., Thomson, M., and Afzal, M., Garlic and onions: Their effect on eicosanoid mretabolism and its clinical relevance, *Prost. Leuk. Essent. Fatty Acids,* 62:55–73, 2000.

Belman, S., Onion and garlic oils inhibit tumor promotion, *Carcinogenesis,* 4:1063–1065, 1983.

Bordia, A., Bansal, H.C., Arora, S.K., and Singh, S.V., Effect of essential oils of garlic and onion on alimentary hyperlipemia, *Atherosclerosis,* 21:15–19, 1975.

Bordia, A., Verma, S.K., Vyas, A.K., Khabya, B.L., Rathore, A.S., Bhu, N., and Bedi, H.K., Effect of essential oil of onion and garlic on experimental atherosclerosis in rabbits, *Atherosclerosis,* 26:379–386, 1977.

Dorsch, W.V., W., Adam, H.O., Weber, J., and Ziegeltrum, T., Antiasthmatic effects of onion extracts — detection of benzyl- and other isothiocyanates (mustard oils) as antiasthmatic compounds of plant origin, *Eur. J. Pharmacol.,* 107:17–24, 1984.

Glasser, G., Graefe, E.U., Struck, F., Veit, M., and Gebhardt, R., Comparison of antioxidative capacities and inhibitory effects on cholesterol biosynthesis of quercetin and potential metabolites, *Phytomedicine,* 9:33–40, 2002.

Griffiths, G., Trueman, L., Crowther, T., Thomas, B., and Smith, B., Onions — a global benefit to health, *Phytother. Res.,* 16:603–615, 2002.

Hu, J., La Vecchia, C., Nigri, E., Chatenoid, L., Bosetti, C., Jia, X., Liu, R., Huang, G., Bi, D., and Wang, C., Diet and brain cancer in adults: a case controlled study in Northeat China, *Inst. J. Cancer,* 81:2–23, 1999.

Kleijnen, J., Knipschild, P., and Terriet, G., Garlic, onions and cardiovascular risk factors: A review of the evidence from human experiments with emphasis on commercially available preparations, *Br. J. Clin. Pharmacol.,* 28:535–544, 1989.

Knekt, P., Jarvinen, R., Reunanen, A., and Maatela, J., Flavonoid intake and coronary mortality in Finland: A cohort study, *Br. Med. J.,* 312:478–481, 1996.

Kumari, K. and Augusti, K.T., Antidiabetic and antioxidant effects of S-methyl cysteine sulfoxide from onions (Allium cepa Linn) as compared to standard drugs in alloxan diabetic rats, *Ind. J. Exp. Biol.,* 40: 1005–1009, 2002.

Seki, T., Tsuji, K., Hayato, Y., Moritomo, T., and Ariga, T., Garlic and onion oils inhibit proliferation and induce proliferation and induce differentiation of HL60 cells, *Cancer Lett.,* 160:29–35, 2000.

O

Shon. M.-Y., Choi, S.-D., Kahng, G.-G., Nam, S.-H., and Sung, N.-J., Antimutagenic, antioxidant and free radical scavenging activity of ethyl acetate extracts from white, yellow and red onions, *Food Chem. Toxicol.*, 42:659–666, 2004.

Thomson, M., Alnaqeeb, M.A., Bordia, T., Al-Hassan, J., Afzal, M., and Ali, M., Effects of aqueous extract of onion on the liver and lung of rats, *J. Ethnopharmacol.*, 61:91–99, 1998.

Wagner, H., Dorsch, W., Bayer, Th., Breu, W., and Willer, F., Antiasthmatic effects of onions: Inhibition of 5-lipoxygenase and cyclooxygenase *in vitro* by thiosulfinates and cepaenes, *Prostagland. Leuk. Essent. Fatty Acids*, 39:59–62, 1990.

Oolong tea (*Camelia sinensis*) Oolong tea, one of three types of tea manufactured from tea leaves, is considered a functional food because of its antioxidant, hypocholesterolemic, and antiobesity properties (Yang and Koo, 1997; Benzie and Szeto, 1999; Han et al., 1999). It is produced from green tea by heating and fermentation and contains more than 70 different compounds, such as oolonghomobisflavan A, B[1], and theasinensin, formed from epigallocatechin gallate. Mihara and coworkers (2004) recently identified a novel acylated quercetin tetraglycoside in oolong tea extracts, 3-*O*-(2^G-p-coumaroyl-3^G-*O*-β-L-arabinosyl-3^R-*O*-D-glucosylrutinoside (compound 1). These researchers also found that compound 1 was a good antioxidant but not quite as strong as quer-

cetin (Table O.50). Unlike quercetin, the acylated quercetin tetraglycoside (compound 1) was soluble in water, which suggested it might be a better antioxidant, as it would be absorbed more easily.

Yang and coworkers (2001) compared green-, oolong-, and black-tea extracts for their ability to modulate lipid metabolism in hyperlipidemia rats maintained on a high-sucrose diet. Oolong tea reduced food intake, while both oolong and black teas significantly decreased body weight gain and food efficiency. Although green and oolong teas had similar catechins, green tea still exerted a greater antihyperlipidemic effect. Kuihara et al. (2002) showed oolong tea alleviated the stress-induced

TABLE O.50
Antioxidant Activity of Compound 1

	EC$_{50}$ (nmol/mL)[1]
Compound 1	16.2
Quercetin	8.6
p-Coumaric acid	377.8
α-Tocopherol	27.4

[1] The effective concentration of antioxidant needed to decrease the initial DPPH radical by 50 percent.

Source: From Mihara et al., *Tetrahedron Lett.*, 45:5077–5080, 2004. With permission.

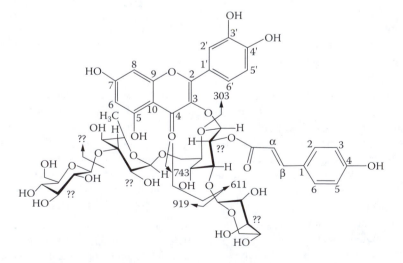

Compound 1. (From Mihara et al., *Tetrahedron Lett.*, 45:5077–5080, 2004. With permission.)

decrease in the rate of blood-lipid metabolism in mice. Reduction in plasma-triacylglycerol levels by oolong tea in the stressed mice was attributed to the antistress and antioxidant properties of its polyphenols and saponins, theasaponins E1 and E2 (Okuda and Han, 2001).

Shimada et al. (2004) demonstrated, for the first time, that long-term intake of oolong tea (one month) significantly ($p < 0.05$) increased plasma adiponectin levels from 6.26 ± 3.26 µg/mL to 6.88 ± 3.28 µg/mL in patients suffering from coronary artery disease. Adiponectin, a collagen-like plasma protein produced by adipose tissue normally abundant in circulation, is reduced in patients suffering from obesity, type 2 diabetes mellitus, and coronary artery disease (Matsuzawa et al., 1999; Ouchi et al., 1999; Hotta et al., 2000). A significant ($p < 0.01$) increase in LDL particle-size plasma levels from 25.02 ± 0.67 nm to 25.31 ± 0.60 nm was also observed. These effects could slow down the progression of atherosclerosis, as plasma-level LDL particle sizes were shown previously to be lower in patients with coronary artery disease and associated with the etiology of the disease (Lamarche et al., 1998).

References

Benzie, I.F.F. and Szeto, Y.T., Total antioxidant capacity of teas by the ferric reducing/antioxidant power assay, *J. Agric. Food Chem.*, 47:633–636, 1999.

Han, L.K., Takaku, T., Li, J., Kimura, Y., and Okuda, H., Anti-obesity action of Oolong tea, *Int. J. Obes. Reat. Metab. Disord.*, 23:98–115, 1999.

Hotta, K., Funahashi, T., and Arita, Y., et al., Plasma concentrations of a novel, adipose-specific protein, adiponectin, in type 2 diabetic patients, *Arterioscler. Thromb. Vasc. Biol.*, 20:1595–1599, 2000.

Kurihara, H., Fukami, H., Koda, H., Tsuruoka, N., Suguira, N., Shibata, H., and Tanaka, T., Effects of oolong tea on metabolism of plasma fat in mice under restraint stress, *Biosci. Biotechnol. Biochem.*, 66:1955–1958, 2002.

Lamarche, B., Tchernof, A., and Mauriege, P., Fasting insulin and apolipoprotein B levels and low-density lipoprotein particle size as risk factors for ischemic heart disease, *JAMA*, 279:1955–1961, 1998.

Matsuzawa, Y., Funahashi, T., and Nakamura, T., Molecular mechanism of metabolic syndrome X: Contribution of adipocytokines adipocyte-derived bioactive substances, *Ann. N.Y. Acad. Sci.*, 892:146–154, 1999.

Mihara, R., Mitsunaga, T., Fukui, Y., Nakai, M., Yamaji, N., and Shibata, H., A novel acylated quercetin tetraglycoside from oolong tea (*Camelia sinensis*) extracts, *Tetrahedron Lett.*, 45:5077–5080, 2004.

Okuda, H. and Han, L.K., Medicinal plant and its related metabolic modulators, *Nippon Yakurigaku Zasshi*, 118:347–352, 2001.

Ouchi, N., Kihara, S., Arita, Y., et al., Novel modulator for endothelial adhesion molecules: Adipocyte-derived plasma protein adiponectin, *Circulation*, 100:2473–2476, 1999.

Shimada, K., Kawarabayashi, T., Tanaka, A., Fukuda, D., Nakamura, Y., Yoshiyama, M., Takeuchi, K., Sawaki, T., Hosoda, K., and Yoshikawa, J., Oolong tea increases plasma adiponectin levels and low-density lipoprotein particle size in patients with coronary artery disease, *Diab. Res. Clin. Practice*, 65:227–234, 2004.

Yang, M.-H., Wang, C.-H., and Chen, H.-L., Green, oolong and black tea extracts modulate lipid metabolism in hyperlipidemia rats fed high-sucrose diet, *J. Nutr. Biochem.*, 12:14–20, 2001.

Yang, T.T. and Koo, M.W.L., Hypercholesterolemic effects of Chinese tea, *Pharmacol. Res.*, 35:505–512, 1997.

O

Oranges *see* Orange Juice

Orange juice *see also* Hesperidin, Nobiletin, and Tangeretin

Besides being an excellent source of provitamin A carotenoids, orange juice is rich in antioxidant carotenoids. Many of these carotenoids appear to play a role in the reduction of degenerative diseases, such as cancer and heart disease. These include β-carotene, α-carotene, and β-cryptoxanthin, as well as zeaxanthin and lutein. Using the 2,2-diphenyl-1-picrylhydrazyl stable radical-scavenging method, Sanchez-Moreno et al. (2003) found vitamin C was the largest contributor to the antioxidant potential of orange juice, followed by flavonoids and carotenoids.

TABLE O.51
Effect of Orange Juice on Plasma Lipids

Variable	Baseline	1	2	3	Washout
			Dietary Period		
Plasma cholesterol (mmol/L)					
Total	6.3 ± 1.0	6.4 ± 0.9	6.5 ± 1.0	6.5 ± 0.9	6.3 ± 1.0
VLDL	0.8 ± 0.4	1.0 ± 0.6	0.8 ± 0.4	0.9 ± 0.4	0.8 ± 0.4
LDL	3.6 ± 0.7	3.8 ± 0.6	3.7 ± 0.7	3.6 ± 0.7	3.5 ± 0.7
HDL	1.0 ± 0.3	1.0 ± 0.3	1.1 ± 0.3	1.2 ± 0.3[1]	1.3 ± 0.4[1]
Change in HDL (percent)	0	5	7	21	27
LDL:HDL cholesterol	3.8 ± 0.9	3.8 ± 0.9	3.6 ± 1.0	3.1 ± 0.9[1]	3.0 ± 1.0[1]
Change in LDL:HDL cholesterol (percent)	—	0	−4	−16	−20
Total triacylglycerol (mmol/L)	1.6 ± 0.7	1.9 ± 1.0	1.8 ± 0.8	2.0 ± 0.9[1]	1.7 ± 1.0

[1] Significantly different from baseline, $p < 0.05$ (ANOVA followed by Dunnett's test).

Source: From Kurowska et al., *Am. J. Clin. Nutr.,* 72:1095–1100, 2000.

The hypocholesterolemic effect of soybean was attributed to the flavonoid genistein (Anthony et al., 1996). The similarity in structure between genistein and hesperetin in oranges may also make orange juice hypocholesterolemic. This was confirmed by Kurowska and coworkers (2000), who showed a daily minimum consumption of 750 mL of orange juice by hypercholesterolemic individuals significantly increased HDL-cholesterol concentrations by 21 percent and the LDL–HDL cholesterol ratio by 16 percent. No change was observed for LDL-cholesterol and homocysteine levels, while triacylglycerol levels increased 30 percent from 1.6 to 2.0 mmol/L (Table O.51).

Ikegawa et al. (2000) also demonstrated the ability of orange-juice components to inhibit P-glycoprotein in adriamiacyin-resistant human myelogenous leukemia (K562/ADM) cells. P-glycoprotein acts as an energy-dependent drug efflux pump, decreasing the intracellular drug accumulation and the therapeutic effect of many chemotherapeutic agents. All three orange-juice components, tangeretin, nobiletin, and heptamethoxyflavone (HMF), were found to reverse the multidrug resistance (MDR) without inhibiting CYP-3A4.

Sprecher and coworkers (2002) reported a positive effect of dietary intervention of not-from-concentrate orange juice to 24 nondiabetic patients with angiographic CAD on

vascular regulation, which could affect health strategies for reducing blood pressure. A study by Lilja and coworkers (2004) noted that orange juice reduced the bioavailability of celiprolol, a β-adrenergic-blocking agent with vasodilating properties. The negative impact of orange juice with celiprolol must be avoided by patients on this drug.

References

Anthony, M.S., Clarkson, T.B., Hughes, Ch., Jr., Morgan, T.M.. and Burke, C.L., Soybean isoflavones improve cardiovascular risk without affecting the reproductive system of prebuteral Rhesus monkeys, *J. Nutr.,* 126:43–70, 1996.

de Ancos, B., Sgroppo, S., Plaza, L. and Cano, M.P., Possible nutritional and health-related value by high-pressure treatment, *J. Sci Food Agric.,* 82:790–792, 2002.

Ikegawa, T., Ushigome, F., Kobayu, N., Morimoto, S., Shoyama, Y., Naito, M., Tsuruo, T., Ohtani, H., and Sawada, Y., Inhibition of P-glycoprotein by orange juice components, polymethoxyflavones in adriamycin-resistant human myelegenous leukemia (K562/ADM) cells, *Cancer Lett.,* 160:21–28, 2000.

Kurowska, E.M., Spence, J.D., Jordan, J., Wetmore, S., Freeman, D.J., Piche, L.A., and Serratore, P., HDL-cholesterol-raising effect of orange juice in subjects with hypercholesterolemia, *Am. J. Clin. Nutr.,* 72:1095–1100, 2000.

Lilja, J.J., Juntti-Patinen, L., and Neuvonen, P.J., Orange juice substantially reduces the bioavailability of the β-adrenergic-blocking agent celiprolol, *Clin. Pharmacol. Ther.,* 75:184–190, 2004.

Sanchez-Moreno, C., Plaza, L., de Ancos, B., and Cano, M.P., Quantitative bioactive compounds assessment and their relative contribution to theantioxidant capacity of commercial orange juices, *J. Sci. Food Agric.,* 83:430–439, 2003.

Sprecher, D.L., Foody, J.M., Acevedo, M., Scafidi, K.M., Aronow, H., and Pearce, G.L., Dietary intervention with orange juice lowers blood pressure: Pilot study, *JACC,* 39:254–258, 2002.

Oregano (*Origanum vulgare* L.)   Oregano, an aromatic perennial herb, is a member of the *Labiatae* family. The oil from oregano is used for its fragrance in perfumes and for its flavor in seasonings. Health benefits associated with oregano have been attributed to antioxidants in its essential oil and soluble phenols (Engleberger et al., 1988; Peak et al., 1991; Eguchi et al., 1996). Kikuzaki and Nakatani (1988) identified rosmarinic acid as one of the major phenolic compounds in the methanolic extract of oregano leaves. The latter has been reported to exert both antioxidant and anti-inflammatory properties. The variability in the phenolic content of oregano, however, has limited it as a functional food. To overcome the problem of genetic heterogeneity of oregano, clonal selection has been used to ensure consistency in phenolic quantity and quality. Chun et al. (2005) compared a high phenolic clonal line of oregano developed at the University of Massachusetts with a purchased commercial heterogenous line. The clonal line was much higher in total phenolics and antioxidant activity, as well as improved antimicrobial activity against *Helicobacter pylori*, an organism associated with ulcers. The development of high phenolic clonal oregano lines could provide useful functional-food sources of oregano for combating chronic bacterial infections.

References

Chun, S.-S., Vattem, D.A., Lin, Y.-T., and Shetty, K., Phenolic antioxidants from clonal oregano (*Origanum vulgare*) with antimicrobial activity against *Helicobacter pylori*, *Process Biochem.,* 40:809–816, 2005.

Eguchi, Y., Curtis, O.F., and Shetty, K., Interaction of hyperhydricity-preventing *Pseudomonas sp.* with oregano (*Origanum vulgare*) and selection of high phenolics and rosmarinic acid-producing lines, *Food Biotechnol.,* 10:191–202, 1996.

Engleberger, W., Hadding, U., Etschenber, E., Graf, E., Leyck, S., and Winkelmann, J., Rosmarinic acid. A new inhibitor of complement C3-covertase with anti-inflammatory activity, *Int. J. Immunopharmacol.,* 10:721–737, 1988.

Kikuzaki, H. and Nakatani, N., Structure of a new antioxidative phenolic acid from oregano (*Origanum vulgare* L.), *Agric. Biol. Chem.,* 53:519–524, 1988.

Peak, P.W., Pussel, B.A., Martyn, P., Timmermans, V., and Charlesworth, J.A., The inhibitory effect of rosmarinic acid on complement involves the C5 convertase, *Int. J. Immunopharmacol.,* 13:853–857, 1991.

γ-Oryzanol   γ-Oryzanol is a mixture of sterol esters of ferulic acid, found in rice-bran oil (Rogers et al., 1993).

The highest concentration of γ-oryzanol was recently extracted from the rice bran during the shorter milling duration (Rohrer and Siebenmorgen, 2004). Studies showed it lowered blood cholesterol in rats and that the addition of 0.5 percent γ-oryzanol to a cholesterol-enriched diet effectively reduced triacylglycerols, LDL cholesterol, and VLDL cholesterol in the serum, and cholesterol in the liver (Nicolosi et al., 1993; Seetharamaiah and Chandrasekhara, 1993). In addition, γ-oryzanol was also an effective antioxidant, protecting rice-bran oil from oxidation by iron or UV radiation (Jariwalla et al., 2001). Of the three major γ-oryzanol derivatives in rice bran, 24-methylene-cycloartanyl ferulate exhibited the highest antioxidant activity compared to cycloartanyl ferulate or campestryl ferulate.

All three compounds were much stronger antioxidants than any of the vitamin E isomers (Xu et al., 2001). Earlier *in vitro* tests showed γ-oryzanol had superoxide dismutase-like antioxidant activity (Kim et al., 1995). A review by Cicero and Gaddi (2001) discusses some of the health claims made for γ-oryzanol, as well as the pharmacology and toxicology of rice-bran oil.

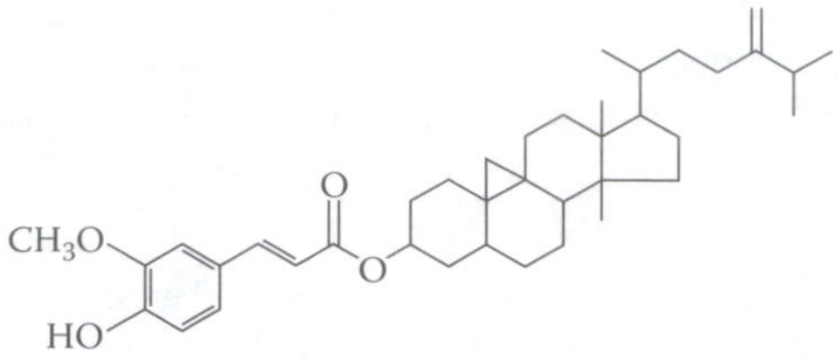

24-Methylene cycloartanyl ferulate

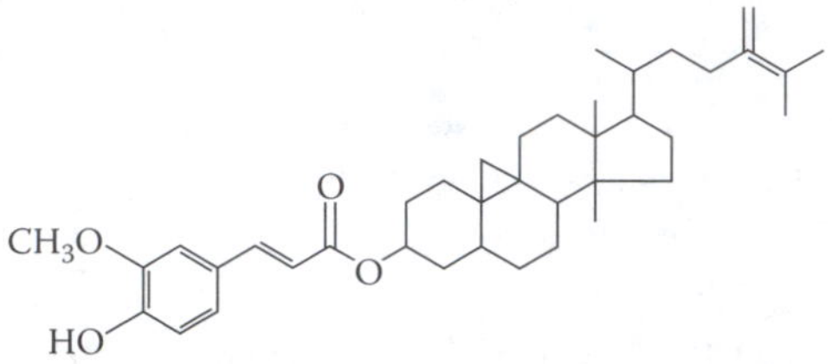

Cycloartanyl ferulate

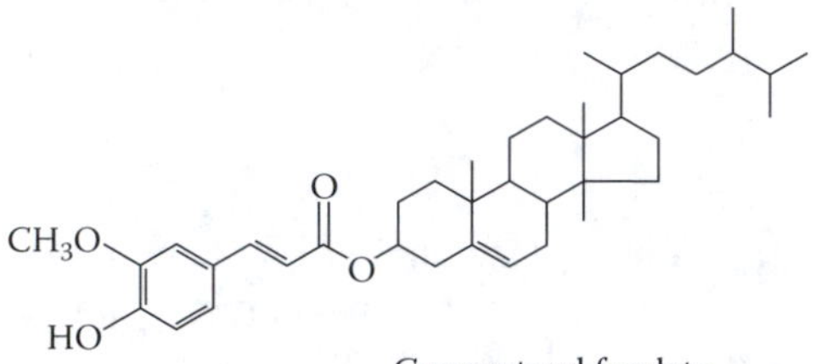

Campesteryl ferulate

Three major γ-oryzanol derivatives in oats. (From Xu et al., 2001. With permission.)

References

Cicero, A.F.G. and Gaddi, A., Rice bran oil and γ-oryzanol in the treatment of hyperlipoproteinaemias and other conditions, *Phytother. Res.*, 15:277–289, 2001.

Jariwalla, R.J., Rice-bran products: Phytonutrients with potential applications in preventive and clinical medicine, *Drugs Under Exp. Clin. Res.*, 217:17–26, 2001.

Kim, S.J., Han, D., Moon, K.D., and Rhee, J.S., Measurement of superoxide-like activity of natural antioxidants, *Biosci. Biotech. Biochem.*, 59:822–826, 1995.

Nicolosi, R.J., Rogers, E.J., Ausman, L.M., and Orthoefer, F.T., Rice bran oil and its health effects, in *Rice Science and Technology*, Marshall, W.E. and Wadsworth, J.I., Eds., Marcel Dekker, New York, 1993, pp. 421–437.

Rogers, E.J., Rice, S.M., Nicolosi, R.J., Carpenter, D.R., McClelland, C.A., and Romanczyk, L.R., Identification and quantitation of gamma-oryzanol components and simultaneous assessment of tocols in

rice oil bran, *J. Am. Oil Chem. Soc.*, 70:301–307, 1993.

Rohrer, C.A. and Siebenmorgen, T.J., Nutraceutical concentrations within the bran of various rice kernel thickness fractions, *Biosyst. Eng.*, 88:453–460, 2004.

Seetharamaiah, G.S. and Chandrasekhara, N., Comparative hypocholesterolemic activities of oryzanol, curcumin and ferulic acid in rats, *J. Food Sci. Technol.*, 30:249–252, 1993.

Xu, Z., Hua, N., and Godber, J.S., Antioxidant activity of tocopherols, tocotrienols, and γ-oryzanol components from rice bran against cholesterol oxidation accelerated by 2,2′-azobis(2-methylpropionamide) dihydrochloride, *J. Agric. Food Chem.*, 49:2077–2081, 2001.

Ovakinin   Ovakinin (2-7) is a novel, antihypertensive peptide produced from ovalbumin by chymotryptic digestion (Matoba et al., 2000). Yamada and coworkers (2002) showed that replacing the C-terminal Phe residue with Tryp improved the antihypertensive activity of ovakinin.

References

Matoba, N., Usui, H., Fujita, H., and Yoshikawa, M., A novel anti-hypertensive peptide derived from ovalbumin induces nitric oxide-mediated vasorelaxation in an isolated SHR mesenteric artery, *FEBS Lett.*, 452:181–184, 1999.

Yamada, Y., Matoba, N., Usui, H., and Onishi, K., Design of a highly potent anti-hypertensive peptide based on ovakinin (2-7), *Biosci. Biotechnol. Biochem.*, 66:1213–1217, 2002.

Oyster mushroom (*Pleurotus ostreatus*) Oyster mushroom is a wood-rotting fungus produced industrially for the food industry on lignocellulose substrates. A pilot study by Bobek and coworkers (1993) showed that oyster mushroms suppressed diet-induced hypercholesterolemia in rats. The mechanisms responsible were shown to be reduced cholesterol absorption and increased excretion of plasma cholesterol (Bobek et al., 1994), reduced activity of 3-hydroxy-3-methylglutaryl CoA reductase, a key enzyme in cholesterol

TABLE O.52
Inhibition of Sarcoma 180 or Hepatoma 22 Growth by POL

Tumor		Control Group ($n = 8$)	Lectin-Treated Group ($n = 8$)
Sarcoma	Tumor weight (g)	0.5774 ± 0.0430	0.0667 ± 0.0021 ($p < 0.002$)
S-180	% Inhibition of tumor growth		88.46
Hepatoma	Tumor weight (g)	0.9928 ± 0.1242	0.2439 ± 0.0004 ($p < 0.002$)
H-22	% Inhibition of tumor growth		75.42

Source: From Wang et al., *Biochem. Biophys. Res. Commun.*, 275:810–816, 2000. With permission.

biosynthesis (Bobek et al., 1995), and a reduction in the production and secretion of very-low-density lipoproteins (VLDL) in hypercholesterolemic rats (Bobek and Ozdin, 1996). Long-term feeding of 5 percent oyster mushrooms to rats by Bobek et al. (1998) significantly reduced serum (31–46 percent) and liver (25–30 percent) cholesterol during the eighth and 28 weeks of feeding. In addition to lowering VLDL, there was a decrease in conjugated dienes in erythrocytes and an increase in reduced glutathione in the liver, accompanied by enhanced catalase and glutathione-peroxidase activity during the last period of the study.

Wang et al. (2000), using a simple procedure, isolated a lectin (POL) from the fresh-fruiting bodies of the edible oyster mushroom (*Pleurotus ostreatum*) that exhibited strong antitumor activity. It proved to be a dimeric lectin composed of two subunits with molecular weights of 40 and 41 kDa, respectively. It was a potent inhibitor of sarcoma S-180 and hepatoma H-22 growth, as evident in Table O.52.

References

Bobek, P. and Galbavy, S., Hypocholesterolemic and antitherogenic effect of oyster mushroom (*Pleurotus ostreatus*) in rabbit, *Nahrung*, 43:339–342, 1999.

Bobek, P., Hromadova, M., and Ozdin, L., Oyster mushroom (*Pleurotus ostreatus*) reduces the activity of 3-hydroxy-3-methylglutaryl CoA reductase in rat liver microsomes, *Experentia.*, 51:589–, 1995.

Bobek, P., Kuniak, L., and Ozdin, L., The mushroom *Pleurotus ostreatus* reduces secretion and accelerates the fractional turnover rate of very low density lipoproteins in rat, *Ann. Nutr. Metab.*, 37:142–145, 1993.

Bobek, P., Ozdin, L, and Galbavy, S., Dose- and time-dependent hypocholesterolemic effect of oyster mushroom (*Pleurotus ostreatus*) in rats, *Nutrition*, 14:282–286, 1998.

Bobek, P. and Ozdin, L., Oyster mushroom (*Pleurotus ostreatus*) reduces the production and secretion of very-low-density lipoproteins in hypercholesterolemic rats, *Z. Ernahrungswiss.*, 35:249, 1996.

Bobek, P., Ozdin, L., and Kuniak, L., Mechanism of hypocholesterolemic effect of oyster mushroom (*Pleurotus ostreatus*) in rats: Reduction of cholesterol absorption and increase of plasma cholesterol removal, *Z. Ernahrungswiss.*, 33:44–50, 1994.

Wang, H., Gao, J., and Ng, T.B., A new lectin with highly potent antihepatoma and antisarcoma activities from the oyster mushroom *Pleurotus ostreatus*, *Biochem. Biophys. Res. Commun.*, 275:810–816, 2000.

O

P

Palatinose® Palatinose® is the commercial product isomaltose, obtained from sucrose by enzymatic rearrangement followed by crystallization (Scheme P.41). It is found naturally in honey (Barez et al., 2000) and products derived from sugar-cane juice, such as treacles and molasses (Takazoe, 1985). Unlike sucrose, a nonreducing disaccharide in which glucose and fructose are linked α-1,2, isomaltose is a reducing disaccharide in which glucose and fructose are linked α-1,6. As a result, palatinose is hardly fermented by oral microbes and appeared to be a suitable noncariogenic sucrose replacement for incorporation into products for diabetics (Kawai et al., 1989).

In vivo studies with rats and pigs showed it is completely hydrolyzed and absorbed in the small intestine. However, the rate of hydrolysis was very slow compared to sucrose or maltose so that in humans the rise of blood glucose and insulin levels after oral administration was slower, reaching lower maxima compared to sucrose. No embryotoxic or teratogenic effects were observed in rat fetuses, nor maternal toxicity at levels up to 7 g/kg body weight/day (Lina et al., 2002). Using the Ames test, they found isomaltose was nonmutagenic and was a safe alternative sugar. Dietary levels of up to 10 percent isomaltose were shown by Jonker et al. (2002) to be well tolerated without any signs of toxicity. The overall intake at this level corresponded to 7.0 and 8.1 g/kg body weight/day in male and female rats, respectively.

Although palatinose appears to be a noncariogenic disaccharide and unable to be utilized by *Streptoccus mutans*, Matsuyama et al. (2003) showed there were still a significant number of bacteria in dental plaque capable of fermenting it. Using the Uchida-Kraepelin psychodiagnostic test, Kashimura et al. (2003) found that 5 g of palatinose enhanced mental concentration by increasing calculation ability.

References

Gomez Barez, J.A., Villanova, R.J.G., Garcia, S.E., Pala, T.R., Paramas, A.M.G., and Sanchez, J.S., Geographical discrimination of honeys through the employment of sugar patterns and common chemical quality parameters, *Eur. Food Res. Technol.*, 210: 437–444, 2000.

Jonker, D., Lina, B.A., and Kozianowski, G., 13-Week oral toxicity study with isomaltulose (Palatinose) in rats, *Food Chem. Toxicol.*, 40:1383–1389, 2002.

Kashimura, J., Nagai, Y., and Ebashi, T., The effect of palatinose on mental concentration in humans, *J. Nutr. Sci. Vitaminol.*, 49:214–216, 2003.

Kawai, K., Yoshikawa, H., Murayama, Y., Okuda, Y., and Yamashita, K., Usefulness of palatinose as a caloric sweetener for diabetic patients, *Horm. Metab. Res.*, 21:338–340, 1989.

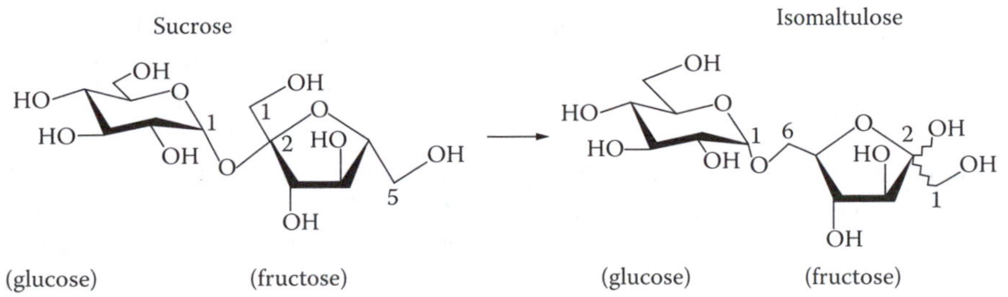

SCHEME P.41 Enzymatic rearrangement of sucrose to isomaltose. (From Lina et al., *Food Chem. Toxicol.*, 40:375–381, 2002. With permission.)

Lina, B.A., Jonker, D., and Kozianowski, G., Isomaltose (Palatinose®): A review of biological and toxicological studies, *Food Chem. Toxicol.*, 40:375–381, 2002.

Matsuyama, J., Sato, T., Hoshino, E., Noda, T., and Takahashi, N., Fermentation of five sucrose isomers by human dental plaque bacteria, *Caries Res.*, 37: 410–415, 2003.

Takazoe, Y., New trends on sweeteners in Japan, *Int. Dental J.*, 35:58–65, 1985.

Palmetto berries   Palmetto berries are obtained from Saw palmetto, an herbal product used to treat symptoms related to benign prostatic hyperplasia. Studies demonstrated the effectiveness of saw palmetto in reducing symptoms associated with benign prostatic hyperplasia (Ernt, 2002; Gordon and Shaughnessy, 2003) and lower urinary-tract symptoms (Wilt et al., 1998; Koch, 2001). The mechanism whereby saw palmetto improves urinary symptoms is unknown (Gerber et al., 2001). There are no known drug interactions with saw palmetto, with reported side effects extremely rare. A six-month study of forty-four men with benign prostatic hyperplasia with a Saw palmetto herbal by Veltri et al. (2002) found an alteration in DNA chromatin structure and organization of prostate epithelial cells. Goldman et al. (2001) reported inhibition of proliferation of a set of prostatic cell lines when dosed with Saw palmetto–berry extract (SPBE) for three days. Reduced cellular activity appeared to be related to decreased expression of COX-2 and possible changes in the expression of Bcl-2. Since an increase in COX-2 expression is associated with an increase in incidence of prostate cancer, its reduction by SPBE suggests its possible use against benign proprostatic hyperplasia and in prostate-cancer prevention. Talpur et al. (2003) showed whole berry and extracts of Saw palmetto influenced hyperplasia via androgen metabolism.

References

Ernst, E., The risk-benefit profile of commonly used herbal therapies: Ginkgo, St. John's wort, ginseng, echinacea, saw palmetto, and kava, *Ann. Intern. Med.*, 136:42–53, 2002.

Gerber, G.S., Kuznetsov, D., Johnson, B.C., and Burstein, J.D., Randomized, double-blind, placebo-controlled trial of saw palmetto in men with lower urinary tract symptoms, *Urology*, 58:960–964, 2001.

Goldmann, W.H., Sharma, A.L., Currier, S.J., Jonston, P.D., Rana, A., and Sharma, C.P., Saw palmetto berry extract inhibits cell growth and COX-2 expression in prostatic cancer cells, *Cell Biol. Int.*, 25: 1117–1124, 2001.

Gordon, A.E. and Shaughnessy, A.F., Saw palmetto for prostate disorders, *Am. Fam. Physician*, 67:1281–1283, 2003.

Koch, E., Extracts from fruits of saw palmetto (*Sabal serrulata*) and roots of stinging nettle (*Urtica dioica*): Viable alternatives in the medical treatment of benign prostatic hyperplasia and associated lower urinary tracts symptoms, *Planta Med.*, 67:489–500, 2001.

Talpur, N., Echard, B., Bagchi, D., Bagchi, M., and Preuss, H.G., Comparison of saw palmetto (extract and whole berry) and cernitin on prostate growth in rats, *Mol. Cell Biochem.*, 250:21–26, 2003.

Veltri, R.W., Marks, L.S., Miller, M.C., Bales, W.D., Fan, J., Macairan, M.L., Epstein, J.I., and Partin, A.W., Saw palmetto alters nuclear measurements reflecting DNA content in men with symptomatic BPH: Evidence for a possible molecular mechanism, *Urology*, 60:617–622, 2002.

Wilt, T.J., Ishani, A., Stark, G., MacDonald, R., Lau, J., and Mulrow, C., Saw palmetto extracts for treatment of benign prostatic hyperplasia: A systematic review, *JAMA*, 280:1504–1609, 1998.

Paprika (*Capsicum annuum* L.)   Carotenoids have been reported to play a role in the prevention of cancer. Oshima et al. (1997) showed that capsanthin, a major carotenoid in paprika (*Capsicum annuum*), was absorbed into the body following ingestion of paprika juice. In addition to capsanthin, 11-*cis*-capsanthin was also identified and could also be important to human health. Narisawa et al. (2000) reported that paprika juice rich in capsanthin (3.54 mg/100 mL) inhibited N-methylnitrosourea-induced colon carcinogenesis in F344 rats. Etoh and coworkers (2000) also reported the absorption of paprika carotenoids following ingestion of paprika juice. The red pigments in paprika, capsanthin, capsorubin, and capsanthin 3,6-epoxide, all possess 3-hydroxy-κ-end groups (Scheme P.42). The antitumor activity of isolated paprika

Capsanthin (1): R_1=H, R_2=H
Capsanthin 3'-ester(2): R_1=H, R_2=Acyl
Capsanthin 3, 3'-diester(3): R_1=Acyl, R_2=Acyl

Capsorubin (4): R_1= H, R_2=H
Capsorubin 3, 3'-diester(5): R_1Acyl, R_2=Acyl

Capsanthin 3, 6-epoxide(6)

Cucurbitaxanthin A 3'-ester (7): R= Acyl

Structures of capsanthin and related paprika carotenoids. (From Maoka et al., *Cancer Lett.*, 172:103–109, 2001. With permission.)

carotenoids associated with these structures was demonstrated by Maoka and coworkers (2001) using an Epstein–Barr virus early antigen (EBV-EA) activation induced by the tumor promoter 12-*O*-tetradecanoylphorbol-13-acetate (TPA) and an *in vitro,* two-stage carcinogenesis assay on mouse skin using 7,12-dimethylbenz[α]anthracene as an initiator and promoter. Strong, antitumor promoting activities were observed for capsanthin and related paprika carotenoids without any significant cytotoxicity to the Raji cells in this assay. Inhibitory activity increased with esterification of the hydroxyl groups with fatty acids, as evident by the increase in inhibitory activity ranging in the order of capsanthin > capsanthin 3′ ester > capsanthin diester > capsorubin diester. This was also evident for inhibition of TPA-induced tumor promotion by capsanthin, capsanthin 3,3″-diester, as shown in Figure P.71.

Sappanen and Csallany (2002) reported *in vivo* antioxidant effects in rats fed vitamin E-deficient diets supplemented with paprika carotenoids (0.5 and 1.0 percent) and β-carotene (1.0 percent) by the lower amount of secondary products from lipid peroxidation in the urine. While the addition of paprika carotenoids could not compensate for the role of vitamin E in normal growth and weight gain, these oxygenated carotenoids, or xanthophylls, were effective by their *in vivo* inhibition of lipid oxidation. Perez-Galvez et al. (2003) showed the availability of carotenoids from paprika oleoresin by the detection of considerable amounts of zeaxanthin, β-cryptoxantin, and β-carotene in the chylomicron fraction.

References

Etoh, H., Utsunomiya, Y., Konori, A., Murakami, Y., Oshima, S., and Inakuma, T., Carotenoids in human blood plasma after ingesting paprika juice, *Biosci. Biotechnol. Biochem.*, 64:1096–1098, 2000.

Maoka, T., Michida, K., Kozuka, M., Ito, Y., Fujiwara, Y., Hashimoto, K., Enjo, F., Ogata, M., Nobukuni, Y., Tokuda, H., and Nishino, H., Cancer chemopreventive activity of carotenoids in the fruits of red paprika *Capsicum annuum* L., *Cancer Lett.*, 172:103–109, 2001.

Narisawa, T., Fukaura, Y., Hasebe, M., Nomura, S., Oshima, S., and Inakuma, T., Prevention of *N*-methylnitrosourea-induced colon carcinogenesis in rats by oxygenated carotenoid capsanthin and capsanthin-rich paprika juice, *Proc. Soc. Exp. Biol. Med.*, 224:116–122, 2000.

Oshima, S., Sakamoto, H., Ishiguro, Y., and Teraom, J., Accumulation and clearance of capsanthin in blood plasma after ingestion of paprika juice in men, *J. Nutr.*, 127:1475–1479, 1997.

Parez-Galvez, M., Martin, H.D., Sies, H., and Stahl, W., Incorporation of carotenoids from paprika oleoresin into human chylomicrons, *Br. J. Nutr.*, 89:787–793, 2003.

Seppanen, C.M. and Csallany, A.S., The effect of paprika carotenoids on *in vivo* lipid peroxidation measured by urinary excretion of secondary oxidation products, *Nutr. Res.*, 22:1055–1065, 2002.

P

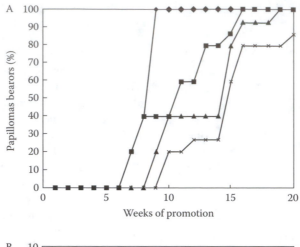

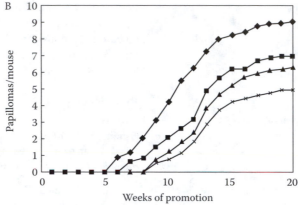

FIGURE P.71 Inhibition of TPA-induced tumor promotion by multiple applications of capsanthin, capsanthin 3′ ester, and capsanthin diester. All mice were initiated with DMBA (390 nmol) and promoted with TPA (1.7 nmol) twice weekly starting at one week after initiation. (A) Percentage of mice bearing papillomas; (B) Average number of papillomas per mouse. (♦), Control TPA alone; (■) TPA + 85 nmol capsanthin; (▲), TPA + 85 nmol capsanthin 3′ ester; (×), TPA + 85 nmol capsanthin 3,3′-diester. (From Maoka et al., *Cancer Lett.,* 172:103–109, 2001. With permission.)

Parsley (*Petroselinium crispum*)   Parsley has a long tradition in folk medicine as a stomachic, carminative, emmenagogue, and abortifacient (Anderson et al., 1996; Robbers and Tyler, 1999; Tyler, 1993). As an herb, it is widely recognized as a diuretic, which could account for its hypotensive properties (Leung, 1980). The mechanism of its diuretic effect appears to be mediated through inhibition of the Na+ K+ pump that leads to a reduction in Na+ and K+ reabsorption, resulting in an osmotic water flow into the lumen and diuresis (Kreydiyyeh and Usta, 2002). Earlier work by Kreydiyyeh et al.

(2001) confirmed the laxative role of parsley by its inhibition of sodium and subsequent water absorption through its inhibition of the Na+ K+ pump, and by stimulating of the NaKCl transporter and increasing electrolyte and water secretion.

Yoshikawa et al. (2000) found the methanolic extract from the aerial parts of parsley had potent estrogenic activity. This was attributed to several flavone glycosides, including a new flavone glycoside, 6″-acetylapiin, together with a new monoterpene, petroside.

Manderfeld et al. (1997) demonstrated the antibacterial properties of parsley leaves. The photoactive furocoumarins extracted from the leaves inhibited human pathogens, *E. coli* and *Lesteria monocytogenes*, and the spoilage organisms, *Erwinia carotovora* and *Listeria innocua*. Flavones, apigenin, luteolin, and chrysoeriol, and flavonols, quercetin and isorhamnetin, isolated from illuminated parsley-cell suspension culture, increased the antioxidative capacity in the plasma of rats (Hempel et al., 1999). Parsley is one of the medicinal herbs used by diabetics in Turkey and is reported to reduce blood pressure (Tunali et al., 1999).

References

Anderson, L.A., Nevall, C.A., and Phillipson, J.D., *Herbal Medicine/A Guide for Health-Care Professionals*, The Pharmaceutical Press, London, 1996, pp. 203–204.

Hempel, J., Pforte, H., Raab, B., Engst, W., Bohm, H., and Jacobasch, Flavonols and flavones of parsley cell suspension culture change the antioxidative capacity of plasma in rats, *Nahrung*, 43:201–204, 1999.

Kreydiyyeh, S.I. and Usta, J., Diueretic effect and mechanism of action of parsley, *J. Ethnopharmacol.*, 79:353–357, 2002.

Kreydiyyeh, S.I., Usta, J., Kaouk, A., and Al-Sadi, R., The mechanism underlying the laxative properties of parsley extract, *Phytomedicine*, 8:382–388, 2001.

Leung, A.Y., *Encyclopedia of Common Natural Ingredients Used in Food, Drugs and Cosmetics*, John Wusket & Sons, New York, 1980, p. 409.

Manderfeld, M.M., Schafer, H.W., Davidson, P.M., and Zottola, E.A., Isolation and identification of antimicrobial furocoumarins from parsley, *J. Food Prot.*, 60:72–77, 1997.

Robbers, J.E. and Tyler, V.E., *Tyler's Herbs of Choice, The Therapeutic Use of Phytochemicals*, Haworth Herbal Press, New York, 1999.

Tunali, T., Yarat, A., Yanardag, R., Ozcelik, F., Ozsoy, O., Ergenekon, G., and Emekeli, N., Effect of parsley (*Petroselinum crispum*) on the skin of STZ-induced diabetic rats, *Phytother. Res.*, 13:138–141, 1999.

Tyler, V.E., The Honest Herbalist, third ed., Pharmaceutical Products Press, New York, London, Norwood, pp. 235–236, 1993.

Yoshikawa, M., Uemura, T., Shimoda, H., Kishi, A., Kawahara, Y., and Matsuda, H., Phytoestrogens from aerial part of *Petroselinum crispum* Mill. (parsley) and structures of 6″-acetylapiin and a new monoterpene glycoside, petroside, *Chem. Pharm. Bull.*, 48: 1039–1044, 2000.

Palm oil   Palm oil, a yellowish, fatty oil obtained from the crushed nuts of the African palm (*Elaeis guineensis*), is used in the manufacture of soaps, chocolates, cosmetics, and candles. The oil contains 50 percent saturated fatty acids, 40 percent unsaturated fatty acids, and 10 percent polyunsaturated fatty acids but does not promote atherosclerosis and arterial thrombosis. The saturated to unsaturated fatty-acid ratio of palm oil is close to one with oleic acid, predominantly at the sn2-position in the main triacylglycerols (Ong and Goh, 2002). Palm oil also contains a large amount of antioxidants, β-carotene, and vitamin E (Ebong et al., 1999). The fruit of palm also contains other components that could enhance the nutritional and health benefits. These include phytonutrients, such as sterols (sitosterol, stigmasterol, and campesterol), phospholipids, glycolipids, and squalene. In addition, it was recently reported that water-soluble, powerful antioxidants, phenolic acids, and flavonoids can be recovered from the palm oil mill effluent (Wattanapenpaiboon and Wahlqvist, 2003).

The benefits of palm oil to health include reduction in the risk of arterial thrombosis and atherosclerosis (Van Jaarsvels et al., 2002), inhibition of endogenous cholesterol biosynthesis, platelet aggregation, lowering of blood triglycerides (or reduced fat storage) as compared with polyunsaturated fat diets (Ong and Goh, 2002), retarding oxidation of low-density lipoproteins, promoting vascular relaxation (Abeywardena et al., 2002), and reduction in blood pressure. Lipolysis of palm-oil triacylglycerols containing oleic acid mainly at the sn-2 position and palmitic and stearic acids at sn 1 and 3 positions allows for the ready absorption of the 2-monoacylglycerols, while the saturated fatty acids are poorly absorbed (Ong and Goh, 2002). Unlike fresh palm oil, oxidized palm (resulting from processing for culinary purposes) induces an adverse lipid profile, reproductive toxicity, and toxicity of the kidney, lung, liver, and heart (Edem, 2002).

P

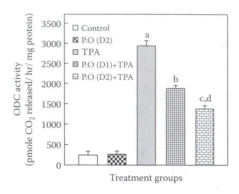

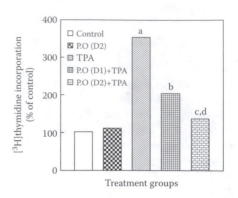

FIGURE P.72A Effect of pretreatment of palm oil on TPA-mediated epidermal ODC activity. Each value represents the mean DNA ±SE of six animals. (a) Significantly different ($p < 0.001$) compared with the acetone-treated control. (b) Significantly different ($p < 0.01$) compared with the TPA-treated group. (c) Significantly different ($p < 0.001$) compared with the TPA-treated group. (d) Significantly different ($p < 0.01$) compared with the P.O. (D1) + TPA-treated group. P.O. (D1), significantly palm oil (100 L); P.O. (D2), palm oil (150 L). (From Kausar et al., *Cancer Lett.*, 192:151–160, 2003. With permission.)

FIGURE P.72B Effect of pretreatment of palm oil on TPA-mediated [³H]thymidine incorporation in epidermal. The data represent the percentage of the acetone-treated control value. The actual acetone-treated control value is 5.00 ± 8.46 DPM/mg DNA. The TPA-treated control is 186 ± 9.66 DPM/mg DNA. The values represent the mean ± six animals. (a) Significantly different ($p < 0.001$) compared with the acetone-treated control. (b) Different ($p < 0.05$) when compared with the TPA-treated group. (c) Significantly different ($p < 0.01$) compared with the TPA-treated group. (d) Significantly different ($p < 0.05$) when compared with the P.O.(D1) + TPA-treated group. P.O. (D1), palm oil (100 L); P.O. (D2), palm oil (150 L). (From Kausar et al., *Cancer Lett.*, 192:151–160, 2003. With permission.)

Red palm oil is a rich source of β-carotene, α-carotene, and tocotrienols (Ong and Goh, 2002). Solomon (1998) showed that β-carotene in red palm oil can be used as a supplement to restore and preserve vitamin A in school children. Radhika et al. (2003) reported red-palm-oil supplementation significantly improved maternal and neonatal vitamin A status and reduced the prevalence of maternal anemia. The effect of palm-oil carotene supplementation was shown by Nesaretman et al. (2002) to modulate the immune system by increasing peripheral blood NK cells and B-lymphocytes and suppress the growth of MCF-7 human breast-cancer cells. The antitumor properties of palm oil (P.O.) were examined by Kausar et al. (2003) against 12-*O*-tetradecanoyl-phorbol-13-acetate (TPA)-induced skin tumorigenesis in Swiss albino mice. The antiskin-tumor effects of palm oil (P.O.) involved inhibition of ornithine decarboxylase (ODC) and [(3)H]thymidine incorporation, conventionally used markers for skin-tumor promotion and cutaneous oxidative stress (Figure P.72A, B).

Other studies showed the tocotrienol-rich fraction (TRF) of palm oil inhibited cell growth and induced apoptosis in both preneoplastic and neoplastic cells. Argawal et al. (2004) suggested that the mechanism of TRF-induced apoptosis in colon carcinoma cells was mediated by p53 signaling network independently of cell-cycle association.

References

Abeywardena, M., Runnie, I., Nizar, M., Momamed, S. and Head, R., Polyphenol-enriched extract from oil palm fronds (*Elaies guineensis*) promotes vascular relaxation via endothelium-dependent mechanisms, *Asian Pacific J. Clin Nutr.,* 11 (Suppl.): S467–S472, 2002.

Argawal, M.K., Argawal, M.L., Athar, M., and Gupta, S., Tocotrienol-rich fraction of palm oil activates p53, modulates Bax/Bcl2 ratio and induces apoptosis independent of cell cycle association, *Cell Cycle*, 3:205–211, 2004.

Cottrell, R.C., Introduction: Nutritional aspects of palm oil, *Am. J. Clin. Nutr.,* 53:9895–10095, 1991.

Ebong, P.E., Owu, D.U., and Isong, E.U., Influence of palm oil (*Elaesis guineensis*) on health, *Plant Foods Hum. Nutr.,* 53:209–222, 1999.

Edem, D.O., Palm oil: Biochemical, physiological, nutritional, hematological, and toxicological aspects: A review, *Plant Foods Hum. Nutr.,* 57:319–341, 2002.

Kausar, H., Bhasin, G., Zargar, M.A., and Athar, M., Palm oil alleviates 12-*O*-tetradecanoyl-phorbol-13-acetate-induced tumor promotion response in murine skin, *Cancer Lett.,* 192:151–160, 2003.

Nesaretnam, K., Radhakrishnan, A., Selvaduray, K.R., Reimann, K., Pailoor, J., Razak, G., Mahmood, M.M., and Dahliwal, J.S., Effect of palm oil carotene on breast cancer tumorigenicity in nude mice, *Lipids,* 37:557–560, 2002.

Ong, A.S.H. and Goh, S.H., Palm oil: A healthful and cost-effective dietary component, *Food Nutr. Bull.,* 23:11–22, 2002.

Radhika, M.S., Bhaskaram, P., Balakrishna, N., and Ramalakshmi, B.A., Red palm oil supplementation: A feasible diet-based approach to improve vitamin A status of pregnant women and their infants, *Food Nutr. Bull.,* 24:208–217, 2003.

Solomons, N.W., Plant sources of vitamin A and human nutrition: Red palm oil does the job, *Nutr. Rev.,* 56:309–311, 1998.

Van Jaarsveld, P.J., Smuts, C.M., and Benade, A.J.S., Effect of palm olein in a moderate-fat diet on plasma lipoprotein profile and aortic atherosclerosis in non-human primates, *Asia Pac. J. Clin. Nutr.,* 11(Suppl. 7):S424–S432, 2002.

Wattanapenpaiboon, N. and Wahlqvist, M.L., Phytonutrient deficiency: the place of palm fruit, *Asia Pac. J. Clin. Nutr.,* 12:363–368, 2003.

Pau d'arco   *Tabebuia* trees are native to the tropical rain forests in Central and South America. A commercial product, lapacho, obtained from its bark, is also known as Pau d'arco, Taheebo, and ipe-roxo. The main species used in folk medicine is *Tabebuia impetiginosa.* Pau d'arco has been used for many years as an anticancer, antifungal, antibacterial, and antiinflammatory drug (Zani et al., 1991). A number of naphthoquinones identified in *Tabebuia* included lapachol and dehydro-α-lapachol, together with α- and β-lapachones (Burnett and Thomson, 1967; Steinert et al., 1995).

Lapachol was reported to be effective against a number of tumors, as well as exhibited antiiflammatory activity (Subramanian et al., 1998; Almeida et al., 1990). The most extensively studied component in the heartwood of *T. impetiginosa* is β-lapachone, whose antitumor properties appear to involve the production of reactive-oxygen species (Portela and Stoppani, 1996). In addition, β-lapachone has been found to induce apoptosis in tumor cells (Chau et al., 1998), as well as topoisomerase II-mediated DNA cleavage (Frydman et al., 1997). Further work by Muller et al. (1999) identified a number of lapacho compounds that were potent inhibitors of human keratinocyte growth of which naphtho[2,3-*b*]furan-4.9-diones were considered the most effective ingredients for treating psoriasis.

Anesini and Perez (1993) screened 132 extracts from Argentine folk-medicinal plants for antimicrobial activity using a penicillin-resistant strain of *Staphyloccocus aureus, Escherichia coli,* and *Aspergillus niger.* Of these, *Tabebuia impetiginosa* produced some of the more active extracts against these organisms.

Koyama et al. (2000) isolated two cyclopenetene dialdehydes from the bark of *Tabebuia.* They were characterized as 2-formyl-5-(4′-methoxybenzoyloxy)-3-methyl-2-cyclopentene-1-acetaldehyde (1) and 2-formyl-5-(3′,4′-dimethoxybenzoyloxy)-3-methyl-2-cyclopentene-1-acetaldehyde (2). Both compounds

P

Structure of lapacho compounds. (From Muller et al., *J. Nat. Prod.,* 62:1134–1136, 1999.)

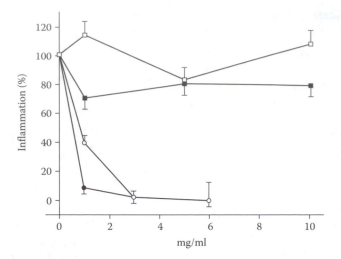

FIGURE P.73 Anti-inflammatory activities of 1 and 2 in the TPA-activated human PMN compared with alkylated benzoic acids. ○ 1; ● 2; □ 4-methoxybenzoic acid; ■ 3,4-dimethoxybenzoic acid. (From Koyama et al., *Phytochemistry,* 53:869–872, 2000. With permission.)

exhibited potent anti-inflammatory activity against 12-*O*-tetradecanoylphorbol (TPA)-activated human PMN compared to alkylated benzoic acids (Figure P.73).

The major volatile constituents of *T. impetiginosa* with antioxidant activity were shown by Park et al. (2003) to be 4-methoxybenzaldehyde, 4-methoxyphenol, 5-allyl-1,2,3-trimethoxybenzene (elimicin), 1-methoxy-4-(1E)-1-propenylbenzene (*trans*-anaethole), and 4-methoxybenzyl alcohol. These volatiles were found to be as effective as α-tocopherol and BHT in their ability to inhibit the formation of conjugated diene hydroperoxides from methyl linoleate and the oxidation of hexanal.

Warashina et al. (2004) recently reported the presence of 19 glycosides in the bark of *Tabebuia impetiginosa*. These included four iridoid glycosides, two lignan glycosides, two isocoumarin glycosides, three phenylethanoid glyosides, and eight phenolic glycosides.

References

Anesini, C. and Perez, C., Screening of plants in Argentine folk medicine for antimicrobial activity, *J. Ethnopharmacol.,* 39:119–128, 1993.

Burnett, A.R. and Thomson, R.H., Naturally occurring quinones, X. Quinonoid constituents of *Tabebuia avellanedae, J. Chem. Soc.,* C:2100–2104, 1967.

Chau, Y.-P., Shiah, S.-C., Don, M.-J., and Kuo, M.-L., Involvement of hydrogen peroxide in topoisomerase inhibitor β-lapachone-induced apoptosis and differentiation in human leukemia cells, *Free Rad. Biol. Med.,* 24:660–770, 1998.

de Almeida, E.R., da Silva Filho, A.A., dos Santos, E.R., and Lopes, C.A.C., Anti-inflammatory action of lapachol, *J. Ethnopharmacol.,* 29:239–241, 1990.

Frydman, B., Marton, L.J., Sun, J.S., Neder, K., Witiak, D.T., Liu, A.A., Wang, H.M., Mao, Y., Wu, H.Y., Sanders, M.M., and Liu, L.F., Induction of DNA topoisomerase II-mediated DNA cleavage by β-lapachone and related naphthoquinones, *Cancer Res.,* 57:620–627, 1997.

Koyama, J., Morita, I., Tagahara, K., and Hirai, K., Cyclopentene dialdehydes from *Tabebuia impetiginosa, Phytochemistry,* 53:869–872, 2000.

Muller, K., Sellmer, A., and Wiegrebe, W., Potential antipsoriatic agents: Lapacho compounds as potent inhibitors of HaCaT cell growth, *J. Nat. Prod.,* 62:1134–1136, 1999.

Park, B.S., Lee, K.G., Shibamoto, T., Lee, S.E., and Takeoka, G.R., Antioxidant activity and characterization of volatile constituents of Taheebo (*Tabebuia impetiginosa* Martinus ex DC), *J. Agric. Food Chem.,* 51:295–300, 2003.

Portela, M.P.M. and Stopani, A.O.M., Redox cycling of β-lapachone and related *O*-naphthoquinones in the presence of dihydrolipoamide and oxygen, *Biochem. Pharmacol.,* 51:275–283, 1996.

Steinert, J., Khalaf, H., and Rimpler, M., HPLC separation and determination of naphtho[2,3-b]furan-4,9-diones and related compounds in extracts of *Tabebuia avellanedae* (Bignoniaceae), *J. Chromatogr. A,* 693:281–287, 1995.

Subramanian, S., Ferreira, M.M.C., and Trsic, M., A structure-activity relationship study of lapachol and some derivatives of 1,4-naphthoquinones against carcinosarcoma walker 256, *Struct. Chem.,* 9:47–57, 1998.

Warashina, T., Nagatani, Y., and Noro, T., Constituents from the bark of *Tabebuia impetiginosa, Phytochemistry,* 65:2003–2011, 2004.

Zani, C.L., de Oliviera, A.B., and de Oliviera, G.G., Furanonaphthoquinones from Tabebuia ochracea, *Phytochemistry,* 30:2379–2381, 1991.

Pears   Pears are a good source of vitamin C (3.8 mg/100 g), vitamin K (4.5 mg/100 g), and dietary fiber (4 g/100 g). The average concentration of phenolic compounds in pears harvested at commercial maturity stage is 3.7 g/kg fresh pulp. The predominant phenolics are procyanidins (96 percent), together with hydroxycinnamic acids (2 percent), arbutin (0.8 percent), and catechins (0.7 percent). Sun-drying causes a decrease of 64 percent (on a dry-pulp basis) in the total amount of native phenolic compounds (Fereira et al., 2002). A comparison of different pear cultivars showed a wide range in both phenolic content (272 to 475 mg of CtE/100 g fresh fruit) and *in vitro* antioxidant activity in the order of Forelle > Taylor > Peckham > Conference. A later study by Sanchez et al. (2003) compared six pear cultivars and found most of the phenolics were located in the peel, ranging from 1235 to 2005 mg/kg compared to 28–81 mg/kg for the corresponding flesh. Vitamin C was also higher in the peels, accounting for 116 to 228 mg/kg compared to 28–53 mg/kg in the flesh. A correlation of r = 0.46 was evident between antioxidant capacity and chlorogenic acid, with vitamin C only making a small contribution. Tanrioven and Eksi (2004) recently showed pear juice from seven different varieties ranged in total polyphenolics from 196 to 457 mg/L. Chlorogenic acid, the main phenolic, accounted for 73.1 to 249 mg/L,

followed by epicatechin, which ranged from 11.9 to 81.3. The two remaining polyphnols were caffeic and p-coumaric acids, each accounting for 2.4–11.4 and 0.0–3.0 mg/L, respectively.

Leontowicz et al. (2002) examined the bioactive compounds in apples, peaches, and pears and their effect on lipids and antioxidant capacity in rats. Diets supplemented with apples and, to a lesser extent, with peaches and pears, improved lipid metabolism and plasma-antioxidant potential. They attributed the antioxidant properties of apples and pears to their polyphenols, phenolic acids, and flavonoids, with the peels being significantly higher ($p < 0.05$) than the pulp. Diets supplemented with fruit peels with added cholesterol exercised a significantly positive influence on rat plasma lipids, with pear peel being less effective than apple peel. The ability to counteract hypercholesterolemia and oxidative stress was consistent with a previous study using lyophilized apple by Aprikan et al. (2002). Because peels were much richer in polyphenols, the washed whole fruit was recommended.

References

Aprikian, O., Busserolles, J., Manach, C., Mazur, A., Morand, C., Davicco, M.J., Besson, C., Rayssiguier, Y., Remesy, C., and Demigne, C., Lyophilized apple counteracts the development of hypercholesterolemia, oxidative stress, and renal dysfunction in Zucker rats, *J. Nutr.,* 132:1969–1976, 2002.

Fereira, D., Guyot, S., Marnet, N., Delgadillo, I., Renard, C.M.G.C., and Coimbra, M.A., Composition of phenolic compounds in a Portuguese pear (*Pyrus communis* L. var. S. Bartolomeu) and changes after sun-drying, *J. Agric. Food Chem.,* 50:4537–4544, 2002.

Leontowicz, H., Gorinstein, S., Lojek, A., Leontowicz, M., Ciz, M., Soliva-Fortuny, R., Park, Y.S., Jung, S.T., Trakhtenberg, S., and Martin-Belloso, O., Comparative content of some bioactive compounds in apples, peaches and pears and their influence on lipids and antioxidant capacity in rats, *J. Nutr. Biochem.,* 13:603–610, 2002.

Sanchez, A.C.G., Gil-Izquierdo, A.G., and Gil, M.I., Comparative study of six pear cultivars in terms of their phenolic and vitamin C contents and antioxidant capacity, *J. Sci. Food Agric.,* 83:995–1003, 2003.

P

Tanrioven, D. and Eksi, A., Phenolic compounds in pear juice from different cultivars, *Food Chem.*, 93: 89–93, 2005.

Pectin   Pectin, the main component of primary plant cell walls of all land plants, encompasses a range of galacturonic acid-rich polysaccharides. Three major pectic polysaccharides, homogalacturonan (HGA), rhamnogalacturonan-I (RG-I), and rhamnogalaturonan-II (RG-II), are present in all primary cell walls, together with cellulose, hemicellulose, and protein (Perez et al., 2003). The "canonical" primary structure of pectins is depicted in Scheme P.42. Pectin is used extensively in the food, pharmaceuticals, and related industries. The importance of pectin is related to its ability to form a gel in the presence of Ca^{2+} ions or a solute at low pH (Thakur et al., 1997).

The quality of fibrin networks and the concentration of fibrinogen are both thought to contribute to increasing the risk of cardiovascular disease. Veldman et al. (1999) showed pectin influenced the fibrin-network architecture in hypercholesterolemic men without causing any changes in fibrinogen concentration. The beneficial effects of pectin appeared to be mediated by acetate as it is fermented in the gastrointestinal tract to acetate, proprionate, and butyrate. Only acetate, however, reaches circulation in humans beyond the liver.

Vergara-Jimeneza et al. (1999) demonstrated that pectin reversed hyperlipidemia associated with high-fat sucrose diets and had a potential antioxidant effect on circulating LDL. The protective effect of pectin on cardiovascular disease was shown by Park and coworkers (2000) to be due to an increase in fecal excretion of neutral sterols and hepatic microsomal fluidity. However, pectin increased risk factors for colon cancer by increasing the production of secondary bile acids and short-chain fatty acids in the colon. Rats fed low-molecular-weight pectin were found by Grizard et al. (2001) to significantly decrease triacylglycerols, total cholesterol,

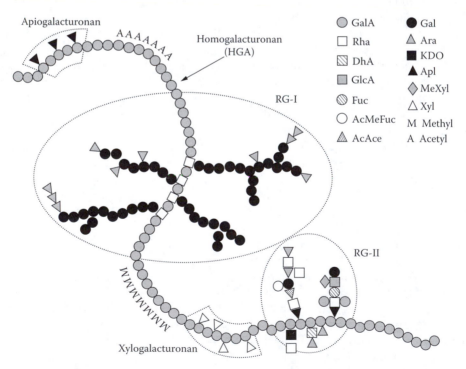

SCHEME P.42 Schematic representation of the "canonical" primary structure of pectins. For the sake of simplicity, their schematic representations of HGA, RG-I, and RG-II are given, assuming that these three domains are covalently linked, although this point is not firmly established. (From Perez et al., *Biochimie*, 85: 109–121, 2003. With permission.)

and insulin concentrations without changing postprandial blood-glucose levels.

Pectins also activate *in vitro* macrophages to be cytotoxic against tumor cells and microbial infections. Modifying citrus pectin, by enzymatic treatment to changes to the molecular structure of the long pectin chain, also inhibited metastases in animals with prostate cancer. Spontaneous lung metastases were also reduced by 60 percent if rats consumed 1 percent citrus pectin in their diets. Hayashi et al. (2000) reported that a pH-modified citrus pectin (MCP) significantly reduced the tumor size of colon-25 solid tumor implants in balb c mice. Rats receiving a low dose of (0.8 mg/mL) MCP produced a 38 percent ($p < 0.02$) decrease in tumor size compared to an impressive 70 percent ($p < 0.001$) reduction when animals were maintained on a high-dose (1.6 mg/mL) of MCP.

New developments with pectin-based formulations, particularly in the area of colon-specific drug-delivery systems, found that pectin showed great promise in engineering drug-delivery systems for oral drug delivery (Liu et al., 2003). Recent work by Liu et al. (2004) showed that composite matrices of pectin/poly(lactide-co-glycolide) had great potential for biomedical applications.

References

Grizard, D., Dalle, M., and Barthomeuf, C., Changes in insulin and corticosterone levels may partly mediate the hypolipidemic effect of guar gum and low-molecular weight pectin in rats, *Nutr. Res.*, 21:1185–1190, 2001.

Hayashi, A., Gillen, A.C., and Lott, J.R., Effects of daily oral administration of quercetin chalcone and modified citrus pectin on implanted colon-25 tumor growth in Balb-c mice, *Altern. Med. Rev.*, 5:546–552, 2000.

Hurd, L., Modified citrus pectin enhances the immune system, *Total Health*, 21:0274–6743, 1999.

Liu, L.S., Fishman, M.L., Kost, J., and Hicks, K.B., Pectin based systems for colon-specific drug delivery via oral route, *Biomaterials*, 24:3333–3343, 2003.

Liu, L.S., Won, Y.J., Cooke, P.H., Coffin, D.R., Fishman, M.L., Hicks, K.B., and Ma, P.X., Pectin/poly(lactide-co-glycolide) composite matrices for biomedical applications, *Biomaterials*, 25:3201–3210, 2004.

Park, H.S., Choi, J.S., and Kim, K.H., Docosahexaenoic acid-rich fish oil and pectin have a hypolipidemic effect, but pectin increases risk factor for colon cancer in rats, *Nutr. Res.*, 20:1783–1794, 2000.

Perez, S., Rodriguez-Carvajal, M.A., and Doco, T., A complex plant cell wall polysaccharide: Rhamnogalacturonan II, a structure in quest of a function, *Biochimie*, 85:109–121, 2003.

Thakur, B.R., Singh, R.K., and Handa, A.K., Chemistry and uses of pectin, *CRC Rev. Food Sci. Nutr.*, 37:47–73, 1997.

Veldman, F.J., Nair, C.H., Vorster, H.H., Vermaak, W.J.H., Jerling, J.C., Oosthuizen, W., and Venter, C.S., Possible mechanisms through which dietary pectin influences fibrin network architecture in hypercholesterolaemic subjects, *Thrombosis Res.*, 93:253–264, 1999.

Vergara-Jimeneza, M., Furra, H., and Fernandeza, M.L., Pectin and psyllium decrease the susceptibility of LDL to oxidation in guinea pigs, *J. Nutr. Biochem.*, 10:118–124, 1999.

Peony   Peonies, herbaceous cultivars of *Paeoniae alba* Radix (red peony root), the dried root of *Paeoniae lactiflora* Pallas or *Paeoniae veitchii* Lynch, originated in China more than 2,000 years ago. The root extract of peony was shown by Sakai et al. (1990) to inhibit the mutagenicity of benzo[a]pyrene-(B[a])p metabolites. Tsuda et al. (1997) found one of the bioactives in peony root extract (*Paeoniae radix*), gallotannin, partially protected neuron damage in the hippocampus of 7-week-old Wistar rats induced by the cobalt focus epilepsy model, while paeoniflorin, a second bioactive, had no effect. However, when both bioactives were combined, they provided complete protection, similar to the whole peony-root extract. Treatment with paeoniflorin was shown by Tabata et al. (2000) to reverse the suppressive effects of scopolamine and prenzepine (muscarinic receptor-antagonists) on long-term potentiation. Tabata et al. (2001) also found paeoniflorin ameliorated memory disruption mediated by the adenosine A1 receptor, which had a beneficial effect on learning and memory impairment in rodents.

The active principal of peony roots that lowered total and LDL cholesterol was identified

P

by Shibata et al. (1963) as paeoniflorin. This water-soluble bioactive is pharmacologically active as an anti-inflammatory and antiallergic (Yamahara et al., 1982), antihyperglycemic (Hsu et al., 1997), and analgesic (Sugishita et al., 1984). More recent studies showed additional

Paeoniflorin. (From He et al., *J. Nat. Prod.*, 62:1134–1136, 1999. With permission.)

pharmacological effects, including antithrombosis (Ye et al., 2001), antihypotension (Cheng et al., 1999), and enhanced glucose uptake (Tang et al., 2003).

Yang et al. (2004) recently isolated paeoniflorin from the methanol extract of *Paeonia lactiflora* and examined its effect as an antihyperlipidemic agent. When 200 and 400 mg/kg of paeoniflorin were fed to experimentally induced hyperlipidemic adult male Wistar rats, plasma total-cholesterol levels were lowered significantly by 19.1 percent and 28.7 percent, respectively, in a dose-dependent manner. Under the same conditions, lovastatin, at a dose of 10 mg/kg, reduced plasma total cholesterol by 25.8 percent. Marked decreases in plasma triglycerides and LDL levels of 51.4 percent and 59.3 percent and 69.3 percent and 80.5 percent were also observed for the two doses of paeoniflorin, respectively. In contrast to lovastatin, which lowered HDL very slightly, paeoniflorin increased HDL by 14.9 percent and 6.3 percent for the two doses, respectively.

Chen et al. (1999, 2002) examined the pharmacokinetics of paeoniflorin in normal, healthy animals, while Ye and coworkers (2004) studied the effect of disease state on its pharmacokinetics. Using rats suffering from cerebral ischemia-reperfusion, they found marked differences in the pharmacokinetics of paeoniflorin between normal and diseased animals. For example, elimination of paeoniflorin slowed down in the ischemic-reperfusion rats, pointing to its accumulation in the pathological

state. This information will ensure greater safety and efficacy when using paeoniflorin in clinical applications.

References

Chen, L.C., Lee, M.H., Chou, M.H., Lin, M.F., and Yang, L.L., Pharmacokinetic study of paeoniflorin in mice after oral administration of *Paeoniae* Radix extract, *J. Chromatogr. B*, 735:33–40, 1999.

Chen, L.C., Chou, M.H., Lin, M.F., and Yang, L.L., Pharmacokinetics of paeoniflorin after oral administration of Shao-yao Gan-chao Tang in mice, *Jpn. J. Pharmacol.*, 88:250–255, 2002.

Cheng, J.T., Wang, C.J., and Hsu, F.L., Paeoniflorin reverses guanethidine-induced hypotension via activation of central adenosine A1 receptors in Wistar rats, *Clin. Exp. Pharmacol. Physiol.*, 26:815–816, 1999.

He, X., Xing, D., Ding, Y., Li, Y., Xu, Y., and Du, L., Effects of cerebral ischemia-reperfusion on pharmacokinetic fate of paeoniflorin after intravenous administration of *Paeoniae* Radix extract in rats, *J. Ethnopharmacol.*, 94: 339–344, 2004.

Hsu, F.L., Lai, C.W., and Cheng, J.T., Antihyperglycemic effects of paeoniflorin and 8-debenzoylpaeoniflorin, glucosides from the root of *Paeonia lactiflora*, *Planta Med.*, 63:323–325, 1997.

Sakai, Y., Nagase, H., Ose, Y., Kito, H., Sato, T., Kawai, M., and Mizuno, M., Inhibitory action of peony root on the mutagenicity of benz[*a*]pyrene, *Mutat. Res. Lett.*, 244:129–134, 1990.

Shibata, S., Nakahara, M., and Aimi, N., Studies on the constituents of Japanese and Chinese crude drugs, VIII. Paeoniflorin, a glucoside of Chinese peony root (1), *Chem. Pharma. Bull.*, 11:372–378, 1963.

Sugishita, S., Amagaya, S., and Ogihara, Y., Studies on the combination of *Glycyrrhizal* Radix in Shakuyakukanzo-To, *J. Pharmacobio-dynamics*, 7:427–435, 1984.

Tabata, K., Matsumoto, K., Murakami, Y., and Watanabe, H., Ameliorative effects of paeoniflorin, a major constituent of peony root, on adenosine A1 receptor-mediated impairment of passive avoidance performance and long-term potentiation in the hippocampus, *Biol. Pharm. Bull.*, 24:496–500, 2001.

Tabata, K., Matsumoto, K., and Watanabe, H., Paeoniflorin, a major constituent of peony root, reverses muscarinic M1-receptor antagonist-induced suppression of long-term potentiation in the rat hippocampal slice, *Jpn. J. Pharmacol.*, 83:25–30, 2000.

Tsuda, T., Sugaya, A., Oghuchi, H., Kishida, N., and Sugaya, E., Protective effects of peony root extract and its components on neuron damage in the hippocampus induced by cobalt focus epilepsy model, *Exp. Neurol.*, 146:518–525, 1997.

Yamahara, J., Yamada, T., Kimura, H., Sawada, T., and Fujimura, H., Biologically active principles of crude drugs, II. Anti-allergic principles in "Shoseiryu-To" anti-inflammatory properties of paeoniflorin and its derivatives, *J. Pharmaco-biodynamics*, 5:921–929, 1982.

Yang, H.O., Ko, W.K., Kim, J.Y., and Ro, H.S., Paeoniflorin: An antihyperlipidemic agent from *Paeonia lactiflora*, *Fitoterapia*, 75:45–49, 2004.

Ye, J., Daun, H., Yang, X., Yan, W., and Zheng, X, Anti-thrombosis effect of paeoniflorin: Evaluated in a photochemical reaction thrombosis model *in vivo*, *Planta Med.*, 67:766–767, 2001.

Peppermint (*Mentha piperita*) Peppermint is a very popular herb with a unique flavor. The oil from peppermint is currently used in cosmetic formulations as a fragrance component. Both peppermint and peppermint oil have psychoactive properties and are believed to be effective for treating nervous disorders and mental fatigue (Tisserand, 1993). The oil is composed primarily of menthol and menthone. Other possible constituents include pulegone, menthofuran, and limone. Because of the toxicity of pulegone, this constituent is limited to

(–)-Menthone   (–)-Menthol

Adapted from Hall, *Eur. J. Pharmacol.*, 506:9–16, 2004.

< or = 1 percent (Nair et al., 2001). Other microelements and macroelements measured in peppermint were As, Cd, Cu, Fe, Mg, Pb, and Zn (Fijalek et al., 2003). Peppermints also contain antioxidants (i.e., > 75 mmol/100 g) (Dragland et al., 2003). They are usually taken after a meal because of their ability to reduce indigestion and colonic spasms by reducing the gastrocolic reflex. It was recently shown that peppermint has a potential role in the management of certain procedures, such as colonoscopy (Spirling and Daniels, 2001) and during upper endoscopy (Hiki et al., 2003). The oil is harmless and acts locally in the stomach and duodenum to produce smooth-muscle relaxation in healthy volunteers (Micklefield et al., 2003).

May and coworkers (2003) demonstrated good tolerability and a favorable risk–benefit ratio of a fixed combination of 90 mg peppermint oil and 50 mg caraway oil for the treatment of functional dyspepsia. Pittler and Ernst (1998) reviewed clinical trials using peppermint extracts and were unable to establish beyond a reasonable doubt the efficacy of peppermint as a symptomatic treatment for irritable bowel syndrome.

A recent study by Norrish and Dwyer (2005) showed peppermint diminished daytime sleepiness, normally associated with sitting in a dark room. The invigorating effects of peppermint oil could enable people to remain awake, such as during the night shift.

References

Dragland, S., Senoo, H., Wake, K., Holte, K., and Blomhoff, R., Several culinary and medicinal herbs are important sources of dietary antioxidants, *J. Nutr.*, 133:1286–1290, 2003.

Fijalek, Z., Soltyk, K., Lozak, A., Kominek, A., and Ostapczuk, P., Determination of some micro- and macroelements made from peppermint and nettle leaves, *Pharmazie*, 58:480–482, 2003.

Hall, A.C., Turcotte, C.M., Betts, B.A., Yeung, W-Y., Agyeman, A.S. and Burk, L.A., Modulation of human $GABA_A$ and glycine receptor currents by menthol and related monoterpenoids, *Eur. J. Pharmacol.*, 506:9–16, 2004.

Hiki, N., Kurosaka, H., Tatsutomi, Y., Shimoyama, S., Tsuji, E., Kojima, J., Shimizu, N., Ono, H., Hirooka, T., Noguchi, C., Mafune, K., and Kaminishi, M., Peppermint oil reduces gastric spasm during upper endoscopy: A randomized, double-blind, double-dummy controlled trial, *Gastrointest. Endosc.*, 57:475–482, 2003.

May, B., Funk, P., and Schneider, B., Fixed peppermint oil/caraway oil combination in functional dyspepsia-efficacy unaffected by *H. pylori* status, *Aliment Pharmacol. Ther.*, 17:975–976, 2003.

P

Micklefield, G., Jung, O., Greving, I., and May, B., Effects of intraduodenal application of peppermint oil (WS® 1340) and caraway oil (WS® 1520) on gastroduodenal motility in healthy volunteers, *Phytother. Res.,* 17:135–140, 2003.

Nair, B., Final report on the safety assessment of *Mentha piperita* (peppermint) oil, *Mentha piperita* (peppermint) leaf extract, *Mentha piperita* (peppermint) leaf, and *Mentha piperita* (peppermint) leaf water, *Health,* 121(Suppl. 3):61–73, 2001.

Norrish, M.I. and Dwyer, K.L., Preliminary investigation of the effect of peppermint oil as an objective measure of daytime sleepiness, *Int. J. Psychophysiol.,* 55:291–298, 2005.

Pittler, M.H. and Ernst, E., Peppermint oil for irritable bowel syndrome: A critical review and metaanalysis, *Am. J. Gastroenterol.,* 93:1131–1135, 1998.

Spirling, L.I. and Daniels, I.R., Botanical perspectives on health peppermint: More than just an after-dinner mint, *J.R. Soc. Health,* 121:62–63, 2001.

Tisserand, R., *The Art of Aromatherapy,* C.W. Daniel, Essex, U.K., 1999.

Peppers *see also* **Capsaicin, Chili peppers, and Red peppers** Peppers (*Capsicum anuum* L.) are good sources of provitamin carotenoids, α-carotene, β-carotene, and crypto-zanthin and a wide array of neutral and acidic phenolic compounds. As peppers mature, the concentrations of these carotenoids increase, together with phenolic acids, capxanthin, and zeaxanthin (Howard et al., 2000). Lutein, on the other was shown to decline. Peppers contain high levels of L-ascorbic acid and carotenoids at maturity, contributing 124–338 percent of the RDA for vitamin C and 0.33–336 RE/100 g provitamin A carotenoids. Peppers also contain oxygenated carotenoids or xanthophylls, which do not possess vitamin A activity but are still effective free-radical scavengers and may help to prevent age-related macular degeneration and cataracts.

Jimeneze et al. (2003) reported that antioxidant capacity and ascorbate content were higher in red peppers than green peppers and that storage increased ascorbate content in both green and red fruits.

The concentration of capsaicinoids in fresh peppers was variable, depending on the relative pungency of the pepper type and geographical origin of the pepper (Reilly et al., 2001). The health-related properties are discussed under capsaicin. Fresh, whole, homogenized peppers have characteristic volatile components, including hydrocarbons, terpenes, alcohols, phenols, ethers, aldehydes, ketones, esters, pyrroles, pyrazines, and sulfurous compounds (Oruna-Concha et al., 1998).

References

Howard, L.R., Talcott, S.T., Brenes, C.H., and Villalon, B., Changes in phytochemical and antioxidant activity of selected pepper cultivars (*Capsicum* species) as influenced by maturity, *J. Agric. Food Chem.,* 48:1713–1720, 2000.

Jimenez, A., Romojaro, F., Gomez, J.M., Llanos, M.R., and Sevilla, F., Antioxidant systems and their relationship with the response of pepper fruits to storage at 20 degrees C, *J. Agric. Food Chem.,* 51: 6293–6299, 2003.

Oruna-Concha, M.J., Lopez-Hernandez, J., Simal-Lozano, J.A., Simal-Gandara, J., Gonzalez-Castro, M.J., and de la Cruz Garcia, C., Determination of volatile components in fresh, frozen, and freeze-dried Padron-type peppers by gas chromatography-mass spectrometry using dynamic headspace sampling and microwave desorption, *J. Chromatogr. Sci.,* 36:583–588, 1998.

Reilly, C.A., Crouch, D.J., and Yost, G.S., Quantitative analysis of capsaicinoids in fresh peppers, oleoresin capsicum and pepper spray products, *Forensic. Sci.,* 46:502–509, 2001.

Peptides *see* **Biopeptides**

Perilla Perilla (*Perrilla frutescens* L.), a common annual weed in the Eastern United States, is a commercial crop in Asia. It is a member of the mint family, and its leaves are used for medicinal purposes. Asian herbalists prescribe perilla for cough and lung afflictions, influenza prevention, etc. Volatile components in perilla oil include an aldehyde chemotype that is the basis of Japanese Ao-shiso, a medicine with an agreeable fragrance (Koezuka et al., 1986). In addition, a perilla ketone was shown to be a very effective laxative without causing diarrhea in laboratory mice (Koezuka et al., 1985). The leaves of perilla have been used for centuries in Chinese medicine for treating a variety of diseases. Chen and coworkers (2003) identified three bioactive triterpenes in perilla leaves as tormentic acid (TA), oleanolic acid (OA), and ursolic acid (UA).

Structure of perilla leaf bioactive triterpenes. (From Chen et al., *J. Pharm. Biomed. Anal.*, 32:1175–1179, 2003. With permission.)

TA: $R_1 = R_3 = OH$, $R_2 = CH_3$, $R_4 = H$
OA: $R_1 = R_2 = R_3 = H$, $R_4 = CH_3$
UA: $R_1 = R_3 = R_4 = H$, $R_2 = CH_3$

The major polyphenol in perilla-leaf extract, rosmarinic acid, was shown by Osakabe et al. (2002) to reduce liver damage induced by lipopolysaccharides and D-galactosamine by scavenging or reducing the activities of superoxide or peroxynitrite.

Perilla-seed oil is used extensively for cooking in Asian countries. It is one of the richest sources of alpha linolenic acid, reported to prevent atherosclerosis and chemically induced cancer, as well as improves immune and mental function (Yamamoto et al., 1987; Shoda et al., 1995; Sadi et al, 1996; Onogi et al., 1996). The hypolipidemic effect of perilla oil was recently demonstrated by Kim et al. (2004), who showed that feeding rats a diet rich in perilla oil suppressed hepatic fatty-acid synthase, which significantly lowered plasma triacylglycerol levels.

Rosmarinic acid. (From Osakabe et al., *Free Rad. Biol. Med.*, 33:798–806, 2002. With permission.)

References

Chen, J.H., Xia, Z.H., and Tan, R.X., High-performance liquid chromatographic analysis of bioactive triterpenes in Perilla frutescens, *J. Pharm. Biomed. Anal.*, 32:1175–1179, 2003.

Kim, H.-K., Choi, S., and Choi, H., Suppression of hepatic fatty acid synthase by feeding a-linolenic acid rich perilla oil lowers plasma triacylglycerol level in rats, *J. Nutr. Biochem.*, 15:485–492, 2004.

Koezuka, L.A., Honda, G., and Tabata, M., An intestinal propulsion promoting substance from *Perilla frutescens* and its mechanism of action, *Planta Med.*, 39:228–231, 1985.

Koezuka, L.A., Honda, G., and Tabata, M., Genetic control of the chemical composition of volatile oils in *Perilla frutescens*, *Phytochemistry*, 25:2085–2087, 1986.

Onogi, N., Okuno, M., Komaki, C., Marikawi, H., Kawamori, T., Tanaka, T., Mori, H., and Muto, Y., Suppressing effect of perilla oil on azoxymethane-induced foci of colonic aberrant crypts in rats, *Carcinogenesis*, 17:1291–1296, 1996.

Osakabe, N., Yasuda, A., Natsume, M., Sanbong, C., Kato, Y., Osawa, T., and Yoshikawa, T., Rosmarinic acid, a major polyphenolic component of *Perilla* frutescens reduces lipopolysaccharide (LPS)-induced liver injury in D-galactosamine (D-GalN)-sensitized mice, *Free Rad. Biol. Med.*, 33:798–806, 2002.

Sadi, A.M., Toda, T., Oku, H., and Hokama, S., Dietary effects of corn oil, oleic acid, perilla oil, and primrose oil on plasma and hepatic lipid level and therosclerosis in Japanese quail, *Exp. Anim.*, 45:55–62, 1996.

Shoda, R., Matsueda, K., Yamato, S., and Umeda, N., Therapeutic efficacy of n-3 polyunsaturated fatty acid in experimental Crohn's disease, *J. Gastroenterol.*, 30(Suppl. 8):98–101, 1995.

Yamamoto, N., Hashimoto, A, Takemoto, Y., Akuyama, H., Nomura, M., Kitajima, R., Togashi, T., and Tamai, Y., Effects of dietary α-linolenate/linoleate balance on lipid components and learning ability of rats, *J. Lipid Res.*, 29:1013–1021, 1988.

Perillyl alcohol and Perillaldehyde

Perillyl alcohol is a naturally occurring monoterpene in citrus fruits, herbs, and spices with anticancer properties (Gould, 1995). Several animal-tumor models reported the anticancer action of perillyl alcohol in breast, liver, colon, and prostate cancer (Haag and Gould, 1994; Mills et al., 1995; Kelloff et al., 1996). Samouti et al. (1999) found

CH$_2$OH

Perillyl alcohol. (Adapted from Zhang et al., *J. Chromatrgr.* B., 728:85–98, 1999.

perillyl alcohol induced transient expression of the *c-jun* and *c-fos* genes, as well as phosphorylation of *c-jun* protein-cultured breast-cancer cell. Both events are associated with activation of an activator protein (AP)-1-dependent reporter gene. These changes are associated with perillyl alcohol's ability to induce apoptosis, or cell death. Phase I human clinical trials with perillyl alcohol indicated it is a relatively nontoxic compound for treating certain human tumors (Hudes et al., 2000; Ripple et al., 2000). Bardon and coworkers (2002) established the molecular mechanisms of perillyl alcohol and its major metabolite, perillic acid (PA), as antiproliferative agents using human colon-cancer cells. These monoterpenes arrested the growth of cancer cells by increasing the expression of the cdk inhibitor p21$^{Waf1/Cip1}$ and decreasing the expression of cyclin D1 and its partner, cdk4. The effect of perillyl alcohol on two human lung-cancer cell lines, H383, nonsmall cell lung cancer cells derived from adenocarcinoma and H322, bronchioloalveolar carcinoma cells, was reported recently by Xu and coworkers (2004). Perillyl alcohol stimulated or sensitized lung-tumor cells to apoptosis via activation of caspase-3, a key executioner of apoptosis. This is evident in Figure P.74 where the highest dose of perillyl alcohol (1.5 mM) significantly decreased cell proliferation in H322 and H838 cells by 83% and 70%, respectively. The increased sensitivity of perillyl-alcohol-treated cells suggested it could be combined with other drugs to maximize chemotherapeutic effects. Ahn et al. (2003) showed the anticancer properties of perillyl alcohol on SCK mammary carcinoma cells of female A/J mice was significantly enhanced by hypothermia. The latter is used for treating certain human tumors, so that the synergism observed in this study could lead to a combination of perillyl alcohol and hyperthermia.

In vitro studies with human carcinoma cell lines (BroTo and A5459) by Elgebede and coworkers (2003) found perillaldehyde only weakly induced apoptosis compared to perillyl alcohol, which probably involved a different mechanism.

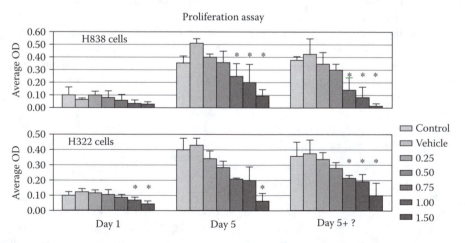

FIGURE P.74 Perillyl alcohol inhibition of cell proliferation. H322 and H838 cells were treated with either 0.06% ethanol (vehicle controls) or perillyl alcohol at concentrations ranging from 0.25 to 1.5 mM for 1 and 5 days. Untreated cells served as an additional negative control. The sulforhodamine B (SRB) cell proliferation assay was performed. The individual bars represent the mean values ± standard deviation of three individual experiments performed in triplicate. Asterisks (*) indicate values that are statistically signifcant at a minimal of *p* < 0.05 relative to vehicle control (Xu, *Toxicol. Applied Pharmacol.*, 195:232–246, 2004).

References

Ahn, K.-J., Lee, C.K., Choi, E.K., Griffin, R., Song, C.W., and Park, H.J., Cytoxicity of perillyl alcohol against cancer cells is potentiated by hyperthermia, *Int. J. Radiat. Oncol. Biol. Phys.,* 57:813–819, 2003.

Bardon, S., Foussard, V., Fournel, S., and Loubat, A., Monoterpenes inhibit proliferation of human colon cancer cells by modulating cell cycle-related protein expression, *Cancer Lett.,* 181:187–194, 2002.

Elgebede, J.A., Flores, R., and Wang, R.C., Perillyl alcohol and perillaldehyde induced cell cycle arrest and cell death in Bro To and A549 cells cultured *in vitro, Life Sci.,* 73:2831–2840, 2003.

Gould, M.N., Prevention and therapy of mammary cancer by monoterpenes, *J. Cell. Biochem.,* 59 (Issue S22):139–144, 1995.

Haag, J.D. and Gould, M.N., Mammary carcinoma regression induced by perillyl alcohol, a hydroxylated analog of limonene, *Cancer Chemother. Pharmacol.,* 34:477–483, 1994.

Hudes, G.R., Szarka, C.W., Adams, A., Ranganathan, S., McCauley, R.A., Weiner, L.M., Langer, C.J., Litwin, S., Yeslow, G., Halberr, T., Qian, M., and Gallo, J.M., Phase I Pharmacokinetic study of perillyl alcohol (NSC 641066) in patients with refractory solid malignancies, *Clin. Cancer. Res.,* 6:3071–3080, 2000.

Kelloff, G.J., Crowell, J.A., Hawk, E.T., Steele, V.E., Lubet, R.A., Boone, C.W., Covey, J.M., Doody, L.A., Omenn, G.S., Greenwald, P., Hong, W.K., Parkinson, D.R., Bagheri, D., Baxter, G.T., Blunden, M., Doeltz, M.K., Eisenhauer, K.M., Johnson, K., Longfellow, D.G., Knapp, G.G., Malone, W.F., Nayfield, S.G., Seifried, H.E., Swall, L.M., and Sigman, C.C., Strategy and planning for chemopreventive drug development. Clinical development plans: l-Perillyl alcohol, *J. Cell. Biochem.,* 26S:137–148, 1996.

Mills, J.J., Chari, R.S., Boyer, I.J., Gould, M..N. and Jirtle, R.L., Induction of aoptosis in liver tumors by the monoterpene perillyl alcohol, *Cancer Res.,* 55: 979–983, 1995.

Ripple, G.H., Gould, M.N., Arzoomanian, R.Z., Alberti, D., Feierabend, C., Simon, K., Binger, K., Tutsch, K.D., Pomplun, M., Wahamaki, A., Marnocha, R., Wilding, G., and Bailey, H.H., Phase I clinical and pharmacokinetic study of perillyl alcohol administered four times a day, *Clin. Cancer. Res.,* 6:390–396, 2000.

Satomi, Y., Miyamoto, S., and Gould, M.N., Induction of AP-1 activity by perillyl alcohol in breast cancer cells, *Carcinogenesis,* 20:1957–1961, 1999.

Xu, M., Floyd, H.S., Greth, S.M., Chang, W.-C.L., Lohman, K., Stoyanova, R., Kucera, G.L., Kute, T.E., Willingham. M.C., and Miller, M.S., Perillyl alcohol-mediated inhibition of lung cancer cell line proliferation: Potential mechanisms for its chemotherapeutic effects, *Toxicol. Appl. Pharmacol.,* 195:232–246, 2004.

Persimmon   Persimmon (*Diospyros khaki*) is grown in Asia, where the leaves are brewed into a tea for its health benefits, such as homeostasis, diuretic, constipation, and hypotension. These properties reflect the health-promoting effects of flavonoids, such as kaempferol, and the higher total, soluble, and insoluble dietary fibers, total phenols, epicatechin, gallic, and p-coumaric acids, as well as minerals Na, K, Mg, Ca, Fe, and Mn compared to apples (Gorinstein et al., 2001).

In vitro and *in vivo* studies with persimmon and grape extracts by Ahn et al. (2002) showed both were potent antioxidants. Using DPPH, both extracts exhibited similar free-radical-scavenging activities of around 87–88 percent, which was attributed to their high tannin contents. *In vivo* studies with Sprague–Dawley rats resulted in a significant inhibition of lipid peroxidation. However, Figure P.75 shows that the persimmon extract was more effective in lowering hepatic TBARS, secondary oxidation products, than the grape-seed extract. In addition, there was a corresponding reduction in hepatic lipid-peroxide levels accompanied by an increase in catalase and superoxide dismutase (SOD) levels.

References

Ahn, H.S., Jeon, T.I., Lee, J.Y., Hwang, S.G., Lim, Y., and Park, D.K., Antioxidative activity of persimmon and grape seed extract: *In vitro* and *in vivo, Nutr. Res.,* 22:1265–1273, 2002.

Gorinstein, S., Zachwieja, Z., Folta, M., Barton, H., Piotrowicz, J., Zenser, M., Weisz,M., Trahktenbergh, S., and Belloso, O., Comparative content of dietary fibre, total phenolics, and minerals in persimmons and apples, *J. Agic. Food Chem.,* 49:952–957, 2001.

P

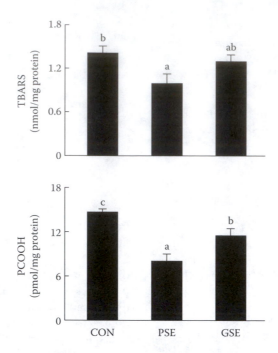

FIGURE P.75 Effects of PSE compared to GSE on the amount of thiobarbituric-acid reactive substances (TBARS; top panel) and phosphatidylcholine hydroperoxide (PCOOH; bottom panel) in the liver of rats. Each bar represents the means ± SEM of five rats. Mean values with different superscripts are significantly different ($p < 0.05$). CON, control; PSE, persimmon seed extract; GSE, grape-seed extract. (From Ahn et al., *Nutr. Res.,* 22:1265–1273, 2002. With permission.)

Phenols *see also* **Flavonoids**   Phenols and polyphenols are ubiquitous in plant foods and, depending on their bioavailability, may play an important role as antioxidants. A number of comprehensive reviews on the health aspects of polyphenols are recommended to the reader (Mahmoud et al., 2000; Zheng and Ramirez, 2000; Parr and Bolwell, 2000; Hollman, 2001). A large variety of plant phenols are synthesized via phenylpropanoid pathways, as shown in Scheme P.43. One of these, the flavonoids, consists of six different classes that account for more than 4,000 different compounds (see Flavonoids). The overall beneficial activities of phenols and polyphenols include their potent antioxidant activity, preventing oxidative damage to DNA, lipids, and proteins associated with prevention of chronic diseases. The inverse association between flavonol intake and cardiovascular disease points to their preventive role in atherosclerosis. The bioavailability of flavonoids in humans is only around 1 percent, and recent work by Lotito and Frei (2004) suggested that the increased plasma antioxidant capacity recorded in humans following apple consumption may not be due to apple-derived flavonoids but to the effect of fructose on urate.

References

Hollman, P.C.H., Evidence for health benefits of plant phenols: Local or systemic effects? *J. Sci. Food Agric.,* 81:842–852, 2001.

Lotito, S.B. and Frei, B., The increase in human plasma antioxidant capacity after apple consumption is due to the metabolic effect of fructose on urate, not apple-derived antioxidant flavonoids, *Free Rad. Biol. Med.,* 37:251–258, 2004.

Mahmoud, N.N., Carothers, A.M., Grunberger, D., Bilinski, R.T., Churchill, M.R., Martucci, C., Newmark, H.L., and Bertagnolli, M.M., Plant phenolics decrease intestinal tumors in an animal model of familial adenomatous polyposis, *Carcinogenesis,* 21: 921–927, 2000.

Parr, A.J. and Bolwell, G.P., Phenols in the plant and in man, the potential for possible nutritional enhance-

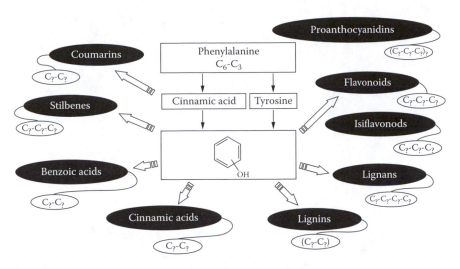

SCHEME P.43 Most plant phenols are synthesized via the phenylpropanoid pathway and share a common building block, the C_6-C_3 unit. (From Hollman, *J. Sci. Food Agric.*, 81:842–852, 2001. With permission.)

ment of the diet by modifying the phenols content or profile, *J. Sci. Food Agric.*, 80:985–1012, 2000.

Zheng, J. and Ramirez, V.D., Inhibition of mitochondrial proton F0F1-ATPase/ATPsynthase by polyphenolic phytochemicals, *Br. J. Pharmacol.*, 130:1115–1123, 2000.

2-Phenylethyl isothiocyanate (PEITC)

2-Phenylethyl isothiocyanate (PEITC) is formed in some *Brassica* species, such as watercress, by the action of myrosinase on its precursor gluconasturtiin (2-phenylethyl glucosinolate) (Scheme P.44). This occurs by chewing or in food preparation. PEITC is recognized as one of the most effective anticancer agents (Huang et al., 1998) by inhibiting phase I enzymes and activating phase II enzymes (Hecht et al., 1999). In addition, *in vitro* and *in vivo* studies showed PEITC had therapeutic value by inducing apoptosis in cells resistant to

chemotherapy due to mutation of p53 (Huang et al., 1998; Xiao and Singh, 2002; Yang et al., 2002). Hu and coworkers (2003) reported induction of apoptosis in human HT-29 colon adenocarcinoma cells by PEITC was both time-dependent and dose-dependent, mediated via the mitochondrial caspase cascade, with activation of the mitogen-activated kinase JNK critical for initiation of the process. Using isolated hepatocyte mitochondria from rat hepatoma HepG2 cells, Rose et al. (2005) showed that decreased cell viability by PEITC was concentration dependent with an IC_{50} of 20 mM (Figure P.76). The inability of pharmacological inhibitors of mitochondrial permeability, cyclosporine A, trifluoperazine, and Bongkrekic acid, to prevent PEITC-induced apoptosis of HepG2 cells suggested the key target was the mitochondria. Apoptosis of HeG2 cells by PEITC appeared to be via the pore-forming ability of proapoptotic Bax.

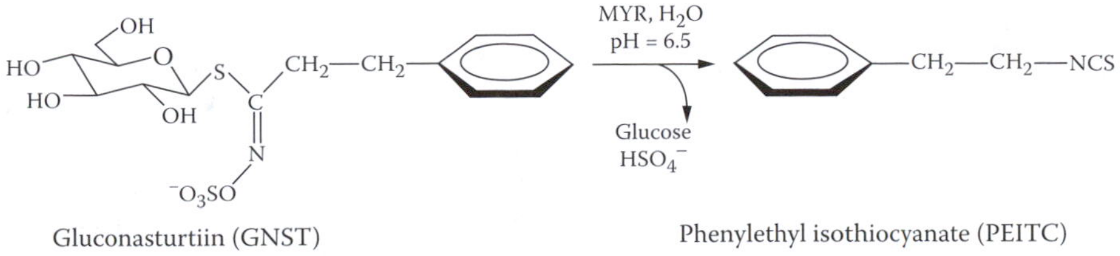

SCHEME P.44 Generation of the phenylethyl isothiocyanate (PEITC) from gluconasturtiin (GNST) by myrosinase (MYR) action. (From Canistro et al., *Mutat. Res.*, 545:23–35, 2004. With permission.)

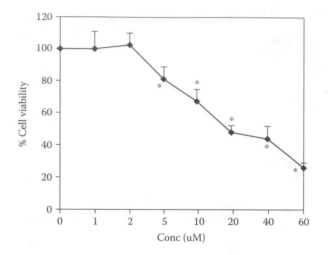

FIGURE P.76 Concentration-dependant effects of PEITC on HepG2 cells as determined at 24 h using the crystal violet viability assay. Data are representative of three separate experiments (means ± SD). (From Rose et al., *Int. J. Biochem. Cell Biol.,* 37:100–119, 2005. With permission.)

References

Canistro, D., Della Croce, C., Iori, R., Barilla, J., Bronzetti, G., Poi, G., Cini, M., Caltavuturo, L., Perocco, P., and Paolini, M., Genetic and metabolic effects of gluconasturtiin, a glucosinolate derived from cruciferae, *Mutat. Res.,* 545:23–35, 2004.

Hecht, S.S., Carmella, S.G., and Murphy, S.E., Effects of watercress consumption in urinary metabolites of nicotine in smokers, *Cancer Epidemiol. Biomark. Prevent.,* 8:907–913, 1999.

Hu, R., Kim, B.R., Chen, C., Hebbar, V., and Kong, A.-N.T., The roles of JNK and apoptotic signaling pathways in PEITC-mediated responses in human HT-29 colon adenocarcinoma cells, *Carcinogenesis,* 24:1361–1367, 2003.

Huang, C., Ma, W.Y., Li, J., Hecht, S.S., and Dong, Z., Essential role of p53 in phenylethyl isothiocyanate-induced apoptosis, *Cancer Res.,* 58:4102–4108, 1998.

Rose, P., Armstrong, J.S., Chua, Y.L., Ong, C.N., and Whiteman, M., β-Phenylethyl isothiocyanate mediated apoptosis: Contribution of Bax and the mitochondrial death pathway, *Int. J. Biochem. Cell Biol.,* 37:100–119, 2005.

Xiao, D. and Singh, S.V., Phenethyl isothiocyanate-induced-apoptosis in p53-deficient PC-3 human prostate cancer cell line is mediated by extracellular signal-regulated kinases, *Cancer Res.,* 62:3615–3619, 2002.

Yang, Y.M., Conaway, C.C., Chiao, J.W., Wang, C.X., Amin, S., Whysner, J., Dai, W., Reinhardt, J., and Chung, F.L., Inhibition of benzo(*a*)pyrene-induced lung tumorigenesis in A/J mice by dietary

N-acetylcysteine conjugates of benzyl and phenylethyl isothiocyanates during the potentiation phase is associated with activation of mitogen-activated protein kinases and p-53 activity and induction of apoptosis, *Cancer Res.,* 62:2–7, 2002.

Pheophytin and Pheophorbide   *see also* **Chlorophyll and Chlorophyllin**   The methanol extracts from eight Japanese edible seaweeds were found to suppress genotoxin-induced *umu* C gene expression in *Salmonella typhimurium*. The edible seaweeds with strong antigenotoxic properties were *Porphyra tenera* and *Enteromorpha prolifera* (Okai et al., 1994). The bioactives identified in *P. tenera* extracts were β-carotene, lutein, and chlorophyll *a* (Okai et al., 1996). Further work by Okai and Higashi-Okai (1997a) showed pheophytin *a*, a degradation product of chlorophyll *a*, was responsible for these suppressor effects. Pheophytin *a* and *b* were also identified as potent as antigenotoxic compounds in the nonpolyphenolic fraction of green tea, capable of suppressing the *umu* C gene (Okai and Higashi-Okai, 1997b). Subsequent work by Higashi-Okai et al. (1998) reported the antitumor suppressors in the nonphenolic fraction from green tea. Using a *Salmonella typhimurium* strain TA100, Chernomorsky and coworkers (1999) found the antimutagenic properties of chlorophyll derivatives, pheophytin, pyropheophytin, and pheophorbide,

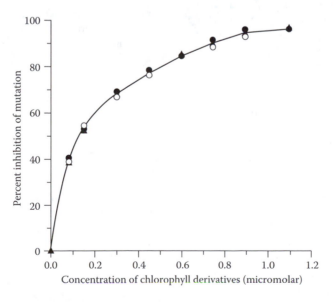

Structure of chlorophyll derivatives. (From Chernomorsky et al., *Teratogenesis Carcinogen. Mutagen.,* 19:313–322, 1999. With permission.)

Pheophytin *a*; $R_1 = CH_3$, $R_2 = C_{20}H_{39}$
Pyropheophytin *a*; $R_1 = H$; $R_2 = C_{20}H_{39}$
Pheophorbide *a*; $R_1 = CH_3$; $R_2 = H$

against the indirect-acting mutagen 3-methylcholanthrene, showed a similar dose–response pattern (Figure P.77). However, in the presence of the direct-acting mutagen, N'-nitro-N'-nitrosoguanidine, derivatives acted quite differently, with the phytol-containing derivatives (pheophytin and pyropheophytin) being far more effective than pheophorbide, which lacked the phytol group. Thus, food sources containing these chlorophyll derivatives may have a role in cancer prevention.

Using yeast cells (*Saccaromyces cerevisiae*), Okai and Higashi-Okai (2001) reported that chlorophyll *a* and pheophytin *a* from green tea were both more effective than chlorophyllin in preventing the endocrine disruptor, p-nonylphenol, from suppressing cell growth and cellular respiration. The antioxidant properties of chlorophyll *a* and pheophytin *a* reported previously by Endo et al. (1985) and Higashi-Okai et al. (2000), could explain, in part, the mechanism involved, as well as their ability to adsorb or bind p-nonylphenol.

References

Chernomorsky, S., Poretz, R., and Segelman, A., Effect of dietary chlorophyll derivatives on mutagenesis and tumor cell growth, *Teratogenesis Carcinogen. Mutagen.,* 7:313–322, 1999.

Endo, Y., Usuki, R., and Kaneda, T., Antioxidant effects of chlorophyll and pheophytin on the autoxidation of oils in the dark, I, Comparison of the inhibitory effects, *J. Am. Oil Chem. Soc.,* 62:1375–1387, 1985.

Higashi-Okai, K., Otani, S., and Okai, Y., Potent suppressor of pheophytin a and b from the non-polyphenolic fraction of green tea (*Camellia sinensis*) against tumor promotion in mouse skin, *Cancer Lett.,* 129:223–228, 1998.

FIGURE P.77 Antimutagenic activity of pheophytin *a* (●), pyropheophytin *a* (▲), and pheophorbide *a* (○) against 3-methylcholanthrene. (From Chernomorsky et al., *Teratogenesis Carcinogen. Mutagen.,* 19:313–322, 1999. With permission.)

Higashi-Okai, K., Taniguchi, M., and Okai, Y., Potent antioxidative activity of non-polyphenolic fraction of green tea (*Camellia sinensis*)-association with pheophytins *a* and *b*, *J. Sci. Food Agric.*, 80:117–120, 2000.

Okai, Y. and Higashi-Okai, K., Pheophytin *a* is a potent suppressor against genotoxin-induced *umu* C gene expression in *Salmonella typhimurium* (TA 1535/pSK 1002), *J. Sci. Food Agric.*, 74:531–535, 1997a.

Okai, Y. and Higashi-Okai, K., Potent suppressing activity of the non-polyphenolic fraction of green tea (*Camellia sinensis*) against genotoxin-induced umu C gene expression in *Salmonella typhymurium* (TA 1535/pSK 1002)-association with pheophytins *a* and *b*, *Cancer Lett.*, 120:117–123, 1997b.

Okai, Y. and Higashi-Okai, K., Protective effects ofchlorophyll a and pheophytin a derived from green tea (*Camellia sinensis*) on p-nonylphenol-induced cell growth inhibition and oxygen radical generation in yeast (*Saccharomyces cerevisiae*), *J. Sci. Food Agric.*, 81:1443–1446, 2001.

Okai, Y., Higashi-Okai, K., Nakamura, S., Yano, T., and Otani, S., Suppressive effects of the extracts of Japanese edible seaweeds on mutagen-induced *umu* C gene expression in *Salmonella typhimurium* (TA 1535/pSK 1002) and tumor promoter-dependent ornithin decarboxylase induction in BALB/c3T3 fibroblast cells, *Cancer Lett.*, 87:25–32, 1994.

Okai, Y., Higashi-Okai, K., Yano, Y., and Otani, S., Identification of antimutagenic substances in an extract of edible red alga, *Porphyra tenera* (Asausanori), *Cancer Lett.*, 100:235–240, 1996.

P

Phloretin *see also* **Phloridzin** Phloretin, a polyphenolic compound found in the root bark of apple trees, is the aglycone of phloridzin. It was recently found to enhance skin permeation of a number of drugs (Valenta et al., 2001; Valenta and Nowak, 2001; Auner et al., 2003a, b). Research by Curtis-Prior et al. (1980) showed that phloretin derivatives were antagonists of prostaglandins, which pointed to their therapeutic potential as anti-inflammatory agents. Auner and Valenta (2004) confirmed the ability of phloretin to increase lidocaine skin permeation. The effect of lidocaine, a local anesthetic used to suppress burning, itching, surgical operations, injections, and dermatological

Phloretin. (From Valenta et al., *Eur. J. Pharmaceut. Biopharmaceut.*, 57:329–336, 2004. With permission.)

diseases, was enhanced 1.39-fold in a hydrophilic formulation and 1.25 and 1.76 in lipophilic formulations.

Valenta and coworkers (2004) studied the mechanism of phloretin and 6-ketocholestanol interaction with the lipid layer which decreased the lipid phase transition temperature of 1,2-dimyristyl-*sn*-3-phosphocholine (DMPC) and 1,2-palmitoyl-*sn*-glycero-3-phosphocholine (DPPC) liposomes, resulting in a higher fluidity of the membrane. Phloretin modified the binding and translocation rates of hydrophobic ions in lipid-vesicle systems, resulting in lowering and raising of the internal dipole potential (Franklin and Cafiso, 1993).

References

Auner, B.G. and Valenta, C., Influence of phloretin on the skin permeation of lidocaine from semisolid preparations, *Eur. J. Pharm. Biopharm.*, 57:307–312, 2004.

Auner, B.G., Valenta, C., and Hadgraft, J., Influence of lipophilic counter-ions in combination with phloretin and 6-ketocholestanol on the skin permeation of 5-aminolevulinic acid, *Int. J. Pharm.*, 255:109–113, 2003a.

Auner, B.G., Valenta, C., and Hadgraft, J., Influence of phloretin and 6-ketocholestanol on the skin permeation of sodium-fluorescein, *J. Control Rel.*, 89: 321–328, 2003b.

Curtis-Prior, P.P., Oblin, A.P., Bennet, A., Parkinson, N.A., and Orloff, A.M., Polyphloretin phosphate (PPP) antagonists of prostaglandin action also inhibits prostaglandin biosynthesis *in vitro*, *J. Pharm. Pharmacol.*, 42:660–662, 1990.

Franklin, J.C. and Cafisco, D.S., Internal electrostatic potentials in bilayers: Measuring and controlling dipole potentials in lipid vesicles, *Biophys. J.,* 65: 289–299, 1993.

Valenta, C., Cladera, J., O'Shea, P., and Hadgraft, J., Effect of phloretin on the percutaneous absorption of lignocaine across human skin, *J. Pharm. Sci.,* 90: 485–492, 2001.

Valenta, C., Nowak, M., and Hadgraft, J., Influence of phloretin and 6-ketocholestanol on the permeation of progesterone through porcine skin, *Int. J. Pharm.,* 217:79–86, 2001.

Valenta, C., Steininger, A., and Auner, B.G., Phloretin and 6-ketocholestanol: Membrane interactions studied by a phospholipid/polydiacetylene colorimetric assay and differential scanning calorimetry, *Eur. J. Pharmaceut. Biopharmaceut.,* 57:329–336, 2004.

Phloridzin *see also* Apples and Phloretin

Phloridzin, a polyphenol found in apples, has been used to inhibit the intestinal Na+/glucose transporter (SGLT1) (Hirayama et al., 1998). Mizuma and Awazu (1998) reported phloridzin was metabolized to its aglycone, phloretin, with both inhibiting glucuronidation of p-nitrophenol, acetaminophen, and 1-naphthol in rats. Inhibition of glucuronidation metabolism improves the intestinal absorption of those drugs susceptible to glucuronidation. A recent study by Andlauer and coworkers (2004) found phloridzin amplified the absorption of the isoflavone, genistin, 2.5-fold. Isoflavones are generally poorly absorbed so that a high intake is normally required to ensure their chemoprevention effects. A combination of nutraceuticals, such as genistin, with functional phloridzin-

Phloridzin. (From Valenta et al., *Eur. J. Pharmaceut. Biopharmaceut.,* 57:329–336, 2004.)

containing foods provides a novel way of enhancing genistin absorption and increasing its efficacy in cancer prevention.

The antioxidant and radical-scavenging activities of polyphenols, including phloridzin and 3-hydroxy-phloridzin, was reported in apple pomace, the waste product produced in the processing of apple juice. The health-protecting properties of apples may be attributed to these compounds, as Hertog and coworkers (1993) provided data that suggested that men who ate 110 g of apple or day had a 49 percent lower risk factor for heart attack compared to those eating much less (18 g).

References

Andlauer, W., Kolb, J., and Furst, P., Phloridzin improves absorption of genistin in isolated rat small intestine, *Clin. Nutr.,* 23:989–995, 2004.

Hertog, M.G.L., Feskens, E.J.M., Kromhout, D., Hollman, P.C.H., Hertog, M.G.L., and Katan, M.B., Dietary antioxidant flavonids and risk of coronary heart disease: The Zutphen elderly study, *Lancet,* 342:1007–1012, 1993.

Hirayama, B.A., Lostao, M.P., Panayotova-Heiermann, M., Loo, D.D.F., Turk, E., and Wright, E.M., Kinetic and specificity differences between rat, human, and rabbit Na_1-glucose co-transporters (SGLT-1), *Am. J. Physiol.,* 270:G919–926, 1998.

Mizuma, T. and Awazu, S., Inhibitory effect of phloridzin and phloretin on glucuronidation of p-nitrophenol, acetaminophen and 1-napthol: Kinetic administration of the influence of glucuronidation metabolism on intestinal absorption in rats, *Biochem. Biophys. Acta,* 1425:398–404, 1998.

Valenta, C., Steininger, A., and Auner, B.G., Phloretin and 6-ketocholestanol: Membrane interactions studied by a phospholipid/polydiacetylene colorimetric assay and differential scanning calorimetry, *Eur. J. Pharmaceut. Biopharmaceut.,* 57:329–336, 2004.

Phosphatides *see also* Phosphatidylcholine and Phosphatidylserine

These include numerous lipids in which phosphoric acid, as well as fatty acids, are esterified to glycerol and are found in all living cells and in bilayers of plasma membranes. Phospholipids have been associated with a number of health benefits. A glycerol-free phospholipid analogue, hexade-cyl-phosphocholine (HePC), was shown by Wieder et al. (1996) to exhibit antitumor prop-erties using cultured human breast fibroblasts. The antitumor activity appeared to be related to activation of cellular phospholipase D.

References

Wieder, T., Zu-Chuan, Z., Geilen, C.C., Orfanosa, C.E., Giulianob, A.E., and Cabot, M.C., The antitu-mor phospholipid analog, hexadecylphosphocholine, activates cellular phospholipase D, *Cancer Lett.,* 100:71–79, 1996.

Phosphatidylcholine   Phosphatidylcholine (PC), or lecithin, constitutes a major portion of cellular phospholipids and displays unique molecular species in different cell types and tissues. PC is also the major delivery form of the essential nutrient choline and is involved in the hepatic form, which is involved in the hepatic export of very-low-density lipoproteins. The main roles of PC are the flow of informa-tion within cells from DNA to RNA to proteins and the formation of cellular energy and intra-cellular communication or signal transduction. PC also has a marked fluidizing effect on cel-lular membranes. Decreased cell-membrane fluidization and breakdown of cell-membrane integrity, as well as impairment of cell-mem-brane repair mechanisms, are associated with a number of disorders, including liver disease, neurological diseases, various cancers, and cell death.

Many agents that perturb PC homeostasis also induce cell death, but the signaling path-ways that mediate this cell death have not been well defined (Cui and Houweling, 2002). PC is absorbed into the mucosal cells of the small intestine, mainly in the duodenum and upper jejenum, following some digestion by the pan-creatic enzyme phospholipase, producing lyso-phosphatidylcholine, which is transported by the lymphatics in the form of chylomicrons to the blood. PC is transported in the blood in various lipoprotein particles, including very-low-density lipoproteins (VLDL), low-density lipoproteins (LDL), and high-density lipopro-teins (HDL), and is then distributed to various tissues in the body. Some PC is incorporated into cell membranes and some is metabolized to choline, fatty acids, and glycerol.

PC may have a beneficial effect by restoring liver function in a number of disorders (Hatashi et al., 1999), including alcoholic fibrosis and possibly viral hepatitis (Canty and Zeisel, 1994). Dietary lecithin (a complex mixture of phospholipids and other lipids) has been used in emergencies and in the treatment of atheroma plaques in cardiac diseases. It promotes a return to normal of the plasma lipoprotein-distribution profile and the removal of lipid from established atherosclerotic plaques in Dutch-Belted rabbits (Hunt and Duncan, 1985). Recently, PC was used to treat localized fat deposits, such as lower eyelid fat pads (Hexsel et al., 2003; Ablon and Rotunda, 2004).

Some studies found PC had a positive effect on memory (Ladd et al., 1993; Chung et al., 1995). Masuda and coworkers (1998) found egg PC, together with vitamin B_{12}, improved mem-ory impairment of rats with nucleus basalis Magnocellularis (NBM) lesions. PC has also been used to treat manic conditions (Cohen et al., 1982) and in some tardive dyskinesia (Gelenberg et al., 1989). PC has even been eval-uated in Parkinson's disease (Tweedy and Gar-cia, 1982). Cytidine 5′-diphosphocholine, an essential intermediate in the biosynthetic path-way of PC, was reported to be effective as cotherapy for Parkinson's disease (Secades and Frontera, 1995) and was recently shown to have a positive effect on memory, with demonstrated hippocampal morphology resembling that of younger animals (Crespo et al., 2004). There is some inconclusive evidence that PC may be useful in managing Alzheimer's disease and some cognitive disorders (Higgins and Flicker, 2003; McDaniel et al., 2003).

A possible future role for PC suggested by Gallo et al. (2003) is in cancer therapy. A com-plex of silybin/phosphatidylcholine (IdB 1016) appeared to have clinical potential in the man-agement of recurrent ovarian cancer.

References

Ablon, G., and Rotunda, A.M., Treatment of lower eyelid fat pads using phosphatidylcholine: Clinical trials and review, *Dermatol. Surg.,* 30:422–427, 2004.

P

Canty, D.J. and Zeisl, S.H., Lecithin and choline in human health and disease, *Nutr. Rev.,* 52:327–339, 1994.

Chung, S.Y., Moriyama, T., Uezu, E., Uezu, K., Hirata, R., Yohena, N., Masuda, Y., Kokubu, T., and Yamamoto, S., Administration of phosphatidylcholine increases brain acetylcholine concentration and improves memory in mice with dementia, *J. Nutr.,* 125:1484–1489, 1995.

Cohen, B.M., Lipinski, J.F., and Altesman, R.I., Lecithin in the treatment of mania: Double-blind, placebo-controlled trials, *Am. J. Psychiatry,* 139:1162–1164, 1982.

Crespo, D., Megias, M., Fernandez-Viadero, C., and Verguda, R., Chronic treatment with a precursor of cellular phosphatidylcholine ameliorates morphological and behavioral effects of aging in the rat hippocampus, *Ann. N.Y. Acad. Sci.,* 1019:41–43, 2004.

Cui, Z. and Houweling, M., Phosphatidylcholine and cell death, *Biochem. Biophys. Acta,* 1585:87–96, 2002.

Gallo, D., Giacomelli, S., Ferlini, C., Raspaglio, G., Apollonio, P., Prislei, S., Riva, A., Morazzoni, P., Bombardelli, E., and Scambia, G., Antitumor activity of the silybin-phosphatidylcholine complex, IdB 1016, against human ovarian cancer, *Eur. J. Cancer,* 39:2403–2410, 2003.

Gelenberg, A.J., Wojcik, J., Falk, W.E., Bellinghausen, B., and Joseph, A.B., CDP-choline for the treatment of tardive dyskenisia: A small negative series, *Compr. Psych.,* 30:1–4, 1989.

Hayashi, H., Tanaka, Y., Hibino, H., Umeda, Y., Kawamitsu, H., Fujimoto, H., and Amakawa, T., Beneficial effect of salmon roe phosphatidylcholine in chronic liver disease, *Curr. Med. Res. Opin.,* 15: 177–184, 1999.

Hexsel, D., Serra, M., Mazzuco, R., Dal'Forno, T., and Zechmeister, D., Phosphatidylcholine in the treatment of localized fat, *J. Drugs Dermatol.,* 2: 511–518, 2003.

Higgins, J.P. and Flicker, L., Lecithin for dementia and cognitive impairment, *The Cochrane Database Syst. Rev.,* 3:CD001015, 2003.

Hunt, C.E. and Duncan, L.A., Hyperlipoproteinaemia and atherosclerosis in rabbits fed low-level cholesterol and lecithin, *Br., J. Exp. Pathol.,* 66:35–46, 1985.

Ladd, S.L., Sommer, S.A., LaBerge, S., and Toscano, W., Effect of phosphatidylcholine on explicit memory, *Clin. Neuropharmacol.,* 16:540–549, 1993.

Masuda, Y., Kokubu, T., Yamashita, M., Ikeda, H., and Inoue, S., EFF phosphatidylcholine combined with vitamin B12 improved memory impairment following lesioning of nucleus basalis in rats, *Life Sci.,* 62:813–822, 1998.

McDaniel, M.A., Maier, S.F., and Einstein, G.O., Brain-specific nutrients: A memory cure? *Nutrition,* 19:957–975, 2003.

Secades, J.J. and Frontera, G., CDP-choline: Pharmacological and clinical review, *Methods Find Exp. Clin. Pharmacol.,* 17(Suppl. B):1–54, 1995.

Tweedy, J.R. and Garcia, C.A., Lecithin treatment of cognitively impaired Parkinson's patients, *Eur. J. Clin. Invest.,* 12:87–90, 1982.

Phosphatidylserine Phosphatidylserine (PS), a natural component of the brain cortex, is the major phospholipid in the outer surface of brain-synaptic membranes. It plays an important role in signal transduction, secretory-vesicle release, and cell-to-cell communication (Nishizuka, 1984; Blokland et al., 1999). PS may be the signal by which apoptotic cells are recognized and phagocytosed (Brauer, 2003). Studies with geriatric patients suffering from Alzheimer's or Parkinson's disease or arteriosclerotic encephalopathy suggested that prolonged treatment with PS particularly improved attention, memory, withdrawal and apathy, sleep disturbances, and mood (Maggioni et al., 1990). A significant improvement in depressive symptomatology in patients with major depressive disorders was found in subsequent studies, also with PS administration compared to controls (Brambilla et al., 1996; Brambilla and Maggioni, 1998). Crook et al. (1991) treated patients with age-associated memory impairment with a daily dose of PS (100 mg/day tid) over 12 weeks and found improved performance tests related to learning and memory tasks of daily life compared to those receiving the placebo. Castilho et al. (2004) found PS exerted an antidepressive effect in rats using the forced swimming test but did not act as a cognitive enhancer, as it was ineffective in the water-maze test.

References

Blokland, A., Honig, W., Brouns, F., and Jolles, J., Cognition-enhancing properties of subchronic phosphatidylserine (PS) treatment in middle-aged rats: Comparison of bovine cortex PS with egg PS and soybean PS, *Nutrition,* 15:778–783, 1999.

Brambilla, F. and Maggioni, M., Blood levels of cytokines in elderly patients with major depressive disorders, *Acta Psychiatr. Scand.,* 97:309–313, 1998.

Brambilla, F., Maggioni, M., Panerai, A.E., Sacerdote, P., and Cenacchi, T., Beta-endorphin concentration in peripheral blood mononuclear cells of elderly depressed patients — effects of phosphatidylserine therapy, *Neuropsychobiology,* 34:18–21, 1996.

Brauer, M., *In vivo* monitoring of apoptosis, *Prog. Neuro-Psychopharmacol. Biol. Psychiatry,* 27:323–33, 2003.

Castilho, J.C., Perry, J.C., Andreatini, R., and Vital, M.A.B.F., Phosphatidylserine: An antidepressive or a cognitive enhancer? *Prog. Neuro-Psychopharmacol. Biol. Psychiatry,* 28:731–738, 2004.

Crook, T.H., Tinklelberg, J., Yesavage, J., Petrie, W., Nunzi, M.G., and Massari, D.C., Effects of phosphatidylserine in aged-associated memory impairment, *Neurology,* 41:644-649, 1991.

Maggioni, M., Picotti, G.B., Bondiolotti, G.P., Panerai, A., Cenacchi, T., Nobile, P., and Brambilla, F., Effects of phosphatidylserine therapy in geriatric patients with depressive disorders, *Acta Psychiatr. Scand.,* 81:265–270, 1990.

Nishizuka, Y., Turnover of inositiol phospholipids and signal transduction, *Science,* 225:1365–1370, 1984.

Phospholipids *see* **Phosphatides, Phosphatidyl choline, and Phosphatidylserine**

Phosvitin Phosvitin, a phosphoprotein known as an iron-carrier in egg yolk, binds almost all of the yolk iron. The formation of phosvitin-Fe complex promotes the precipitation of Fe in the small-intestinal tract, which may be responsible for the poor iron availability of egg and egg yolk (Sato et al., 1984). Ishakawa et al. (2004) reported that phosvitin acts as a natural antioxidant by chelating iron ions. It accelerates Fe(II) autoxidation and thus decreases the availability of Fe(III) for participation in the OH-generating Fenton reaction. These results provide insight into the mechanism of protection of the developing embryo against iron-dependent oxidative damage. Phosvitin was found to be more effective in cooked ground pork compared with uncooked, salted ground pork (Lee et al., 2002). Kobayashi et al. (2004) demonstrated that the role of phosvitin in bone formation was to enhance nucleation of hydroxyapatite crystals on collagen in the same way as that observed in human bone.

References

Ishikawa, S., Yano, Y., Arihara, K., and Itoh, M., Egg yolk phosvitin inhibits hydroxyl radical formation from the Fenton reaction, *Biosci. Biotechnol. Biochem.,* 68:1324–1331, 2004.

Kobayashi, N., Onuma, K., Oyane, A., and Yamazaki, A., The role of phosvitin for nucleation of calcium phosphates on collagen, *Key Eng. Materials,* 254–256:537–540, 2004.

Lee, S.K., Han, J.H., and Decker, E.A., Antioxidant activity of phosvitin in phosphatidylcholine liposomes and meat model, *J. Food Sci.,* 67:37–41, 2002.

Sato, R., Lee, Y.S., Noguchi, T., and Naito, H., Iron solubility in the small intestine of rats fed egg yolk protein, *Nutr. Rep. Intern.,* 30:1319–1326, 1984.

Phyllanthus Plants of the genus *Phyllanthus* (family Euphorbiaceae) are found in most tropical and subtropical countries. They have been used in folk medicine to treat kidney and urinary-bladder disturbances, intestinal infections, diabetes, and hepatitis B. Studies conducted on extracts and purified compounds from these plants by Calixto and coworkers (1998) confirmed their

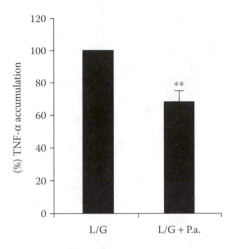

FIGURE P.78 *In vivo* inhibition of TNF-α production by *P. amarus* extract (P.a.). Male BalbA2 mice received either 45 mg/kg *Phyllanthus* extract or saline/DMSO i.p. 30 min later, mice were injected with 500 mg/kg galactosamine i.p., and immediately afterwards with 1.5 mg/kg of LPS(L/G). After 90 min, a serum sample was obtained by tail bleeding and murine TNF-α was determined by ELISA. Three independent experiments were carried out with four animals each. TNF-α level of the respective control group was normalized to 100 percent. Data are expressed as means ± SEM. **$p < 0.01$ represents statistical differences from animals treated with LPS/galactosamine only. (From Kiemer et al., *J. Hepatol.*, 38:289–297, 2003. With permission.)

efficacy as an antiviral, as well as in the treatment of genitourinary disorders, and as antinociceptive agents. They also found that *Phyllanthus* had potential therapeutic benefits in the management of hepatitis *B. nefrolitase* and in painful disorders. The leaves of *Phyllanthus* were shown earlier by Ihantola-Vormisto et al. (1997) to exert inhibitory activity on human polymorphonuclear leukocytes and antipyretic and platelets, which confirmed their anti-inflammatory and antipyretic properties for use in traditional medicine. The anti-inflammatory properties of standardized *Phyllanthus* extracts were demonstrated by Kiemer and coworkers (2003) by their ability to inhibit induction of endoxin-unduced nitric-oxide synthase (iNOS), cyclooxygenase (COX-2), and TNF-α production in rat Kuppfer cells, in RAW264.7 macrophages, and in human whole blood. The significant inhibition of TNF-α in Male BalbA2 mice in the presence of the *Phyllanthis* extract is shown in Figure P.78.

Huang et al. (2004) recently demonstrated the anticancer properties of *Phyllanthus urinaria* on human myeloid leukemia (HL-60) cells, which appeared to be mediated via a ceramide-related pathway. An increase in the inhibition of HIV-1 reverse transcriptase was reported by Wagner and Notka (2002) to be linear, with increasing concentrations of gallo-tannins extracted from *Phyllanthus*, suggesting its potential for preventing and treating retrovirus-related diseases, such as human immunodeficiency virus (HIV).

References

Calixto, J.B., Santo, A.R.S., Filho, C.V., and Yunes, R.F., A review of the plants from the genus *Phyllanthus*: Their chemistry, pharmacology, and therapeutic potential, *Med. Res. Rev.*, 18:225–258, 1998.

Huang, S-T., Yang, R.-C., Chen, M.-Y., and Pang, J.-H. S., *Phyllanthus urinaria* induces the Fas receptor/ligand expression and ceramide-mediated apoptosis in HL-60 cells, *Life Sci.*, 75:339–351, 2004.

Ihantola-Vormusto, A., Summanen, J., Kankaanranta, H., Vuorela, H., Asmawi, Z.M., and Moilanen, E., Anti-inflammatory activity of extracts from leaves of Phyllanthus emblica, *Planta Med.*, 63:518–524, 1997.

Kiemer, A.K., Hartung, T., Huber, C., and Vollmar, A.M., *Phyllanthis amarus* has anti-inflammatory potential by inhibition of iNOS, COX-2, and cytokines via the NF-κB pathway, *J. Hepatol.*, 38:289–297, 2003.

Wagner, R. and Notka, F., *Phyllanthus*-derived compounds for the prevention and/or treatment of diseases associated with a retrovirus, *PCT Int. Appl.*, 35 p., 2002.

Phytic acid   Phytic acid (*myo*-inositol hexaphosphate, IP$_6$) is the major storage form of phosphorus and accounts for 1–5 percent by weight of edible legumes, cereals, and oilseeds (Graf and Eaton, 1995). Historically, phytic acid was considered to be an antinutrient because of its ability to bind divalent cations,

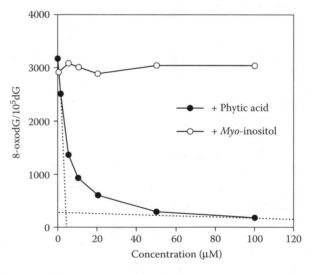

Pi=OPO$_3$H$_2$

Structure of phytic acid. (From Chen and Li, *J. Chromatogr. A.,* 1018:41–52, 2003. With permission.)

such as calcium, magnesium, zinc, and iron, reducing their bioavailability (Reddy et al., 1989). However, it has since been recognized as an antioxidant because of its potent inhibi-

tion of iron-catalyzed hydroxyl-radical formation (Rimbach and Pallauf, 1998). In addition, phytic acid has also been shown to have anticarcinogenic (Shamsuddin et al., 1996), as well as hypoglycemic and hypolipidemic, (Rickard and Thompson, 1997) properties.

Obata (2003) examined the effect of phytic acid on the neurotoxin 1-methyl-4-phenylpyridinium (MPP$^+$), a potent Parkinson-causing reagent formed in the brain from 1-methyl-4-phenyl-1,2,3,6-tetrahydropyridine (MPTP). Phytic acid suppressed the ability of this neurotoxin to induce hydroxyl-radical generation by chelating the required iron, suggesting its clinical potential as an antioxidant.

Phytic acid was shown earlier by Midorikawa et al. (2001) to prevent the formation of reactive-oxygen species, such as 8-oxodG, in cultured cells treated with an H$_2$O$_2$-generating system. The dramatic reduction in the formation of oxidative DNA damage in the presence of phytic acid is evident from Figure P.79 compared to the inability of *myo*-inositol

FIGURE P.79 Formation of 8-oxodG in calf thymus DNA induced by H$_2$O$_2$ and Cu(II) in the presence of phytic acid or *myo*-inositol. Calf thymus DNA fragments (100 μM/base) were incubated with 20 μM CuCl$_2$, 100 μM H$_2$O$_2$, and indicated concentrations of phytic acid (closed circles) or *myo*-inositol (open circles) at 37°C for 15 min. After ethanol precipitation, the DNA was digested into nucleosides with nuclease P1 and calf-intestine phosphatase and analyzed with an HPLC-ECD system. Intersection of dotted lines showed the concentration of phytic acid to inhibit 8-oxodG formation. (From Midorikawa et al., *Biochem. Biophys. Res. Commun.,* 288:552–557, 2001. With permission.)

to inhibit 8-oxodG formation. The antioxidant properties of phytic acid were due to its ability to chelate transition metal ions. The possible role of phytic acid in cancer prevention was further confirmed by Muraoka and Miura (2004), who showed that phytic acid, and not *myo*-inositol, inhibited xanthine oxidase, the enzymatic source of superoxide (O_2^-). In addition, phytic acid also prevented the formation of ADP-iron-oxygen complexes. The potential of phytic acid to prevent the formation of oxygen radicals in the intestine could prevent the development of chronic diseases, such as cancer.

A systematic review of phytic acid as a novel broad-spectrum, antineoplastic agent by Fox and Eberl (2002) suggested its role in cancer prevention warranted phase I and phase II human clinical trials.

References

Chen, Q.-C. and Li, B.W., Separation of phytic acid and other related inositol phosphates by high-performance ion chromatography and its applications, *J. Chromatogr. A.*, 1018:41–52, 2003.

Fox, C.H. and Eberl, M., Phytic acid (IP6), a novel broad spectrum anti-neoplastic agent: A systematic review, *Comp. Ther. Med.*, 10:229–234, 2002.

Graf, E. and Eaton, J.W., Antioxidant function of phytic acid, *Free Rad. Biol. Med.*, 8:61–69, 1990.

Midorikawa, K., Murata, M., Oikawa, S., Hiraku, Y., and Kawanishi, S., Protective effect of phytic acid on oxidative DNA damage with reference to cancer chemoprevention, *Biochem. Biophys. Res. Commun.*, 288:552–557, 2001.

Muraoka, S. and Miura, M., Inhibition of xanthine oxidase by phytic acid and its antioxidative action, *Life Sci.*, 74:1691–1700, 2004.

Obata, T., Phytic acid suppresses 1-methyl-4-phenylpyridinium ion-induced hydroxyl radical generation in rat striatum, *Brain Res.*, 978:241–244, 2003.

Reddy, N.R., Pierson, M.D., Sathe, S.K., and Salunkhe, D.K., *Phytates in Cereals and Legumes*, CRC Press, Boca Raton, Florida, 1989, p. 152.

Rickard, S.E. and Thompson, L.U., Interactions and biological effects of phytic acid, in *Antinutrients and Phytochemicals in Food*, ACS symposium series No. 662, Shahidi, F., Ed., American Chemical Society, Washington, D.C., 1997, pp. 294–312.

Rimbach, G. and Pallauf, J., Phytic acid inhibits free radical formation *in vitro* but does not affect liver oxidant or antioxidant status in growing rats, *J. Nutr.*, 128:1950–1955, 1998.

Shamsuddin, A.M., Yang, G.Y., and Vucenik, I., Novel anti-cancer functions of IP6: growth inhibition and differentiation of human mammary cancer cell lines *in vitro*, *Carcinogenesis*, 16:3287–3292, 1996.

Phytoestrogens *see also* **Genistein, Daidzein, and Matairesinol**   Phytoestrogens are a group of plant compounds that exert both estrogenic and antiestrogenic properties. The four separate plant families of phenolic compounds recognized as phytoestrogens are isoflavonoids, stilbenes, lignans, and coumestans (Scheme P.45). The richest plant sources are isoflavones in soybeans and lignans in flaxseed products (Tham et al., 1998). The anticancer properties of both isoflavonoids and lignans are thought to be responsible for the low incidence of prostate cancers by influencing both endocrine and growth-factor signaling pathways. Phytoestrogens from soybean, genistein and daidzein, were both found by Karamsetty and coworkers (2001) to restore the impaired-relaxation response to nitric-oxide release in pulmonary arteries isolated from chronically hypoxic rats. The latter condition is associated with pulmonary hypertension. For an excellent review of this subject, the article by Cornwell and coworkers (2004) is recommended.

References

Cornwell, T., Cohick, W., and Raskin, I., Dietary phytoesterogens and health, *Phytochemistry*, 65:995–1016, 2004.

Karamsetty, M.R., Klinger, J.R., and Hill, N.S., Phytoestrogens restore nitric oxide-mediated relaxation in isolated pulmonary arteries from chronically hypoxic rats, *Pharmacol. Exp. Ther.*, 297:968–974, 2001.

Tham, D.M., Gardner, C.D. and Haskell, W.L., Potential health benefits of dietary phytoestrogens: A review of the clinical, epidemiological, and mechanistic evidence. *J. Clin. Endocrinol. Metab.*, 83:2223–2235, 1998.

P

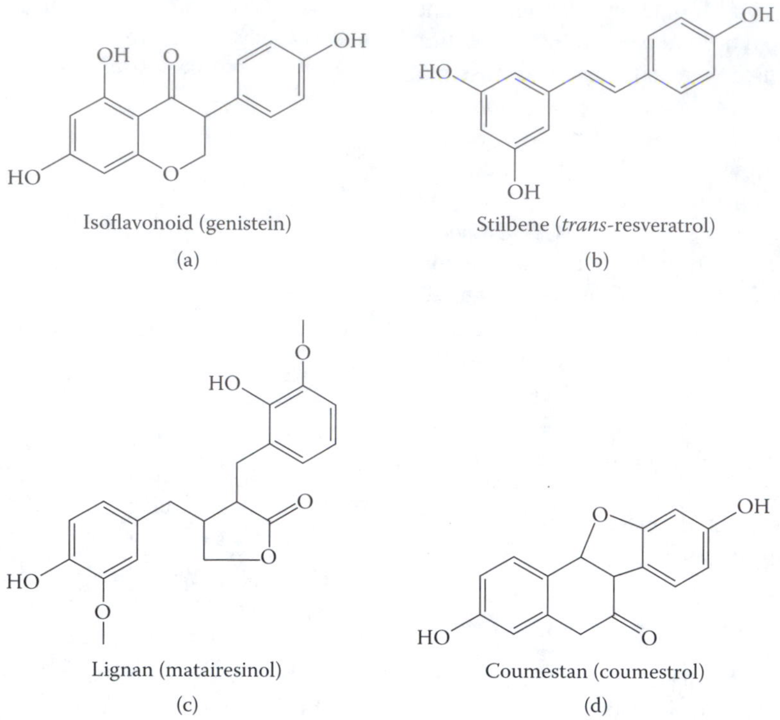

Isoflavonoid (genistein)

(a)

Stilbene (*trans*-resveratrol)

(b)

Lignan (matairesinol)

(c)

Coumestan (coumestrol)

(d)

SCHEME P.45 Structure of phytoestrogens, genistein, coumestrol, trans-resveratrol, and matairesinol. (From Cornwell et al., *Phytochemistry,* 65:995–1016, 2004. With permission.)

Phytohemagglutinins *see also* **Lectins**

Phytohemagglutinins (PHA), or lectins, are proteins that bring about the agglutination of red blood cells. They are heat-labile and readily destroyed during normal food processing. Previous studies showed that a diet containing lectin a phytohemagglutinins from raw kidney bean markedly diminished the growth of Krebs II non-Hodgkin lymphoma (NHL) tumors in NMRI mice (Pryme et al., 1994, 1996, 1998). The reduced rate of growth was dose-dependent within the range of 0.45–3.5 mg/g of PHA in the diet (Pryme et al., 1996). Pryme and coworkers (1999) allowed the NMRI mice to develop non-Hodgkin lymphoma tumors for five days prior to feeding different levels of PHA to determine whether feeding the raw kidney lectin was also effective in reducing tumor growth. These researchers found that including PHA in the diet five days after injecting NHL tumors still reduced the progression of tumor development. This work suggested that further reduction in tumor proliferation might be achieved through manipulation of the diet with PHA and reduced protein.

References

Pryme, I.F., Bardocz, S., Grant, G., Pusztai, A., and Pfuller, A., The plant lectins PHA and ML-1 suppress the growth of a lymphosarcoma tumor in mice, in *Effects of Antinutrients on the Nutritional Value of Legume Diets,* Cost 98 vol. 5, Bardocz, S., Pfuller, U., and Pusztai, A., Eds., EC Publications, Luxemberg, 1998, pp. 86–90.

Pryme, I.F., Pusztai, A., and Bardocz, S., A diet containing the lectin phytohaemagglutinin (PHA) slows down the proliferation of Krebs II cell tumors in mice, *Cancer Lett.,* 76:133–137, 1994.

Pryme, I.F., Bardocz, S., Pusztai, A., and Ewen, S.W.B., The growth of an established murine non-Hodgkin lymphoma tumor is limited by switching to a phytohaemagglutinin-containing diet, *Cancer Lett.,* 146:87–91, 1999.

Pryme, I.F., Pusztai, A., and Bardocz, S., Phyto-hemagglutinin-induced gut hyperplasia and the growth of a mouse lymphosarcoma, *J. Exp. Ther. Oncol.,* 1:171–176, 1996.

Phytosterols Phytosterols are plant sterols differing very slightly in structure from cholesterol by the presence of an ethyl or methyl group at C-24 in the side chain (Scheme P.46). There are more than 100 different phytosterols, but the major ones are β-sitosterol, campesterol, and stigmasterol. Phytosterols stabilize the phospholipid bilayers in plant-cell membranes, as cholesterol does in animal-cell membranes. The fully saturated form of phytosterols (containing no double bond at the 5,6 position) are the phytostanols, which are present in only trace amounts but can also be formed by hydrogenation of phytosterols. On average, we consume approximately 250 mg per day of phytosterols from vegetable oils, cereals, fruits, and vegetables (Hicks and Moreau, 2001; Conner, 1968). In comparison, we consume around 25 mg per day of phytostanols (Conner, 1968; Cerqueira et al., 1979). The ability of phytosterols to lower cholesterol has been well documented (Pollak and Kritchevsky, 1981; Ling and Jones, 1995; Jones et al., 1997; Moghadasian and Frolich, 1999; Law, 2000). In fact, sitosterol was marketed as a drug for lowering cholesterol during the 1950s, but its poor solubility and bioavailability, plus the introduction of "statin" drugs, rapidly diminished its use. Scientists in Finland, however, improved the solubility of phytosterols by esterification which resulted in the first commercial production of phytosterol-containing margarines (Miettinen et al., 1996). Research subsequently showed that 2–3 g/day of phytostanyl ester-containing margarine consistently reduced LDL-cholesterol levels.

Clinical studies on the cholesterol-lowering properties of esterified phytosterols have shown they consistently lower serum LDL cholesterol. Miettingen et al. (1995) showed that consumption of around 23 g/day of a fat spread enriched with 10 percent hydrogenated sterols lowered LDL-cholesterol levels by 10–14 percent. A randomized, double-blind, placebo-controlled crossover study by Neil et al. (2003) showed patients with heterozygous familial hypercholesterolemia fed a vegetable-oil enriched fat spread reduced LDL cholesterol by 10–15 percent. Mussner and coworkers (2002) found that patients with mild to moderate hypercholesterolemia all had reduced LDL-cholesterol levels

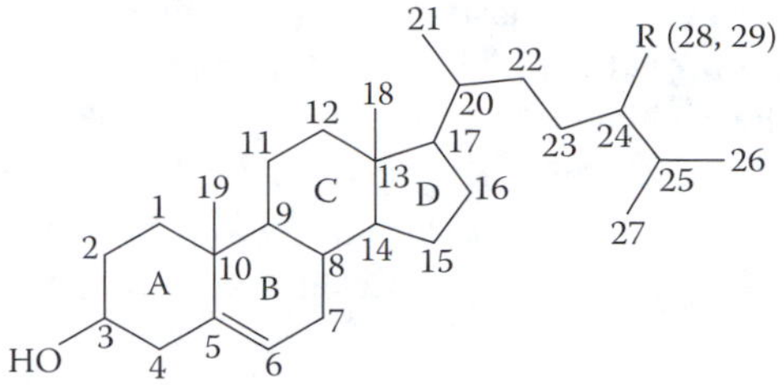

SCHEME P.46 Structure of cholesterol and phytosterols. (From Lea et al., *Food Chem. Toxicol.*, 42: 771–783, 2004. With permission.)

when fed a 1.83-g/day dosage of phytosterol esters. The most marked reduction in LDL-cholesterol levels, however, were observed in subjects with a high intake of cholesterol, energy, total fat, and saturated fat and with a high baseline absorption of cholesterol. Bourque and coworkers (2003) showed a combination of dietary ingredients (medium-chain triacylglycerols, phytosterols, and w-3 fatty acids), referred to as a functional oil, significantly lowers total plasma cholesterol and LDL-cholesterol levels in overweight women by 9.1 percent and 16.0 percent, respectively, compared to a beef-tallow-based diet.

The main mechanism responsible for the ability of free and esterified phytosterols to lower cholesterol is inhibition of cholesterol absorption (Trautwein et al., 2003). A recent survey of 9581 participants in Finland by De Jong et al. (2004) showed that of the 31 percent with high cholesterol, 19 percent used cholesterol-lowering drugs, 11 percent used phytosterol-containing spreads, while 5 percent used a combination of both therapies.

Several epidemiological and animal studies indicated that phytosterols may suppress the growth of colonic tumors (Carbin et al., 1990). A randomized, placebo-controlled, double-blind study of 53 men found phytosterols alleviated the symptoms of prostate cancer over a three-month period (Carbin, et al. 1990). A multicentric, placebo-controlled, double-blind clinical trial involving 177 patients showed β-sitosterol as an effective option for treating benign prostatic hyperplasia. Several mechanisms were proposed based on animal-model studies in which phytosterols suppressed the metabolism and growth of the prostate by inhibiting prostatic 5α-reductase and aromatase activities (Mettlin, 1997; Awad et al., 1998). Inhibition of tumor growth was also explained by the effect of phytosterols on sphingosine metabolism in the membrane, increasing ceramide production with possible alteration of the signal-transduction pathways (Hannun and Linardic, 1993; Wollf et al., 1994). A systematic review of papers published between 1968 and 1998 on the efficacy of β-sitosterol for treating benign prostatic hyperplasia in men by Wilt et al. (1999) showed improvements in urological systems and flow measures. However, these studies were all of short duration, pointing to the need for more long-term studies to assess the efficacy and safety of β-sisterol treatment.

Possible adverse effects of high concentrations of phytosterols could result in cell fragility, particularly in patients suffering from phytosterolemia, a rare genetic disorder with very high concentrations of plasma sitosterols (Patel et al., 2004; Wang et al., 1981). Phytosterols, however, were given generally regarded as safe (GRAS) status in the U.S.A. with the Food and Drug Administration approving fat spreads containing up to 20 percent of either steryl or stanyl esters. For a more detailed discussion of phytosterols, reviews by Moghadasian (2000), Moreau et al. (2002), Tapiero et al. (2003), and Quilez et al. (2003) should be consulted.

References

Awad, A.B., Hartati, M.S., and Fink, C.S., Phytosterol feeding induces alteration in testosterone metabolism in rat tissues, *J. Nutr. Biochem.*, 9:712–717, 1998.

Bourque, C., St-Onge, M.P., Papamandjaris, A.A., Cohn, J.S., and Jones, P.H.J., Consumption of an oil composed of median chain triacylglycerols, phytosterols, and n = 3 fatty acid improves cardiovascular risk profile of overweight women, *Metab.*, 52:771–777, 2003.

Carbin, B.E., Larsson, B., and Lindahl, O., Treatment of benign prostatic hyperplasia with phytosterols, *Br. J. Urol.*, 66:639–641, 1990.

Cerqueira, M.T., Fry, M.M., and Conner, W.E., The food and nutrient intakes of the Tarahumara Indians of Mexico, *Am. J. Clin. Nutr.*, 32:905–915, 1979.

Conner, W.E., Dietary sterols: Their relationship to atherosclerosis, *J. Am. Diet. Assoc.*, 52:202–208, 1968.

de Jong, N., Simojoki, M., Laatikainen, T., Tapanainen, H., Valsta, L., Lahti-Koski, M., Uutela, A., and Vartjainen, E., The combined use of cholesterol-lowering drugs and cholesterol-lowering bread spreads: Health behavior data from Finland, *Prev. Med.*, 39:849–855, 2004.

Hannun, Y.A. and Linardic, C.M., Spingomyelin breakdown products: Anti-proliferative and tumor suppressor lipids, *Biochem. Biophys. Acta*, 1154:223–236, 1993.

Hicks, K.B. and Moreau, R.A., Phytosterols and phytostanols: Functional food cholesterol busters, *Food Technol.*, 55(1):63–67, 2001.

Jones, P.J.H., MacDougall, D.E., Ntanios, F., and Vanstone, C.A., Dietary phytosterols as cholesterol-lowering agents in humans, *Can. J. Physiol. Pharmacol.*, 75:217–227, 1997.

Law, M., Plant sterol and stanol margarines and health, *Br. Med. J.*, 320:861–864, 2000.

Lea, L.J., Hepburn, P.A., Wolfreys, A.M., and Baldrick, P., Safety evaluation of phytosterol esters, part 8. Lack of genotoxicity and subchronic toxicity with phytosterol oxides, *Food Chem. Toxicol.*, 42:771–783, 2004.

Ling, W.H. and Jones, P.J.H., Dietary phytosterols: A review of metabolism, benefits and side effects, *Life Sci.*, 57:195–206, 1995.

Mettlin, C., Clinical oncology update: Prostate cancer, recent developments in the epidemiology of prostate cancer, *Eur. J. Cancer*, 33:340–347, 1997.

Miettinen, T.A., Puska, P., Gylling, H., Vanhanen, H.T., and Vartianen, E., Reduction of serum cholesterol with sitostanol-ester margarine in a mildly hypercholesterolemic population, *N. Eng. J. Med.*, 333:1308–1312, 1995.

Moghadasian, M.H., Pharmacological properties of plant sterols: *In vivo* and *in vitro* observations, *Life Sci.*, 67:605–615, 2000.

Moghadasian, M.H. and Frolich, J.J., Effects dietary phytosterols on cholesterol metabolism and atherosclerosis: Clinical and experimental evidence, *Am. J. Med.*, 107:588–594, 1999.

P

Moreau, R.A., Whitaker, B.D., and Hicks, K.B., Phytosterols, phytostanols, and their conjugates in foods: Structural diversity, quantitative analysis, and health-promoting properties, *Prog. Lipid Res.,* 41:457–500, 2002.

Mussner, M.-J., Pashofer, K.G., von Bergmann, K., Schwandt, P., Broedl, U., and Otto, C., Effects of phytosterol ester-enriched margarine on plasma lipoproteins in mild to moderate hypercholesterolemia are related to basal cholesterol and fat intake, *Metab.,* 51:189–194, 2002.

Neil, H.A.W., Huxley, R.R., Hawkins, M.M., Durrington, P.N., Betteridge, D.J., Humphries, S.E., and Simon Broome Hyperlipidemia Register Group and Scientific Steering Committee, Comparison of the risk of fatal coronary heart disease in treated xanthomatous and non-xanthomatous heterozygous familial hypercholesterolaemia: A prospective registry study, *Atherosclerosis,* 170:73–78, 2003.

Patel, S.B., Klett, E.L., Anh, G.-S., Yu, H., Chen, J., Pandit, B., Lee, M.-H., and Salen, G., Sitosterolemia; of mice and man, *Intern. Cong. Series,* 1262:300–304, 2004.

Pollack, O.J. and Kritchevsky, D., *Sitosterol, Monographs on Atherosclerosis,* Vol. 10, Krager, Basel, New York, 1981.

Quilez, J., Garcia-Lorda, P., and Salas-Salvado, J., Potential uses and benefits of phytosterols in diet: Present situation and future directions, *Clin. Nutr.,* 22:343–351, 2003.

Tapiero, H., Townsend, D.M., and Tew, K.D., Phytosterols in the prevention of human pathologies, *Biomed. Pharmacother.,* 57:321–325, 2003.

Trautwein, E.A., Duchateau, G.S.M.J.E., Lin, Y., Mel'nikov, S.M., Molhuizen, H.O.F., and Ntanios, F.Y., Proposed mechanisms of cholesterol-lowering action of plant sterols, *Eur. J. Lipid Sci. Technol.,* 105:171–185, 2003.

Wang, C., Lin, H.J., Chan, T., Salen, G., Chan, W.C. and Tse, T.F., A unique patient with coexisting cerebrotendinosus xanthomatosis and β-sitosterolemia, *Am. J. Med.,* 71:313–319, 1981.

Wilt, TJ., MacDonald, R., and Ishani, A., Beta-sitosterol for the treatment of benign prostatic hyperplasia: A systematic review, *Br. J. Urol. Int.,* 83:976–983, 1999.

Wolff, R.A., Dobrowsky, R.T., Bielawski, A., Obeid, L.M., and Hannun, Y.A., Role of ceramide-activated protein phosphatase in ceramide mediated signal transduction, *J. Biol. Chem.,* 269:19607–19609, 1999.

Pine *see also* **Pycnogenol**   Pine bark is a medicinal plant used primarily for its proanthocyanidin content. Proanthocyanidins are bioflavonoids with demonstrated antioxidant properties and taken for arthritis, bruises, phlebitis, ulcers, varicose veins, and other vascular problems (Rohdewald, 2002). A pilot study by Shand et al. (2003) showed dietary supplementation with enzogenol, a flavonoid extract from pine bark, was safe and well-tolerated with a number of beneficial effects, including lowering cardiovascular risk factors. Devaraj et al. (2002) reported an increase in plasma antioxidant capacity and favorable effects on the lipid profile of human subjects treated with extract from pine bark. Pine bark antioxidants may also be helpful in treating hypoxia from arteriosclerosis, inflammation, and cardiac or cerebral infarction (Rohdewald, 2002).

Pycnogenol, a procyanidin extracted from pine bark, is a trademarked, highly standardized extract of pine bark. Supplementation of pycnogenol to patients with conventional diabetes treatment lowered glucose levels and improved endothelial function (Liu et al., 2004). Kim et al. (2004) reported that *Pinus densiflora* bark extracts (out of 1400 tested plants) were the strongest inhibitors of several carbohydrate-hydrolyzing enzymes, with potential as an antihyperglycemic drug. In mildly hypertensive patients, pycnogenol also significantly reduced the dose of the calcium antagonist nifedipine (Liu et al., 2004).

Roseff (2002) demonstrated pycnogenol therapy improved capacitated sperm morphology and increased the function of normal sperm, suggesting a less invasive and less expensive fertility-promoting procedure. Pycnogenol also proved a useful dietary supplement for *C. pavum*-infected patients, affording some positive health benefits, while significantly reducing oocyst shedding (Kim and Healey, 2001).

References

Devaraj, S., Vega-Lopez, S., Kaul, N., Schonlau, F., Rohdewald, P. Nd Jialal, I., Supplementation with pine bark extract rich in polyphenols increases plasma antioxidant capacity and alters the plasma lipoprotein profile, *Lipids,* 37:931–934, 2002.

Kim, Y.M., Wang, M.H., and Rhee, H.I., A novel alpha-glucosidase inhibitor from pine bark, *Carbohydr. Res.*, 339:715–717, 2004.

Kim, H.C. and Healy, J.M., Effects of pine bark administered to immunosuppressed adult mice infected with *Cryptosporidium pervum*, *Am. J. Chem. Med.*, 29:469–75, 2001.

Liu, X., Wei, J., Tan, F., Zhou, S., Wurthwein, G., and Rohdewald, P., Pycnogenol®, French maritime pine bark extract, improves endothelial function of hypertensive patients, *Life Sci.*, 74:855–862, 2004.

Rohdewald, P., A review of the French maritime pine bark extract (Pycnogenol), an herbal medication with a diverse clinical pharmacology, *Int. J. Clin. Pharm. Ther.*, 40:158–168, 2002.

Roseff, S.J., Improvement in sperm quality and function with French maritime pine tree bark extract, *J. Reprod. Med.*, 47:821–824, 2002.

Shand, B., Strey, C., Scott, R., Morrison, Z., and Gieseg, S., Pilot study on the clinical effects of dietary supplementation with Enzogenol®, a flavonoid extract of pine bark and vitamin C, *Phytother. Res.*, 17:490–494, 2003.

Pinto beans   Pinto beans are excellent sources of fiber. In addition to lowering cholesterol (Bazzano et al., 2003), their high-fiber content prevents blood-sugar levels from rising too rapidly after a meal, making pinto beans a good choice for individuals with diabetes, insulin resistance, or hypoglycemia (McIntosh and Miller, 2001).The ability of pinto beans to bind bile acids *in vitro* suggests that they may have important, health-promoting properties by lowering cholesterol and the risk of coronary heart disease (Kahlon and Woodruff, 2002).

Marzo and coworkers (2002) showed extrusion cooking significantly ($p < 0.01$) decreased the antinutrients, phytic acid, condensed tannins, α-amylase inhibitors, and hemagglutinnins. Pretreatment of pinto beans by extrusion cooking improved food intake and utilization in rats by gaining body weight.

Ye and Ng (2001) isolated peptides from pinto beans with a molecular weight of 5 kDa and an N-terminal sequence similar to cowpea 10-kDa protein precursor. In addition to possessing potent antifungal activity against

Botyris cinerea, Mycospaerella arachidicola, and *Fusarium oxysporum*, they also had mitogenic activity toward mouse splenocytes and inhibited HIV-1 reverse transcriptase.

References

Bazzano, L.A., He, J., Ogden, L.G., Loria, C.M., and Whelton, P.K., Dietary fiber intake and reduced risk of coronary heart disease in U.S. men and women: The National Health and Nutrition Examination Survey I Epidemiologic Follow-up Study, *Arch. Intern. Med.,* 163:1897–1904, 2003.

Kahlon, T.S. and Woodruff, C.L., *In vitro* binding of bile acids by soy protein, pinto beans, black beans and wheat gluten, *Food Chem.*, 79:425–429, 2002.

Marzo, F., Alonso, R., Urdaneta, E., Arricibita, F.J., and Ibanez, F., Nutritional quality of extruded kidney bean (*Phaseolus vulgaris* L. var. Pinto) and its effect on growth and skeletal muscle nitrogen fractions in rats, *J. Anim. Sci.*, 80:875–879, 2002.

McIntosh, M. and Miller, C., A diet containing food rich in soluble and insoluble fiber improves glycemic control and reduces hyperlipidemia among patients with type 2 diabetes mellitus, *Nutr. Rev.*, 59:52–55, 2001.

Ye, X.Y. and Ng, T.B., A new antifungal protein and a chitinase with prominent macrophage-stimulating activity from seeds of *Phaseolus vulgaris* cv. pinto, *Biochem. Biophs. Res. Commun.*, 290:813–819, 2002.

Piperine   Piperine is the major alkaloid component of black (*Piper nigrum* Linn) and long pepper (*Piper longum* Linn). Previous studies using animal models showed piperine inhibited several cytochrome p450-mediated pathways

Structure of piperine. (From Bajad et al., *J. Chromatogr. B.*, 776:245–249, 2002. With permission.)

and phase II reactions (Atal et al., 1986; Singh et al., 1986). Rodents treated with piperine were found to have an increase in plasma levels of theophylline, phenytoin, rifampin, and propanolol (Atal et al., 1986; Velpandian et al.,

---

TABLE P.53
Effect of Piperine on the IL-1β, IL-6, GM-CSF, and TNF-α Production by B16F-10 Melanoma Cells

Cytokine	Control	Piperine (10 µg/mL)
IL-1β	185 ± 8.16 pg/mL	51.66 ± 6.23 pg/mL*
IL-6	203 ± 12.47 pg/mL	58.33 ± 6.28 pg/mL*
GM-CSF	96 ± 6.97 pg/mL	27.33 ± 2.49 pg/mL*
TNF-α	191.66 ± 13.12 pg/mL	53.66 ± 4.92 pg/mL*

Note: B16F-10 melanoma cells were incubated for 24 h in the presence or absence of piperine (10 mg/mL). Concentrations of IL-1b, IL-6, GM-CSF, and TNF-α were determined by quantitative ELISA. All experiments were repeated thrice. Values are the means ± S.D. *Statistically significant from the untreated control: $p < 0.001$.

Source: From Pradeep and Kuttan, *Int. Immunipharmacol.*, 4: 1795–1803, 2004. With permission.

2001). Rifampin and phenytoin are both substrates of the drug transporter P-glycoprotein (Schinkel et al., 1996; Schuetz et al., 1996). Bhardwaj and coworkers (2002) showed piperine inhibited both the drug transporter P-glycoprotein and the major drug-metabolizing enzyme CYP3A4. These researchers felt that further work was needed to clarify the impact of piperine on drug disposition in humans.

The anti-inflammatory effect of piperine was shown by Pradeep and Kuttan (2004) by its ability to significantly reduce proinflammatory cytokines, IL-1β, IL-6, TNF-α, and GM-CSF in B16-10 melanoma cells, as summarized in Table P.53. This was reflected by a marked inhibition of nuclear translocation of c-Fos, ATF-2, and CREB by 28.74 percent, 46.89 percent, and 64.31 percent, respectively. These results suggest that piperine prevents metastasis by targeting transcription factors.

References

Atal, C.K, Dubey, R.K., and Singh, J., Biochemical basis of enhanced drug bioavailability by piperine: Evidence that piperine is a potent inhibitor of drug metabolism, *J. Pharmacol. Exp. Ther.*, 232:258–262, 1985.

Bajad, S., Singla, A.K., and Bedi, K.L., Liquid chromatographic method for determination of piperine in rat plasma: Application to pharmacokinetics, *J. Chromatogr. B.*, 776:245–249, 2002.

Bhardwaj, R.K., Glaeser, H., Becquemont, L., Klotz, U., Gupta, S.K., and Fromm, M.F., Piperine, a major constituent of black pepper, inhibits human P-glycoprotein and CYP3A4, *J. Pharmacol. Exp. Ther.*, 302: 645–650, 2002.

Pradeep, C.R. and Kuttan, G., Piperine is a potent inhibitor of nuclear factor-κB (NF-κB), c-Fos, CREB, ATF-2 and proinflamatory cytokine gene expression in B16F-10 melanoma cells, *Inter. Immunopharmacol.*, 4:1795–1803, 2004.

Schinkel, A.H., Wagenaar, E., Mol, C.A.A.M., and van Deemter, L., P-glycoprotein in the blood–brain barrier in mice influences the brain penetration and pharmacological activity of many drugs, *J. Clin. Invest.*, 97:2517–2524, 1996.

Schuetz, E.G., Schinkel, A.H., Relling, M.V., and Schuetz, J.D., P-glycoprotein: A major determinant of rifampicin-inducible expression of cytochrome P4503A in mice and humans, *Proc. Natl. Acad. Sci U.S.A.*, 93:4001–4005, 1996.

Singh, J., Dubey, R.K., and Atal, C.K., Piperine-mediated inhibition of glucuronidation activity in isolated epithelial cells of the guinea pig small intestine: Evidence that piperine lowers endogenous UDP-glucuronic acid content, *J. Pharmacol. Exp. Ther.*, 236:488–493, 1986.

Velpandian, T., Jasuja, R., Bhardwaj, R.K., Jaiswal, J., and Gupta, S.K., Piperine in food: Interference in the pharmacokinetics of phenytoin, *Eur. J. Drug. Metab. Pharmacokinet.*, 26:241–247, 2001.

P

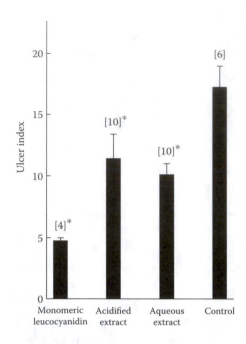

FIGURE P.80 Acute aspirin-induced lesions. The antiulcerogenic potential of the monomeric leucocyanidin (5 mg/day), acidified aqueous extract, and active aqueous extract were derived from 5 g unripe plantain banana. Ulcer index values (Best et al., 1984) are given as the mean ± SEM, with the number of repetitions in parentheses. Significant differences between treatments and control diets determined using the Wilcoxon rank sum test (*$p < 0.05$). (From Lewis et al., *J. Ethnopharmacol.,* 65:283-288, 1999. With permission.)

Plantain (*Musa sapientum* L. var. *paradisiaca*)

Plantain bananas, grown extensively in tropical and subtropical countries, can be eaten raw or cooked. Early studies by Elliot and Heward (1976) suggested bananas were antiulcerogenic. Subsequent work confirmed this property in plantain bananas (Best et al., 1984; Goel et al., 1989). Best and coworkers (1984) showed unripe plantain banana protected the gastric mucosa from aspirin-induced damage and that the active agent was polar and readily extracted with warm water or aqueous alcohol. Lewis and coworkers (1999) identified the antiulcerogenic agent in unripe plantain banana as the natural flavonoid, leucocyanidin. Addition of extracted and purified synthetic leucocyanidin in the diet of male Wistar rats significantly ($p- < 0.05$) protected them from aspirin-induced lesions (Figure P.80). Unfortunately, these beneficial prophylactic effects are lost when plantains are cooked.

Leucocyanidin (3,3′,4,4′,5,7-hexahydroxyflavan). (From Lewis et al., *J. Ethnopharmacol.,* 65:283-288, 1999. With permission.)

References

Best, R., Lewis, D.A., and Nasser, N., The antiulcerogenic activity of the unripe plantain banana, *Br. J. Pharmacol.,* 82:107–116, 1984.

Elliot, R.C. and Heward, G.J.F., The effect of banana-supplemented diet on garlic ulcer in mice, *Pharmacol. Res. Commun.,* 8:167–171, 1976.

Goel, R.K., Tavares, I.A., and Bennett, A., Stimulation of gastric and colonic mucosal eicosanoid synthesis by plantain banana, *J. Pharm. Pharmacol.*, 41: 747–750, 1989.

Lewis, D.A., Fields, W.N., and Shaw, G.P., A natural flavonoid present in unripe plantain pulp (*Musa sapientum* L. var. *paradisiaca*) protects the gastric mucosa from aspirin-induced erosions, *J. Ethnopharmacol.*, 65:283-288, 1999.

Platycodon (Platycodon grandiflorum)

Platycodon is an essential herb and a favored ingredient in Chinese medicine. The roots of *Plactycodon grandiflorum* have been used as a food or as a traditional oriental medicine for treating bronchitis, asthma, pulmonary tuberculosis, hyperlipidemia, diabetes, and inflammatory diseases (Takagi and Lee, 1972; Lee, 1973). Subsequent studies by Nagao et al. (1986) identified its immunopharmacological properties, while others identified some active compounds, including saponins (Ishii et al., 1984) and triterpenoids (Nikaido et al., 1999). A wide variety of compounds were reported in *Platycodon grandiflorum* by Kim et al. (2000) that exhibited these immunopharmacological properties. Several active compounds, platycodin D (PD) and D3 (PD3) related to oleanolic acid, were isolated from *P. grandiflorum* roots (Tada et al., 1975; Ishii et al., 1978). Using a rabbit macrophage-like cell line, RAW 264.7

cells, Wang et al. (2004) reported both these glycosides were powerful regulators of inflammation by reducing nitric oxide and possessed antitumor activities by stimulating TNF-α synthesis or inhibiting TNF-α mRNA degradation. (See structure for Platycodon on the next page.) Yoon and coworkers (2004) showed that a polysaccharide isolated from *P. grandiflorum* activated macrophages in RAW 264.7 cells, mediated, in part, by mitogen-activated protein kinases (MAPKs) and activator protein-1 (AP-1).

A crude petroleum-ether extract from *P. grandiflorum* was shown by Lee et al. (1998) to be a much stronger inhibitor of human cancer-cell growth compared to an aqueous extract. Further fractionation of this petroleum-ether extract by Lee and coworkers (2004a) separated five fractions (I–V) on a silica-gel column. The phenolic content ranged from 1.66 to 4.80 mg/g, with fraction II containing the highest level. Comparison of their antioxidant activities, based on the formation of TBA, showed that with the exception of fraction I, all other fractions were significantly different ($p < 0.01$) from the control (Figure P.81). Fraction II was the next most effective antioxidant after BHA, with fractions II–IV all exhibiting greater antioxidant activity than α-tocopherol. These data strongly correlated with antioxidant measurements using the ferric-thiocyanate test in which fraction II also proved to be the strongest antioxidant. Using the DPPH free-radical-scavenging test also confirmed FII to be the most potent

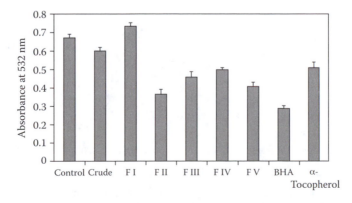

FIGURE P.81 Absorbance at 532 nm of the fractions (F1–V) from *P. grandiflorum* extract by TBA method compared with BHA and α-tocopherol. (From Lee et al., *J. Ethnopharmacol.*, 93:409–415, 2004a. With permission.)

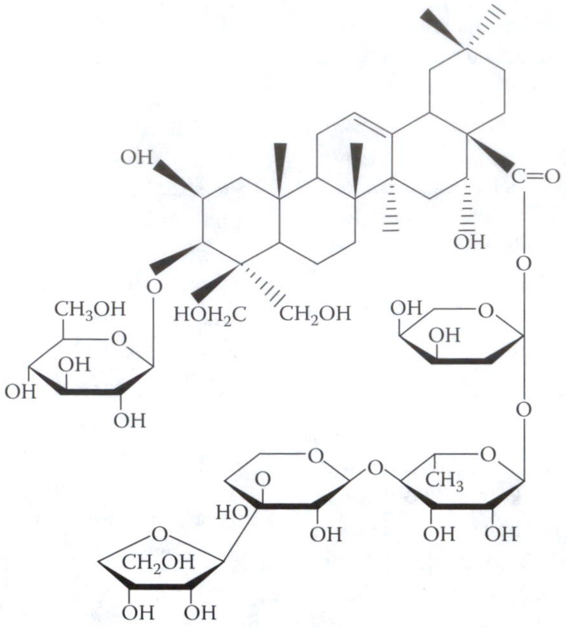

Platycodon D

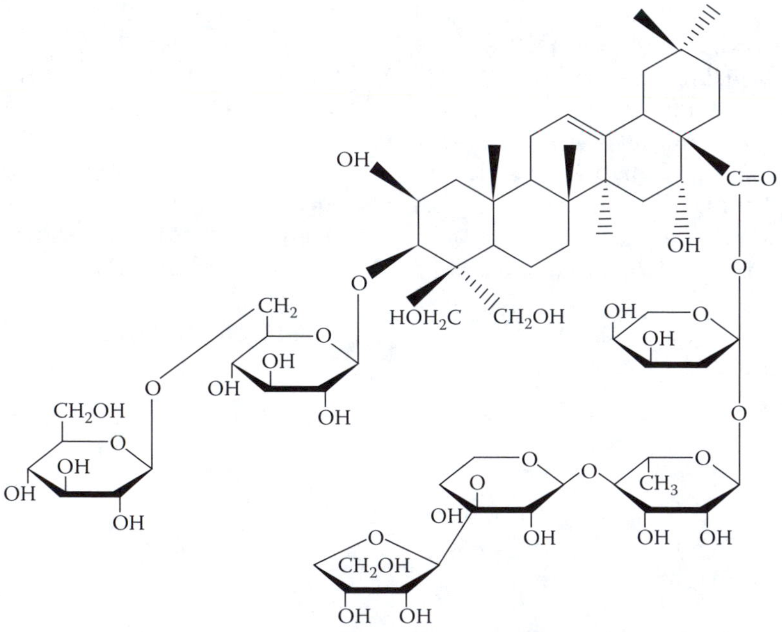

Platycodon D₃

Platycodon D and platycodon D$_3$. (Wang et al., *Int. Immunopharmacol.*, 4:1039–1049, 2004. With permission.)

P

DPPH scavenger when present at 100 and 200 mg/mL, followed by FIII. A comparison of their cytotoxicity using three human cancer lines, HT-29, HepG2, and HRT-18, showed fraction III was the most potent inhibitor. Further work by Lee et al. (2004b) identified coniferyl alcoholic esters of palmitic and oleic acids in fraction II, which may account for its antioxidant properties.

References

Ishii, H., Tori, T., Tozyo, T., and Yoshimura, Y., Structures of polgalacin D and D2, platycodon D determined by 13C nuclear magnetic resonance spectroscopy, *Chem. Pharm. Bull*, 26:674–677, 1978.

Ishii, H., Tori, K., Tozyo, T., and Yoshimura, Y., Saponins from roots of *Platycodon grandiflorum*, part 2, isolation and structure of new triterpene glycosides, *J. Chem. Soc. Perkin. Trans.*, 1:661–668, 1984.

Kim, K., Seo, E., Lee, Y-C., Lee, T-K., Cho, Y-W., Ezaki, O., and Kim, C-H., Effect of dietary *Platycodon grandiflorum* on improvement of insulin resistance in obese Zucker rats, *J. Nutr. Biochem.*, 11: 420–424, 2000.

Lee, E.B., Pharmacological studies on *Platycodon grandiflorum* A. DC, IV, a comparison of experimental pharmacological effects of crude platycodin with clinical indications of Platycodi radix, *Yakugaku Zasshi*, 93:1188–1194, 1973.

Lee, J.Y., Hwang, W.I., and Lim, S.T., Effect of *Platycodon grandiflorum* extract on cancer cell lines, *Korean J. Food Sci. Technol.*, 30:13–21, 1998.

Lee, J.Y., Hwang, W.I., and Lim, S.T., and anticancer activities of organic extracts from *Platycodon grandiflorum* A. De Candolle roots, *J. Ethnopharmacol.*, 93:409–415, 2004a.

Lee, J-N., Yoon, J-Y., Kim, C-T., and Lim, S-T., Antioxidant activity of phenylpropanoid esters isolated and identified from *Platycodon grandiflorum* A.DC, *Phytochemistry*, 63:3033–3039, 2004b.

Nagao, T., Matsuda, H., Namba, K., and Kubo, M., Immune pharmacological studies on platicodi radix (II): Antitumor activity of insulin from platicodi radix, *Shoykagaku Zasshi, J. Pharm. Soc. Jpn.*, 40: 375–380, 1986.

Nikaido, T., Koike, K., Mitsunaga, K., and Sacki, T., Two new triterpenoid saponins from *Platycodon grandiflorum*, *Chem. Pharm. Bull.*, 47:903–904, 1999.

Tada, A., Kaneiwa, Y., Shoji, J., and Shibata, S., Studies on the saponins of the roots of *Platycodon grandiflorum* A. DC CANDOLLE I: Isolation and structure of Platycodon-D, *Chem. Pharm. Bull.*, 23: 2965–2972, 1975.

Takagi, K. and Lee, E.B., Pharmacological studies on *Platycodon grandiflorum* A. DC, activities of crude platycodin on respiratory and circulatory systems and its pharmacological activities, *Yakugaku Zasshi*, 92:969–973, 1972.

Wang, C., Schuller Levis, G.B., Lee, E.B., Levis, W.R., Lee, D.W., Kim, B.S., Park, S.Y., and Park, E., Platycodin D and D3 isolated from the root of *Platycodon gradiflorum* modulate the production of nitric oxide and secretion of TNF-α in activated RAW 264.7 cells, *Int. Immunopharmacol.*, 4:1039–1049, 2004.

Yoon, Y.D., Kang, J.S., Han, S.B., Park, S.-K., Lee, H.S., Kang, J.S., and Kim, H.M., Activation of mitogen-activated protein kinases and AP-1 by polysaccharide isolated from the radix of Platycodon gradiflorum in RAW 264.7 cells, *Int. Immunopharmacol.*, 4:1477–1487, 2004.

Polydextrose Polydextrose, a nondigestible polysaccharide, is prepared by bulk-melt polycondensation of glucose and sorbitol, together with small amounts of food-grade acid *in vacuo* (Flood et al., 2004). The overall product resulting from this random polymerization is a polymer with an average degree of polymerization of 12 with 1,6 glucosidic bonds predominating (Scheme P.47). It was approved as an additive by the FDA in 1982 and is used as a low-calorie bulking agent, replacing sugar in reduced-calorie foods (Mitchell et al., 2001). Polydextrose is often referred to as a resistant oligosaccharide or resistant polysaccharide. As a dietary fiber, it is fermented in the lower gastrointestine, producing short-chain fatty acids (SCFA), fecal bulking, reduced transit time, and glucose homeostasis (Pfizer, Inc., 1978).

Studies on the physiological effects of dietary polydextrose found it increased calcium absorption (Hara et al., 2000) and retarded lipid transport into the lymph (Ogata et al., 1997). Ishizuka and coworkers (2003) showed ingestion of polydextrose (30 mg/kg) significantly ($p < 0.05$) suppressed formation of aberrant crypt foci (ACF) in the rat colorectum induced by 1,2-dimethylhydrazine (DMH) compared to the fiber-free diet. The earlier the animals were started on polydextrose, the more effective was the treatment in suppressing ACF development (Table P.54).

Flood and coworkers (2004) showed polydextrose was well tolerated and unlikely to induce diarrhea in adults taking less than 50 g per day. The mean laxative threshold dose for

P

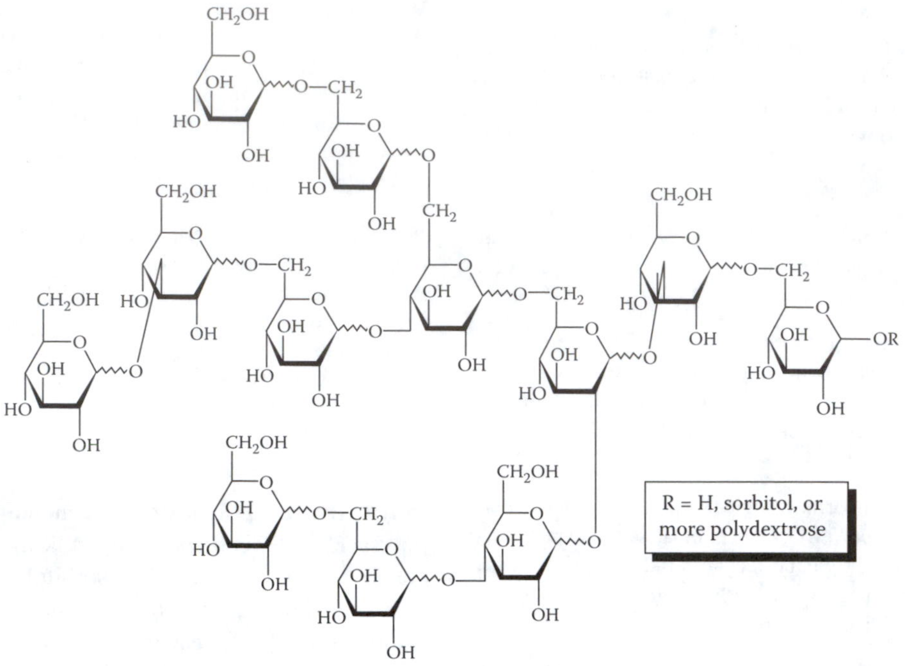

SCHEME P.47 A representative structure for polydextrose. (From Craig et al., *Cereal Foods World*, 43:370–375, 1998. With permission.)

TABLE P.54
Effect of Polydextrose Ingestion on the Number of ACF in the Rat Colorectum Induced by DMH at Five Weeks After Injection[1,2]

	Proximal colon	Distal colon	Rectum	Total Colorectum
Fiber-free	ND	29 ± 5	12 ± 2	42 ± 7
Polydextrose A	ND	21 ± 3	5 ± 1*	26 ± 4*
Polydextrose B	ND	24 ± 3	7 ± 1*	30 ± 4
Polydextrose C	0.14 ± 0.14	29 ± 5	7 ± 2*	37 ± 4
Polydextrose D	0.14 ± 0.14	31 ± 4	9 ± 2	40 ± 5

[1] Values expressed as mean ± SEM (n = 7).
[2] Polydextrose A rats were started eight days prior to DMH injection. Polydextrose B rats were started one day prior to DMH injection. Polydextrose C rats were started one day after DMH injection. Polydextrose D rats were started seven days after DMH injection.
* Significantly different from fiber-free-fed group ($p < 0.05$).

Source: From Ishizuka et al., *Nutr. Res.,* 23:117–123, 2003. With permission.

---

polydextrose (90 g/d or 1.3 g/kg bw) was higher than almost all of the low-caloric carbohydrates on the market.

References

Anonymous, *Polydextrose Food Additive Petition* #9A3441, Zpfizer, 1978.

Craig, S.A., Holden, J.F., Auerbach, M.H., and Frier, H.I., Polydextrose as soluble fiber: Physiological and analytical aspects, *Cereal Foods World*, 43:370–375, 1998.

Flood, M.T., Auerbach, M.H., and Craig, S.A.S., A review of the clinical toleration studies of polydextrose in foods, *Food Chem. Toxicol.*, 42:1531–1542, 2004.

Hara, H., Suzuki, T., and Kasai, T., Ingestion of the soluble dietary fibre polydextrose, increases calcium absorption and bone mineralization in normal and total-gastrectomized rats, *Br. J. Nutr.,* 84:655–661, 2000.

Ishizuka, S., Nagai, T., and Hara, H., Reduction of aberrant crypt foci by ingestion of polydextrose in rat colorectum, *Nutr. Res.,* 23:117–123, 2003.

Mitchell, H., Auerbach, M.H., and Moppett, F.K., Polydextrose, in *Alternative Sweeteners,* 3rd edition, Nabors, L.O., Ed., Marcel Dekker, New York, 2001, chap. 26, pp. 499–518.

Ogata, S., Fujimoto, K., Iwakiri, R., Matsunaga, C., Ogawa, Y., Koyama, T., and Sakai, T., Effect of poly-dextrose on absorption of triglyceride and cholesterol in mesenteric lymph-fistula rats, *Proc. Soc. Exp. Biol. Med.,* 215:53–58, 1997.

Pfizer Inc., Polydextrose food addtive petition. New York: Pfizer Inc. (FDA petition 9A344), 1978.

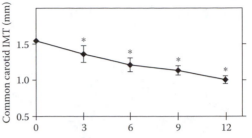

FIGURE P.82 The effect of pomegranate-juice con-sumption by patients with carotid-artery stenosis on carotid mean intima-media thickness (IMT). Ten patients with severe carotid-artery stenosis were sup-plemented with pomegranate juice for up to one year, with carotid IMT measured in the patients' left and right carotid arteries before treatment (Baseline) and during pomegranate-juice consumption. (From Avi-ram et al., *Clin. Nutr.,* 23:423–433, 2004. With per-mission.)

Pomegranate (*Punica granatum*)   The peel of pomegranates was reported to contain large amounts of polyphenols and is used in tinctures, cosmetics, therapeutic formulations, and food recipes (Ben Nasr et al., 1996). The juice of pomegranates was also a rich source of antiox-idants (Gil et al., 2000), which accounted for its antiatherogenic effects in humans and ani-mals (Aviram et al., 2000). Using *in vitro* mod-els, Singh et al. (2002) determined the antiox-idant activity of ethyl acetate, methanol, and water extracts of pomegranate peels and seeds. Of these, the methanol extract exhibited the greatest antioxidant activity. A recent study by Negi and coworkers (2003) prepared dried pow-ders from peeled pomegranates by Soxhlet extraction with ethyl acetate, acetone, metha-nol, and water and tested each one for antioxi-dant and antimutagenic activities. All peel extracts showed potent antioxidant capacity, with the water extract being the lowest. With respect to their antimutagenicity using the Ames test, the order of activity was water extract > acetone > ethyl acetate > methanol. These results suggested pomegranate-peel extracts have considerable potential as nutra-ceuticals. This was confirmed by Aviram and coworkers (2004) who fed pomegranate juice

for a year to 10 patients suffering from carotid-artery stenosis, with five of them continuing on for up to three years. In contrast to patients with severe carotid-artery stenosis not consuming pomegranate juice, there was a significant ($p < 0.01$) decrease in the mean intima-media thick-ness of the left and right common carotid arter-ies of 13 percent, 22 percent, 26 percent, and 35 percent after 3, 6, 9, and 12 months con-sumption of pomegranate juice compared to a 9 percent increase for the control (Figure P.82). A significant ($p < 0.05$) decrease in systolic pressure also accompanied pomegranate-juice consumption, with a reduction of 7 percent, 11 percent, 10 percent, 10 percent, and 12 percent after 1, 3, 6, 9, and 12 months of consumption. No significant changes were observed on the patients' diastolic pressure.

Kulkarni et al. (2004) recently isolated and characterized the phenolic compound, puni-calagin, from the methanol extract of the pith and carpellary membrane of pomegranate fruit. This compound exhibited potent DPH radical-scavenging activity by donating electrons to free radicals. They suggested that the waste material (pith and carpellary membrane) in pomegranate could be a viable source of this natural and potent antioxidant.

P

Punicalagin. (From Kularni et al., *Food Chem.,* 87: 551–557, 2004. With permission.)

References

Aviram, M., Dornfeld, L., Rosenblat, M., Volkova, N., Kaplan, M., Coleman, R., Hayek, T., Presser, D., and Fuhrman, B., Pomegranate juice consumption reduces oxidative stress, atherogenic modifications to LDL, and platelet aggregation: studies in humans and atherosclerotic apolipoprotein E-deficient mice, *Am. J. Clin. Nutr.,* 71:1062–1076, 2000.

Aviram, M., Rosenblat, M., Gaitini, D., Nitecki, S., Hoffman, A., Dornfield, L., Volkova, N., Presser, D., Attias, J., Liker, H., and Hayek, T., Pomegranate juice consumption for 3 years by patients with carotid artery stenosis reduces common carotid intima-media thickness, blood pressure and LDL oxidation, *Clin. Nutr.,* 23:423–433, 2004.

Ben Nasr, C.B., Ayed, N., and Metche, M., Quantitative determination of the polyphenolic content of pomegranate peel, *Z. Lebensm Unters Forsch,* 203: 374–378, 1996.

Gil, M.I., Tomas-Barberan, F.A., Hess-Pierce, B., Holcroft, D.M., and Kader, A.A., Antioxidant activity of pomegranate juice and its relationship with phenolic composition and processing, *J. Agric. Food Chem.,* 48:4581–4589, 2000.

Kulkarni, A.P., Aradhya, S.M., and Divakar, S., Isolation and identification of a radical scavenging antioxidant-punicalagin from pith and carpellary membrane of pomegranate fruit, *Food Chem.,* 87: 551–557, 2004.

Negi, P.S., Jayaprakasha, G.K., and Jena, B.S., Antioxidant and antimutagenic activities of pomegranate peel extracts, *Food Chem.,* 80:393–397, 2003.

Singh, R.P., Murthy, K.N.C., and Jayaprakasha, G.K., Studies on the antioxidant activity of pomegranate (*Punica granatum*) peel and seed extract using *in vitro* models, *J. Agric. Food Chem.,* 50:81–86, 2002.

Poppy The opium poppy, *Papaver somniferum*, is one of man's oldest medicinal plants. Today, opium poppy is a commercial source of narcotic analgesics, morphine and codeine. Along with two morphinans, opium poppy produces approximately 80 alkaloids belonging to various tetrahydrobenzylisoquinoline derivatives. These morphinan alkaloids accumulate in the latex of opium poppy (Weid et al., 2004).

Originally, opium poppies were grown for the pharmaceutical industry for morphine production. However, morphine-free varieties were developed for baking and confectionery purposes. Poppy seeds contain up to 50 percent of a high-quality, semi-drying oil, containing 72 percent linoleic acid, used in artists' paints (Table P.55).

Raw opium contains approximately 25 different alkaloids by weight, depending on the variety. The major alkaloids are morphine (4–21 percent), codeine (0.8–2.5 percent), thebaine (0.5–2.0 percent), papaverine (0.5–2.5 percent), noscapine (0.5–2.5 percent), and meconic acid (3–5 percent). Interaction of poppy alkaloid opioids with endogenous opiate receptors in the

TABLE P.55
Fatty-Acid Composition of Poppy Oil

Fatty Acid	%
Palmitic (C16:0)	10
Stearic (C18:0)	2
Oleic (C16:1)	11
Linoleic (C18:2)	72
Linolenic (C18:3)	5

Source: Adapted from Serpico and White, *Ancient Egyptian Materials and Technology,* Cambridge University Press, Cambridge, UK, 2000.

brain is recognized by clinical pharmacologists for such plants with a long-established medicinal use (Perry et al., 1999). Poppy seeds from *Papaver somniferum* L. were found to contain total morphine (free and bound) in the range of 58.4 to 52.2 micrograms/g of seed and total codeine (free and bound) in the range of 28.4 to 54.1 micrograms/g of seed (Lo and Chua, 1992). Thus, a positive result for morphine in oral fluid may be due to ingestion of poppy seeds (Rohrig and Moore, 2003). However, poppy seeds can also induce immediate-type allergic reactions, ranging from mild, local symptoms to severe anaphylactic reactions, by cross-reacting with other plant-derived allergens (Jensen-Jarolim et al., 1999).

References

Jensen-Jarolim, E., Gerstmayer, G., Kraft, D., Scheiner, O., Ebner, H., and Ebner, C., Serological characterization of allergens in poppy seeds, *Clin. Exp. Allergy*, 29:1075–1079, 1999.

Lo, D.S. and Chua, T.H., Poppy seeds: Implications of consumption, *Med. Sci. Law*, 32:296–302, 1992.

Perry, E.K., Pickering, A.T., Wang, W.W., Houghton, P.J., and Perry, N.S., Medicinal plants and Alzheimer's disease from ethnobotany to phytotherapy, *J. Pharm. Pharmacol.*, 51:527–534, 1999.

Rohrig, T.P. and Moore, C., The determination of morphine in urine and oral fluid following ingestion of poppy seeds, *J. Anal. Toxicol.*, 27:449–452, 2003.

Serpico, M. and White, R., Oil, fat, and wax in *Ancient Egyptian Materials and Technology*, P. Nicholson and I. Shaw, Eds., Cambridge University Press, Cambridge, UK., pp. 390–429, 2000.

Weid, M., Ziegler, J., and Kutchan, T.M., The roles of latex and the vascular bundle in morphine biosynthesis in the opium poppy, *Papaver somniferum*, *Proc. Natl. Acad. Sci. U.S.A.*, 101:13957–13962, 2004.

Pot marigold   Pot marigold (*Calendula officinalis*) is an annual herb with many pharmacological properties. It is used to treat skin disorders and as a bactericide, antiseptic, and anti-inflammatory. The butanol extract of *Calendula officinalis* was shown to have significant radical-scavenging activity (Cordova et al., 2002), which may explain part of its therapeutic efficacy. Dichloromethane extracts of its flowers were shown to contain eight known bioactive triterpenoid monoesters (Neukirch et al., 2004). Faradiol 3-*O*-laurate, palmitate, and myristate were identified as the major anti-inflammatory triterpenoid esters in the flower heads of *Calendula officinalis* (Hamburger et al., 2003).

The main carotenoids found in the petals and pollens of *Calendula officinalis* were flavoxanthin and astaxanthin, while the stems and leaves contained mostly lutein and β-carotene (Bako et al., 2002). Calendasaponins A, B, C, and D, ionone glucosides (officinosides A and B), and sesquiterpene oligoglycosides (officinosides C and D) were all isolated from the flowers of Egyptian *Calendula officinalis* exhibiting hypoglycemic, gastric emptying inhibitory, and gastroprotective effects (Yoshikawa et al., 2001).

Perez-Carreon et al. (2002) demonstrated the chemopreventive properties of *Calendula officinalis* extracts by their antigenotoxic effects on rat liver cell cultures treated with diethylnitrosamine. At higher concentrations, however, they proved genotoxic. In a phase III randomized trial, Pommier et al. (2004) found *Calendula officinalis* was an effective, nonsteroid topical agent for preventing acute dermatitis during adjuvant radiotherapy for breast carcinoma compared to the drug trolamine. They proposed its use for patients undergoing postoperative irradiation for breast cancer.

References

Bako, E., Deli, J., and Toth, G., HPLC study on the carotenoid composition of *Calendula* products, *J. Biochem. Biophys. Methods*, 53:241–250, 2002.

Cordova, C.A., Siqueira, I.R., Netto, C.A., Yunes, R.A., Volpato, A.M., Cechinel, Filho, V., Curi-Pedrosa, R., and Creczynski-Pasa, T.B., Protective properties of butanoilic extract of the *Calendula officinalis* L. (marigold) against lipid peroxidation of rat liver microsomes and action as free radical scavenger, *Redox Rep.*, 7:95–102, 2002.

Hamburger, M., Adler, S., Baumann, D., Forg, A., and Weinreich, B., Preparative purification of the major anti-inflammatory triterpenoid esters from marigold (*Calendula officinalis*), *Fitoterapia*, 74:328–338, 2003.

Neukirch, H., D'Ambrosio, M., Dalla Via, J., and Guerriero, A., Simultaneous quantitative determination of eight triterpenoid monoesters from flowers of 10 varieties of *Calendula officinalis* L. and characterization of a new triterpenoid monoester, *Phytochem. Anal.*, 15:30–35, 2004.

Perez-Carreon, J.I., Cruz-Jimenez, G., Licea-Vega, J.A., Arce Popoca, E., Fattel Fazenda, S., and Villa-Trevino, S., Genotoxic and anti-genotoxic properties of *Calendula officinalis* extracts in rat liver cultures treated with diethylnitrosamine, *Toxicol. In Vitro*, 16: 253–258, 2002.

Pommier, P., Gomez, F., Sunyach, M.P., D'Hombres, A., Carrie, C., and Montbarbon, X., Phase III randomized trial of *Calendula officinalis* compared with trolamine for the prevention of acute dermatitis during irradiation for breast cancer, *J. Clin. Oncol.*, 22: 1447–1453, 2004.

Yoshikawa, M., Murakami, T., Kishi, A., Kageura, T., and Matsuda, H., Medicinal flowers III. Marigold. (1): hypoglycemic, gastric emptying inhibitory, and gastroprotective principles and new oleanane-type triterpene oligoglycosides, calendasaponins A, B. C, and D from Egyptian *Calendula officinalis*, *Chem. Pharm. Bull.*, 49:863–870, 2001.

Potato   Antioxidant activity in potatoes is supported by the findings of free and bound phenolics (Chu et al., 2002). In particular, potato peel, a waste product from potato processing, was found to be rich in phenolic acids (Lisinska and Leszczynski, 1987) and later shown to be a source of antioxidants in food systems (Rodriguez et al., 1994). Rehman et al. (2004) recently examined a petroleum-ether extract from potato peels that exhibited strong antioxidant activity and enhanced the shelf life of soybean oil. The free-radical-scavenging activity of a freeze-dried aqueous extract of potato peel was confirmed by Singh and Ranjini (2004) using 1,1-diphenyl-2-picrylhydrazine) (DPPH). They also reported it strongly inhibited lipid peroxidation of rat liver homogenates induced by the $FeCl_2$-H_2O_2 system. Further work is needed to ensure the safety and efficacy of the antioxidants from potatoes and potato peels in relation to their potential as sources of nutraceuticals.

Morita et al. (1997) reported lower serum total-cholesterol concentrations in rats fed potato proteins compared to those fed casein. Schafer et al. (2003) later showed potatoes, as a carbohydrate source, elicited significantly better glycemic and insulinemic responses in patients with type 2 diabetes compared to dried peas.

References

Chu, Y-F., Sun, J., Wu, X., and Liu, R.H., Antioxidant and antiproliferative activities of common vegetables, *J. Agric. Food Chem.*, 50:6910–6916, 2002.

Lisinska, G. and Leszczynski, W., Potato tubers as raw materials for processing and nutrition, in *Potato Science and Technology*, Lisinska, G., and Leszczynski, W., Eds., Elsevier Applied Science, London, 1987, chap. 2, pp. 34–38.

Morita, T., Oh-hashi, A., Takei, K., Ikai, M., Kasaoka, S., and Kiriyama, S., Cholesterol-lowering effects of soybean, potato and rice proteins on their low methionine contents in rats fed a cholesterol-free purified diet, *J. Nutr.*, 127:470–477, 1997.

Rehman, Z.-U., Habib, F., and Shah, W.H., Utilization of potato peels extract as a natural antioxidant in soybean oil, *Food Chem.*, 85:215–220, 2004.

Rodriguez de Sotillo, D., Hadley, M., and Holm, E.T., Potato peel waste: Stability and antioxidant activity of freeze-dried extract, *J. Food Sci.*, 59: 1031–1033, 1994.

Schafer, G., Schenck, U., Ritzel, U., Ramadori, G., and Leonhardt, U., Comparison of the effects of dried peas with those of potatoes in mixed meals on postprandial glucose and insulin concentrations in patients with type 2 diabetes, *Am. J. Clin. Nutr.*, 78: 99–103, 2003.

Singh, N. and Rajini, P.S., Free radical scavenging activity of an aqueous extract of potato peel, *Food Chem.*, 85:611–616, 2004.

Prebiotics *see also* **Acacia gum, Arabinoxylan, Fructooligosaccharides, and Inulin**   Prebiotics are oligosaccharides that promote the growth of beneficial bacteria in the GI tract. These include inulin-type fructans, which include native inulin, hydrolyzed inulin, or oligofructose and synthetic fructooligosaccharides (Roberfroid, 1998; Roberfroid et al., 1998).

Human milk oligosaccharides represent the first prebiotics in humans, as they are only partially digested in the small intestine. Once they reach the colon, they selectively stimulate the development of the bifidogenic flora (Coppa et al., 2004). A bovine-milk formula supplemented with a prebiotic mixture of galactooligosaccharides and fructooligosaccharides can stimulate an intestinal flora, similar to that of

P

breast-fed infants. Several biota, whose growth is enhanced by this prebiotic mixture, represent important factors in the postnatal development of the immune system (Boehm et al., 2004).

Dietary modulation of the gut microflora by prebiotics is designed to improve health by stimulating the numbers and activities of the bifidobacteria and lactobacilli. Having an "optimal" gut microflora can increase resistance to pathogenic bacteria, lower blood ammonia, increase stimulation of the immune response, and reduce the risk of cancer (Manning and Gibson, 2004). Thus, the physiological consequences of prebiotic consumption are evaluated in terms of potential to reduce risk for disease. Most research has been done with $\beta(2\text{-}1)$ fructans as an example of prebiotics. These results are relevant in the fields of gut function, lipid metabolism, mineral absorption, bone formation, immunology, and cancer (Van Loo, 2004).

References

Boehm, G., Jelinek, J., Stahl, B., van Laere, K., Knol, J., Fanaro, S., Moro, G., and Vigi, V., Prebiotics in infant formulas, *J. Clin. Gastroenterol.,* 38(Suppl. 6): S76–S79, 2004.

Coppa, G.V., Bruni, S., Morelli, L., Soldi, S., and Gabrielli, O., The first prebiotics in humans: Human milk oligosaccharides, *J. Clin. Gastroenterol.,* 38(Suppl. 6):S80–S83, 2004.

Manning, T.S. and Gibson, R.R., Prebiotics, *Best Pract. Res. Clin. Gastroenterol.,* 18:287–298, 2004.

Roberfroid, M.B., Dietary fructans, *Ann. Rev. Nutr.,* 18:117–143, 1998.

Roberfroid, M.B., Van Loo, J.A.E., and Gibson, G.R., The bifidogenic nature of chicory inulin and its hydrolyzed products, *J. Nutr.,* 128:11–19, 1998.

Van Loo, J.A., Prebiotics promote good health: The basis, the potential, and the emerging evidence, *J. Clin. Gastroenterol.,* 38(Suppl. 6):S70–S75, 2004.

Probiotics   Probiotics are bacteria that keep disease-causing organisms in check. For example, *Lactobacillus acidophilus* is added to yogurt while *Lactobacillus reuteri* and *Lactobacillus bifidus* also promote health. Probiotics are viable microbial food ingredients that have a beneficial effect on the intestinal tract of their host (Salimen et al., 1998). Most probiotics are lactobacilli and bifidobacteria, presently consumed almost exclusively as fermented dairy products, such as yogurts or freeze-dried cultures. These probiotics survive the digestive process and become established in the large bowel with recognized benefits (Sanders, 1993; Marteau and Rambaud, 1993; Salimen et al., 1996). Studies have shown probiotics may be effective in reducing diarrhea (Isolauri et al., 1991; Corthier, 1997; Allen et al., 2004). Other studies suggest probiotics could help in managing clinical inflammatory-bowel disease (Fedorak and Madsen, 2004) and in treating functional abdominal bloating (Di Stefano et al., 2004).

Steatohepatitis is recognized as the leading cause of cryptogenic cirrhosis, although the pathogenesis of this disease is not fully understood. Nevertheless, among various factors implicated, intestinal bacterial overgrowth may be involved. Thus, probiotic treatment may be beneficial (Nardone and Rocco, 2004).

Studies examining the use of probiotics in food allergy, atopic dermatitis, and in the primary prevention of atopy found probiotic therapy alleviated allergic inflammation by controlling symptoms and reducing local and systemic inflammatory markers (Miraglia del Giudice and De Luca, 2004).

Probiotics may also improve lactose absorption and *Helicobacter pylori* eradication and constipation. In animal models with colorectal cancer, treatment with probiotics reduces the prevalence of this disease, while in humans, the amount of genotoxic substances in the feces are reduced (Goossens et al., 2003).

In summary, the potential benefits of probiotics include: adherence to cells; exclusion or reduction of pathogenic adherence; production of acids, hydrogen peroxide, and bacteriocins antagonistic to pathogen growth; safe, noninvasive, noncarcinogenic, and nonpathogenic characteristics; and congregate to form a more balanced intestinal flora (Otles et al., 2003).

References

Allen, S.J., Okobo, B., Martinez, E., Gregorio, G., and Dans, L.F., Probiotics for treating infectious diarrhoea, *Cochrane Database Syt. Rev.,* CD003048, 2004.

Corthier, G., Antibiotic-associated diarrhoea and pseudomembranous colitis, in *Probiotics 2: Applications and Practical Aspects,* Fuller, R., Ed., Chapman & Hall, London, 1997, pp. 40–64.

Di Stefano, M., Miceli, E., Armellini, E., Missanelli, A., and Corazza, G.R., Probiotics and functional abdominal bloating, *J. Clin. Gastroenterol.,* 38(Suppl. 6):S102–S103, 2004.

Fedorak, R.N. and Madsen, K.L., Probiotics and the management of inflammatory bowel disease, *Inflamm. Bowel Dis.,* 10:286–299, 2004.

Goossens, D., Jonkers, D., Stobberingh, E., van den Bogaard, A., Russel, M., and Stockbrugger, R., Probiotics in gastroenterology: Indications and future perspectives, *Scand. J. Gastroenterol.,* 38(Supp. 239):15–23, 2003.

Isolauri, E., Juntunen, M., Rautanen, T., Sillanaukee, P., and Koivula, T., A human Lactobacillus strain (*Lactobacillus casei* strain CG) promotes recovery of acute diarrhea in children, *Pediatrics,* 88:90–97, 1991.

Marteau, P. and Rambaud, J.C., Potential of using lactic acid bacteria for therapy and immunomodulation in man, *FEMS Microbiol. Rev.,* 12:202–220, 1993.

Miraglia del Giudice, M. and De Luca, M.G., The role of probiotics in the clinical management of food allergy and atopic dermatitis, *J. Clin. Gastroenterol.,* 38:S84–S85, 2004.

Nardone, G. and Rocco, A., Probiotics: A potential target for the prevention and treatment of steatohepatitis, *J. Clin. Gastroenterol.,* 38:S121–S122, 2004.

Otles, S., Cagindi, O., and Akcicek, E., Probiotics and health, *Asian Pac. J. Cancer Prev.,* 4:369–372, 2003.

Salimen, S., Bouley, C., Boutron-Ruault, M.C., Cummings, J.H., Franck, A., Gibson, G.R., Isolauri, E., Moreau, M-C., Roberfroid, M., and Rowlands, J., Functional food science and gastrointestinal physiology and function, *Br. J. Nutr.,* 80 (Suppl. 1): S147–171, 1988.

Salimen, S., Isolauri, E., and Salimen, E., Clinical uses of probiotics for stabilizing the gut micosal barrier: Successful strains and future challenges, *Antonie Van Leeuwenhok,* 70:347–358, 1996.

Sanders, M.E., Summary of the conclusions from a consensus panel of experts on health attributes of lactic cultures: significance to fluid milk products containing cultures, *J. Dairy Sci.,* 76:1819–1828, 1993.

Propolis or bee glue Propolis or bee glue, a resinous plant material collected by honeybees from the buds and bark of certain plants and trees, may serve as a defense for their hives (Ghisalberti, 1979). A number of health benefits have been ascribed to propolis, including anti-cancer (Matsuno, 1995), antimicrobial (Koo et al., 2000), anti-inflammatory, and antibiotic (Bianchini and Bendendo, 1998) properties. Propolis contains many different types of fla-vonoids and cinnamic-acid derivatives, some of which are known antitumor agents. One of the components identified by Matsuno et al. (1997) was artepillin C (3,5-diprenyl-4-hydroxycin-namic acid). This compound was shown to reduce tumors in experimental-animal models

Artepillin C. (From Uto et al., *J. Org. Chem.,* 67: 2355–2357, 2002.)

(Kimoto et al., 2000, 2001). The antimutagenic properties of an ethanol extract of bee glue or propolis (EEGB) against a number of environmental mutagens was demonstrated by Jeng and coworkers (2000). These researchers reported EEGB suppressed the mutagenicity of two direct mutagens, 4-nitro-*O*-phenylenediamine (4-NO) and 1-nitropyrene (1NP), and two indirect mutagens, 2-amino-3-methylimidazo[4.5-*f*] quinoline (IQ) and benzo[α]pyrene (B[a]P in a dose-dependent manner. Sugimoto et al. (2003) recently examined the inhibitory effects of propolis granular A.P.C., an extract containing more than 35.8 µg artepillin C/g, on female A/J mice lung tumors induced by 4-(methylni-trosamino)-1-(3-pyridyl)-1-butanone (NNK), one of the most potent carcinogens among tobacco-specific nitrosamines. While lung-tumor incidence was not affected by propolis, tumor multiplicity was significantly ($p < 0.01$) reduced by 72 percent. No adverse effects were

TABLE P.56
Lipid Levels in Serum of Rats Given Alcohol and
Alcohol + Propolis for 15 Days

Parameters	Groups		
	Control	Alcohol	Alcohol + Propolis
HDL (mg/dL)	37.0 ± 0.96	7.85 ± 3.7[a]	29.8 ± 1.1[a]
LDL (mg/dL)	5.8 ± 0.73	19.0 ± 4.17[a,b]	4.28 ± 1.44
VLDL (mg/dL)	21.5 ± 1.43	29.3 ± 4.03	22.7 ± 2.94
Cholesterol (mg/dL)	62.6 ± 1.83	53.8 ± 1.19[a,b]	49.0 ± 1.54[a]
Triglyceride (mg/dL)	148 ± 7.66	146 ± 20.2[b]	114 ± 14.8[a]

[a] Significantly different from control group ($p \leq 0.05$).
[b] Significantly diferent from propolis group ($p \leq 0.05$).

Source: From Kolankaya et al., *Food Chem.*, 78:213–217, 2002. With permission.

observed from propolis granular A.P.C., suggesting possible clinical applications. Further research is warranted to substantiate the role of artepillin C and other components in the antitumor properties of propolis A.P.C.

Kolankaya and coworkers (2002) reported that Turkish *Castenea sativa* propolis exerted a protective effect against degenerative diseases and alcohol-induced oxidative stress. In the presence of propolis treatment, the alcohol-induced oxidative stressed male rats had increased HDL and decreased the LDL levels compared to the alcohol-induced stressed animals (Table P.56).

In addition, the activity of LDH enzyme increased in the presence of propolis compared to the control. These researchers suggested that propolis exerted its protective effect against degenerative diseases through its protection against free radicals.

Matsui and coworkers (2004) showed a single, oral administration of propolis extract to Sprague–Dawley rats had a potent antihyperglycemic effect, with a significant reduction of 38 percent at a dose of 20 mg/kg compared to the control. Among the active compounds isolated from this fraction, 3,4,5-tri-*O*-caffeoylquinic acid, proved to be most prominent.

References

Bianchini, L. and Bedendo, I.P., Antibiotic effect of propolis against plant pathogenic bacteria, *Scienta Agricola*, 55:149–152, 1998.

Ghisalberti, E.L., Propolis: A review, *Bee World*, 60: 59–84, 1979.

Jeng, S.N., Shih, M.K., Kao, C.M., Liu, T.Z., and Chen, S.C., Antimutagenicity of ethanol extracts of bee glue against environmental mutagens, *Food Chem. Toxicol.*, 38:893–897, 2000.

Kimoto, T., Koya, S., Hino, K., Yamamoto, Y., Nomura, Y., Micallef, M.J., Hanaya, T., Arai, S., Ikeda, M., and Kurimoto, M., Renal carcinogenesis induced by ferric nitriloacetate in mice, and protection from its Brazilian propolis and artepillin C, *Pathol. Int.*, 50:670–680, 2000.

Kimoto, T., Koya-Miyata, S., Hino, K., Micallef, M.J., Hanaya, T., Arai, S., Ikeda, M., and Kurimoto, M., Pulmonary carcinogenesis induced by ferric nitriloacetate in mice and protection from it by Brazilian propolis and artepillin C, *Virchows Arch.*, 438: 259–270, 2001.

Kolankaya, D., Selmanoglu, G., Sorkun, K., and Salih, B., Protective effects of Turkish propolis on alcohol-induced serum lipid changes and liver injury in male rats, *Food Chem.*, 78:213–217, 2002.

Koo, H., Gomes, B.P.F.A., Rosalen, P.L., Ambrosano, G.M.B., Park, Y.K., and Cury, J.A., *In vitro* antimicrobial activity of propolis and *Arnica montana* against oral pathogens, *Arch. Oral Biol.*, 45: 141–148, 2000.

Matsui, T., Ebuchi, S., Fujise, T., Abesundara, K.J., Doi, S., Yamada, H., and Matsumoto, K., Strong antihyperglycemic effects of water-soluble fraction from Brazilian propolis and its bioactive constituent, 3,4,5-tri-*O*-caffeoylquinic acid, *Biol. Pharm. Bull.*, 27:1797–1803, 2004.

P

Matsuno, T., A new clerodane diterpenoid isolated from propolis, *Z. Naturforsch.*, 50c:93–97, 1995.

Matsuno, T., Kung, S.K., Matsumoto, Y., Saito, M., and Morikawa, J., Preferential cytoxicity to tumor cells of 3.5-diprenyl-4-hydroxycinnamic acid (artepillin C) isolated from propolis, *Anticancer Res.*, 17:3565–3568, 1997.

Nagai, T., Inoue, R., Inoue, H., and Suzuki, N., Preparation and antioxidant properties of water extract of propolis, *Food Chem.*, 80:29–33, 2003.

Pascual, C., Gonzalez, R., and Torricella, R.G., Scavenging action of propolis extract against oxygen radicals, *J. Ethnopharmacol.*, 41:9–13, 1994.

Sugimoto, Y., Iba, Y., Kayasuga, R., Kirino, Y., Nishiga, M., Hossen, M.A., Okihara, K., Sugimoto, H., Yamada, H., and Kamei, C., Inhibitory effects of propolis granular A.P.C on 4-(methylnitrosamino)-1-(3-pyridyl)-1-butanone-induced lung tumorigenesis in A. J. mice, *Cancer Lett.*,193:155–159, 2003.

Uto, Y., Hirata, A., Fujita, T., Takubo, S., Nagasawa, H., and Hitoshi, H., First total synthesis of artepillin C established by *o,o′*-diprenylation of p-halophenols in water, *J. Org. Chem.*, 67:2355–2357, 2002.

Walker, P. and Crane, E., Constituents of propolis, *Apidologie*, 18:327–334, 1987.

Prostaglandins   Prostaglandins are bioactive lipids produced from arachidonic acid. They are found in many vertebrate tissues, where they act as messengers involved in reproduction and inflammatory response to infection. They exert an autocrine-paracrine function by attaching to specific prostanoid G protein-coupled receptors to activate intracellular signaling and gene transcription. For many years, prostaglandins were recognized as key molecules in reproductive biology by regulating ovulation, endometrial physiology, and proliferation of endometrial glands and menstruation (Sales and Jabbour, 2003). More recently, a role in reproductive-tract pathology was reported, including carcinomas, menorrhagia, dysmenorrhoea, and endometriosis. Although the mechanism by which prostaglandins modulate these pathologies is still unclear, a large body of evidence supports a role for them in angiogenesis, apoptosis and proliferation, tissue invasion, and

metastases and immunosuppression (Martel-Pelletier et al., 2004).

Prostaglandins thus act on a variety of cells, such as vascular smooth muscle cells, causing constriction and dilation, on platelets causing aggregation or disaggregation, and on spinal neurons causing pain. Other effects can be calcium movement, hormone regulation, and cell-growth control. Certain prostaglandins are involved with induction of labor and other reproductive processes. For example, PGE2 causes uterine contractions and has been used to induce labor. Prostaglandins are also involved in several other organs, such as the gastrointestinal tract (inhibiting acid synthesis and increasing secretion of protective mucus), increases blood flow in the kidneys, and leukotrienes, which promote constriction of bronchi associated with asthma. A recent review by Prisk and Huard (2004) examines the role of prostaglandins and their potential for therapeutic interventions.

References

Martel-Pelletier, J., Pelletier, J.P., and Fahmi, H., New insights into prostaglandin biology, *J. Rheumatol.*, 31:14–16, 2004.

Prisk, V. and Huard, J., Muscle injuries and repair: The role of prostaglandins and inflammation, *Histol. Histopathol.*, 18:1243–1256, 2003.

Jabbour, H.N. and Sales, K.J., Prostaglandin receptor signaling and function in human endometrial pathology, *Trends Endocrinol. Metab.*, 15:398–404, 2004.

Protease inhibitors *see* **Bowman-Birk protease inhibitor and Trypsin inhibitors**

Proteins *see* **Amaranth, Casein, Quinoa, and Soybean**

Prunes   Prunes (*Prunus domestica* L.) are a good source of dietary fiber, as well as phenolic compounds, ascorbic acid, and carotenoids (Bravo, 1998). The dietary fiber in prunes is

TABLE P.57
Proximate Analysis of Prune Powder

Component	Amount Per 100 Gram Portion
Protein	3.0
Fat	0.5
Total carbohydrates	80.0
Total dietary fiber	9.0

Source: Adapted from Lucas et al., *J. Nutr. Biochem.*, 11: 255–259, 2000.

composed mainly of pectin (60 percent). The major components of prune powder are shown in Table P.57. Lucas et al. (2000) reported that inclusion of 25 percent prunes in the diets of ovariectomy-induced hypercholesterolemic rats prevented a rise in serum, total, and non-HDL cholesterol concentrations.

Prunes are particularly well known for their laxative action, which is explained by their high sorbitol content. They are also a good source of energy in the form of simple sugars but do not mediate a rapid rise in blood sugar, possibly because of their high fiber, fructose, and sorbitol content. The large amounts of phenolic compounds (184 mg/kg) in prunes may aid their laxative action and delay glucose absorption (Kikuzaki et al., 2004). Phenolic compounds in prunes have also been found to inhibit human LDL oxidation *in vitro*, and thus might serve as preventive agents against chronic diseases, such as heart disease and cancer (Kayano et al., 2003). In addition, the high potassium content of prunes (745 mg/100 g) might be beneficial for cardiovascular disease. Dried prunes are also an important source of boron, which is postulated to play a role in the prevention of osteoporosis (Stacewicz-Sapuntzakis et al., 2001).

References

Bravo, L., Polyphenols: Chemistry, dietary sources, metabolism and nutritional significance, *Nutr. Rev.*, 56:317–333, 1998.

Kayano, S., Yamada, N.F., Suzuki, T., Ikami, T., Shioaki, K., Kikuzaki, H., Mitani, T., and Nakatani, N., Quantitative evaluation of antioxidant components in prunes (*Prunus domestica* L.), *J. Agric. Food Chem.*, 51:1480–1485, 2003.

Kikuzaki, H., Kayano, S., Fukutsuka, N., Aoki, A., Kasamatsu, K., Yamasaki, Y., Mitani, T., and Nakatani, N., Abscisic acid related compounds and lignans in prunes (*Prunus domestica* L.) and their oxygen radical absorbance capacity (ORAC), *J. Agric. Food Chem.*, 52:344–349, 2004.

Lucas, E.A., Juma, S., Stoecker, B.J., and Arjmandi, B.H., Prune suppresses ovariectomy-induced hypercholesterolemia in rats, *J. Nutr. Biochem.*, 11:255–259, 2000.

Stacewicz-Sapuntzakis, M., Bowen, P.E., Hussain, E.A., Damayanti-Wood, B.I., and Farnsworth, N.R., Chemical composition and potential health effects of prunes: A functional food? *Crit. Rev. Food Sci. Nutr.*, 41:251–286, 2001.

Pseudopterosins Pseudopterosins are diterpeneglycosides isolated from the Caribbean sea whip *Pseudopterogorgia elisabethae* (Octocrallia, Cnidaria). They have been shown to possess anti-inflammatory and analgesic properties (Look et al., 1986). Pseudopterosin A, a C-9 xylose glycoside isolated from the marine gorgonian *Pseudopterogorgia elisabethae*, was found to be effective in reducing PMA-induced mouse-ear edema when administered topically. Mayer et al. (1998) showed it inhibited prostaglandin ER2 and leukotriene C4 production in zymosan-stimulated murine peritoneal macrophages, suggesting pseudopterosin A mediated anti-inflammatory effects by inhibiting ecosanoid release from inflammatory cells. The nonsteroidal, anti-inflammatory, and analgesic properties of pseudopterosins were shown to be greater than the industry standard drug, indomethacin. This led investigators to examine the biosynthesis and enzymology of these compounds to develop a biotechnology production method (Kohl et al., 2003). Ata and coworkers (2003) identified a number of new pseudopterosins and seco-pseudopterosins from marine gorgonian *Pseudoprerogorgia elisabethae*, as well as a novel hydroxyquinone, elisabethadione. The anti-inflammatory properties of the latter, however, proved more potent than either pseudopterosin A or E. Seven new pseudopterosins, P–V, were identified recently by Duque et al. (2004) from gorgonian octocoral

P

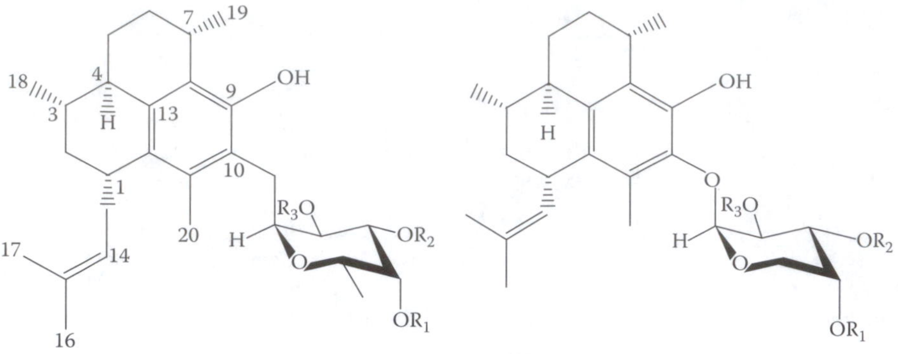

1: $R_1, R_2, R_3 = H$
2: $R_1 = Ac, R_2, R_3 = H$
3: $R_2 = Ac, R_1, R_3 = H$
4: $R_3 = Ac, R_1, R_2 = H$

5: $R_1, R_2, R_3 = H$
6: $R_1 = Ac, R_2, R_3 = H$
7: $R_2 = Ac, R_1, R_3 = H$

SCHEME P.48 New pseudopterosins isolated from *Pseudopterogorgia elisabethae* from Providencia island, Colombian Caribbean. (From Duque et al., *Tetrahedron*, 60:10627–10635, 2004. With permission.)

Pseudopterogorgia elisabethae from Providencia Island in the Colombian Caribbean, as shown in Scheme P.48. However, their health-related properties still remain to be studied.

References

Atta, A., Kerr, R.G., Moya, C.E., and Jacobs, R.S., Identification of anti-inflammatory diterpenes from the marine gorgonian *Pseudopterogorgia elisabethae*, *Tetrahedron*, 59:4215–4222, 2003.

Duque, C., Puyana, M., Narvaez, G., Osorno, O., Hara, N., and Fujimoto, Y., Pseudopterosins P–V, new compounds from gorgonian octocoral *Pseudopterogorgia elisabethae* from Providencia island, Columbian Caribbean, *Tetrahedron*, 60: 10627–10635, 2004.

Kohl, A.C., Ata, A., and Kerr, R.G., Pseudopterosin biosynthesis — pathway elucidation, enzymology, and a proposed production method for anti-inflammatory metabolites from *Pseudopterogorgia elisabethae*, *J. Ind. Microbiol. Biotechnol.*, 30:495–499, 2003.

Look, S.A., Fenical, W., Jacobs, R.S., and Clardy, J., The pseudopterosins: Anti-inflammatory and analgesic natural products from the sea whip *Pseudopterogorgia elisabethae*, *Proc. Natl. Acad. Sci. U.S.A.*, 83:6238–6340, 1986.

Mayer, A.M., Jacobson, P.B., Fenical, W., Jacobs, R.S., and Glaser, K.B., Pharmacological characterization of the pseudopterosins: Novel anti-inflammatory natural products isolated from the Caribbean soft coral, *Pseudopterogorgia elisabethae*, *Life Sci.*, 62:PL401–PL407, 1998.

Psyllium Psyllium is the mucilage obtained from the seed coat (husk or hull) of the plant genus *Plantago*. It has a long history of medicinal use because of its cholesterol-lowering, laxative, gastro-hypoacidity, and possibly weight-control properties (Anderson et al., 1990; Arjmandi et al., 1992; Hara et al., 1996; Park et al., 1997). A meta-analysis of 12 studies involving 404 adults with mild to moderate hypercholesterolemia by Olson et al. (1997) concluded that psyllium reduced total and LDL cholesterol by 5 percent and 9 percent, respectively. A study on 125 patients with type 2 diabetes by Rodriguez-Moran et al. (1998) found that treatment with 5 grams of psyllium t.i.d. over six weeks significantly reduced ($p < 0.05$) fasting plasma glucose (Figure P.83), as well as total plasma cholesterol, LDL cholesterol, and triglycerides, while significantly increasing ($p < 0.01$) HDL cholesterol.

Fang (2000) showed that psyllium improved the serum-lipid profiles in Sprague–Dawley rats by reversing the hypercholesterolemic effects of *trans* fatty acids. Recently, Marlett and Fischer (2003) reported that a gel-forming component in psyllium seeds, which was not fermented, was responsible for its laxative and cholesterol-lowering properties. The active fraction was a highly branched arabinoxylan consisting of a xylose backbone and arabinose- and xylose-containing side chains.

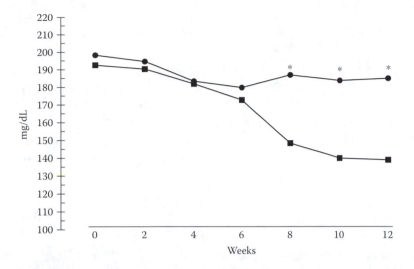

FIGURE P.83 Mean plasma-glucose levels. In the period of diet counseling (weeks 0–6), there were mild but not significant variations on glucose levels for both groups. The treatment beginning at week 6, and during all this period (to week 12), the patients on psyllium group (■) showed a greater and statistically significant reduction in plasma-glucose levels compared to the placebo group (●). Asterisk indicates a significant difference at $p < 0.01$. (From Rodriguez-Moran et al., *J. Diab. Comp.*, 12:273–278, 1998. With permission.)

Psyllium was shown to improve glucose homeostasis and the lipid and lipoprotein profiles in obese children and adolescents with abnormalities in carbohydrate and lipid metabolism (Moreno et al., 2003). Beneficial, therapeutic effects reported for psyllium include the metabolic control of type 2 diabetes, as well as lowering the risk of coronary heart disease (Sierra et al., 2002).

The synergistic effect of wheat bran and psyllium was shown by Albaster et al. (1993) to inhibit the early phases of carcinogenesis. Cohen et al. (1996) also reported the effects of wheat bran and psyllium diets in reducing *N*-methylnitrosourea-induced mammary tumorigenesis in F344 rats. The antitumor activity of psyllium was recently demonstrated by Nakamura et al. (2004), who showed it restored normal gap junctional intercellular communication (GJIC) and anchorage-independent growth (AIG) by reversing two tumor-cell phenotypes induced by the *Ha-ras* oncogene.

While no adverse effects have been associated with psyllium intake, nevertheless some individuals may be allergic to it (James et al., 1991). In addition, Luccia and Kunkel (2002) showed that an increase in soluble fiber from sources such as psyllium reduced calcium bioavailability in weanling Wistar rats, as well as had negative effects on bone composition. The increased consumption of psyllium, however, has since led to its recognition as an emerging food allergen (Khalili et al., 2003)

References

Alabaster, O., Tang, Z.C., Frost, A., and Shivapurkar, N., Potential synergism between wheat bran and psyllium: Enhanced inhibition of colon cancer, *Cancer Lett.,* 75:53–58, 1993.

Anderson, J., Deakins, D.A., Floore, T.L., Smith, B.M., and Whitis, S.E., Dietary fiber and coronary heart disease, *Crit. Rev. Food Sci. Nutr.,* 29:95–146, 1990.

Arjmandi, B.H., Craig, J., Nathani, S., and Reeves, R.D., Soluble dietary fiber and cholesterol influence *in vivo* hepatic intestinal cholesterol biosynthesis in rats, *J. Nutr.,* 122:1559–1565, 1992.

Cohen, L.A., Zhao, Z., Zang, E.A., Wynn, T.T., Simi, B., and Rivenson, A., Wheat bran and psyllium diets: Effects on *N*-methylnitrosourea-induced mammary tumorigenesis in F344 rats, *J. Natl. Cancer Inst.,* 88: 899–907, 1996.

Fang, C., Dietary psyllium reverses hypercholesterolemic effect of *trans* fatty acids in rats, *Nutr. Res.,* 20:695–705, 2000.

Hara, H., Suzuki, K., Koyabashi, S., and Kasai, T., Fermentable property of dietary fiber may not determine cecal and colonic mucosal growth in fiber-fed rats, *J. Nutr. Biochem.*, 7:549–554, 1996.

James, J.M., Cooke, S.K., Barnett, A., and Sampson, H.A., Anaphylactic reactions to psyllium-containing cereal, *J. Allergy Clin. Immunol.*, 88:402–408, 1991.

Khalili, B., Bardana, E.J., Jr., and Yunginger, J.W., Psyllium-associated anaphylaxis and death: A case report and review of the literature, *Ann. Allergy Asthma Immunol.*, 91:579–584, 2003.

Luccia, B.D.H. and Kunkel, M.E., Psyllium reduces calcium bioavailability and induces negative changes in bone consumption in weanling Wistar rats, *Nutr. Res.*, 22:1027–1040, 2002.

Marlett, J.A. and Fischer, M.H., The active fraction of psyllium seed husk, *Proc. Nutr. Soc.*, 62:207–209, 2003.

Moreno, L.A., Tresaco, B., Bueno, G., Fleta, J., Rodriguez, G., Garagorri, J.M., and Bueno, M., Psyllium fibre and the metabolic control of obese children and adolescents, *J. Physiol. Biochem.*, 59:235–242, 2003.

Nakamura, Y., Trosko, J.E., Chang, C.-C., and Upham, B.L., Psyllium extracts decreased neoplastic phenotypes induced by the *Ha-Ras* oncongene transfected into a rat liver oval cell line, *Cancer Lett.*, 203:13–24, 2004.

Olson, B.H., Anderson, S.M., Becker, M.P., Anderson, J.W., Hunninghake, D.B., Jenkins, D.J.A., Larosa, J.C., Rippe, J.M., Roberts, D.C.K., Stoy, D.B., Summerbell, C.D., Truswell, A.S., Wolever, T.M.S., Morris, D.H., and Fulgoni, V.L., Psyllium-enriched cereals lowers blood total cholesterol and LDL cholesterol, but not HDL cholesterol, in hypercholesterolemic adults: Results EF a meta-analysis, *J. Nutr.*, 127:1973–1980, 1997.

Park, H., Seib, P.A., and Chung, O.K., Fortifying bread with a mixture of wheat fiber and psyllium husk fiber plus three antioxidants, *Cereal Chem.*, 74:207–211, 1997.

Rodriguez-Moran, M., Guerrero-Romero, F., and Lazcano-Burciaga, G., Lipid- and glucose-lowering efficacy of Plantago psyllium in type II diabetes, *J. Diab. Comp.*, 12:273–278, 1998.

Sierra, M., Garcia, J.J., Fernandez, N., Diez, M.J., and Calle, A.P., Therapeutic effects of psyllium in type 2 diabetic patients, *Eur. J. Clin. Nutr.*, 56:830–842, 2002.

Pulses *see also* **Beans, Lentils, and Soybeans**   Pulses are the health-promoting, edible seeds of leguminous plants grown for food and include peas, beans, and lentils (Messina et al., 1999). The nonnutrient, bioactive agents in pulses were reviewed by Champ (2002). While many were considered antinutritional factors, subsequent research suggests many of these compounds may play a role in the prevention of chronic diseases. A list of these compounds can be found in Table P.58.

Anderson and Major (2002) reviewed both the epidemiological and clinical data, which supported the hypocholesterolemic effect of soybean and pulses. In addition, they performed a meta-analysis of 11 clinical trials that showed pulses decreased cholesterol and LDL cholesterol while increasing HDL cholesterol. These effects were attributed to the presence of soluble dietary fiber, protein, oligosaccharides, isoflavones, phospholipids, fatty acids, and

TABLE P.58
Major Nonnutrient Bioactive Pulse Compounds

Bioactive Component	Possible Beneficial Effects
Amylase inhibitors	Diabetes treatment
Lectins	Obesity and tumors
Phenolic compounds	
Flavonoids, isoflavones	Menopause and anticancer
Lignans (phytoestrogens)	Menopause
Protease inhibitors	Anticarcinogenic
Saponins	Hypocholesterolemic, anticancer

Source: Adapted from Champ, *Br. J. Nutr.*, 88:S307–S319, 2002.

saponins. Additional benefits included reduction in blood pressure, glycemia, and the risk for obesity.

References

Anderson, J.W. and Major, A.W., Pulses and lipaemia, short- and long-term effect: Potential prevention of cardiovascular disease, *Br. J. Nutr.,* 88(Suppl. 3):S263–S271, 2002.

Champ, M. M.-J., Non-nutrient bioactive substances of pulses, *Br. J. Nutr.,* 88(Suppl. 3):S307–S319, 2002.

Messina, M.J., Legumes and soybeans: An overview of their nutritional profiles and health effects, *Am. J. Clin. Nutr.,* 70:439S–450S, 1999.

Purple corn color   Purple corn color (PCC) is a natural anthocyanin pigment that was found by Hagiwara and coworkers (2001) to have anticancer properties. When fed at a dietary level of 5 percent to male F344/DuCrj rats, pretreated with 1,2-dimethylhydrazine (DMH) to develop colorectal carcinogenesis, it suppressed lesions, as well as decreased the induction of aberrant crypts by the presence of 2-amino-1-methyl-6-phenylimidazo[4,5-*b*]pyridine (PhIP) in the diet.

References

Hagiwara, A., Miyashita, K., Nakanishi, T., Sano, M., Tamano, S., Kadota, T., Koda, T., Nakamura, M., Imaida, K., Ito, N., and Shirai, T., Pronounced inhibition by a natural anthocyanin, purple corn color, of 2-amino-1-methyl-6-phenylimidazo[4,5-*b*]pyridine (PhIP)-associated colorectal carcinogenesis in male F344 rats pretreated with 1,2-dimethylhydrazine, *Cancer Lett.,* 171:17–25, 2001.

Pycnogenol   Pycnogenol is a mixture of oligomeric and monomeric procyandins isolated from the bark extract of French maritime pine (*Pinus pinaster*) (Masquelier, 1997). Composed of water-soluble procyanidins, catechin, taxofolin, and phenolcarbonic acid, it is used as a dietary supplement. Hosseini et al. (2001) showed Pycnogenol® (200 mg/day) lowered diastolic blood pressure, but not statistically, in mildly hypertensive patients. However, serum-thromboxane levels were reduced significantly during treatment.

Using a rat pheochromocytoma (PC12) cell line, Peng et al. (2002) found Pycnogenol® protected neurons from amyloid-β peptide-induced apoptosis, one of the pathological features associated with Alzheimer's disease. Pycnogenol decreased the percentage of apoptotic cells and inhibited caspase-3 activation, DNA fragmentation, and poly(ADP-ribase) polynerase (PARP) cleavage. The possible involvement of oxidative stress was evident by Pycnogenol®'s suppression of amyloid-β peptide's generation of reactive-oxygen species (ROS), as evident in the presence of vitamin E. Thus, the antioxidant properties of Pycnogenol® appeared partly responsible for reducing these cells from amyloid-β peptide's neurotoxicity. Huang et al. (2005) recently reported Pycnogenol® induced differentiation and apoptosis in human promyeloid leukemia HL-60 cells, suggesting it could act as a potent cancer chemopreventive or chemotherapeutic agent.

The role of ROS in inflammatory processes, such as rheumatic diseases, led to a recent study by Grimm et al. (2004) on matrix-degrading enzymes, matrix metalloproteinases (MMPs). MMPs are a family of zinc-dependent proteolytic enzymes activated by ROS that contribute to the inflammatory network (Visse and Nagase, 2003; Rajagopalan et al., 1996). Two major metabolites of the standardized pine-bark extract Pycnogenol®, M1 and M2, were identified by Grosse-Duweler and Rohdewald (2000), with strong reducing power (Scheme P.49). Grimm et al. (2004) showed M1 and M2 strongly inhibited matrix metalloproteinase MMP-1, as shown in Figure P.84. Similar inhibitory effects were also observed on MMP-2 and MMP-9. M1 proved a more effective scavenger of superoxide than (+)-catechin, ascorbic acid, and trolox, while M2 had no scavenging activity. These results point to the potential prophylaxis and therapeutic uses of Pycnogenol® in disorders resulting from an imbalance or excess of metalloproteinase activity.

Recent research by Liu et al. (2004a) suggested that supplementation of mildly hypertensive patients with Pycnogenol® significantly reduced the dosage of the antihypertensive drug, nidipine. A double-blind, placebo-controlled, randomized, multicenter study by Liu et al. (2004b) on 77 diabetes type 2 patients

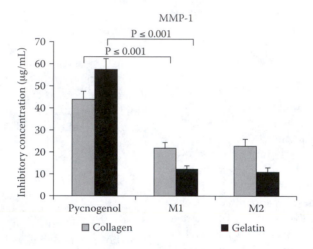

M1
*-(3,4-dihydroxyphenyl)-(-valerolactone)

M2
*-(3,4methoxy-4-hydroxyphenyl)-(-valerolactone)

SCHEME P.49 The two main metabolites of Pycnogenol® identified in human urine. (From Grosse-Duweler and Rohdewald, *Pharmazie*, 55:364–368, 2000. With permission.)

FIGURE P.84 Mean concentrations of Pycnogenol®, M1, and M2 that produced 50 percent inhibition of MMP-1 activity toward degradation of collagen or gelatin, respectively. Each column represents the mean and SD of six independent experiments. Statistically significant differences between compounds are shown only for metabolite M1 (ANOVA with subsequent Tukey test). (From Grimm et al., *Free Rad. Biol. Med.*, 36:811–822, 2004. With permission.)

also showed multiple benefits were derived from supplementation with 100 mg Pycnogenol® over 12 weeks, including significantly lowering of plasma-glucose levels. Other benefits included inhibiting endothelin-1 production, expression of adhesion molecules, and platelet aggregation.

Durackova et al. (2003) found Pycnogenol® was beneficial in the treatment of erectile dysfunction, as well as improving the atherogenic factor of lipoproteins and antioxidant status of plasma. Mantle et al. (2005) recently noted pycnogenol was part of a nutritional supplement that included calcium, carnitine, coenzyme Q_{10}, glucosamine, magnesium, methyl sulfonyl methane, silica, vitamin C, and vitamin K, which proved effective in treating Ehlers–Dantos

syndrome, a rare, inherited disorder of the connective tissue.

References

Durackova, Z., Trebaticky, B., Novotny, V., Zitnanova, I., and Breza, J., Lipid metabolism and erectile function improvement by Pycnogenol® extract from the bark of *Pinus pinaster* in patients suffering from erectile dysfunction — a pilot study, *Nutr. Res.*, 23:1189–1198, 2003.

Grimm, T., Schafer, A., and Hogger, P., Antioxidant activity and inhibition of matrix metalloproteinases by metabolites of maritime pine bark extract (Pycnogenol), *Free Rad. Biol. Med.*, 36:811–822, 2004.

Grosse-Duweler, K.G. and Rohdewald, P., Urinary metabolites of French maritime pine bark extract in humans, *Pharmazie*, 55:364–368, 2000.

Hosseini, S., Lee, J., Sepulveda, R.T., Rohdewald, P., and Watson, R.R., A randomized, double-blind, placebo-controlled, prospective, 16 week crossover study to determine the role of Pycnogenol in modifying blood pressure in mildly hypertensive patients, *Nutr. Res.,* 21:1251–1260, 2001.

Huang, W.W., Yang, J.S., Lin, C.F., Ho, W.J., and Lee, M.R., Pycnogenol induces differentiation and apoptosis in human promyeloid leukemia HL-60 cells, *Leukemia Res.,* 29:685–692, 2005.

Liu, X., Wei, J., Tan, F., Zhou, S., Wurthwein, G., and Rohdewald, P., Pycnogenol®, French maritime pine bark extract, improves endothelial function of hypertensive patients, *Life Sci.,* 74:855–862, 2004a.

Liu, X., Wei, J., Tan, F., Zhou, S., Wurthwein, G., and Rohdewald, P., Antidiabetic effect of Pycnogenol® French maritime pine bark extract in patients with diabetes type II, *Life Sci.,* 75:2505–2513, 2004b.

Mantle, D., Wilkins, R.M., and Preedy, V., A novel therapeutic strategy for Ehlers-Danlos syndrome based on nutritional supplements, *Med. Hypotheses,* 64:279–283, 2005.

Masquelier, J., Plant extract with a proanthcyanidins content as therapeutic agent having radical scavenging effect and use thereof, U.S. patent 4,698,360, 1987.

Peng, Q.L., Buz'Zard, A.R., and Lau, B.H.S., Pycnogenol® protects neurons from amyloid-β peptide-induced apoptosis, *Mol. Brain Res.,* 104:55–65, 2002.

Rajagopalan, S., Meng, X.P., Ramasamy, S., Harrison, D.G., and Galis, Z.S., Reactive oxygen species produced by macrophage-derived foam cells regulate the activity of vascular matrix metalloproteinases *in vitro*: Implications for atherosclerotic plaque stability, *J. Clin. Invest.,* 98:2572–2579, 1996.

Visse, R. and Nagase, H., Matrix metalloproteinases and tissue inhibitors of metaloproteinases: Structure, function, and biochemistry, *Circ. Res.,* 92:827–839, 2003.

P

Q

Quercetin Quercetin (3,3′,4′,5,7-pentahy-droxyflavone) is one of the most abundant bioflavonoids in edible fruits and vegetables, with an estimated daily intake of 25–50 mg (Formica and Regelson 1995). It is associated with little toxicity when administered orally or

Quercetin. (From Igura et al., *Cancer Lett.,* 171:11–16, 2001. With permission.)

intravenously. Quercetin is a potential antican-cer agent through its cell-cycle regulation, inter-action with type II estrogen-binding sites (Shenouda et al., 2004), and inhibition of tyrosine kinase. *In vitro* studies showed quer-cetin inhibited tumor growth and proliferation of tumor cells by reducing the number of aber-rant crypt foci (Lamson and Brignall, 2000). A possible mechanism is that quercetin upregu-lates expression of several tumor-suppressor genes (Nair et al., 2004; Van Erk, 2004). A recent study by Mertens-Talcott and Percival (2005) reported a synergistic interaction between quercetin and ellagic acid with resver-atrol in the induction of apoptosis and cell-cycle kinetics in a human leukemia-cell line (MOLT-4). For example, caspase-3 activation, which precedes apoptosis, was induced in 35 percent of the treated cells (EC_{35}) by 12.8 mmol/L for quercetin, 54.0 mmol/L for resveratrol, and 68.4 mmol/L for ellagic acid (Figure Q.85A). The EC_{35} for the combinations of quercetin:res-veratrol and ellagic acid:resveratrol were 6.4 mol/L and 16.9 mol/L, respectively (Figure Q.85B).

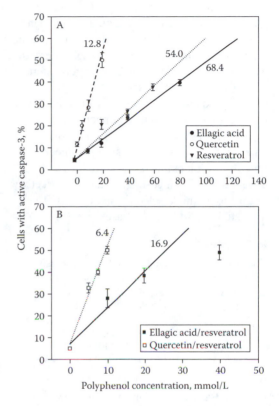

FIGURE Q.85 Caspase-3 activity in MOLT-4 cells after 10 h of treatment with ellagic acid, quercetin, or resveratrol (A) and 1:1 combinations of these (B). Values are means + SEM, n = 4. Numbers above each data line represent the EC_{35}, as determined by linear regression. *The line was generated from the linear portion of the curve; therefore, the value induced by the highest concentration was not included in the calculation. (From Mertens-Talcott and Percival, *Cancer Lett.,* 218:141–151, 2005. With permission.)

Epidemiological studies point to a crucial role for quercetin in the prevention of cardio-vascular disease. There is an inverse relation-ship between dietary flavonoids, particularly quercetin, and the risk of cardiovascular disease (Hertog et al., 1993). This protective effect is attributed to quercetin's antioxidant capacity and its inhibition of LDL oxidation *in vitro*

(Janisch et al., 2004). The antiproliferative and antimutagenic activities of quercetin *in vitro* have made it a candidate for clinical trials in cancer therapy (Hertog, 1996).

Cornish et al. (2002) showed quercetin played a possible role in reducing the incidence of cataracts by inhibiting oxidative damage in rat lenses. Using the LOCH model, quercetin was converted by catechol-*O*-methyltransferase (COMT) in the rat lenses to its metabolite, 3-*O*-methyl quercetin, both of which inhibited hydrogen peroxide-induced opacification.

Muthian and Bright (2004) found quercetin ameliorated experimental allergic encephalomyelitis by blocking IL-12 signaling and Th1 differentiation, suggesting it may be effective in treating multiple sclerosis and other Th1-cell-mediated autoimmune diseases.

References

Cornish, K.M., Williamson, G., and Sanderson, J., Quercetin metabolism in the lens: Role in inhibition of hydrogen peroxide induced cataract, *Free Rad. Biol. Med.,* 33:63–70, 2002.

Formica, J.V. and Regelson, W., Review of the biology of quercetin and related bioflavonoids, *Food Chem. Toxicol.,* 33:1061–1080, 1995.

Hertog, M.G.L., Feskens, E.J.M., Hollman, P.C.H., Katan, M.B., and Kromhout, D., Dietary antioxidant flavonoids and risk of coronary heart disease — the Zutphen elderly study, *Lancet,* 342:1007–1011, 1993.

Hertog, M.G.L. and Hollman, P.C., Potential effect of the dietary flavonol quercetin, *Eur. J. Clin. Nutr.,* 50:63–71, 1996.

Igura, K., Ohta, T., Kuroda, Y., and Kaji, K., Resveratrol and quercetin inhibit angiogenesis *in vitro*, *Cancer Lett.,* 171:11–16, 2001.

Janisch, K.M., Williamson, G., Needs, P., and Plumb, G.W., Properties of quercetin conjugates: Modulation of LDL oxidation and binding of human serum albumin, *Free Rad. Res.,* 38:877–884, 2004.

Lamson, D.W. and Brignall, M.S., Antioxidants and cancer, Part 3. Quercetin, *Altern. Med. Rev.,* 5:196–208, 2000.

Mertens-Talcott, S.U. and Percival, S.S., Ellagic acid and quercetin interact synergistically with resveratrol in the induction of apoptosis and cause transient cell cycle arrest in human leukemia cells, *Cancer Lett.,* 218:141–151, 2005.

Muthian, G. and Bright, J.J., Quercetin, a flavonoid phytoestrogen, ameliorates experimental allergic encephalomyelitis by blocking IL-12 signaling through JAK-STAT pathway in T lymphocyte, *J. Clin. Immunol.,* 24:542–552, 2004.

Nair, H.K., Rao, K.V.K., Aalinkeel, R., Mahajan, S., Chawda, R., and Schwartz, S.A., Inhibition of prostate cancer cell colony formation by the flavonoid quercetin correlates with modulation of specific regulatory genes, *Clin. Diagn. Lab Immunol.,* 11:63–69, 2004.

Shenouda, N.S., Zhou, C., Browning, J.D., Ansell, P.J., Sakla, M.S., Lubahn, D.B., and Macdonald, R.S., Phytoestrogens in common herbs regulate prostate cancer cell growth *in vitro*, *Nutr. Cancer*, 49:200–208, 2004.

Van Erk, M.J., Roepman, P., Van Der Lende, T.R., Stierum, R.H., Aarts, J.M., Van Bladeren, P.J., and Van Ommen, B., Integrated assessment by multiple gene expression analysis of quercetin bioactivity on anticancer-related mechanisms in colon cancer cells *in vitro*, *Eur. J. Nutr.,* 30:1–14, 2004.

Quinic acid *see also* **Cat's claw** Quinic acid, a water-soluble, organic acid, is a metabolite of the shikimic-acid pathway in plants. Akesson et al. (2005) identified quinic acid as the active component in the hot-water extract (C-Med-100®)

Quinic acid. (Adapted from Banwell et al., *Org. Lett.,* 6:2737–2740, 2004.)

from the bark of Cat's Claw (*Uncaria tomentosa*). The water extract from *U. tomentosa* has been associated with the anti-inflammatory properties of Cat's Claw (Aquino et al., 1991; Lemaire et al., 1999). While the content of free quinic acid was low in the water extract, it was present in the form of esters. Quinic acid was shown to inhibit NF-κB in cells grown in tissue culture *in vitro* by a different mechanism than C-Med-100®. Recent work by Sheng and

TABLE Q.59
The Coupling of the Disappearance of *In Vitro* Biological Efficacy of C-Med-100 Assessed in HL-60 and HML Cells to a Corresponding Disappearance in CAE Content Analyzed as QA Esters by the Bartos Reaction

Compound	HL-60 MTT IC_{50} (µg/mL)	HML MTT 2x #cells (µg/mL)	%QA est. (Bartos)	QA est. TLC Identical
QA	2300	>2300	0	++++
QAL	2300	>2300	100	0
QAL + 2MNaOH, 2 h	1900	>2300	35	++
C-Med-100 (no base hydrolysis)	536	500	4.7	±
C-Med-100 (M NaOH for 2 h)	900	1200	2.5	++

Source: From Sheng et al., *J. Ethnopharmacol.*, 96:577–584, 2005. With permission.

coworkers (2005) showed the active ingredients in C-Med 100® were carboxyl alkyl esters (CAEs), that enhance DNA repair and immune cell responses. Their disappearance was responsible for the loss in biological efficacy of C-Med-100®. Thus the data presented in Table Q.59, in which quinic-acid lactone (QAL) and C-Med-100® preparations were far more effective in reducing the growth of human leukemic cells (HL-60) and human mononuclear leukocytes (HML). This was assessed using the MTT vital staining colorimetric bioassay, which is only taken up by the viable cells but cannot distinguish between those replicating and not replicating.

References

Akesson, C., Lindgren, H., Pero, R.W., Leanderson, T., and Ivars, F., Quinic acid is a biologically active component of the *Uncaria tomentosa* extract C-Med-100®, *Int. Immunopharmacol.*, 5:219–229, 2005.

Aquino, R., De Feo, V., De Simona, F., Pizza, C., and Cirino, G., Plant metabolites. New compounds and anti-inflammatory activity of *Uncaria tomentosa*, *J. Nat. Prod.*, 54:453–459, 1991.

Banwell, M.G., Hungerford, N.L., and Jolliffe, K.A., Synthesis of the sialic acid (–)-KDN and certain epimers from (–)-3-dehydroshikimic acid or (–)-quinic acid, *Org. Lett.*, 6:2737–2740, 2004.

Lemaire, I., Assinewe, V., Cano, P., Awang, D.V., and Arnason, J.T., Stimulation of interleukin-1 and -6 production in alveolar macrophages by the neotropical liana, *Uncaria tomentosa* (Una de Gato), *J. Ethnopharmacol.*, 64:109–115, 1999.

Sheng, Y., Akesson, C., Holmgren, K., Bryngelsson, C., Giamapa, V., and Pero, R.W., An active ingredient of Cat's Claw water extracts. Identification and efficacy of quinic acid, *J. Ethnopharmacol.*, 96:577–584, 2005.

Quince   Quince (*Cyndonia oblonga* Miller) is a pome fruit of a deciduous tree of the *Rosaceae* family. The fruit is inedible due to its hardness, bitterness, and astringency and is generally processed and used for its jam, called "marmaleda" (Silva et al., 2005).

The antioxidant activity of quince was examined by Silva et al. (2004). The wide array of phenolic compounds identified in quince fruit and jam are shown in Scheme Q.50. In addition, seven organic acids were also identified, including ascorbic, shikimic, quinic, oxalic, citric, malic, and fumaric acids. The strongest antioxidant activity was observed in the peel, while the pulp and seed exhibited lower but similar activities. The peel and seed extracts, however, both had the strongest antiradical activity compared to the pulp. This study suggested that quince fruit and jam were a rich and inexpensive source of antioxidants, which could play a role in the prevention of free-radical-related chronic diseases. The antioxidant activity was attributed primarily to the presence of phenolic compounds.

References

Silva, B.M., Andrade, P.B., Martins, R.C., Valentao, P., Ferreres, F., Seabra, R.M., and Ferreira, M.A., Quince (*Cyndonia oblonga* Miller) fruit characterization using

Q

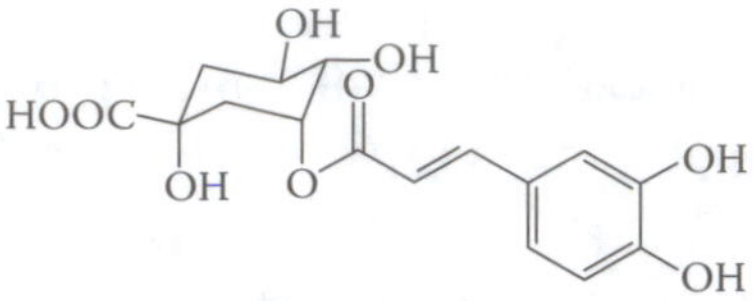

3-*O*-caffcoylquinic acid

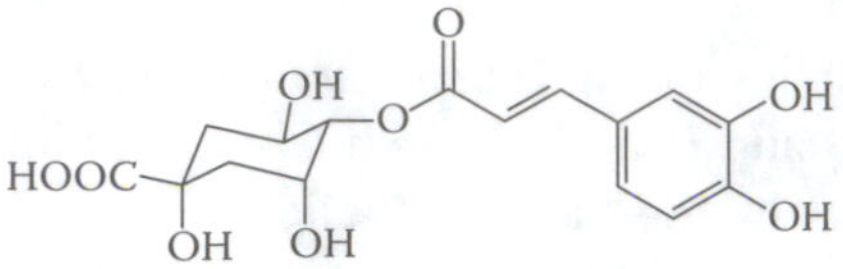

4-*O*-caffcoylquinic acid

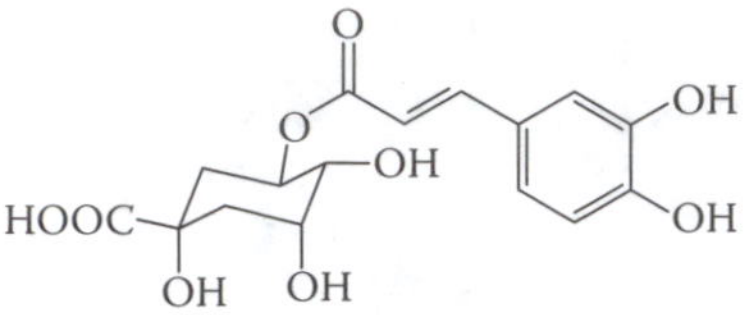

5-*O*-caffcoylquinic acid

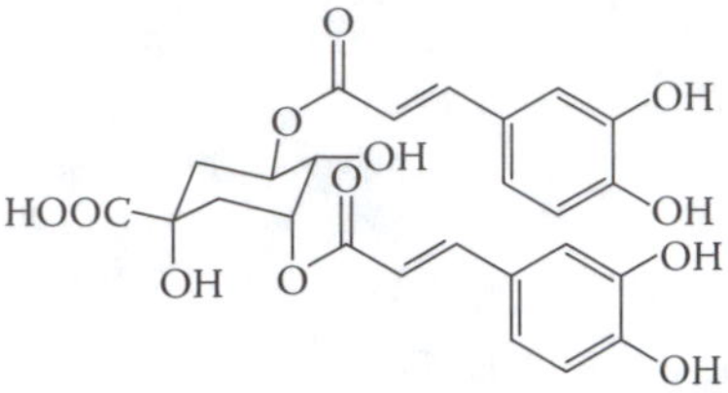

3, 5-*O*-dicaffcoylquinic acid

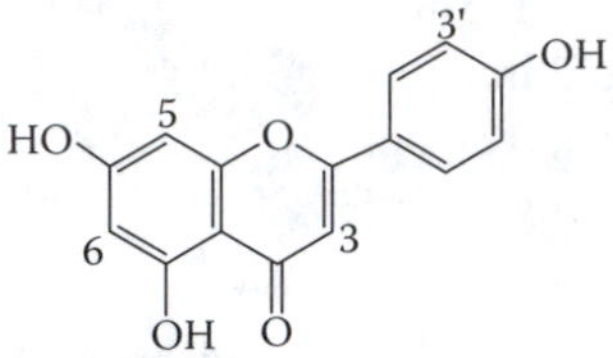

Compound	3	6	8	3′
Quercetin 3-galactoside	O-Galactose	H	H	OH
Rutin	O-Rutinose	H	H	OH
Kaempferol 3-glucoside	O-Glucose	H	H	H
Kaempferol 3-rutinoside	O-Rutinose	H	H	H
Vicenin-2	H	Glucose	Glucose	H
Isoschaftoside	H	Arabinose	Glucose	H
Schaftoside	H	Glucose	Arabinose	H
Lucenin-2	H	Glucose	Glucose	OH
Stellarin-2	H	Glucose	Glucose	OCH$_3$
6-*C*-pentosyl-8-*C*-glucoside of chrysoeriol	H	Pentose	Glucose	OCH$_3$
6-*C*-glucosyl-8-*C*-pentoside of chrysoeriol	H	Glucose	Pentose	OCH$_3$

SCHEME Q.50 Phenolic compounds of quince fruit and jam. (From Silva et al., *J. Agric. Food Chem.,* 52: 4705–4712, 2004. With permission.)

principal component analysis, *J. Agric. Food Chem.,* 53:111-122, 2005.

Silva, B.C., Andrade, P.B., Valentao, P., Ferreres, F., Seabra, R.M., and Ferreira, M.A., Quince (*Cyndonia oblonga* Miller) fruit (pulp, peel, and seed) and jam: Antioxidant activity, *J. Agric. Food Chem.,* 52:4705–4712, 2004.

Quinoa Quinoa (*Chenopodium quinoa*) is a hardy and nutritious Latin American pseudocereal (Ahamed et al., 1998). The seeds contain 15.6 percent crude protein, 7.7 percent fat, 69.5 percent carbohydrate, and 2.5 percent crude fiber (Chauhan et al., 1993). It has a high proportion of D-xylose (120.0 mg/100 g sample) and maltose (101.0 mg/100 g sample), and a low content of glucose (19.0 mg/100 g sample) and fructose (19.6 mg/g sample) (Ogungbenle, 2003). In general, the content of essential amino acids in quinoa is higher than in common cereals. Animal experiments showed NPU values of 75.7 and a biological value of 82.6 for the protein in raw quinoa. *In vitro* enzymatic methods showed that the digestibility of protein in quinoa was comparable to other high-quality food proteins (Chauhan et al., 1999; Ruales and Nair, 1992).

At least 16 saponins were detected in the seeds of *Chenopodium quinoa* exhibiting antifungal activity against *Candida albicans* and hemolytic activity on erythrocytes (Woldemichael and Wink, 2001). Estrada and coworkers (1998) reported earlier that saponins extracted from quinoa enhanced both systemic and mucosal antigen-specific antibody (IgG and IgA) responses in mice following intragastric or intranasal immunization with cholera toxin or ovalbumin. By increasing the permeability of the membrane, the quinoa saponins allowed a greater uptake of the antigen, making them a valuable adjuvant for generating systemic and mucosal responses.

Studies on minor cereals and pseudocereals without celiac activity, to meet the needs of individuals affected by celiac disease, showed the glycemic index (GI) for quinoa was slightly lower than that of gluten-free (GF) pasta and bread. In addition, quinoa induced lower free fatty-acid levels than GF pasta, and significantly lower triglyceride concentrations compared to GF bread. Thus, quinoa was a potential alternative to traditional foods demonstrating hypoglycemic effects (Berti, 2004).

Dini et al. (2004) identified a number of polyphenols in *Kancolla*, a sweet variety of *Chenopodium quinoa*. Five kaempferol and quercetin glycosides, as well as a glucoside of vanillic acid, were reported. Zhu and coworkers (2001) identified five ecdysteroids in quinoa seeds for the first time. These phytoecdysteroids were shown by Miller et al. (1985) to inhibit hypercholesterolemia and hyperglyceridimia in rats.

References

Ahamed, N.T., Singhal, R.S., Kulkarni, P.R., and Pal, M., A lesser-known grain, *Chenopodium quinoa*: Review of the chemical composition of its edible parts, *Food. Nutr. Bull.,* 19:61–70, 1998.

Berti, C., Riso, P., Monti, L.D., and Porrini, M., *In vitro* starch digestibility and *in vivo* glucose response of gluten-free foods and their gluten counterparts, *Eur. J. Nutr.,* 43:198–204, 2004.

Chauhan, G.S., Eskin, N.A.M., and Tkachuk, R., Nutrients and antinutrients in quinoa seed, *Cereal Chem.,* 69:85–88, 1992.

Chauhan, G.S., Eskin, N.A.M., and Mills, P.A., Effect of saponin extraction on the nutritional quality of quinoa (*Chenopodium quinoa* Willd.) proteins, *J. Food Sci. Technol.,* (India). 36:123–126, 1999.

Dini, I., Tenore, G.C., and Dini, A., Phenolic constituents of *Kencolla* seeds, *Food Chem.,* 84:163–168, 2004.

Estrada, A., Li, B., and Laarveld, B., Adjuvant action of *Chenopodium quinoa* saponins on the induction of antibody responses to intragastric and intranasal administered antigens in mice, *Com. Immun. Microbiol. Infect. Dis.,* 21:225–236, 1998.

Miller, R., Clardy, J., Koslowski, J., Mikolajcak, K.L., Plattner, R.D., Powell, R.G., Smith, C.R., Weisleder, D., and Zheng, Q.T., Phytoecdysteroids of *Diplolisia glaucescens* seeds, *Planta Med.,* 51:40–42, 1985.

Ogunbenle, H.N. Nutritional evaluation and functional properties of quinoa (*Chenopodium quinoa*) flour, *Int. J. Food Sci. Nutr.,* 54:153–158, 2003.

Ruales, J. and Nair, B.M., Nutritional quality of the protein in quinoa (*Chenopodium quinoa*, Willd.) seeds, *Plant Fds. Hum. Nutr.,* 42:1–11, 1992.

Woldemichael, G.M. and Wink, M., Identification and biological activities of triterpenoid saponins from *Chenopodium quinoa*, *J. Agric. Food Chem.,* 49:2327–2332, 2001.

Zhu, N., Kikuzaki, H., Vastano, B.C., Nakatani, N., Karwe, M.Y., Rosen, R.T., and Ho, C.-T., Ecdysteroids in quinoa seeds (*Chenopodium quinoa* Willd.), *J. Agric. Food Chem.,* 49:2576–2578, 2001.

Q

R

Radish (*Raphanus sativus*)   Unlike the West, where the radishes are small-rooted vegetables, the Far East grows them as large-rooted vegetables (Curtis, 2003). They are cultivated for their fleshy, pungent, edible roots, which are usually reddish but sometimes white or black. The leaves and roots have been used in various parts of the world to treat cancer or as antimicrobial, antifungal, and antiviral agents (Terras et al., 1993; Gutierrez and Perez, 2004). Isothiocyanates present as thioglucoside conjugates in radish were shown to inhibit the development of tumors in many experimental models investigated (Conaway et al., 2002). Radishes are recognized as a food remedy for stones, gravel, and scorbutic conditions. The juice has been used for treating gall stones (choleithiasis) and for preventing the formation of biliary caculi. Kumar (2004) showed a diet containing radishes increased excretion of calcium oxalate compared to a self-selected diet, with the crystal count significantly higher in both genders.

Glucoraphanin, the natural precursor of sulforaphane found mostly in cruciferous vegetables, but also in radishes, is known for maintaining good heath (West et al., 2004).

Using the bleomycin-Fe(III) method, the methanolic extract from radish sprouts (*Raphanus sativus*) was shown by Takaya et al. (2003) to be the most potent hydroxyl-radical scavenger of 11 commonly used vegetables, with close to double that of L-ascorbic acid (Figure R.86). This activity was attributed to the presence of various sinapic acid esters and flavonoids.

Matsufuji et al. (2003) attempted to isolate and characterize the reaction products of 12 acylated anthocyanins from red radish (*Raphanus sativus*) by reacting with 2,2′-azobis(2-amidinopropane) dihydrochloride (AAPH) to generate peroxyl radicals. A number of products were isolated, and their chemical structures determined by preparative HPLC to be *p*-hydroxybenzoic acid, 6-*O*-(*E*)-*p*-coumaroyl-2-*O*-β-D-glucopyranosyl-α-D-glucopyrano-side,

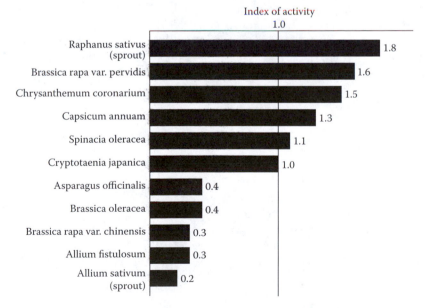

FIGURE R.86 Antioxidant activity of vegetables expressed as index of activity compared to ascorbic acid (1.0). (From Takaya et al., *J. Agric. Food Chem.,* 51:8061–8066, 2003. With permission.)

p-coumaric acid, 6-*O*-(*E*)-feruloyl-2-*O*-β-D-glucopyranosyl-α-D-glucopyranoside, and ferulic acid.

References

Curtis, I.S., The noble radish: Past, present and future, *Trends Plant Sci.,* 8:305–307, 2003.

Conoway, C.C., Yang, Y.M., and Chung, F.I., Isothiocyanates as cancer chemopreventive agents: Their biological activities and metabolism in rodents and humans, *Curr. Drug. Metab.,* 3:233–255, 2002.

Gutierrez, R.M. and Perez, R.L., *Raphanus sativus* (Radish): Their chemistry and biology, *Curr. Drug. Metab.,* 3:233–255, 2004.

Kumar, A., Influence of radish consumption on urinary calcium oxalate excretion, *Nepal. Med. Coll. J.,* 6:41–44, 2004.

Matsufuji, H., Otsuki, T., Takeda, T., Chino, M., and Takeda, M., Identification of reaction products pf acylated anthocyanins from red radish with peroxyl radicals, *J. Agric. Food Chem.,* 51:3157–3161, 2003.

Takaya, Y., Kondo, Y., Furukawa, T., and Niwa, M., Antioxidant constituents of radish sprouts (Kaiware-daikon), *Raphanus sativus* L., *J. Agric. Food Chem.,* 51:8061–8066, 2003.

Terras, F.R.G., Torrekens, S., Van Leuven, B.P.A.F., Osborn, R.W., Vanderleyden, J., Cammue, B.P., and Broekaert, W.T., A new family of basic cysteine-rich plant antifungal proteins from Brassicaceae species, *FEBS Lett.,* 316:233–240, 1993.

West. L.G., Meyer, K.A., Balch, B.A., Rossi, F.J., Schultz, M.R., and Haas, G.W., Glucoraphanin and 4-hydroxyglucobrassicin contents in seeds of 59 cultivars of broccoli, raab, kohlrabi, radish, cauliflower, Brussels sprouts, kale, and cabbage, *J. Agric. Food Chem.,* 52:916–926, 2004.

Rapeseed *see also* **Canola** Rapeseed, known scientifically as *Brassica napus* or *Brassica rapa*, is cultivated in northern climates primarily for animal feed and vegetable oil for human consumption and for biodesel. According to the USDA, rapeseed is the third leading source of vegetable oil in the world in 2000 after soy and palm. Canola, a specific variety of rapeseed bred to have a low erucic-acid content (2.0 percent) in the oil and a low glucosinolate content (< 18 mmol/g) in the meal, is grown in Canada, with related varieties grown in Europe. Barrett

et al. (1998) showed that cruciferous seed meals that include rapeseed exerted protective effects against tumor formation and growth. Four potent, angiotensin-converting, enzyme-inhibitory peptides were isolated by Marczak et al. (2003) from subtilisin digestion of rapeseed protein. They lowered blood pressure in spontaneously hypertensive rats, suggesting the digest may be a promising functional food for preventing and treating hypertension. Del Mar Yust et al. (2004) recently treated rapeseed protein hydrolysates with the food-grade endoprotease, alcalase, and identified two fractions rich in HIV-protease inhibitors.

Thiyam et al. (2004) recently examined the antioxidant potential of rapeseed oil by-products and found the meal contained significant amounts of phenolic compounds. Of these, the major one was sinapic acid, and in the form of its esters and glucosides. These antioxidants could make a significant contribution to the meal industry.

The genotoxin potential of rapeseed oil cooking fumes was studied by Chen et al. (1992). The cooking fumes contained mutagenic activity, suggesting Chinese women exposed to such fumes were at high risk for lung cancer. However, it should be pointed out that the rapeseed grown in China is high in glucosinolates, resulting in much higher levels of sulfur in the oil and not characteristic of canola oil. In addition, many of the homes are poorly ventilated.

References

Barret, J.E., Klopfenstein, C.F., and Leipold, H.W., Protective effects of cruciferous seed meal and hulls against colon cancer in mice, *Cancer Lett.,* 127:83–88, 1998.

Chen, H., Yang, M., and Ye, S., A study on genotoxicity of cooking fumes from rapeseed oil, *Biomed. Environ. Sci.,* 5:229–235, 1992.

del Mar Yust, M., Pedroche, J., Megias, C., Giron-Calle, J., Alaiz, M., Millan, F., and Vioique, J., Rapeseed protein hydrolysates: A source of HIV protease peptide inhibitors, *Food Chem.,* 87:387–392, 2004.

Marczak, E.D., Usui, H., Fujita, H., Yang, Y., Yokoo, M., Lipkowski, A.W., and Yoshikawa, New antihypertensive peptides isolated from rapeseed, *Peptides,* 24:791–798, 2003.

R

Thiyam, U., Kuhlmann, A., Stockmann, H., and Schwartz, K., Prospects of rapeseed oil by-products with respect to antioxidative potential, *C.R. Chemie,* 7:5611–5616, 2004.

Raspberry (*Rubus idaes*)   Raspberry is an aggregate fruit that is fleshy and contains seeds. It grows best in climates with cool summers and mild winters (Duel, 1996). Ethanol extracts from raspberry fruits showed *in vitro* anticancer activity on cervical- and breast-cancer cell lines (Wedge, 2001). Haung and coworkers (2002) proposed that the ability of black raspberries to inhibit the development of chemically induced esophageal and colon cancer in rodents and to inhibit benzo(a)pyrene-induced cell transformation *in vitro* may be mediated by impairing signal-transduction pathways, leading to activation of AP-1 and NF-κB, known to be involved in tumor promotion/progression.

The fruits and leaves from red raspberry (*Rubus idaeus* L.) and black raspberry (*Rubus occidentalis* L.) plants were reported to be high in phenolics, with the highest antioxidant activity found at the ripe stage. Total anthocyanin content increased with maturity, with the leaves being higher in antioxidant activity than the fruits (Wang et al., 2000). The bright color of red raspberries is due to the presence of two anthocyanins, cyanidin-3-glucoside and cyanidin-3-sophoroside (Scheme R.51) (van Elbe and Schwartz, 1996).

Juranic and coworkers (2005) correlated the antiproliferative activity of the water extracts from the seed or pulp of five raspberry cultivars on malignant human colon carcinoma LS174 cells with ellagic acid content.

Raspberry leaves are also high in tannins and, like its relative the blackberry, may relieve acute diarrhea (Tyler, 1994). The antimicrobial properties of raspberry juice, raspberry-leaf extract, and a commercial brand of raspberry-leaf tea were investigated against five human pathogenic bacteria and two fungi. Raspberry juice was found to significantly reduce the growth of several species of bacteria, including *Salmonella*, *Shigella*, and *E. coli*. No antimicrobial activity was detected in the leaf extract or tea (Ryan et al., 2001). Lin et al. (2005) recently demonstrated the potential of enriching

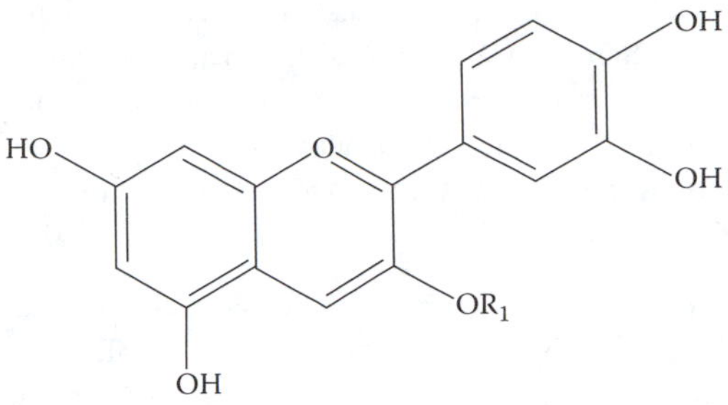

Cyanidin-3-glucoside (R_1 = glucose)
Cyanidin-3-sophoroside (R_1 = sophoroside)

SCHEME R.51 Anthocyanins of red raspberry. (From Suthanthangjai et al., 2005)

wine or vodka with phenolics to inhibit *H. pylori* in laboratory medium. Raspberry-, cinnamon-, and peppermint-enriched wines all exhibited high antimicrobial activity, while raspberry-enriched vodka proved the most potent inhibitor of *H. pylori*.

Tea made from the leaves of *Rubus idaeus* L. (raspberry) has been used for centuries as a uterine relaxant in folk medicine. Rojas-Vera et al. (2002) reported that methanol extracts of dried raspberry have relaxant activity on transmurally stimulated guinea-pig ileum. Many women consume the raspberry leaf herb during their pregnancy, believing that it shortens labor and makes labor "easier." Simpson and coworkers (2001) undertook a double-blind, randomized, placebo-controlled trial with 192 low-risk women who birthed their babies between May 1999 and February 2000. Raspberry leaf, consumed in tablet (2 × 1.2 g per day) from 32 gestation week until labor, was found to cause no adverse effects for mother or baby, but contrary to popular belief, did not shorten the first stage of labor. The only clinically significant findings were a shortening of the second stage of labor (mean difference = 9.59 minutes) and a lower rate of forceps deliveries between the treatment group and the control group (19.3 percent vs. 30.4 percent) (Wang and Lin, 2000).

References

Duel, C.L., Strawberries and raspberries, in *Processing Fruits: Science and Technology; Major Processed Products*, vol. 2, Somogyi, L.P., Barrett, D.M., and Hui, Y.U., Eds., Technomic Pub. Co., New York, 1996, pp. 157–177.

R

Huang, C., Huang, Y., Li, J., Hu, W., Aziz, R., Tang, M.S., Sun, N., Cassady, J., and Stoner, G.D., Inhibition of benzo(a)pyrene diol-epoxide-induced trans-activation of activated protein 1 and nuclear factor κB by black raspberry extracts, *Cancer Res.*, 62: 6857–6863, 2002.

Juranic, Z., Zizak, Z., Tasic, S., Petrovic, S., Nidzovic, S., Leposavic, A., and Stanojkovic, T., Antiproliferative action of water extracts of seeds or pulp of five different raspberry cultivars, *Food Chem.*, 93: 39–45, 2005.

Lin, Y.T., Dhiraj Vattem,. Labbem R.G., and Shetty, K., Enhancement of antioxidant activity and inhibition of Helicobacter pylori by phenolic phytochemical-enriched alcoholic beverages, *Process Biochem.*, 40:2059–2065, 2005.

Rojas-Vera, J., Patel, A.V., and Dacke, C.G., Relaxant activity of raspberry (*Rubus idaeus*) leaf extract in guinea-pig ileum *in vitro*, *Phytother. Res.*, 16:665–668, 2002.

Ryan, T., Wilkinson, J.M., and Cavanagh, H.M., Antibacterial activity of raspberry cordial *in vitro*, *Res. Vet. Sci.*, 71:155–159, 2001.

Simpson, M., Parsons, M., Greenwood, J., and Wade, K., Raspberry leaf in pregnancy: Its safety and efficacy in labor, *J. Midwifery Womens Health*, 46:51–59, 2001.

Suthanthangjai, W., Kajda, P., and Zabetakis, I., The effect of high hydrostatic pressure on the anthocyanins of raspberry (*Rubus ideaus*), *Food Chem.*, 90: 193–197, 2005.

Tyler, V.E., *Herbs of Choice: The Therapeutic Use of Phytomedicinals,* Pharmaceutical Products Press, Binghamton, New York, 1994, pp. 52, 139.

Von Elbe, J.H. and Schwartz, S.J., Colorants, in *Food Chemistry,* Fennema, O.R., Ed., Marcel Dekker, New York, 1996, pp. 611–722.

Wang, S.Y. and Lin, H-S., Antioxidant activity in fruits and leaves of blackberry, raspberry, and strawberry varies with cultivar and developmental stage, *J. Agric. Food Chem.*, 48:140–146, 2000.

Wedge, D.E., Meepagala, K.M., Magee, J.B., Smith, S.H., Huang, G., and Larcom, L.L., Anticarcinogenic activity of strawberry, blueberry, and raspberry extracts to breast and cervical cancer cells, *J. Med. Food,* 4:49–51, 2001.

Red clover   Red clover is a perennial herb that commonly grows wild in meadows throughout Europe and Asia, and has now been naturalized to grow in North America. The red flowers at the end of the branched stems are considered to be the source of its medicinal properties and are usually dried for therapeutic use. Red-clover (*Trifolium pratense*) extracts are becoming increasingly popular, primarily for the treatment of menopausal symptoms (Fugh-Berman and Kronenberg, 2001). Although promoted as a phytoestrogen source similar to soybeans, red clover is a medicinal herb, not a food, and traditionally has not been used for long term. Formononentin and biochanin A are the principal isoflavones of red clover, and are known to help

Biochanin A

Formononentin

(Adapted from Hurr and Rafii, FEMS *Microbiol Lett.* 192:21–25, 2000.)

with hot flushes, which are a common menopausal complaint. The conflicting data on randomized, controlled trials of red clover for the control of menopausal symptoms are encouraging and suggest that phytoestrogens are a treatment modality that needs pursuing (Pitkin, 2004; Barentsen, 2004).

Current research has focused on a red-clover extract high in isoflavones as a possible treatment for symptoms associated also with cardiovascular health. Isolated isoflavones from red clover enriched in biochanin lowered LDL-C in men (Nestel et al., 2004). Campbell and coworkers (2004) recently reported that one-month supplementation with red clover isoflavones had a positive effect on HDL cholesterol. Mean daytime systolic and diastolic blood pressures were significantly lowered during isoflavone therapy, compared to placebo, and forearm vascular endothelial function was significantly greater during isoflavone than placebo supplementation in postmenopausal, type 2 diabetic women. These data suggest that isoflavone supplementation from red clover may favorably influence blood pressure and endothelial function in postmenopausal, type 2 diabetic women (Howes et al., 2003).

Various studies also suggest that red-clover isoflavones may help prevent cancer. Jarred and coworkers (2003) found red-clover-derived isoflavones had a significant effect on prostatic growth, reducing the enlarged, nonmalignant prostate phenotype of the adult aromatase knock-out mouse, by acting as antiandrogenic agents rather than weak, estrogenic substances. Isoflavones in red clover significantly reduced the synthesis of prostaglandin E2 and thromboxane B2 ($p < 0.001$ to $p < 0.05$) in the murine macrophage cell line, indicating COX inhibition. Thus, it is possible that the lower rate of some cancers in populations with a high intake of dietary isoflavones may be linked to their inhibition of COX activity. In mice fed a diet supplemented with red-clover isoflavones, the prostatic epithelium displayed a significant increase in the production of estrogen-receptor beta and the adhesion protein E-cadherin, but a decrease in transforming growth factor beta1. This study suggested that red-clover isoflavones represent a nontoxic dietary treatment for prostatic hyperplasia, reducing the potential for neoplastic transformation (Slater et al., 2002).

The activity of alkaline phosphatase increased following incubation of osteosarcoma cells (HOS58) with red-clover-chloroform extracts, suggesting a role for red-clover isoflavonoids in the stimulation of osteoblastic-cell activity.

References

Barentsen, R., Red clover isoflavones and menopausal health, *J. Br. Menopause Soc.,* 1:4–7, 2004.

Campbell, M.J., Woodside, J.V., Honour, J.W., Morton, M.S., and Leatham, A.J.C., Effect of red clover-derived isoflavone supplementation on insulin-like growth factor, lipid and antioxidant status in healthy female volunteers: A pilot study, *Eur. J. Clin. Nutr.,* 58:173–179, 2004.

Fugh-Berman, A. and Kronenberg, F., Red clover (*Trifolium pratense*) for menopausal women: Current state of knowledge, *Menopause,* 8:333–337, 2001.

Howes, J.B., Tran, D., Brillante, D., and Howes, L.G., Effects of dietary supplementation with isoflavones from red clover on ambulatory blood pressure and endothelial function in postmenopausal type 2 diabetes, *Diabetes Obes. Metab.,* 5:25–332, 2003.

Hur, H.-G. and Rafii, F., Biotransformation of the isoflavonoids biochanin A, formononentin, and glycitein by *Eubacterium limosum, FEMS Microbiol. Lett.,* 192:21–25, 2000.

Jarred, R.A., McPherson, S.J., Jones, M.E.E., Simpson, E.R., and Risbridger, G.P., Anti-androgenic action by red clover-derived dietary isoflavones reduces non-malignant prostate enlargement in aromatase knockout (ArKo) mice, *Prostate,* 56:54–64, 2003.

Lam, A.N., Demasi, M., James, M.J., Husband, A.J., and Walker, C., Effect of red clover isoflavones on COX-2 activity in murine and human monocyte/macrophage cells, *Nutr. Cancer,* 49:89–93, 2004.

Nestel, P., Cehun, M., Chronopoulos, A., DaSilva, L., Teede, H., and McGrath, B., A biochanin-enriched isoflavone from red clover lowers LDL cholesterol in men, *Eur. J. Clin. Nutr.,* 58:403–408, 2004.

Pitkin, J., Red clover isoflavones in practice: A clinician's view, *J. Br. Menopause Soc.,* 10:7–12, 2004.

Slater, M., Brown, D., and Husband, A., In the prostatic epithelium, dietary isoflavones from red clover significantly increase estrogen receptor β and E-cadherin expression but decrease transforming growth factor β1, *Prostate Cancer Prostatic Dis.,* 5:16–21, 2002.

Wende, K., Krenn, L., Unterrieder, I., and Lindequist, U., Red clover extracts stimulate differentiation of human osteoblastic osteosarcoma HOS58 cells, *Planta Med.,* 70:1003–1005, 2004.

R

Red wines *see also* **Wines**   Polyphenols, mainly flavonoids, exert protective effects on the cardiovascular system (Wollin and Jones, 2001), as well as exhibit anticancer (Bianchini and Vainio, 2003), antiviral, and antiallergic properties (Bhat et al., 2001). In coronary heart disease, the protective effects of flavonoids are antithrombic, antioxidant, antiischemic, and vasorelaxant properties (de Lorimier, 2000). It has been hypothesized that the phenomenon of a low incidence of coronary heart disease in French people may be partially related to the pharmacological properties of polyphenolic compounds included in red wine (Zenebe and Pechanova, 2002). The mechanisms underlying CHD protective benefits of red wine have not been elucidated. Recently, the polyphenol res-veratrol (3,5,4'-trihydroxy-*trans-stilbene*), known to be abundantly present in red wine compared to white wine, beer, or spirits, has been demonstrated to elicit a broad spectrum of biological responses in *in vitro* and in animal studies, including effects that are compatible with the cardioprotective roles proposed for red wine. Other studies relate exposure to wine/res-veratrol with reduction in myocardial damage during ischemia-reperfusion, modulation of vascular cell functions (Wu et al., 2001), inhibition of LDL oxidation, and suppression of platelet aggregation (Halpern et al., 1998; Wu et al., 2001; Wollin and Jones, 2001). Grapes contain a variety of antioxidants, including res-veratrol, catechin, epicatechin, and proanthocy-anidins. Of these, resveratrol is present mainly in grape skin, while proanthocyanidin is present in the seeds. Das and coworkers (1999) demonstrated that red-wine extract, as well as res-veratrol and proanthocyanidins, are equally effective in reducing myocardial ischemic reperfusion injury, which suggests that these red-wine polyphenolic antioxidants play a crucial role in cardioprotection.

Schafer and Bauersachs (2002) reported that red wine may beneficially affect the development of high-altitude pulmonary edema, which is the predominant cause of death due to high-altitude illness. Two cellular mechanisms have been described for the altitude-related reduction in barometric pressure: enhanced endothelin 1 production and the increased generation of reactive-oxygen species. Both were suppressed by red wine.

References

Bhat, K.P.L., Kosmeder, II, J.W., and Pezzuto, J.M., Biological effects of resveratrol, *Antioxid. Redox Signal,* 3:1041–1064, 2001.

Bianchini, F. and Vainio, H., Wine and resveratrol: Mechanisms of cancer prevention? *Eur. J. Cancer Prev.,* 12:417–425, 2003.

Das, D.K., Sato, M., Ray, P.S., Maulik, G., Engelman, R.M., Bertelli, A.A., and Bertelli, A., Cardioprotection of red wine: Role of polyphenolic antioxidants, *Drugs Exp. Clin. Res.,* 25:115–120, 1999.

de Lorimier, A.E., Alcohol, wine, and health, *Am. J. Surg.,* 180:357–361, 2000.

Halpern, M.J., Dahlgren, A.L., Laakso, I., Seppanen-Laakso, T., Dahlgren, J., and McAnulty, P.A., Red-wine polyphenols and inhibition of platelet aggregation: Possible mechanisms, and potential use in health promotion and disease prevention, *J. Int. Med. Res.,* 26:171–180, 1998.

Schafer, A. and Bauersachs, J., High-altitude pulmonary edema: Potential protection by red wine, *Nutr. Metab. Cardiovasc. Dis.,* 12:306–310, 2002.

Wollin, S.D. and Jones, P.J., Alcohol, red wine and cardiovascular disease, *J. Nutr.,* 131:1401–1404, 2001.

Wu, J.M., Wang, Z.R., Hsieh, T.C., Bruder, J.L., Zou, J.G., and Huang, Y.Z., Mechanism of cardioprotection by resveratrol, a phenolic antioxidant present in red wine (review), *Int. J. Mol. Med.,* 8:3–17, 2001.

Zenebe, W. and Pechanova, O., Effects of red wine polyphenolic compounds on the cardiovascular system, *Bratisl. Lek. Listy.,* 103:159–165, 2002.

Rehmannia   Rehmannia refers to the root of *Rehmannia glutinosa*, an herb of the Scrophu-lariaceae family. The species name *glutinosa*

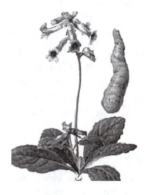

comes from glutinous, referring to the sticky nature of the root. Another name for rehmannia is Chinese foxglove.

Rehmannia is a Chinese herb that is often combined with other herbs to treat anemia (Yuan et al., 1998; Zee-Cheng, 1992), cancer (Wei and Ru, 1997; Kamei et al., 2000), constipation, and diabetes. It has been mainly used to treat broken bones and severed sinews from falls. Oh and coworkers (2003) reported recently that *Rehmannia glutinosa* Libosch extracts stimulate the proliferation and activities of osteoblasts, while inhibiting the generation and resorptive activities of osteoclasts. It also shows preventive effects on osteoporotic bone loss induced by an ovariectomy. Other uses include the treatment of fatigue (Zee-Cheng, 1992) and high blood pressure (Yi et al., 1965). Rehmannia may be applied to the skin to treat eczema or psoriasis (Prieto et al., 2003) and may be beneficial in the regulation of immediate-type allergic reaction (Kim et al., 1998). It may also be used to treat cuts and wounds (Luo, 1993).

In modern times, rehmannia is especially used for treating hormonal disorders, such as menopause, thyroid imbalance, and adrenal insufficiency (Shan, 1994; Chao et al., 2003).

The main components of rehmannia are simple sugars (including glucose, galactose, fructose, sucrose, and mannitol), which make the root sticky and give it the sweet taste. About half the content of dried rehmannia is stachyose and verbascose, polysaccharides that are difficult to digest. The stachyose extract from *Rehmannia glutinosa* Libosch had a significant, hypoglycemic effect in glucose- and adrenaline-induced hyperglycemic and alloxan-induced diabetic rats (Zhang et al., 2004).

The major active constituents of rehmannia are iridoid glycosides. In a study of several samples of rehmannia, Luo et al. (1994) found that catalpol made up about 3–11 percent of the undried root content. The pharmacological action of catalpol and related iroids involved

Catalpol. (Adapted from Li et al., *Brain Res.*, 1029: 179–185, 2004.)

production of adrenal cortical hormones (Hson-Mou and Pui-Hay, 1986). These hormones have anti-inflammatory action (explaining the claimed benefits of rehmannia for asthma, skin diseases, and arthritis) and are also involved in the production of sex hormones (explaining the claimed benefit of treating menopause, impotence, and other signs of hormone deficiency). Recent research by Li et al. (2004) suggested catalpol were a potential neuroprotective agent, and its neuroprotective effects were achieved, at least partly, by promoting endogenous anti-oxidant enzymatic activities and reducing the formation of nitric oxide. Kim and coworkers (1999) suggested rehmannia may inhibit TNF-α secretion by inhibiting IL-1 secretion and has an anti-inflammatory activity in the central nervous system, curing some pathological-disease states.

References

Anh, N.T., Sung, T.V., Franke, K., and Wessjohann, L.A., Phytochemical studies of *Rehmannia glutinosa* rhizomes, *Pharmazie,* 58:593–595, 2003.

Chao, S.L., Huang, L.W., and Yen, H.R., Pregnancy in premature ovarian failure after therapy using Chinese herbal medicine, *Chang Gung Med. J.,* 26:449–452, 2003.

Hson-Mou, C. and Pui-Hay, P.B., Eds., *Pharmacology and Applications of Chinese Materia Medica,* (2 vols.), World Scientific, Singapore, 1986.

Kamei, T., Kumano, H., Iwata, K., Nariai, Y., and Matsumoto, T., The effect of a traditional Chinese prescription for a case of lung carcinoma, *J. Altern. Complement Med.,* 6:557–559, 2000.

Kim, H.M., An, C.S., Jung, K.Y., Choo, Y.K., Park, J.K., and Nam, S.Y., *Rehmannia glutinosa* inhibits tumor necrosis factor-alpha and interleukin-1 secretion from mouse astrocyte, *Pharmacol. Res.,* 40:171–176, 1999.

Kim, H.M., Lee, E.H., Lee, S.J., Shin, T.Y., Kim, Y.J., and Kim, J.B., Effect of *Rehmannia glutinosa* on immediate type allergic reaction, *Int. J. Immunopharmacol.,* 20:231–240, 1998.

Li, D.-Q., Bao, Y.-M., Zhao, J.-J., Liu, C.-P., Liu, Y., and An, L.-J., Neuroprotective properties of catalpol in transient global cerebral ischemia in gerbils: Dose–response, therapeutic time-window and long-term efficacy, *Brain Res.,* 1029:179–185, 2004.

Luo, Y., Determination of catalpol in rehmannia root by high performance liquid chromatography, *Chinese Pharm. J.,* 29: 8–40, 1994.

Luo, Z.H., The use of Chinese traditional medicines to improve impaired immune functions in scald mice, *Zhonghua Zheng Xing Shao Shang Wai Ke Za Zhi,* 9:56–58, 80, 1993.

R

Oh, K-O., Kim, S-W., Kim, J-Y., Ko, S-Y., Kim, H-M., Baek, J-H., Ryoo, H-M., and Kim, J-K., Effect of *Rehmannia glutinosa* Libosch extracts on bone metabolism, *Clin. Chim. Acta,* 334:185–195, 2003.

Prieto, J.M., Recio, M.C., Giner, R.M., Manez, S., Giner-Larza, E.M., and Rios, J.L., Influence of traditional Chinese anti-inflammatory medicinal plants on leukocyte and platelet functions, *J. Pharm. Pharmacol.,* 55:1275–1282, 2003.

Shan, J.C., Determination of hepatocyte adrenergic alpha 1 receptor and study on actions of nourishing yin and replenishing qi drugs in experimental hyperthyroid rats, *Zhongguo Zhong Xi Yi Jie He Za Zhi,*14:96–98, 69–70, 1994.

Wei, X.L. and Ru, X.B., Effects of low-molecular-weight *Rehmannia glutinosa* polysaccharides on p53 gene expression, *Zhongguo Yao Li Xue Bao,* 18:471–474, 1997.

Yi, N.Y., Chu, W., and Koang, N.K., Pharmacologic studies on liu wei di huang t'ang (decoction of Rehmannia with 6 components): its action on kidney function and blood pressure of rats with renal hypertension, *Chin. Med. J.,* 84:433–436, 1965.

Yuan, A., Liu, C., and Huang, X., Treatment of 34 cases of chronic aplastic anemia using prepared Rehmannia polysaccharide associated with stanozolol, *Zhongguo Zhong Xi Yi Jie He Za Zhi,* 18:351–353, 1998.

Zee-Cheng, R.K., Shi-quan-da-bu-tang (ten significant tonic decoction), SQT, a potent Chinese biological response modifier in cancer immunotherapy, potentiation and detoxification of anticancer drugs, *Exp. Clin. Pharmacol.,* 14:725–736, 1992.

Zhang, R.X., Jia, Z.P., Kong, L.Y., Ma, H.P., Ren, J., Li, M.X., and Ge, X., Stachyose extract from *Rehmannia glutinosa* Libosch to lower plasma glucose in normal and diabetic rats by oral administration, *Pharmazie,* 59:552–556, 2004.

Resistant starch Resistant starch is starch that resists digestion by enzymes in the small intestine. It is found naturally in many cereals and grains, as well as in some processed foods, such as extruded cereals (Brown, 2004). Resistant starch functions like a fiber in the diet, as it plays a role in gut health (Asp et al., 1996). In humans, resistant starch lowers fecal bile-acid excretion (Langkilde et al., 1998). In their review, Young and Leu (2004) showed that the consumption of resistant starch dramatically affected the colonic luminal environment by facilitating apoptotic deletion of genetically damaged cells in the colon, several of which are considered to be biomarkers associated with risk for colorectal cancer. In addition, its ability to lower colonic pH is usually considered beneficial for cancer prevention, as well for mineral biovailability in the colon (Champ, 2004). Cheng and Lai (2000) showed that resistant rice starch was fermented to produce proprionic acid, which resulted in reduction in serum total cholesterol, serum LDL cholesterol, hepatic cholesterol, and hepatic triglycerides in rats. Foods in this class also have a low glycemic index and reduce postprandial-insulin levels and increase HDL cholesterol levels (Kendall et al., 2004; Park et al., 2004). Other researchers found that retrograded resistant starch was a very potent butyrate producer (Bird et al., 2000; Topping and Bird, 1999). In a recent review, Brouns and coworkers (2002) highly recommend resistant starch in relation to butyrate. Higgins et al. (2004) reported that replacement of 5.4 percent of the total dietary carbohydrate with resistant starch increased postprandial lipid oxidation significantly and therefore might decrease fat accumulation in the long term.

The protective effect of high-amylose cornstarch ingestion on trinitrobenzene sulfonic acid-induced colitis suggested to Morita et al. (2004) that it altered the colonic mucosa, possibly due to the production of cecal short-chain fatty acids.

In summary, resistant-starch intake seems to decrease postprandial glycemic and insulinemic responses, lower plasma cholesterol and triglyceride concentrations, improve whole-body insulin sensitivity, increase satiety, and reduce fat storage. These properties make resistant starch an attractive dietary target for the prevention of diseases associated with dyslipidemia and insulin resistance, as well as the development of weight-loss diets and dietary therapies for the treatment of type 2 diabetes and coronary heart disease (Higgins, 2004).

References

Asp, N.G., van Amelsvoort, J.M.M., and Hautvast, J.G.A.J., Nutritional implications of resistant starch, *Nutr. Res. Rev.,* 9:1–31, 1996.

Bird, A.R., Brown, I.L., and Topping, D.L., Starches, resistant starch, the gut microflora and human health, *Curr. Issues Intest. Microbiol.,* 1:25–27, 2000.

Brouns, F., Kettlitz, B., and Arrigoni, E., Resistant starch and "the butyrate revolution," *Trends Food Sci. Technol.,* 13:251–261, 2002.

Brown, I.L., Applications and uses of resistant starch, *J. AOAC Int.,* 87:727–732, 2004.

Champ, M-J., Physiological aspects of resistant starch and *in vivo* measurements, *J. AOAC Int.,* 87: 749–755, 2004.

Cheng, H.-H. and Lai, M.-H., Fermentation of resistant rice starch produces proprionate reducing serum and hepatic cholesterol in rats, *J. Nutr.,* 130:1991–1995, 2000.

Higgins, J.A., Higbee, D.R., Donahoo, W.T., Brown, I.L., Bell, M.L., and Bessesen, D.H., Resistant starch consumption promotes lipid oxidation, *Nutr. Metab.,* 1:8, 2004.

Higgins, J.A., Resistant starch: metabolic effects and potential health benefits, *J. AOAC Int.,* 87:761–768, 2004.

Kendall, C.W.C., Emam, A., Augustin, L.S.A., and Jenkins, D.J.A., Resistant starches and health, *J. AOAC Int.,* 87:769–774, 2004.

Langkilde, A.M., Ekwall, H., Bjork, I., Asp, N.-G., and Andersson, H., Retrograded high-amylose corn starch reduces cholic acid excretion from the small bowel in ileostomy subjects, *Eur. J. Clin. Nutr.,* 52: 790–795, 1998.

Morita, T., Tanabe, H., Sugiyama, K., Kasaoka, S., and Kiriyama, S., Dietary resistant starch alters the characteristics of colonic mucosa and exerts a protective effect on trinitrobenzene sulfonic acid-induced colitis in rats, *Biosci. Biotechnol. Biochem.,* 68:2155–2164, 2004.

Park, O.J., Kang, N.E., Chang, M.J., and Kim, W.K., Resistant starch supplementation influences blood lipid concentrations and glucose control in overweight subjects, *J. Nutr. Sci. Vitaminol.,* 50:93–99, 2004.

Topping, D.L. and Bird, A.R., Foods, nutrients and digestive health, *Aust. J. Nutr. Dietet.,* 56(Suppl. 3): 522–534, 1999.

Young, G.P. and Le Leu, R.K., Resistant starch and colorectal neoplasia, *J. AOAC Int.,* 87:775–786, 2004.

Resveratrol Resveratrol is a trihydroxystilbene in the skins of grapes and in wine. It is a powerful phytoestrogen with a wide range of pharmacological and therapeutic health benefits. The beneficial effects of wine on cardiovascular health include prevention of oxidative

Resveratrol. (From Li et al., *Free Rad. Biol. Med.,* 38:243–257, 2005. With permission.)

damage, vasodilation, and prevention of platelet aggregation. Laden and Porter (2001) showed it was resveratrol that inhibited purified human squalene monooxygenase, a rate-limiting enzyme in cholesterol biosynthesis. Thus, protection by resveratrol is related to inhibition of cholesterol synthesis. Other mechanisms for the protection of the cardiovascular system by resveratrol include defense against ischemic-reperfusion injury, promotion of vasorelaxation, protection and maintenance of intact endothelium, antiatherosclerotic properties, inhibition of low-density lipoprotein oxidation, suppression of platelet aggregation, and estrogen-like actions (Hao and He, 2004). Gusman and coworkers (2001) reappraised the chemopreventive and chemotherapeutic properties of resveratrol. The literature confirmed the ability of resveratrol to inhibit activation of carcinogenic compounds, stimulate detoxification, prevent interaction with DNA, and, finally, to suppress tumor progression (Teel and Huynh, 1998). Bhat and Pezzuto (2001) reported that resveratrol exerted antiproliferative effects in cultured human endometrial adenocarcinoma (Ishikawa) cells involving either both estrogen-dependent and estrogen-independent mechanisms. Resveratrol has been shown to significantly alter the cellular physiology of tumor cells, as well as block initial and progression of the tumors. Zoberi et al. (2002) showed that resveratrol altered both cell-cycle progression and cytotoxic response to ionizing radiation in two cervical

TABLE R.60
Mechanisms of Resveratrol in Cells *In Vitro* Related to Cancer Chemoprevention

Mechanism	Experimental system	"Efficacious" concentrations (μM)[a]
Inhibition of growth	Multiple cell lines	~5–10
Induction of apoptosis	Leukemia cells	32–100
Induction of p53-independent apoptosis	Colon tumor cells	100
Estrogen agonism	Mammary cells	10–25
Antiestrogenicity	Mammary cells	0.1–1
Inhibition of oxygen radical formation nitric oxide production	Macrophages	~30
Inhibition of cytochrome P450 enzymes: CYP1A1 CYP1B1, CYP3A4	Liver cells, microsomes, recombinant enzyme	1–20
Activation of p53	Mouse epidermal cells	20
Activation of c-jun kinase	Mouse epidermal cells	10–40
Decrease in COX-2 expression	Mammary epithelial cells	~5
Increase in p21/Cip1, cyclins D1, D2, E; decrease in cdks 2, 4, 6	Epidermoid carcinoma cells	~10
Increase in cyclins A, B1, and cdks 1 and 2	Colon tumor cells	30
Inhibition of protein kinase C activity	Gastric cells	50
Inhibition of protein kinase D activity	Fibroblasts	>100
Inhibition of NF-κB[b] activation	Monocytes, macrophages	30
Inhibition of NF-κB and AP-1 activation	Myeloid, lymphoid, epithelial cells	5

[a] Lowest concentrations at which reproducible changes have been observed, or IC_{50} or EC_{50}, if provided.
[b] NF-κB, nuclear factor κB.

Source: From Gescher and Steward, *Cancer Epidemiol. Biomarkers Prev.,* 12:953–957, 2003. With permission.

tumor cell lines. Resveratrol was also shown by Niles and coworkers (2003) to inhibit growth and induce apoptosis in two human melanoma-cell lines. Thus, resveratrol could be effective as a therapeutic or chemopreventive agent against melanoma.

Pharmacokinetic studies revealed that the target organs of resveratrol are liver and kidney, where it is concentrated after absorption, and is mainly converted to a sulfated form and a glucuronide conjugate. *In vivo*, resveratrol blocks the multistep process of carcinogenesis at various stages: it blocks carcinogen activation by inhibiting aryl hydrocarbon-induced CYP1A1 expression and activity, and suppresses tumor initiation, promotion, and progression. Besides chemopreventive effects, resveratrol appears to exhibit therapeutic effects against cancer (Aggarwal et al., 2004). Kundu and Surh (2004) reviewed the molecular mechanisms underlying chemoprevention by resveratrol, with special focus on its effect on cellular-signaling cascades mediated by NF-κB and AP-1. The

various mechanisms associated with cancer prevention by resveratrol are listed in Table R.60.

Mertens-Talcott and Percival (2005) recently reported that ellagic acid and quercetin both interacted synergistically with resveratrol, inducing apoptosis and causing transient cell-cycle arrest in human leukemia cells (MOLT-4).

Liu and Liu (2004) showed both resveratrol and its analogue, isorhapontigenin, inhibited oxidation of LDL and the generation of reactive-oxygen species. Li and coworkers (2005) recently reported that isorhapontigenin prevented cardiac hypertrophy, a major cause of morbidity and

Isorhapontigenin. (From Li et al., *Free Rad. Biol. Med.,* 38:243–257, 2005. With permission.)

mortality worldwide. As an antioxidant, the mechanism involved inhibition of intracellular signaling transduction pathways.

The ability of resveratrol to protect against age-related macular degeneration (AMD) was recently demonstrated by King et al. (2005), who showed resveratrol significantly reduced cell proliferation of a human retinal epithelium cell line (ARPE-19). At a concentration of 100 μmol/L, resveratrol inhibited H_2O_2-induced intracellular oxidation and protected retinal pigment epithelium from H_2O_2-induced cell death.

References

Aggarwal, B.B., Bhardwa, A., Aggarwal, R.S., Seeram, N.P., Shishodia, S., and Takada, Y., Role of resveratrol in prevention and therapy of cancer: preclinical and clinical studies, *Anticancer Res.*, 24: 2783–2840, 2004.

Bhat, K.P.L. and Pezzuto, J.M., Resveratrol exhibits cytostatic and antiestrogenic properties with human endometrial adenocarcinoma (Ishkawa) cells, *Cancer Res.*, 61:6137–6144, 2001.

Gescher, A.J. and Steward, W.P., Relationship between mechanisms, bioavailability, and preclinical chemopreventive efficacy of resveratrol: a conundrum, *Cancer Epidemiol. Biomarkers Prev.*, 12:953–957, 2003.

Gusman, J., Malonne, H., and Atassi, G., A reappraisal of the potential chemopreventive and chemotherapeutic properties of resveratrol, *Carcinogenesis*, 22:1111–1117, 2001.

Hao, H.D. and He, L.R., Mechanisms of cardiovascular protection by resveratrol, *J. Med. Food*, 7:290–298, 2004.

King, R.E., Kent, K.D., and Bomser, J.A., Resveratrol reduces oxidation and proliferation of human retinal pigment epithelial cells via extracellular signal-regulated kinase inhibition, *Chemico-Biol. Interact.*, 151:142–149, 2005.

Kundu, J.K. and Surh, Y-J., Molecular basis of chemoprevention by resveratrol: NF-κB and AP-1 as potential targets, *Mutat. Res.*, 555:65–80, 2004.

Laden, B.P. and Porter, T.D., Resveratrol inhibits human squalene monooxygenase, *Nutr. Res.*, 21: 747–753, 2001.

Li, H.-L., Wang, A.-B., Huang, Y., Liu, D.-P., Wei, C., Williams, G.M., Zhang, C.-N., Liu, G., Liu, Y.-Q., Hao, D.-L., Hui, R.-T., Lin, M., and Liang, C.-C., Isorhapontigenin, a new resveratrol analog, attenuates cardiac hypertrophy via blocking signaling transduction pathways, *Free Rad. Biol. Med.*, 38: 243–247, 2005.

Liu, Y. And Liu, G. , Isorhapontigenin and resveratrol suppress oxLDL-induced proliferaton and activation of ERK1/2 mitogen-activated protein kinase of bovine aortic smooth muscle cells, *Biochem. Pharmacol.*, 67:777–785, 2004.

Mertens-Talcott, S.U. and Percival, S.S., Ellagic acid and quercetin interact synergistically with resveratrol in the induction of apoptosis and cause transient cell cycle arrest in human leukemia cells, *Cancer Lett.*, 218:141–151, 2005.

Niles, R.M., McFarland, M., Weimer, M.B., Redkar, A., Fu, Y.-M., and Meadows, G.G., Resveratrol is a potent inducer of apoptosis in human melanoma cells, *Cancer Lett.*, 190:157–163, 2003.

Pervaiz, S., Resveratrol: from grapevines to mammalian biology, *FASEB J.*, 17:1975–1985, 2003.

Teel, R.W. and Huynh, H., Modulation by phytochemicals of cytochrome P450-linked enzyme activity, *Cancer Lett.*, 133:135–141, 1998.

Zoberi, I., Bradbury, C.M., Curry, H.A., Bisht, K.S., Goswami, P.C., Roti Roti, J.L., and Gius, D., Radio sensitizing and anti-proliferative effects of resveratrol in two human cervical tumor cell lines, *Cancer Lett.*, 175:165–173, 2002.

Retinoic acid *see also* **Retinol and Vitamin A**

Retinoic acid (RA), a transcriptionally active metabolite of vitamin A (retinol), activates two families of nuclear-retinoid receptors that have the potential to regulate the expression of a

All-*trans*-retinoic acid (RA). (From Seo et al., *Eur. J. Pharm. Biopharm.*, 58:681–687, 2004. With permission.)

large number of genes (Soprano et al., 2004). Retinoids are essential for normal embryo development and epithelial differentiation (Klug et al., 1989; Gajovic et al., 1998). These compounds are also involved in chemoprevention and differentiation therapy of some cancers (Hayashi et al., 2000; Yang et al., 2002), with particularly impressive results in the management of acute promyelocytic leukemia (Otsuki

R

et al., 2004; Avvisati and Tallman, 2003). RA is derived from retinol by oxidation through retinol and retinal dehydrogenases, and several cytochrome P450S. The mechanisms that serve to adjust the metabolism of vitamin A to maintain retinoid homeostasis and prevent retinoid excess are not well understood, but the diet has some effects (Ross, 2003).

Maden and Hind (2004) have shown that RA is also required during alveologenesis and throughout life for the maintenance of lung alveoli. When rats are deprived of dietary retinol they lose alveoli and show the features of emphysema.

Ping and coworkers (2005) recently examined the effect of all-*trans*-retinoic acid on p62, a tumor-associated autoantigen identified with autoantibodies from patients with hepatocellular carcinoma (Zhang et al., 1999). RA induced apoptosis in a human gastric cancer-cell line BGC-823 by downregulation and translocation of p62.

References

Avvisati, G. and Tallman, M.S., All-*trans* retinoic acid in acute promyelocytic leukaemia, *Best Pract. Res. Clin. Haematol.,* 16:419–432, 2003.

Gajovic, S., Chowdhury, K., and Gruss, P., Genes expressed after retinoic acid-mediated differentiation of embryoid bodies are likely to be expressed during embryo development, *Exp. Cell Res.,* 242:138–143, 1998.

Hayashi, K., Yokozaki, H., Naka, K., Yasui, W., Yajin, K., Lotan, R., and Tahara, E., Effect of 9-*cis*-retinoic acid on oral squamous cell carcinoma cell lines, *Cancer Lett.,* 151:199–208, 2000.

Klug, S., Creech-Kraft, J., Wildi, E., Merker, H.J., Persaud, T.V., Nau, H., and Neubert, D., Influence of 13-*cis* and all-*trans* retinoic acid on rat embryonic development *in vitro*: correlation with isomerisation and drug transfer to the embryo, *Arch. Toxicol.,* 63: 185–192, 1989.

Maden, M. and Hind, M., Retinoic acid in alveolar development, maintenance and regeneration, *Philos. Trans. R. Soc. Lond. B. Biol. Sci.,* 359:799–808, 2004.

Otsuki, T., Sakaguchi, H., Hatayama, T., Wu, P., Takata, A., and Hyodoh, F., Effects of all-*trans* retinoic acid (ATRA) on human myeloma cells, *Leuk. Lymphoma,* 44:1651–1656, 2003.

Ping, S., Wang, S., Zhang, J., and Peng, X., Effect of all-*trans*-retinoic acid on mRNA binding protein p62 in human gastric cancer cells, *Int. J. Biochem. Cell Biol.,* 37:616–627, 2005.

Ross, A.C., Retinoid production and catabolism: role of diet in regulating retinol esterification and retinoic acid oxidation, *J. Nutr.,* 133:291–296, 2003.

Seo, S.J., Kim, S.H., Sasagawa, T., Choi, Y.J., Akaike, T., and Cho, C.S., Delivery of all *trans* retinoic acid (RA) to hepatocyte cell line from RA/galactosyl α-cyclodextrin inclusion compound, *Eur. J. Pharm. Biopharm.,* 58:681–687, 2004.

Soprano, D.R., Qin, P., and Soprano, K.J., Retinoic acid receptors and cancers, *Annu. Rev. Nutr.,* 24:201–221, 2004.

Yang, Q., Sakurai, T., and Kakudo, K., Retinoid, retinoic acid receptor beta and breast cancer, *Breast Cancer Res. Treat.,* 76:167–173, 2002.

Zhang, J.Y., Chan, E.K.L., Peng, X.X., and Tan, E.M., A novel cytoplasmic protein with RNA-binding motifs is an autoantigen in human hepatocellular carcinoma, *J. Exp. Med.,* 189:1101–1110, 1999.

Retinol   *see also* **Retinoic acid, Vitamin A**
Retinol, the alcohol form of vitamin A, is stored as retinyl esters and delivered from liver stores into the bloodstream as retinol bound to a retinol-binding protein. In situations of high vitamin A demand (e.g., inflammation, diseases, prenatal period), this supply can be insufficient because of delayed production of retinol-binding protein, leading to local deficiencies and impairment of structure and function in the respective tissues. This delay may be overcome by cellular-retinyl esters stores that can be enriched by topically applied retinyl esters (Biesalski and Nohr, 2004).

The metabolism of vitamin A (retinol) to retinyl esters by lecithin:retinol acyl-transferase has been found to be substantially reduced in human carcinoma cell lines. Recently, Boorjian and coworkers (2004) tested normal and malignant bladder-tissue specimens from human patients and found a significant reduction in lecithin:retinol acyl-transferase expression in bladder cancer with an inverse correlation between lecithin:retinol acyl-transferase mRNA and protein expression with increasing

16 17 19 20
7 11 15
2 1 6 9 13 CH₂OR
8 10 12 14
3 5
4 18

R=H, Retinol

Retinol structure. (From Choi et al., *Anal. Chim. Acta,* 512:141–147, 2004. With permission.)

tumor stage. These data suggest that loss of lecithin:retinol acyl-transferase expression is associated with invasive bladder cancer.

The all *trans* form of retinol is a naturally occurring form, which can be converted to a corresponding geometrical isomer, 9-*cis*-retinol form. In fact, 9-*cis*-retinol in combination with *cis*-retinol dehydrogenase was found to inhibit breast-cancer cell proliferation by producing retinol metabolites other than 9-*cis*-retinoic acid (Paik et al., 2005). An epidemiological study on postmenopausal women in Sweden revealed that chronic excess of retinol intake (> 1.5 mg/day) decreased bone-mineral density and increased hip-fracture risk (Whiting and Lemke, 1999). Skeletal effects of toxic amounts of vitamin A are known from acute toxic exposure to chronic high-dose intake of vitamin A. Such effects have led experts to speculate that long-term consumption of diets high in vitamin A (retinol) that stimulate bone resorption and inhibit bone formation may contribute to osteoporosis and hip fractures (Genaro Pde and Martini, 2004; Boucher et al., 2003).

References

Biesalski, H.K. and Nohr, D., New aspects in vitamin a metabolism: the role of retinyl esters as systemic and local sources for retinol in mucous epithelia, *J. Nutr.,* 134:3453S–3457S, 2004.

Boucher, B.J., Chandra, R.K., Melhus, H., and Michaelssohn, K., Serum retinol levels and fracture risk, *N. Engl. J. Med.,* 348:1927–1928, 2003.

Boorjian, S., Tickoo, S.K., Mongan, N.P., Yu, H., Bok, D., Rando, R.R., Nanus, D.M., Scherr, D.S., and Gudas, L.J., Reduced lecithin: retinol acyltransferase expression correlates with increased pathologic tumor stage in bladder cancer, *Clin. Cancer Res.,* 10:3429–3437, 2004.

Choi, Y.H., Kim, H.K., Wilson, E.G., Erkelens, C., Trijzelaar, B., and Verpoorte, R., Quantitative analysis of retinol and retinol palmitate in vitamin tablets using ¹H-nuclear magnetic resonance spectroscopy, *Anal. Chim. Acta,* 512:141–147, 2004.

de Souza Genaro, P.S. and Martín, L.A., Vitamin A supplementation and risk of skeletal fracture, *Nutr. Rev.,* 62:65–67, 2004.

Holick, C.N., Michaud, D.S., Stolzenberg-Solomon, R., Mayne, S.T., Pietinen, P., Taylor, P.R., Virtamo, J., and Albanes, D., Dietary carotenoids, serum β-carotene, and retinol and risk of lung cancer in the alpha-tocopherol, beta-carotene cohort study, *Am. J. Epidemiol.,* 156:536–547, 2002.

Paik, J., Blaner, W.S., and Swisshelm, K., *Cis*-retinol dehydrogenase: 9-*cis*-retinol metabolism and its effect on proliferation of human MCF7 breast cancer cells, *Exp. Cell Res.,* 303:183–196, 2005.

Schuurman, A.G., Goldbohm, R.A., Brants, H.A., and van den Brandt, P.A., A prospective cohort study on intake of retinol, vitamins C and E, and carotenoids and prostate cancer risk (Netherlands), *Cancer Causes Con.,* 13:573–582, 2002.

Whiting, S.J. and Lemke, B., Excess retinol intake may explain the high incidence of osteoporosis in northern Europe, *Nutr. Rev.,* 57:192–195, 1999.

R

Rhubarb The rhubarb plant originated in Tibet or Mongolia, and from the 16th to 18th centuries was used medicinally in Europe and Asia. It served as a laxative, antiphlogistic, and

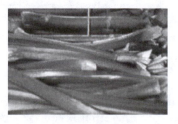

Red rhubarb stalks.

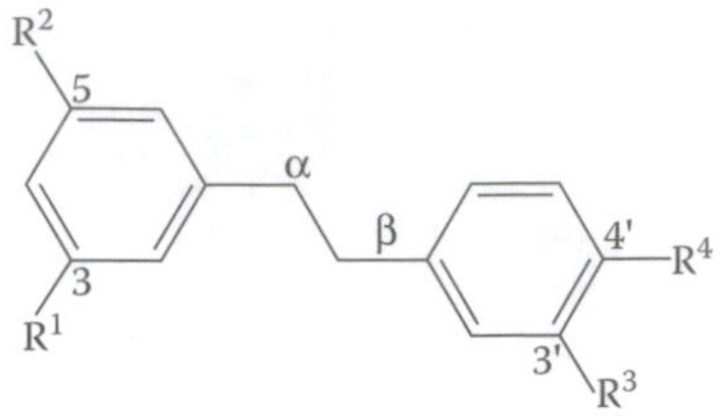

Compound	a-b	R¹	R²	R³	R⁴
Piceatannol	C=C	OH	OH	OH	OH
3,5,4′-Trimethylpiceatannol	C=C	OCH₃	OCH₃	OH	OCH₃
Trimethylresveratrol	C=C	OCH₃	OCH₃	H	OCH₃

SCHEME R.52 Stilbene structures. (Adapted from Matsuda et al., *Bioorg. Med. Chem.,* 12:871–4876, 2004.)

homeostatic in the treatment of constipation, diarrhea, jaundice, gastrointestinal hemorrhage, menstrual disorders, conjunctivitis, traumatic injuries, superficial supportive supperative sores, and ulcers (Peigen et al., 1984; Gu et al., 2000). Chunsheng et al. (2000) suggested rhubarb can ameliorate acute lung injury by inhibiting intercellular adhesion molecule mRNA expression. It can also be applied externally for thermal burns. Chen et al. (2001) reported that rhubarb reduced intestinal juice IgA content in mice caused by burn, which suggested an important mechanism of rhubarb was involved in protecting the muco–membranous barrier.

The edible stalk, about an inch wide, is often more than a foot long and is composed of 95 percent water. It is a fair source of potassium, contributing minor amounts of vitamins, and is low in sodium. Rhubarb's crisp, sour stalks are rich in vitamin C, dietary fiber, and calcium, although the calcium is combined with oxalic acid. Oxalic acid can lead to an increase in urinary-oxalate excretion, which is a risk factor for kidney-stone formation. Rhubarb is somewhat acidic (pH 3.1–3.2), with one cup of diced rhubarb containing about 26 calories.

Stilbenes were isolated from Korean rhubarb by Matsuda et al. (2004) and their antiallergic activities studied *in vitro*. Their results revealed that 3,5,4′-trimethylpiceatannol exhibited the most potent inhibition against β-hexosaminidase release as a marker of degranulation, followed by trimethylresveratrol (Scheme R.52). Piceatannol, 3,5,4′-trimethylpiceatannol, resveratrol, and trimethylresveratrol all signifi-

cantly inhibited antigen-induced release of TNF-α and IL-4.

Iizuka et al. (2004) attempted to estimate the antioxidative activity of rhubarb components on low-density lipoprotein (LDL). They reported a significant, multiple correlation coefficient for antioxidative activities on LDL (R = 0.914, $p < 0.01$) involving five components: aloe-emodin, chrysophanol, emodin 1-O-β-D-glucoside, lindleyin, and 6-hydroxymusizin 8-O-β-D-glucoside.

Rhubarb was also reported to exert protective effects on severe acute pancreatitis, probably by inhibiting inflammation of the pancreas, improving pancreatic microcirculation, and altering exocrine secretion (Zhao et al., 2004). Emodin and rhein isolated from rhubarb were found to be major iNOS inhibitors and may possibly serve as bioactive substances for anti-inflammation effects (Wang et al., 2002).

References

Chen, X.L., Huang, X.L., and Wu, H., Effect of rhubarb on intestinal immune associated secretion in healthy mice and in burn mice, *Zhongguo Zhong Xi Yi Jie He Za Zhi*, 21:754–756, 2001.

Chunsheng, L., Peichun, G., and Xinhua, H., Expression of intercellular adhesion molecule in lung tissues of experimental acute lung injury and the effect of Rhubarb on it, *Chin. Med. Sci. J.,* 15:93–97, 2000.

Gu, J., Zhang, X., Fei, Z., Wen, A., Qin, S., Yi, S., Chen, Y., and Li, X., Rhubarb extracts in treating complications of severe cerebral injury, *Chin. Med. J.,* 113:29–531, 2000.

Iizuka, A., Iijima, O.T., Kondo, K., Itakura, H., Yoshie, F., Miyamoto, H., Kubo, M., Higuchi, M., Takeda, H., and Matsumiya, T., Evaluation of rhubarb using antioxidative activity as an index of pharmacological usefulness, *J. Ethnopharmacol.,* 91:89–94, 2004.

Matsuda, H., Tewtrakul, S., Morikawa, T., and Yoshikawa, M., Anti-allergic activity of stilbenes from Korean rhubarb (*Rheum undulatum* L.): structure requirements for inhibition of antigen-induced degranulation and their effects on the release of TNF-α and IL-4 in RBL-2H3 cells, *Bioorg. Med. Chem.,* 12:871–4876, 2004.

Peigen, X., Liyi, H., and Liwei, W., Ethnopharmacologic study of Chinese rhubarb, *J. Ethnopharmacol.,* 10:275–293, 1984.

Wang, C.C., Huang, Y.J., Chen, L.G., Lee, L.T., and Yang, L.L., Inducible nitric oxide synthase inhibitors of Chinese herbs III, *Rheum palmatum, Planta Med.,* 68:869–874, 2002.

Yamagishi, T., Nishizawa, M., Ikura, M., Hikichi, K., Nonaka, G., and Nishioka, I., New laxative constituents of rhubarb, isolation and characterization of rheinosides A, B, C and D, *Chem. Pharm. Bull.,* 35:3132–3138, 1987.

Zhao, Y.-Q., Liu, X.-H., Ito, T., and Qian, J.M., Protective effects of rhubarb on experimental severe acute pancreatitis, *World J. Gastroenterol.,* 10:1005–1009, 2004.

Rice   Rice (*Oryzae sativum*) is the principal food crop in Asia, where the incidence of breast and colon cancer is markedly below that found in the Western world. Hudson et al. (2000) investigated the potential colon and breast tumor-suppressive properties of rice. Their results suggested that brown rice and bran contain compounds had putative cancer chemopreventive properties. The phenols exhibiting this activity were present in brown-rice bran, such as tricin (Cai et al., 2004). However, they are present at much lower levels in white compared to brown rice. Thus, the consumption of rice bran or brown rice instead of milled white rice may be advantageous with respect to cancer prevention.

While tricin was a potent inhibitor of breast tumor-cell growth *in vitro*, Cai et al. (2004) found it had little effect on nude mice bearing human-derived malignant MDA-MB-468 breast-

Cancertricin structure. (4′,5,7-trihydroxy-3′,5′-dimethoxy-flavone). (From Cai et al., *Br. J. Cancer,* 91:1364–1371, 2004. With permission.)

tumor cells. However, the high levels of tricin in the gastrointestinal tract after dietary intake may prove beneficial in preventing colorectal cancer.

Other investigations of potential beneficial effects of specific rice constituents in terms of prevention or amelioration of malignant disease have been published. These reports suggest that rice constituents counteract chemical-induced mutagenicity (Kang et al., 1996; Nam and Kang, 1997), tumor promotion (Yasukawa et al., 1998), carcinogenicity (Aoe et al., 1993), and established neoplastic growth in rodents (Hayashi et al., 1998; Koide et al., 1996). However, relatively little is known about which specific molecules may be responsible for these activities. Some of the evidence concerning the chemopreventive and antitumor properties of rice suggests that it is predominantly the bran portion of the grain that contains biologically active substances. The preventive potential of rice bran extract against the oxygen radical-related chronic diseases, such as cardiovascular diseases and cancer, antioxidative and antigenotoxic activities of the rice-bran extracts was demonstrated recently by Higashi-Okai et al. (2004).

Rice-bran oil is tenaciously believed to be a healthy vegetable oil in Asian countries. It exerts hypocholesterolemic activity in relation to more commonly used vegetable oils and is characterized by a relatively high content of nonfatty-acid components, some of which are known to have beneficial health effects, such as gamma-oryzanol and tocotrienols that could participate in its hypocholesterolemic effects (Sugano et al., 1999).

R

References

Aoe, S., Oda, T., Tojima, T., Tanaka, M., Tatsumi, K., and Mizutani, T., Effects of rice bran hemicellulose on 1,2-dimethylhydrazine-induced intestinal carcinogenesis in Fischer 344 rats, *Nutr. Cancer*, 20: 41–49, 1993.

Cai, H., Hudson, E.A., Mann, P., Verschoyle, R.D., Greaves, P., Manson, M.M., Steward, W.P., and Gescher, A.J., Growth-inhibitory and cell cycle-arresting properties of the rice bran constituent tricin in human-derived breast cancer cells *in vitro* and in nude mice *in vivo*, *Br. J. Cancer*, 91:1364–1371, 2004.

Hayashi, Y., Nishikawa, Y., Mori, H., Tamura, H., Matsushita, Y.-I., and Matsui, T., Antitumor activity of (10*E*,12*Z*)-9-hydroxy-10,12-octadecadienoic acid from rice bran, *J. Ferment. Bioengineer.*, 86:149–153, 1998.

Higashi-Okai, K., Kanbara, K., Amano, K., Hagiwara, A., Sugita, C., Matsumoto, N., and Okay, Y., Potent antioxidative and antigenotoxic activity in aqueous extract of Japanese rice bran — association with peroxidase activity, *Phytother. Res.*, 18:628–633, 2004.

Hudson, E.A., Dinh, P.A., Kokubun, T., Simmonds, M.S.J., and Gescher, A., Characterization of potentially chemopreventive phenols in extracts of brown rice that inhibit the growth of human breast and colon cancer cells, *Cancer Epidemiol. Biomarkers Prev.*, 9:1163–1170, 2000.

Kang, M.Y., Choi, Y.H., and Nam, S.H., Inhibitory mechanism of colored rice bran extract against mutagenicity induced by chemical mutagen mitomycin C, *Agric. Chem. Biotech.*, 39:424–429, 1996.

Koide, T., Kamei, H., Hashimoto, Y., Kojima, T., and Hasegawa, M., Antitumor effect of hydrolyzed anthocyanin from grape rinds and red rice, *Cancer Biother. Radiopharm.*, 11:73–277, 1996.

Nam, S.H. and Kang, M.Y., *In vitro* inhibitory effect of colored rice bran extracts on carcinogenicity, *Agric. Chem. Biotech.*, 40:307–312, 1997.

Sugano, M., Koba, K., and Tsuji, E., Health benefits of rice bran oil, *Anticancer Res.*, 19:3651–3657, 1999.

Yasukawa, K., Akihisa, T., Kimura, Y., Tamura, T., and Takido, M., Inhibitory effect of cycloartenol ferulate, a component of rice bran, on tumor promotion in two-stage carcinogenesis in mouse skin, *Biol. Pharm. Bull.*, 21:1072–1076, 1998.

Rice starch   Rice starch cannot be completely digested by enzymes in the small intestine. Cheng and Lai (2000) demonstrated that resistant rice starch is fermented to produce propionic acid, which reduced serum total cholesterol, serum LDL cholesterol, hepatic cholesterol, and hepatic triglyceride in rats. Kim et al. (2003) reported that resistant starch from rice could also shorten the intestinal transit time and could lower plasma total lipid and cholesterol concentrations compared to diabetic control.

Rice-starch-based oral rehydration solution (ORS) has been shown to be a suitable alternative to glucose-based ORS in the treatment of both choleragenic and noncholeragenic dehydration in older infants and in children and also in the rehydration of acute diarrheal dehydration in infants below 6 months of age (Iyngkaran and Yadav, 1998).

Rice starch added to bath water was found to have beneficial effects on impaired barrier function, as evaluated by trans-epidermal water-loss measurements. Rice starch in powder or formulated in a bath product is therefore recommended by de Paepe et al. (2002) as a skin-repair bathing additive for barrier-damaged skin, particularly in the case of atopic-dermatitis patients.

References

Cheng, H.H. and Lai, M.H., Fermentation of resistant rice starch produces propionate reducing serum and hepatic cholesterol in rats, *J. Nutr.*, 30:1991–1995, 2000.

de Paepe, K., Hachem, J-P., Vanpee, E., Roseeuw, D., and Rogiers, V., Effect of rice starch as a bath additive on the barrier function of healthy but SLS-damaged skin and skin of atopic patients, *Acta Derm. Venereol.*, 82:184–186, 2002.

Iyngkaran, N. and Yadav, M., Rice-starch oral rehydration therapy in neonates and young infants, *J. Trop. Pediatr.*, 44:199–203, 1998.

Kim, W.K., Chung, M.K., Kang, N.E., Kim, M.H., and Park, O.J., Effect of resistant starch from corn or rice on glucose control, colonic events, and blood lipid concentrations in streptozotocin-induced diabetic rats, *J. Nutr. Biochem.*, 14:166–172, 2003.

Rooibos tea   Rooibos tea is an herbal tea produced from the leaves and fine stems of the South African leguminous shrub *Aspalathus linearis,* also known as Rooibos. The herbal tea is considered a health drink due to the presence of beneficial phenolic antioxidants. The antioxidant properties of Rooibos tea were found to be similar to green, oolong, and black tea (von Gadow et al., 1997a). Rooibos tea, however, contains a unique compound, aspalathin, that mimics superoxide dismutase (SOD) (Yoshikawa et al., 1990; Ito et al., 1991). Compared to BHA, BHT, and α-tocopherol, aspalathin exhibited the highest radical-scavenging activity (von Gadow et al., 1997b). *In vitro* and *in vivo* studies found rooibos tea exhibited antimutagenic properties against aflatoxin B_1 and 2-acetylamino fluorine-induced mutagenesis (Marnewick et al., 2000; Marnewick et al., 2004a). In addition, aqueous extracts of rooibos tea enhanced phase II detoxifying enzymes, glutathione-*S* transferase, and UDP-glucuronyl transferase in rat liver, stabilizing glutathione (GSH) (Marnewick et al., 2003). Ethanol/acetone (E/A)-soluble fractions prepared from methanolic extracts of processed and unprocessed South African herbal teas, rooibos, and honeybush compared to green tea were recently shown by Marnewick and coworkers (2004b) to inhibit tumor promotion in mouse skin. Using the two-stage mouse-skin carcinogenesis assay with the tumor promoter 12-*O*-tetra decanoylphorbol-13-acetate (TPA) on ICR mouse skin initiated with 7,12-dimethyl benz[a]anthracene (DMBA), they found herbal-tea fractions significantly ($p < 0.001$) decreased tumor volume, as well as delayed their development (Figure R.87). Compared to the control, tumors did not appear in the DMBA/TPA-treated mice at 4 and 12 weeks when maintained on processed and unprocessed rooibos, respectively. Green tea exhibited 100 percent

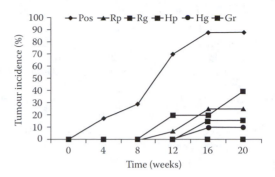

FIGURE R.87 Inhibitory effect of topical application of various E/A polyphenolic fractions on TPA-induced tumor promotion. The percentage of mice with tumors is plotted as a function of the treatment period (weeks). The fractions include Rp, processed rooibos; Rg, unprocessed rooibos; Hp, processed honeybush; Hg, unprocessed honeybush; and Gr, green tea. The number of animals per group = 15–20. (From Marnewick et al., *Cancer Lett.,* 224:193–202, 2005.)

inhibition compared to 90 percent and 84.2 percent inhibition for unprocessed and processed honeybush. While processed and unprocessed rooibos proved to be the least effective, they nevertheless accounted for an impressive 75 percent and 60 percent inhibition of tumor promotion, respectively. The variability in tumor inhibition exhibited by these herbal teas was attributed to differences in their flavonol/proanthocyanidin and flavonol/flavone composition and nonpolyphenolic components.

References

Ito, A., Shinohara, K., and Kator, K., Protective action of Rooibos tea (Aspalathis linearis) extract against inactivation of L5178Y cells by H_2O_2, in *Proceedings of the International Symposium on Tea Science*, Shizuoka, Japan, 1991, pp. 381–384.

Jaganyi, D. and Wheeler, P.J., Rooibos tea: equilibrium and extraction kinetics of aspalathin, *Food Chem.*, 83:121–126, 2003.

R

Aspalathin. (From Jaganyi and Wheeler, *Food Chem.*, 83:121–126, 2003. With permission.)

Marnewick, J.L., Batenburg, W., Wart, P., Joubert, E., Swanevelder, S., and Gelderblom, W.C.A., *Ex vivo* modulation of chemical-induced mutagenesis by sub cellular liver fraction of rats treated with rooibos (*Aspalathus linearis*) tea, honeybush (*Cyclopia intermedia*) tea, as well as green and black (*Camellia sinensis*) teas, *Mutat. Res.*, 558:145–154, 2004a.

Marnewick, J.L., Gelderblom, W.C.A., and Joubert, E., An investigation of the antimutagenic properties of South African herbal teas, *Mutat. Res.*, 471:157–166, 2000.

Marnewick, J., Joubert, E., Joseph, S., Swanevelder, S., Swart, P., and Gelderblom, W., Inhibition of tumor promotion in mouse skin by extracts of rooibos (*Aspalathis linearis*) and honeybush (*Cyclopedia intermedia*), unique South African herbal teas, *Cancer Lett.*, 224:193–202, 2005.

Marnewick, J.L., Joubert, E., Swart, P., Joubert, E., van der Westhuizen, F., and Gelderblom, W.C.A., Modulation of hepatic drug metabolizing enzymes and oxidative status of rooibos (*Aspalathus linearis*) and honeybush (*Cyclopia intermedia*) green and black (*Camellia sinensis*) teas in rats, *J. Agric. Food Chem.*, 51:8113–8119, 2003.

von Gadow, A., Joubert, E., and Hansmann, C.F., Comparison of the antioxidant activity of rooibos tea (*Aspalathus linearis*) with green, Oolong and black tea, *Food Chem.*, 60:73–77, 1997a.

von Gadow, A., Joubert, E., and Hansmann, C.F., Comparison of the antioxidant activity of aspalathin with that of other plant phenols of Rooibos tea (*Aspalathus linearis*), alpha-tocopherol, BHT, and BHA, *J. Agric. Food Chem.*, 45:632–638, 1997b.

Yoshikawa, T., Naito, Y., Oyamada, H., Ueda, S., Tanigawa, S., Takemura, T., Sugino, S., and Kondo, M., Scavenging effect of *Aspalathus linearis* (Rooibos tea) on active oxygen species, in *Antioxidants in Therapy and Preventative Medicine*, Emerit, I., Packer, L., and Auclair, C., Eds., Plenum Press, New York. 1990. pp. 171–174.

Rosemary *see also* **Rosmarinic acid**

Rosemary (*Rosmarinus officinalis* Linn.) is a common household plant. It is used as food flavoring and a beverage drink, as well as in cosmetics. In folk medicine, it is used as an antispasmodic in renal colic and dysmenorrhoea, to relieve respiratory disorders, to stimulate growth of hair, and as a mild analgesic and antimicrobial agent (Newall, 1996). Extract of rosemary relaxes smooth muscles of trachea and intestine, and has choleretic, hepatoprotective, and antitumerogenic activity (Al-Sereiti et al., 1999). The leaves of rosemary contain valuable essential oils rich in mono- and sesquiterpenes, including borneol, camphor, carophyllene, cineol, humulene, linalool, and thujone "salviol." The strong, antioxidant activity associated with rosemary leaves is associated with these phenolic diterpenes.

The most important constituents of rosemary are caffeic acid and its derivatives, such as rosmarinic acid. These compounds and other phenolic diterpenes, flavonoids, and phenolic acids (Ho et al., 2000) have antioxidant effects. Slamenova et al. (2002) also reported that rosemary extract exhibits a protective effect against oxidative damage to DNA as a consequence of scavenging of both OH radicals and singlet oxygen.

Rosmarinic acid, a caffeic-acid derivative, is well-absorbed from the gastrointestinal tract and from the skin. It increases the production of prostaglandin E2 and reduces the production of leukotriene B4 in human polymorphonuclear leucocytes, and inhibits the complement system (Al-Sereiti et al., 1999). It also showed therapeutic potential in treatment or prevention of bronchial asthma, spasmogenic disorders, peptic ulcer, inflammatory diseases, hepatotoxicity, atherosclerosis, ischaemic heart disease, cataract, cancer, and poor sperm motility (Rampart et al., 1986; Al-Sereiti et al., 1999).

(1)   (2)

Rosmarinic acid (1) and caffeic acid (2). (From Wang et al., *Food Chem.*, 87:307–311, 2004.)

Among the antioxidant compounds in rosemary leaves, ~90 percent of the antioxidant activity can be attributed to carnosol and carnosic acid. Topical application of rosemary extract, carnosol, or ursolic acid to mouse skin inhibited the covalent binding of benzo[*a*]pyrene to epidermal DNA, tumor initiation by 7,12-dimethylbenz[*a*]anthracene (DMBA), TPA-induced tumor promotion, ornithine decarboxylase activity, and inflammation (Huang et al., 1994).

Additional studies revealed that carnosic acid and carnosol strongly inhibited phase I enzyme CYP 450 activities and induced the expression of the phase II enzyme, glutathione *S*-transferase (GST) (Mace et al., 1998). These results give insight into different mechanisms involved in the chemopreventive actions of rosemary.

Recently Lo et al. (2002) demonstrated that carnosol can suppress the NO production and iNOS gene expression by inhibiting NF-κB activation, and provide possible mechanisms for its anti-inflammatory and chemopreventive action.

References

Al-Sereiti, M.R., Abu-Amer, K.M., and Sen, P., Pharmacology of rosemary (*Rosmarinus officinalis* Linn.) and its therapeutic potentials, *Indian J. Exp. Biol.*, 37:124–130, 1999.

Ho, C.T., Wang, M., Wei, G.J., Huang, T.C., and Huang, M.T., Chemistry and antioxidative factors in rosemary and sage, *Biofactors*, 13:161–166, 2000.

Huang, M.T., Ho, C.T., Wang, Z.Y., Ferraro, T., Lou, Y.R., Stauber, K., Ma, W., Georgiadis, C., Laskin, J.D., and Conney, A.H., Inhibition of skin tumorigenesis by rosemary and its constituents carnosol and ursolic acid, *Cancer Res.*, 54:701–708, 1994.

Lo, A-H., Liang, Y-C., Lin-Shiau, S-Y., Ho, C-T., and Lin, J-K., Carnosol, an antioxidant in rosemary, suppresses inducible nitric oxide synthase through down-regulating nuclear factor-κB in mouse macrophages, *Carcinogenesis*, 23:983–991, 2002.

Mace, K., Offord, E.A., Harris, C.C., and Pfeifer, A.M., Development of *in vitro* models for cellular and molecular studies in toxicology and chemoprevention, *Arch. Toxicol. Suppl.*, 20:227–236, 1998.

Newall, C.A., *Herbal Medicines — A Guide For Health Care Professionals*, The Pharmaceutical Press, London, 1996.

Rampart, M., Beetens, J.R., Bult, H., Herman, A.G., Parnham, M.J., and Winkelmann, J., Complement-dependent stimulation of prostacyclin biosynthesis: inhibition by rosmarinic acid, *Biochem. Pharmacol.*, 35:1397–1400, 1986.

Slamenova, D., Kuboskova, K., Horvathova, E., and Robichova, S., Rosemary-stimulated reduction of DNA strand breaks and FPG-sensitive sites in mammalian cells treated with H_2O_2 or visible light-excited Methylene Blue, *Cancer Lett.*, 177:145–153, 2002.

Wang, H., Provan, G.J., and Helliwell, P.K., Determination of rosmarinic acid and caffeic acid in aromatic herbs by HPLC, *Food Chem.*, 87:307–311, 2004.

Rosmarinic acid *see also* **Rosemary**   Rosmarinic acid is a phenolic compound widely distributed in *Labiatae* herbs, such as rosemary, sweet basil, and perilla (Scarpati and Oriente, 1958; Makino et al., 1998). This naturally occurring polyphenol exhibits antioxidant

Rosmarinic acid. (From Wang et al., *Food Chem.*, 87:307–311, 2004. With permission.)

(Tada et al., 1996) and anti-inflammatory effects, such as inhibitory effects on a complement-dependent inflammatory process (Peake et al., 1991), 5-lipoxygenase (Yamamoto et al., 1998), and histamine release from mast cells (Rimando et al., 1987). Sanbong et al. (2003) showed that it inhibited diesel-exhaust particles (DEP)-induced lung injury by reducing the expression of the macrophage inflammatory protein-1α.

Toshiaki et al. (2000) reported rosmarinic acid inhibited cytokine-induced mesangial-cell proliferation and suppressed platelet-derived growth factor (PDGF) and c-myc mRNA expression in PDGF-stimulated mesangial

R

cells, all of which suggest that it might be a promising agent to prevent mesangial-cell proliferation.

References

Makino, T., Ono, T., Muso, E., and Honda, G., Inhibitory effect of *Perilla frutescens* and its phenolic constituents on cultured murine mesangial cell proliferation, *Planta Med.*, 64:541–545, 1998.

Peake, P.W., Pussell, B.A., Martyn, P., Timmermans, V., and Charlesworth, J.A., The inhibitory effect of rosmarinic acid on complement involves the C5 convertase, *Int. J. Immunopharmacol.*, 13:853–857, 1991.

Rimando, A.M., Inoshiri, S., Otsuka, H. et al., Screening for mast cell histamine release inhibitory activity of Philippine medicinal plants. Active constituent of *Ehretia microphyll, Shoyakugaku Zasshi,* 41:242–247, 1987.

Sanbongi, C., Takano, H., Osakabe, N., Sasa, N., Natsume, M., Yanagisawa, R., Inoue, K., Kato, Y., Osawa, T., and Yoshikawa, T., Rosmarinic acid inhibits lung injury induced by diesel exhaust particles, *Free Rad. Biol. Med.*, 34:1060–1609, 2003.

Scarpati, M.L. and Oriente, G., Isolation and constitution of rosmarinic acid from *Rosmarinus officinalis, Ricerca Sci.*, 28:2329–2333, 1958.

Tada, M., Matsumoto, R., Yamaguchi, H., and Chiba, K., Novel antioxidants isolated from *Perilla frutescens* Britton var. *crispa* (Thunb.), *Biosci. Biotech. Biochem.*, 60:1093–1095, 1996.

Toshiaki, M., Ono, T., Muso, E., Yosida, H., Honda, G., and Sasayray, S., Inhibitory effects of rosmarinic acid on the proliferation of cultured murine mesangial cells, *Nephrol. Dial. Transplant,* 15:1140–1145, 2000.

Wang, H., Provan, G.J., and Helliwell, P.K., Determination of rosmarinic acid and caffeic acid in aromatic herbs by HPLC, *Food Chem.*, 87:307–311, 2004.

Yamamoto, H., Sakakibara, J., Nagatsu, A., and Sekiya, K., Inhibitors of arachidonate lipoxygenase from defatted perilla seed, *J. Agri. Food Chem.*, 46: 862–865, 1998.

Rosy or Madagascar periwinkle (Other names: Cape Periwinkle, *Catharanthus roseus*, Church Flower, Red Periwinkle)

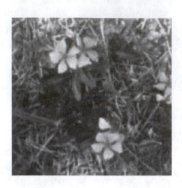

Rosy periwinkle (*Catharanthus roseus*), a medicinal plant found on the island of Madagascar, was used in traditional medicines for the treatment of cancer, Hodgkin's disease, and leukemia in children (Cardinali, 1973). Synthetic vincristine, used to treat leukemia, is only 20 percent as effective as the natural product derived from *Catharanthus roseus*. It was also found to have some potent blood-sugar-lowering activity (Chattopadhyay, 1999). Wang et al. (2004) reported that aqueous extracts of *Catharanthus roseus* significantly inhibited proliferation of cultured bovine aortic endothelial cells at a concentration of 1 g dry herb/mL, suggesting its role as a potential antiangiogenic agent. However, the use of *Catharanthus roseus* is not recommended due to the risk of severe side effects (Carod-Artal, 2003). Chemicals derived from it are used in prescription-only anticancer drugs (Ram and Kumari, 2001). *Catharanthus roseus* and the drugs derived from it have been associated with causing birth defects, neurotoxicity, bone-marrow suppression, and sensitivity to sunlight (Mathur and Chaudan, 1985). In addition, it may also cause gastrointestinal complaints, headache, and muscle weakness.

References

Cardinali, G., Place of *Vinca rosea* alkaloids (*Catharanthus roseus*) in the treatment of Hodgkin's disease, *Haematologica,* 53:51–64, 1973.

Carod-Artal, F.J., Neurological syndromes linked with the intake of plants and fungi containing a toxic component (I), neurotoxic syndromes caused by the

R

ingestion of plants, seeds and fruits, *Rev. Neurol.,* 36: 860–871, 2003.

Chattopadhyay, R.R., A comparative evaluation of some blood sugar lowering agents of plant origin, *J. Ethnopharmacol.,* 67:367–372, 1999.

Mathur, R. and Chaudan, S., Antifertility efficacy of *Catharanthus roseus* Linn: a biochemical and histological study, *Acta Eur. Fertil.,* 16:203–205, 1985.

Ram, V.J. and Kumari, S., Natural products of plant origin as anticancer agents, *Drug News Perspect.,* 14: 465–482, 2001.

Wang, S., Zheng, Z., Weng, Y., Yu, Y., Zhang, D., Fan, W., Dai, R., and Hu, Z., Angiogenesis and antiangiogenesis activity of Chinese medicinal herbal extracts, *Life Sci.,* 74:2467–2478, 2004.

Rye *see also* **Ferulic acid** Rye bran contains, in addition to a high-content dietary fiber, plant lignans and other bioactive compounds, such as alkylresorcinols (AR) (Ross et al., 2004). These are phenolic lipids present in large amounts in the bran fraction of rye (Scheme R.53). They are amphiphilic 1,3-dihydroxybenzene derivatives with an odd-numbered alkyl chain at position 5 in the benzene ring (Kozubek and Tyman, 1999). Early research reported serious growth inhibition and other pathological symptoms in several animal species (Sedlet et al., 1984). Other reports, however, suggest ARs have antibacterial and antifungal properties, as well as antiparasitic, antitumor, and antioxidant properties (Kozubek and Tyman, 1999). Gasiorowski and coworkers (1996) showed AR markedly decreased the mutagenic effects of a number of mutagens using the Ames test. Kamil-Eldin and coworkers (2001) showed AR exhibited antioxidant activity *in vitro,* but it was still poor relative to α-tocopherol.

At present, evidence from studies in human subjects does not warrant the conclusion that rye, whole grains, or phytoestrogens protect against cancer. Some studies, however, have pointed in that direction, especially in relation to cancers of the upper digestive tract and of

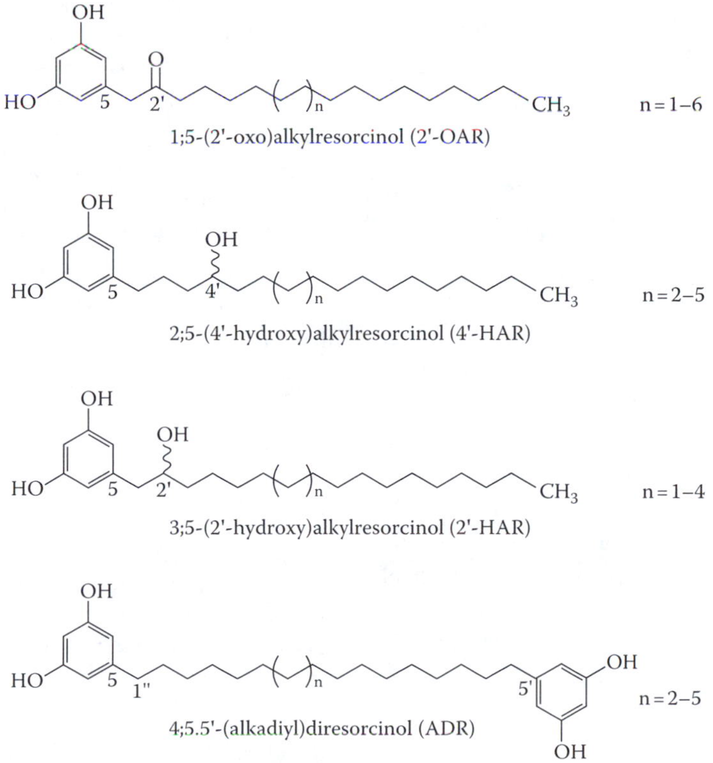

1;5-(2'-oxo)alkylresorcinol (2'-OAR) $n = 1–6$

2;5-(4'-hydroxy)alkylresorcinol (4'-HAR) $n = 2–5$

3;5-(2'-hydroxy)alkylresorcinol (2'-HAR) $n = 1–4$

4;5.5'-(alkadiyl)diresorcinol (ADR) $n = 2–5$

SCHEME R.53 Skeletal structures of alkylresorcinol-related analogs in rye. (From Suzuki et al., *Phytochemistry,* 52:281–289, 1999. With permission.)

the colon (Grasten et al., 2000). Rye foods also improved bowel health, as assessed by relevant markers (McIntyre et al., 1993; McIntosh et al., 2003). In comparison to wheat, rye is a slightly better source of total dietary fiber and is more commonly used in whole-grain food forms, which, together with cellulose, contributes more mixed linked $1{\rightarrow}3,1{\rightarrow}4\,\beta$-glucan and arabinoxylan (Aman et al., 1997). The latter fiber types are of particular interest, because they are present in soluble and insoluble forms, and arabinoxylan is considered to be an optimal substrate for fermentative generation of short-chain fatty acids in particular, and of butyrate in the colon. High concentration of butyrate in the colon is hypothesized to improve bowel health and lower cancer risk by several possible mechanisms (Bach et al., 1997). Ferulic acid, the major phenolic compound in rye bran and an antioxidant *in vitro*, however, did not produce a measurable antioxidative effect on human LDL (Harder et al., 2004).

Ferulic acid. (Adapted from Hynes and O'Coinceanainn, *J. Inorg. Biochem.,* 98:1457–1464, 2004.)

A number of prospective epidemiological studies have clearly shown a protective effect by whole-grain cereals against myocardial infarctions (Pietinen et al., 1996). A corresponding protective effect against diabetes (Leinonen et al., 1999) and ischemic stroke (brain infarct) have also been demonstrated (Hallmans et al., 2003). A high-fiber rye diet decreased insulin secretion, measured as decreased excretion of C-peptide in the urine and decreased plasma insulin peaks at the end of the day, during nibbling regimen (Lundin et al., 2004).

References

Aman, P., Nilsson, M., and Anderson, R., Positive health effects of rye, *Cereal Foods World,* 42:684–688, 1997.

Bach Knudsen, K.E., Johansen, H.N., and Glitso, L., Rye dietary fiber and fermentation in the colon, *Cereal Foods World,* 42:690–694, 1997.

Gasiorowski, K., Szyba, K., Brokos, B., and Kozubek, A., Antimutagenic activity of alkylresorcinols from cereal grains, *Cancer Lett.,* 106:109–115, 1996.

Grasten, S.M., Juntunen, K.S., Poutanen, K.S., Gylling, H.K., Miettinen, T.A., and Mykkanen, H.M., Rye bread improves bowel function and decreases the concentrations of some compounds that are putative colon cancer risk markers in middle-aged women and men, *J. Nutr.,* 130:2215–2221, 2000.

Hallmans, G., Zhang, J.X., Lundin, E., Stattin, P., Johansson, A., Johansson, I., Hulten, K., Winkvist, A., Aman, P., Lenner, P., and Adlercreutz, H., Rye, lignans and human health, *Proc. Nutr. Soc.,* 62:193–199, 2003.

Harder, H., Tetens, I., Let, M.B., and Meyer, A.S., Rye bran bread intake elevates urinary excretion of ferulic acid in humans, but does not affect the susceptibility of LDL to oxidation *ex vivo, Eur. J. Nutr.,* 43:230–236, 2004.

Hynes, M.J. and O'Coinceanainn, M., The kinetics and mechanisms of reactions of iron (III) with caffeic acid, chlorogenic acid, sinapic acid, ferulic acid and naringin, *J. Inorg. Biochem.,* 98:1457–1464, 2004.

Kamil-Eldin, A., Pouru, A., Eliasson, C., and Aman, P., Alkylresorcinols as antioxidants: hydrogen donation and peroxyl scavenging effects, *J. Sci. Food Agric.,* 81:353–356, 2001.

Kozubek, A. and Tyman, J.H.P., Resorcinolic lipids, the natural non-isoprenoid phenolic amphiphiles and their biological activity, *Chem. Rev.,* 99:1–26, 1999.

Leinonen, K., Liukkonen, K., Poutanen, K., Uusitupa, M., and Mykkanen, H., Rye bread decreases postprandial insulin response but does not alter glucose response in healthy Finnish subjects, *Eur. J. Clin. Nutr.,* 53:262–267, 1999.

Lundin, E.A., Zhang, J.X., Lairon, D., Tidehag, P., Aman, P., Adlercreutz, H., and Hallmans, G., Effects of meal frequency and high-fibre rye-bread diet on glucose and lipid metabolism and ileal excretion of energy and sterols in ileostomy subjects, *Eur. J. Clin. Nutr.,* 58:410–1419, 2004.

McIntyre, A., Gibson, P.R., and Young, G.P., Butyrate production from dietary fiber and protection against large bowel cancer in a rat model, *Gut,* 34:386–391, 1993.

McIntosh, G.H., Noakes, M., Royle, P.J., and Foster, P.R., Whole-grain rye and wheat foods and markers of bowel health in overweight middle-aged men, *Am. J. Clin. Nutr.,* 77:967–974, 2003.

Pietinen, P., Rimm, E.B., Korhonen, P., Hartman, A.M., Willett, W.C., Albanes, D., and Virtamo, J., Intake of dietry fibre and risk of coronary heart disease in a cohort of Finnish men, The Alpha-Tocopherol, Beta-Carotene Cancer Prevention Study, *Circulation,* 94:2720–2727, 1996.

Ross, A.B., Kamal-Eldin, A., and Aman, P., Dietary alkylresorcinols: absorption, bioactivities, and possible use as biomarkers of whole-grain wheat- and rye-rich foods. *Nutr. Rev.,* 62:81–95, 2004.

Sedlet, K., Mathias, M., and Lorenz, K., Growth-depressing effects of 5-*n*-pentadecylresorcinol: a model for cereal alkylresorcinols, *Cereal Chem.,* 61: 239–241, 1984.

Suzuki, Y., Esumi, Y., and Yamaguchi, I., Structures of 5-alkylresorcinol-related analogues in rye, *Phytochemistry,* 52:281–289, 1999.

R

S

Saffron *see also* **Crocin** Saffron (*Crocus sativus* L.) is an important spice grown in Greece, Spain, Turkey, Iran, India, and Morocco. In folklore medicine, as well as in modern pharmacy, saffron has been reputed to be useful in treating numerous human diseases, such as cardiovascular diseases (Grisolia, 1974; Abdullaev, 1993) and neurodegenerative disorders accompanying memory impairment (Abe and Saito, 2000). It contains three main, pharmacologically active metabolites: (1) saffron-colored compounds crocins, which are unusual, water-soluble carotenoids. The digentiobiosyl ester of crocetin — α-crocin — is the major component of saffron. (2) Picrocrocin is the main substance responsible for the bitter taste in saffron. (3) Safranal is the volatile oil responsible for the characteristic saffron odor and aroma. Furthermore, saffron contains proteins, sugars, vitamins, flavonoids, amino acids, mineral matter, gums, and other chemical compounds (Rios et al., 1996; Winterhalter and Straubirger, 1971.)

Studies by Escribano and coworkers (1996) found extracts from saffron inhibited cell growth of human tumor cells. Cells treated with crocin proved very effective in inhibiting tumor growth. A growing body of research has demonstrated that the saffron extract itself and its main constituents, the carotenoids, possess chemopreventive properties against cancer. A review by Abdullaev and Espinosa-Aguirre (2004) discusses the recent literature on the anticancer activities of saffron and its main ingredients.

An earlier study by Xuan et al. (1999) on ischemic retinopathy and age-related macular degeneration found that monosaccharide analogues of crocin, because of their ability to significantly increase blood flow to the retina, could be used to alleviate this condition.

Crocetin was found to enhance oxygen diffusivity through liquids, such as the plasma. As a consequence of this property, crocetin has been observed to increase alveolar oxygen transport and to enhance pulmonary oxygenation. It improves cerebral oxygenation in hemorrhaged rats and acts positively in atherosclerosis and arthritis treatment (Giaccio, 2004).

A significant reduction in papilloma formation was found with saffron application in the preinitiation and postinitiation periods. The inhibition appeared to be partly due to the modulatory effects of saffron on some phase II detoxifying enzymes, such as glutathione *S*-transferase, glutathione peroxidase, catalase, and superoxide dismutase (Das et al., 2004).

In a double-blind, randomized clinical pilot trial, Noorbala et al. (2005) showed a hydroalcoholic extract from saffron was as effective as the drug fluoxetine in treating mild to moderate depression (Figure S.88). Based on their results, a larger-scale trial was strongly recommended.

Saffranal (a) picrocrocin (b). (Adapted from Lozano et al., *J. Biochem. Biophys. Methods*, 43:367–378, 2000.)

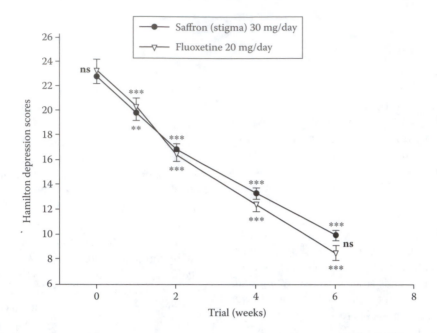

FIGURE S.88 Mean ± S.E.M. scores of two groups of patients on the Hamilton Depression Rating Scale. (ns) Nonsignificant; (**) $p < 0.01$ and (***) $p < 0.001$. The horizontal symbols (** and ***) were used to express statistical significance vs. their respective baseline value, and ns were used for between-group comparisons. (From Noorbala et al., *J. Ethnopharmacol.*, 97:281–284, 2005. With permission.)

References

Abdullaev, F.I., Biological effects of saffron. *BioFactors*, 4:83–86, 1993.

Abdullaev, F.I. and Espinosa-Aguirre, J.J., Biomedical properties of saffron and its potential use in cancer therapy and chemoprevention trials, *Cancer Detect. Prev.*, 28:426–432, 2004.

Abe, K. and Saito, H., Effects of saffron extract and its constituent crocin on learning behaviour and long-term potentiation, *Phytother. Res.*, 14:149–152, 2000.

Das, I., Chakrabarty, R.N., and Das, S., Saffron can prevent chemically induced skin carcinogenesis in Swiss albino mice, *Asian Pac. J. Cancer Prev.*, 5:70–76, 2004.

Escribano, J., Alonso, G.L., Coca-Prados, M., and Fernandez, J.A., Crocin, safranal and picrocrocin from saffron (*Crocus sativus* L.) inhibit the growth of human cancer cells *in vitro*, *Cancer Lett.*, 100:23–30, 1996.

Giaccio, M., Crocetin from saffron: an active component of an ancient spice, *Crit. Rev. Food Sci. Nutr.*, 44:155–172, 2004.

Grisolia, S., Letter: hypoxia, saffron, and cardiovascular disease, *Lancet*, 2(78-71):41–42, 1974.

Lozano, P., Delgado, D., Gomez, D., Rubio, M., and Iborra, J.L., A non-destructive method to determine the safranal content of saffron (*Crocus sativus* L.) by supercritical carbon dioxide extraction combined with high-performance liquid chromatography and gas chromatography, *J. Biochem. Biophys. Methods*, 43:367–378, 2000.

Noorbala, A.A., Akhondzadeh, S., Tahmacebi-Pour, N., and Jamshidi, A.H., Hydro-alcoholic extract of *Crocus sativus* L. versus fluoxetine in the treatment of mild to moderate depression: a double-blind, randomized pilot trial, *J. Ethnopharmacol.*, 97:281–284, 2005.

Rios, J.L., Recio, M.C., Giner, R.M., and Mañez, S., An update review of saffron and its active constituents, *Phytother. Res.*, 10:189–193, 1996.

Winterhalter, P. and Straubinger, M., Saffron — renewed interest in an ancient spice, *Food Rev. Int.*, 16:39–59, 1971.

Xuan, B., Zhou, Y.H., Min, Z.D., and Chiou, G.C., Effects of crocin analogues on ocular blood flow and retinal function, *J. Ocular Pharm. Ther.*, 15:143–152, 1999.

Sage (*Salvia officinalis*)   Sage is a common aromatic and medicinal plant native to Mediterranean countries but now grown throughout Europe and North America. The odor and aromatic taste of sage are due to its volatile oil. The plant's medicinal value resides in its crushed, dried leaves and the oil extracted from its flowers, leaves, and stems. It exhibits antibacterial qualities, inhibits viral and fungal growth (Radulescu et al., 2004), reduces perspiration and other secretions, and acts as an astringent, tightening and drying the tissues (Togel et al., 2002).

Salvia officinalis has been used in herbal medicine for many centuries. It has been suggested, on the basis of traditional medicine and its *in vitro* cholinergic-binding properties and modulation of mood and cognitive performance in humans, that *Salvia officinalis* might potentially provide a novel natural treatment for Alzheimer's disease. A recent study demonstrated the efficacy of *Salvia officinalis* extract in the management of mild to moderate Alzheimer's disease (Akhondzadeh et al., 2003).

Caffeic acid, rosmarinic acid, and oligomers of caffeic acid, with multiple catechol groups, are all constituents of *Salvia officinalis,* with antioxidant potential with regard to their radical-scavenging activity and the stability and structure of the intermediate radicals (Bors et al., 2004). Ursolic acid is the main component in *Salvia officinalis* L. leaves that is involved in sage topical anti-inflammatory activity (Baricevic et al., 2001).

Antimutagenic properties of terpenoid fractions of sage (*Salvia officinalis*) were demonstrated by Vujosevic and Blagojevic (2004) in mammalian system *in vivo*. Sage decreases the frequency of aberrant cells, induced by a potent mutagen. The acidic polysaccharide fractions from the aerial parts of sage were found to exhibit mitogenic activities, indicating that they may have adjuvant properties (Capek and Hribalova, 2004).

Lima and coworkers (2005) recently reported that drinking a water infusion (tea) of common sage (*Salvia officinalis*) improved the liver antioxidant status, measured as GSH content, in mice and rats. Compared to water, drinking sage tea conferred some protection in the hepatocyte cultures exposed to *tert*-butyl hydroperoxide (*t*-BHP). This was particularly evident in the presence of 1 mM *t*BHP (Figure S.89). These results point to the important antioxidant contribution by sage in combating oxidative stress.

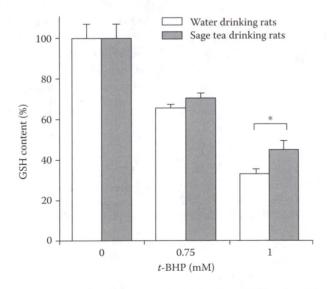

FIGURE S.89 Effect of sage-tea consumption (*in vivo* for 14 days) on *t*-BHP-induced decrease in GSH content of primary hepatocyte cultures, presented as percentage of the control. Values are mean ± S.E.M., n = 4. *$p < 0.05$, significantly different with Student's t-test. (From Lima et al., *J. Ethnopharm.,* 97:383–389, 2005. With permission.)

References

Akhondzadeh, S., Noroozian, M., Mohammadi, M., Ohadinia, S., Jamshidi, A.H., and Khani, M. *Salvia officinalis* extract in the treatment of patients with mild to moderate Alzheimer's disease: a double blind, randomized and placebo-controlled trial, *J. Clin. Pharm. Ther.,* 28:53–59, 2003.

Baricevic, D., Sosa, S., Della Loggia, R., Tubaro, A., Simonovska, B., Krasna, A., and Zupancic, A., Topical anti-inflammatory activity of *Salvia officinalis* L. leaves: the relevance of ursolic acid, *J. Ethnopharmacol.,* 75:125–132, 2001.

Bors, W., Michel, C., Stettmaier, K., Lu, Y., and Foo, L.Y., Antioxidant mechanisms of polyphenolic caffeic acid oligomers, constituents of *Salvia officinalis, Biol. Res.,* 37:301–311, 2004.

Capek, P. and Hribalova, V., Water-soluble polysaccharides from *Salvia officinalis* L. possessing immunomodulatory activity, *Phytochemistry,* 65:1983–1992, 2004.

Lima, C.F., Andrade, P.B., Seabra, R.M., Fernandes-Ferreira, M., and Pereira-Wilson, C., The drinking of a *Salvia officinalis* infusion improves liver antioxidant status in mice and rats, *J. Ethropharm.,* 97:383–389, 2005.

Radulescu, V., Chiliment, S., and Oprea, E., Capillary gas chromatography-mass spectrometry of volatile and semi-volatile compounds of *Salvia officinalis*, *J. Chromatogr. A.,* 1027:121–126, 2004.

Togel, B., Greve, B., and Raulin, C., Current therapeutic strategies for hyperhidrosis: a review, *Eur. J. Dermatol.,* 12:219–223, 2002.

Vujosevic, M. and Blagojevic, J., Antimutagenic effects of extracts from sage (*Salvia officinalis*) in mammalian system *in vivo*, *Acta Vet. Hung.,* 52:439–443, 2004.

Saponins Saponins are a group of surface-active glycosides, produced mainly by plants and some lower marine animals and bacteria (Espada and Riguera, 1997; Yoshiki et al., 1998). They consist of a sugar moiety, such as glucose, galactose, glucuronic acid, xylose, rhamnose, or methylpentose, attached to a hydrophobic aglycone (sapogenin), which can be a triterpenoid or steroid. Triterpenoid saponins are predominant in cultivated crops, while steroid saponins are found in plants used as herbs, particularly for their health-related properties (Fenwick et al., 1991). Some saponins were found by Johnson and coworkers (1986) to increase cell permeability and facilitate the uptake of substances not previously absorbed. For example, Gee and coworkers (1993) showed the ability of quinoa saponins to increase cell permeability, which could be used to enhance drug absorption by patients. In fact, Estrada et al. (1998) found that quinoa saponins could act as adjuvants for mucosally administered vaccines. Saponins from different sources were also shown to lower serum cholesterol levels in a variety of animals and humans (Al-Habori and Raman, 1998) and to have anti-inflammatory (Wei et al., 2004) and antioxidant (Sur et al., 2001) properties. Saponin-based adjuvants stimulated the immune system, as well as enhanced antibody production at low-dose levels (Oda et al., 2000). The adjuvant activity was attributed to branched sugar chains (Bomford et al., 1992) or aldehyde groups (Kensil, 1996). Saponins from different sources were found to inhibit cancer cells *in vitro* (Podolak et al., 1998). Triterpenoid saponins from *Acacia vitoriae* were reported to selectively inhibit the growth of tumor in human breast-cancer cell lines by arresting cell cycle or by apoptosis in leukemia-cell lines (Mujoo et al., 2001). Triterpene saponins also showed a prominent IL-2-inducing activity, which may explain the mechanism involved in their immunomodulatory and anticancer effects (Yesilada et al., 2005). Francis and coworkers (2002) reviewed the biological action of saponins in animal systems. Recently, triterpenoid saponins isolated from the leaves of the Vietnamese medicinal plant *Maesa balansae*, showed *in vitro* and *in vivo* activity against the tropical protozoal parasite *Leishmania infantum* (Scheme S.54) (Germonprez et al., 2005).

References

Al-Habori, M. and Raman, A., Antidiabetic and hypocholesterolaemic effects of fenugreek, *Phytother. Res.,* 12:233–242, 1998.

Bomford, R., Stapleton, M., Winsor, S., Beesley, J.E., Jessup, E.A., Price, K.R., and Fenwick, G.R., Adjuvanticity and ISCOM formation by structurally diverse saponins, *Vaccine,* 10:572–577, 1992.

Espada, A. and Riguera, R., Boussingoside E, a new triterpenoid saponin from the tubers *Boussingaultia baselloides, J. Nat. Prod.,* 60:17–19, 1997.

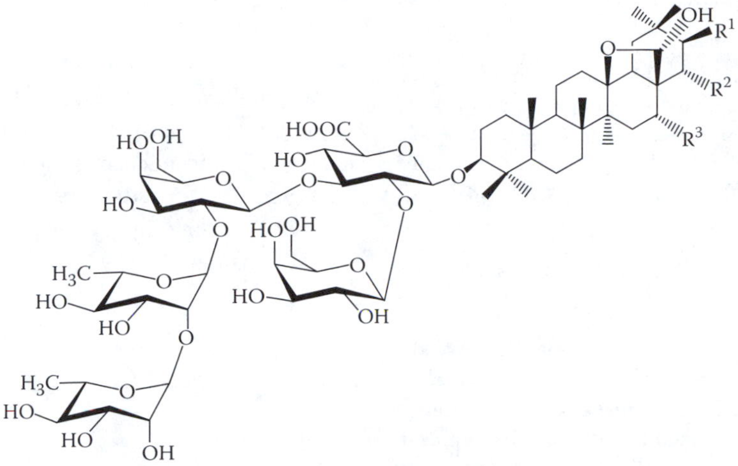

Saponin	R^1	R^2	R^3
1	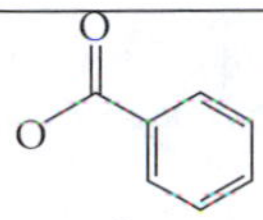	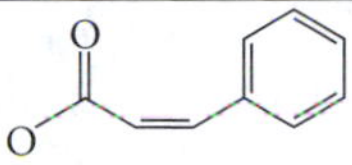	OH
2	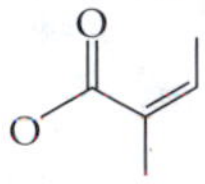	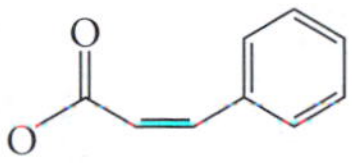	OH
3	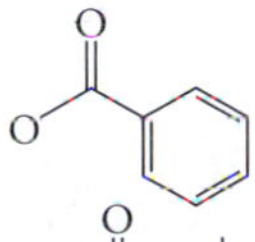	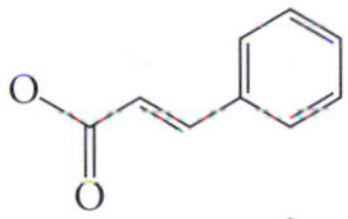	OH
4	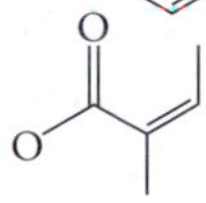	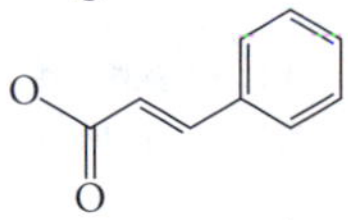	OH
5	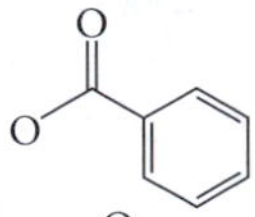	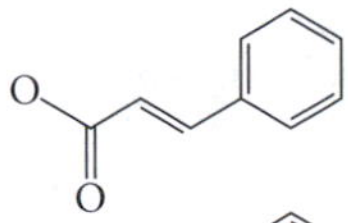	OAc
6	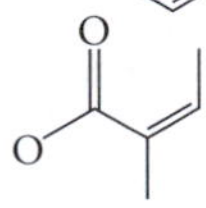	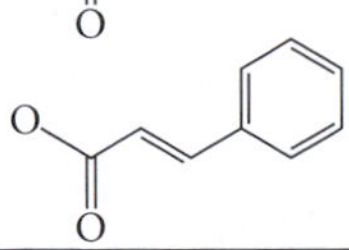	UAc

SCHEME S.54 Six triterpenoid saponins extracted from *Maesa balansae*. (From Leonard et al., *J. Chromatogr. A*, 1012:39–46, 2003. With permission.)

Estrada, A., Li, B., and Laarveld, B., Adjuvant action of *Chenopodium quinoa* saponins on the induction of antibody responses to intragastric and intranasal administered antigens in mice, *Comp. Immunol. Microbiol. Infect. Dis.,* 21:225–236, 1998.

Fenwick, G.R., Price, K.R., Tsukamoto, C., and Okubo, K. Saponins, in *Saponins in Toxic Substances in Crop Plants,* D'Mello, F.J.P., Duffus, C.M., and Duffus, J.H., Eds., Cambridge: The Royal Society of Chemistry, Cambridge, 1991.

Francis, G., Kerem, Z., Makkar, H.P., and Becker, K., The biological action of saponins in animal systems: a review, *Br. J. Nutr.,* 88:587–605, 2002.

Gee, J.M.., Price, K.R., Ridout, C.L., Wortley, G.M., Hurrell, R.F. and Johnson, I.T. , Saponins of quinoa (*Chenopodium quinoa*). Effect of processing in their

S

abundance in quinoa products and their biological effects on intestinal mucosal tissue. *J. Sci. Food Agric.,* 63:201–209, 1993.

Germonprez, N., Maes, L., Van Puyvelde, L., Van Tri, M., Tuan, D.A., and De Kimpe, N., *In vitro* and *in vivo* anti-leishmanial activity of triterpenoid saponins isolated from *Maesa balansae* and some chemical derivatives, *J. Med. Chem.,* 48:32–37, 2005.

Kensil, C.R., Saponins as vaccine adjuvants, *Crit. Rev. Ther. Drug Carrier Sys.,* 13:1–55, 1996.

Leonard, S., Capote, R., Germonprez, N., Puyvelde, L.V., De Kimpe, N., Vermeersch, H., Rosier, J., Maes, L., Roets, E., and Hoeogmartens, J., Liquid chromatographic method for analysis of saponins in *Maesa balansae* extract active against leishmaniasis, *J. Chromatogr. A,* 1012:39–46, 2003.

Mujoo, K., Haridas, V., Hoffman, J.J., Wachter, G.A., Hutter, L.K., Lu, Y., Blake, M.E., Jayatilake, G.S., Bailey, D., Mills, G.B., and Gutterman, J.U., Triterpenoid saponins from *Acacia victoriae* (Bentham) decrease tumor cell proliferation and induce apoptosis, *Cancer Res.,* 61:5486–5490, 2001.

Oda, K., Matsuda, H., Murakami, T., Katamaya, S., Ohgitani, T., and Yoshikawa, W., Adjuvant and haemolytic activities of 47 saponins derived from medicinal and plant foods, *Biol. Chem.,* 381:67–74, 2000.

Podolak, I., Elas, M., and Cieska, K., *In vitro* antifungal and cytotoxic activity of triterpene saponosides and quinoid pigments from *Lysimachia vulgaris* L., *Phytother. Res.,* 12:S70–S73, 1998.

Sur, P., Chaudhuri, T., Vedasiromoni, J.R., Gomes, A., and Ganguly, D.K., Anti-inflammatory and antioxidant property of saponins of tea [*Camellia sinensis* (L) O. Kuntze] root extract, *Phytother. Res.,* 15: 174–176, 2001.

Wei, F., Ma, L.Y., Jin, W.T., Ma, S.C., Han, G.Z., Khan, I.A., and Lin, R.C., Anti-inflammatory triterpenoid saponins from the seeds of *Aesculus chinensis*, *Chem. Pharm. Bull.,* 52:1246–1248, 2004.

Yesilada, E., Bedir, E., Calis, I., Takaishi, Y., and Ohmoto, Y., Effects of triterpene saponins from *Astragalus* species on *in vitro* cytokine release, *J. Ethnopharmacol.,* 96:71–77, 2005.

Yoshiki, Y., Kodov, Y.S. and Okubo, K., Relationship between chemical structures and biological activities of triterpenoid saponins from soybean., *Biosci. Biotechnol Biochem.,* 62:2291–2299, 1998.

Sarcophytol A   Sarcophytol A (SaA) is a cembrane-type diterpene isolated from the marine soft coral *Sarcophyton glaucum*. It showed anticancer and cancer-preventive effects in two animal models: transplanted human pancreatic-cancer cells in nude mice and pancreatic carcinogenesis induced by *N*-nitrobis-(2-hydroxypropyl) amine in Syrian golden hamsters (Yokomatsu et al., 1994).

Sarcophytol A. (From Li et al., *Tetrahedron Lett.,* 40: 965–968, 1999. With permission.)

SaA also provided significant protection against the induction of genetic damage in human lung cells exposed to tobacco-specific nitrosamines (Weitberg and Corvese, 1999).

Recently, the natural cembranolide sarcophine and its lactone ring-opened analogue were oxidized to prepare hydroxylated derivatives, which were shown to have higher activity than the chemopreventive agent sarcophytol A (Katsuyama et al., 2002).

References

Katsuyama, I., Fahmy, H., Zjawiony, J.K., Khalifa, S.I., Kilada, R.W., Konoshima, T., Takasaki, M., and Tokuda, H., Semisynthesis of new sarcophine derivatives with chemopreventive activity, *J. Nat. Prod.,* 65:1809–1814, 2002.

Li, W.-DZ., Li, Y., and Li, Y., Concise and efficient total syntheses of (±)-sacophytols A and B, two antitumor cembrane diterpenoids, by an intramolecular McMurry olefination strategy, *Tetrahedron Lett.,* 40: 965–968, 1999.

Weitberg, A.B. and Corvese, D., The effect of epigallocatechin galleate and sarcophytol A on DNA strand breakage induced by tobacco-specific nitrosamines and stimulated human phagocytes, *J. Exp. Clin. Cancer Res.,* 18:433–437, 1999.

Yokomatsu, H., Satake, K., Hiura, A., Tsutsumi, M., and Suganuma, M., Sarcophytol A: a new chemotherapeutic and chemopreventive agent for pancreatic cancer, *Pancreas,* 9:526–530, 1994.

Saskatoon berry   The Saskatoon (*Amelanchier alnifolia*) is a small to large shrub, or a small

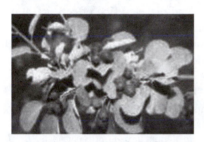

tree, which belongs to the rose family. The Saskatoon, an important food source, was also used as a source wood and a medicinal plant. Today, Saskatoons are used in a wide variety of ways, from pies, jams, jellies, syrups, ice cream toppings, wine, liqueurs, and flavor concentrates to components of baked goods. The methanolic extract of *Amelanchier alnifolia* was found active against an enteric coronavirus, demonstrating antiviral activities at the noncytotoxic concentrations (McCutcheon et al., 1995)

References

McCutcheon, A.R., Roberts, T.E., Gibbons, E., Ellis, S.M., Babiuk, L.A., Hancock, R.E.W., and Towers, G.H.N., Antiviral screening of British Columbian medicinal plants, *J. Ethnopharmacol.,* 49:101–110, 1995.

Savory (*Satureja hortensis* L.)   Savory, an annual herb of the Lamiaceae family, is used as a condiment, as well as in folk medicine, for treating infectious diseases. It contains an essential oil composed of thymol, although the main component is carvacrol, a positional isomer of thymol (30 percent to 45 percent), as well as *p*-cymene (max. 30 percent), γ-terpinene, α-pinene (8 percent), dipentene, borneol, 1-linalool, terpineol, and 1-carvone. Antimicrobial and antioxidant tests by Gulluce

Carvacrol. (From De Vicenzi et al., Fitoterapia, 75: 801-804, 2004. With permission.)

et al. (2003) showed the essential oil exhibited antimicrobial activities against all 23 bacteria and 15 fungi and yeast species tested, while linoleic-acid oxidation was inhibited by 95 percent. The evaluation of antioxidant power of glycosidically bound volatile aglycones from savory showed the antioxidative activity possessed by these compounds was comparable to that of the essential oil (Radonic and Milos, 2003). The antioxidant properties of a crude extract and its purified ethyl acetate-soluble fraction from the aerial material of savory was recently demonstrated by Dorman and Hiltunen (2004) using an Fe(III) reductive and DPPH·, ABTS·+, and hydroxyl free-radical-scavenging assays. Chorianopoulos et al. (2004) reported that essential oils extracted from the *Satureja* species represented an inexpensive source of natural antibacterial compounds for potential use in food systems to prevent the growth of foodborne bacteria and extend the shelf life of the processed food. The antibacterial activity of a number of essential oils, including savory oil, was found to be effective against vaginal microorganisms responsible for infectious gynecological diseases (Arnal-Schnebelen et al., 2004). Other species of savory plants were reported to have antinociceptive (Hajhashemi et al., 2002) and anti-inflammatory (Uslu et al., 2003) effects.

References

Arnal-Schnebelen, B., Hadji-Minaglou, F., Peroteau, J.-F., Ribeyre, F., and de Billerbeck, V.G., Essential oils in infectious gynaecological disease: a statistical study of 658 cases, *Int. J. Aromather.,* 14:192–197, 2004.

S

Chorianopoulos, N., Kalpoutzakis, E., Aligiannis, N., Mitaku, S., Nychas, G-J., and Haroutounian, S.A., Essential oils of *Satureja, Origanum,* and *Thymus* species: chemical composition and antibacterial activities against foodborne pathogens, *J. Agric. Food Chem.,* 52:8261–8267, 2004.

De Vincenzi, M., Stammati, A., De Vincenzi, A., and Silano, M., Constituents of aromatic plants: carvacrol, *Fitoterapia,* 75:801–804, 2004.

Dorman, H.J.D. and Hiltunen, R., Fe(III) reductive and free radical-scavenging properties of summer savory (*Satureja hortensis* L.) extract and subfractions, *Food Chem.,* 88:193–199, 2004.

Gulluce, M., Sokmen, M., Daferera, D., Agar, G., Ozkan, H., Kartal, N., Polissiou, M., Sokmen, A., and Sahin, F., *In vitro* antibacterial, antifungal, and antioxidant activities of the essential oil and methanol extracts of herbal parts and callus cultures of *Satureja hortensis* L., *J. Agric. Food Chem.,* 51: 3958–3965, 2003.

Hajhashemi, V., Ghannadi, A., and Pezeshkian, S.K., Antinociceptive and anti-inflammatory effects of *Satureja hortensis* L. extracts and essential oil, *J. Ethnopharmacol.,* 82:83–87, 2002.

Radonic, A. and Milos, M., Chemical composition and antioxidant test of free and glycosidically bound volatile compounds of savory (*Satureja montana* L. subsp. montana) from Croatia, *Nahrung,* 47:236–237, 2003.

Uslu, C., Murat Karasen, R., Sahin, F., Taysi, S., and Akcay, F., Effects of aqueous extracts of *Satureja hortensis* L. on rhinosinusitis treatment in rabbit, *J. Ethnopharmacol.,* 88:225–228, 2003.

Saw palmetto *see also* **Palmetto berries**
Saw palmetto (*Serenoa repens*) is a North American native plant whose berries are used for medicinal purposes. A letter to the editor by Champault and coworkers in 1984 first highlighted the pharmacological benefits of saw palmetto for the treatment of benign prostatic hyperplasia. It has since become the treatment for enlarged prostate or benign prostatic hyperplasia (BPH) in Europe (Wilt et al., 1998). Using a six-month, randomized trial, Veltri et al. (2002) found that treating men with symptomatic BPH with a saw palmetto herbal blend altered DNA chromatin structure and organization in prostate epithelial cells, suggesting a possible molecular basis for its therapeutic effect. Recent studies in the United States by Gerber et al. (2000) and Gong and Gerber (2004) showed that saw palmetto improved urinary function for those suffering from BPH.

The efficacy of saw palmetto appears to be similar to medications, such as finasteride, but it is better tolerated and less expensive. There are no known drug interactions with saw palmetto, and reported side effects are minor and rare. It was also used to treat chronic prostatitis, but currently there is no evidence of its efficacy (Gordon and Shaughnessy, 2003).

References
Champault, G., Patel, J.C., and Bonnard, A.M., A double-blind trial of an extract of the plant *Serenoa repens* in benign prostatic hyperplasia, *Br. J. Clin. Pharmacol.,* 18:461–462, 1984.

Gerber, G.S., Saw palmetto for the treatment of men with lower urinary tract symptoms, *J. Urol.,* 163: 1408–1412, 2000.

Gong, E.M. and Gerber, G.S., Saw Palmetto and benign prostatic hyperplasia, *Am. J. Chin. Med.,* 32: 331–338, 2004.

Gordon, A.E. and Shaughnessy, A.F., Saw palmetto for prostate disorders, *Am. Fam. Physician,* 67:1281–1283, 2003.

Veltri, R.W., Marks, L.S., Miller, M.C., Bales, W.D., Fan, J., Macairan, M.L., Epstein, J.I., and Partin, A.W., Saw palmetto alters nuclear measurements reflecting DNA content in men with symptomatic BPH: evidence for a possible molecular mechanism, *Urology,* 60:617–622, 2002.

Wilt, T.J., Ishani, A., Stark, G., MacDonald, R., Lau, J., and Mulrow, C., A systematic review: Saw palmetto extracts for treatment of benign prostatic hyperplasia, *JAMA,* 280:1604–1609, 1998.

Sea buckthorn (*Hippophae rhamnoides* L.)
Sea buckthorn, a temperate, hardy bush growing in Central Asia and Europe, produces nutritious and delicious berries (Roussi, 1971). The oil from the berries of sea buckthorn has been used in Chinese medicine for many centuries for treating cardiovascular disease. In fact, sea-buckthorn berries, particularly the alcohol extract of the twigs, was reported to inhibit thrombus

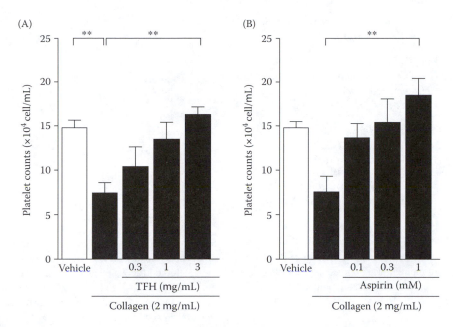

FIGURE S.90 Effects of (A) TFH and (B) aspirin on platelet aggregation induced by collagen (2 µg.mL) in whole blood from five mice. An open column indicates platelet counts in the tubes with added vehicle without collagen. Data are presented as means ± S.E.M. **; $p < 0.01$ by Bonferroni's multiple comparison test. (From Cheng et al., *Life Sci.*, 72:2263–2271, 2003. With permission.)

formation or platelet aggregation (Xu and Chen, 1991). Sea buckthorn is rich in antioxidants, tocopherols (Luhua et al., 2004), carotenoids, and vitamin C, as well as phytosterols, such as sitosterol (Field et al., 1997). In the sea-buckthorn pomace extract, the oligomeric proanthocyanidins accounted for 75 percent of the total antioxidant activity (Rosch et al., 2004). Using a supercritical extract of sea-buckthorn oil, Johansson and coworkers (2000) showed it inhibited platelet aggregation. Cheng and coworkers (2003) reported that a total flavone (TFH) extract from sea buckthorn exhibited a similar inhibitory effect to aspirin on platelet aggregation induced by collagen in mouse femoral artery (Figure S.90). This ability to prevent *in vivo* thrombogenesis, similar to aspirin, suggested sea buckthorn may help prevent cardiac and cerebral thrombosis.

Eccleston et al. (2002) showed sea-buckthorn juice was rich in antioxidants and moderately decreased the susceptibility of LDL to oxidation. An earlier study by Yang and coworkers (1999) found α-linolenic acid in sea buckthorn had a beneficial effect on atopic dermatitis (AD), a condition in which the skin is dry, scaly, and itchy with eczematous inflammation and lesions. Sea buckthorn was also reported to be a hopeful drug for prevention and treatment of liver fibrosis (Gao et al., 2003).

References

Cheng, J., Kondo, K., Suzuki, Y., Ikeda, Y., Meng, X., and Umemura, K., Inhibitory effects of total flavones of *Hippophae rhamnoides* L. on thrombosis in mouse femoral artery and *in vitro* platelet aggregation, *Life Sci.*, 72:2263–2271, 2003.

Gao, Z.L., Gu, X.H., Cheng, F.T., and Jiang, F.H., Effect of sea buckthorn on liver fibrosis: a clinical study, *World J. Gastroenterol.*, 9:1615–7, 2003.

Eccleston, C., Baoru, Y., Tahvonen, R., Kallio, H., Rimbach, G.H., and Minihane, A.M., Effects of an antioxidant-rich juice (sea buckthorn) on risk factors for coronary heart disease in humans, *J. Nutr. Biochem.*, 13:346–354, 2002.

Johansson, A.K., Korte, H., Yang, B., Stanley, J.C., and Kallio, H.P., Sea buckthorn berry oil inhibits platelet aggregation, *J. Nutr. Biochem.*, 11:491–495, 2000.

Luhua, Z., Ying, T., Zhengyu, Z., and Guangji, W., Determination of alpha-tocopherol in the Traditional Chinese Medicinal preparation Sea buckthorn oil

S

capsule by non-aqueous reversed phase-HPLC, *Chem. Pharm. Bull.,* 52:150–152, 2004.

Rosch, D., Mugge, C., Fogliano, V., and Kroh, L.W., Antioxidant oligomeric proanthocyanidins from sea buckthorn (*Hippophae rhamnoides*) Pomace, *J. Agric. Food Chem.,* 52:6712–6718, 2004.

Roussi, A., The genus *Hippophae* L., A taxonomic study, *Ann. Bot. Fennici.,* 8:177–227, 1971.

Xu, Q. and Chen, C., Effects of oil of *Hippophae rhamnoides* on the experimental thrombus formation and blood coagulation system, *Res. Dev. Natu. Prod.,* 3:70–73, 1991.

Yang, B., Kalimo, K.O., Mattila, L.M., Kallio, S.E., Katajisto, J.K., Peltola, O.J., and Kallio, H.P., Effects of dietary supplementation with sea buckthorn (*Hippophae rhamnoides*) seed and pulp oils on atopic dermatitis, *J. Nutr. Biochem.,* 10:622–630, 1999.

Sea cucumbers   Sea cucumbers or *Holothuroida,* are an abundant and diverse group of worm-like, soft-bodied echinoderms. They are ubiquitous in the marine environment but particularly diverse in tropical, shallow-water coral reefs. In the Southeast Asia regions, sea cucumbers are used as food supplements and as traditional remedy for wounds (Perchenik, 1996), parasitic skin infections (Shimada, 1969), and other ailments, such as backache, joint pain, and stomach and mouth ulcers.

Sea cucumber contains a wide range of nutrients, including collagen, marine protein, essential fatty acids, and antioxidants, including vitamin E and minerals (Hawa et al., 1999).

A few species of sea cucumbers showed antibacterial activity (Ridzwan et al., 1995), and glycosphingolipids from the sea cucumber had neuritogenic activity toward the saponin biosynthesis (Kerr and Chen, 1995). Yamada (2002) isolated pheochromocytoma cell line C-type mannan-binding lectins from various species of sea cucumbers exhibiting relatively high agglutinating activity (Bulgakov et al., 2000). Recently, Kariya et al. (2004) isolated two types of fucan sulfates, types A and B, from sea cucumber (*Stichopus japonicus*) that were potent inhibitors of osteoclastogenesis. Type A consisted of a backbone of (163)-linked fucosyl

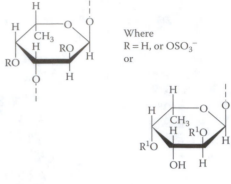

Where
R = H, or OSO_3^-
or

R^1 = H, or OSO_3^-

SCHEME S.55 Hypothetical structures of type A and type B fucan sulfates. Both have a backbone of (1→3)-linked fucose residues substituted with fucosyl residues at C-2 and C-4. Sulfate substitution(s) occur at C-2 and C-4 position(s). (Kariya et al., *Carbohydr. Res.,* 339:1339–1346, 2004. With permission.)

residues substituted at C-4 with the fucosyl residues sulfated at C-2/C-4 (Scheme S.55).

Type B consisted of unbranched (163)-linked fucosyl residues with sulfate substitution(s) at C-2 and/or C-4. The presence of either type A or B inhibited osteoclastogenesis in an *in vitro* osteoclast assay by 99.8 percent and 96.3 percent, respectively, compared to the control (Figure S.91). The potent inhibition of osteoclastogenesis by fucan sulfates points to their potential for treating some of the symptoms associated with osteoporosis and rheumatoid arthritis.

References

Bulgakov, A.A., Nazarenko, E.L., Petrova, I.Y., Eliseikina, M.G., Vakhrusheva, N.M., and Zubkov, V.A., Isolation and properties of a mannan-binding lectin from the coelomic fluid of the holothurian *Cucumaria japonica*, *Biochemistry,* Moscow; 65: 933–939, 2000.

Hawa, I., Zulaikah, M., Jamaludin, M., Zainal Abidin, A.A., Kaswandi, M.A., and Ridzwan, B.H., The potential of the coelomic fluid in sea cucumber as an antioxidant, *Mal. J. Nutr.,* 5:55–59, 1999.

Kariya, Y., Mulloy, B., Imai, K., Tominaga, A., Kaneko, T., Asari, A., Suzuki, K., Masuda, H., Kyogashima, M., and Ishii, T., Isolation and partial characterization of fucan sulfates from the body wall of sea cucumber *Stichopus japonicus* and their ability

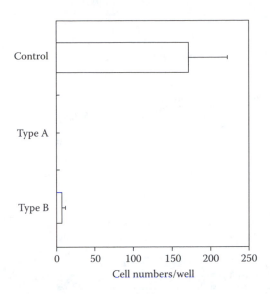

FIGURE S.91 Inhibitory effects of types A and B fucan sulfate on an *in vitro* osteoclast-formation assay system. Data expressed as mean ± SD (n = 3) taking the control as 0 percent. (From Kariya et al., *Carbohydr. Res.,* 339:1339–1346, 2004. With permission.)

to inhibit osteoclastogenesis, *Carbohydr. Res.,* 339: 1339–1346, 2004.

Kerr, R.G. and Chen, Z., *In vivo* and *in vitro* biosynthesis of saponins in sea cucumbers, *J. Nat. Prod.,* 58:172–176, 1995.

Perchenik, J.A., The echinoderms, in *Biology of Invertebrates,* 3rd ed., Dubuque, W.M.C., Ed., Brown Publisher, London, 1996, pp. 445-474.

Ridzwan, B.H., Kaswandi, M.A., Azman, Y., and Fuad, M., Screening for antibacterial agents in three species of sea cucumbers from coastal areas of Sabah, *Gen. Pharmacol.,* 26:1539–1543, 1995.

Shimada, S., Antifungal steroid glycoside from sea cucumber, *Science,* 163:1462, 1969.

Yamada, K., Chemo-pharmaceutical studies on the glycosphingolipid constituents from echinoderm, sea cucumbers, as the medicinal materials, *Yakugaku Zasshi.,* 122:1133–1143, 2002.

Secoisolariciresinol diglycoside *see also* **Lignans** Secoisolariciresinol diglycoside (SDG) is a plant lignan most notably found in flaxseed (linseed). SDG is classified as a phytoestrogen with a weak estrogenic activity. The level of

SDG in flaxseed typically varies between 0.6 percent and 1.8 percent. Following ingestion, SDG is converted to the aglycone secoisolariciresinol, which is then metabolized to the mammalian lignans enterolactone and enterodiol. Most of the effects of oral SDG are mediated by enterolactone and enterodiol.

Secoisolariciresinol diglucoside. (From Coran et al., *J. Chromatogr. A,* 1045:217–222, 2004. With permission.)

SDG, enterolactone, and enterodiol exhibited a number of antioxidant activities (Kitts et al., 1999), including inhibition of lipid peroxidation and scavenging of hydroxy radicals. SDG inhibited mammary-tumor development (Rickard et al., 2000), as well as delayed the progression of dimethylbenz[*a*]anthracene-induced mammary tumorigenesis (Rickard et al., 1999). Supplementation with SDG reduced pulmonary metastasis of mice melanoma cells and inhibited the growth of metastatic tumors formed in the lungs (Li et al., 1999). This was evident by a significant decrease in the mean tumor cross-sectional area and volume in a dose-dependent manner compared to the control (Table S.61).

References

Coran, S.A., Giannellini, V., and Bambagiotti, M., High-performance thin-layer chromatographic-densitometric determination of secoisolariciresinol diglucoside in flaxseed, *J. Chromatogr. A,* 1045:217–222, 2004.

Kitts, D.D., Yuan, Y.V., Wijewickreme, A.N., and Thompson, L.U., Antioxidant activity of the flaxseed lignan secoisolariciresinol diglycoside and its mammalian lignan metabolites enterodiol and enterolactone, *Mol. Cell Biochem.,* 202:91–100, 1999.

S

TABLE S.61
Effect of Dietary Supplementation with SDG on Pulmonary Metastasis of Melanoma Cells in Mice

Group	Mice n	Mice with Lung Tumors 1–50 Tumors	>50 Tumors[a]	Tumors/mouse Median[b]	Mean ± SE	Range
Control	27	11	16	62	64 ± 8	10–180
SDG						
71 µmol/kg	27	19	8	38	43 ± 5	8–117
147 µmol/kg	28	22	6[a]	36	42 ± 4	9–96
293 µmol/kg	27	21	6[a]	29[b]	33 ± 4	4–86

[a] Significantly different from the control, $p < 0.05$. Data were analyzed using Fisher's exact test.
[b] Significantly different from the control, $p < 0.01$. Data were analyzed using the Kruskal–Wallis nonparametric and Dunn's multiple comparison test.

Source: From Li et al., *Cancer Lett.,* 142:91–96, 1999. With permission.

Li, D., Yee, J.A., Thompson, L.U., and Yan, L., Dietary supplementation with secoisolariciresinol diglycoside (SDG) reduces experimental metastasis of melanoma cells in mice, *Cancer Lett.,* 142:91–96, 1999.

Rickard, S.E., Yuan, Y.V., Chen. J., and Thompson, L.U., Dose effects of flaxseed and its lignan on *N*-methyl-*N*-nitrosourea-induced mammary tumorigenesis, *Nutr. Cancer,* 35:50–57, 1999.

Rickard, S.E., Yuan, Y.V., and Thompson, L.U., Plasma insulin-like growth factor I levels in rats are reduced by dietary supplementation of flaxseed or its lignan secoisolariciresinol diglycoside, *Cancer Lett.,* 161:47–155, 2000.

Selenium   Selenium, a trace element essential in small amounts, can be toxic when taken in larger amounts. The levels in the body depend mainly on the amount of selenium in the diet, which is a function of the selenium content of the soil. Selenium is required for the functioning of more than 30 known selenoproteins, essential for normal functioning of the immune system (He et al., 2004), thyroid gland (Zagrodzki et al., 2001), and normal development, growth, metabolism, and defense of the body (Dodig and Cepelak, 2004; Kohrl et al., 2000).

A large number of studies confirmed that selenium supplementation plays a preventive and therapeutic role in diseases, such as male infertility (Foresta et al., 2002), viral infections (Broome et al., 2004), HIV (Kupka et al., 2004), cancer (recently reviewed by Patrick, 2004), and cardiovascular (Alissa et al., 2003) and autoimmune diseases (Gartner and Gasnier, 2003).

Selenium is an essential constituent of a number of enzymes, some of which have antioxidant functions. A deficiency of this element in animals renders them susceptible to injury by certain types of oxidative stress (Burk, 2002). In addition, selenomethionine catalyzes the reduction of peroxynitrite and low-molecular-weight organoselenium, compounds of pharmacologic interest known to catalyze the reduction of hydroperoxides or peroxynitrite with various cellular-reducing equivalents (Klotz et al., 2003). Oxidative stress plays an important role in vascular degenerative lesions observed in diabetes. Selenium is the cofactor of glutathione peroxidase, which is associated with thrombosis and cardiovascular complications of diabetes (Faure, 2003).

Analyses of pooled data from 1763 trial participants showed that statistically, individuals whose blood-selenium values were in the highest quartile (median = 150 ng/mL) had significantly lower odds of developing new adenomas compared with those in the lowest. The inverse association between higher blood-selenium concentration and adenoma risk supports previous

SENEGA 413

findings indicating that higher selenium status may be related to decreased risk of colorectal cancer (Jacobs et al., 2004).

Popova (2002) investigated the influence of neonatal selenium exposure on spontaneous liver-tumor formation in adult mice. Selenium was administered to pregnant CBA mice during their last week of pregnancy and for 10 days following parturition. There was a significant reduction in the incidence of spontaneous hepatomas in the adult male progeny, but not in adult females. This indicated that neonatal selenium altered hepatoma incidence in a sex-dependent manner.

References

Alissa, E.M., Bahijri, S.M., and Ferns, G.A., The controversy surrounding selenium and cardiovascular disease: a review of the evidence, *Med. Sci. Monit.,* 9:RA9–RA18, 2003.

Broome, C.S., McArdle, F., Kyle, J.A.M., Andrews, F., Lowe, N.M., Hart, C.A., Arthur, J.R., and Jackson, M.J., An increase in selenium intake improves immune function and poliovirus handling in adults with marginal selenium status, *Am. J. Clin. Nutr.,* 80:154–162, 2004.

Burk, R.F., Selenium, an antioxidant nutrient (Review), *Nutr. Clin. Care,* 5:75–79, 2002.

Dodig, S. and Cepelak, I., The facts and controversies about selenium, *Acta Pharm.,* 54:261–276, 2004.

Faure, P., Protective effects of antioxidant micronutrients (vitamin E, zinc and selenium) in type 2 diabetes mellitus (Review), *Clin. Chem. Lab. Med.,* 41:995–998, 2003.

Foresta, C., Flohe, L., Garolla, A., Roveri, A., Ursini, F., and Maiorino, M., Male fertility is linked to the selenoprotein phospholipid hydroperoxide glutathione peroxidase, *Biol. Reprod.,* 67:967–971, 2002.

Gartner, R. and Gasnier, B.C., Selenium in the treatment of autoimmune thyroiditis, *Biofactors,* 19:165–170, 2003.

He, S-X., Wu, B., Chang, X-M., Li, H-X., and Qiao, W., Effects of selenium on peripheral blood mononuclear cell membrane fluidity, interleukin-2 production and interleukin-2 receptor expression in patients with chronic hepatitis, *World J. Gastroenterol.,* 10:3531–3533, 2004.

Klotz, L-O., Kroncke, K-D., Buchczyk, D.P., and Sies, H., Role of copper, zinc, selenium and tellurium in the cellular defense against oxidative and nitrosative stress, *J. Nutr.,* 133:1448S–1451S, 2003.

Kohrl, J., Brigelius-Flohe, R., Bock, A., Gartner, R., Meyer, O., and Flohe, L., Selenium in biology: facts and medical perspectives, *Biol. Chem.,* 381:849–864, 2000.

Kupka, R., Msamanga, G.I., Spiegelman, D., Morris, S., Mugusi, F., Hunter, D.J., and Fawzi, W.W., Selenium status is associated with accelerated HIV disease progression among HIV-1-infected pregnant women in Tanzania, *J. Nutr.,* 134:2556–2560, 2004.

Jacobs, E.T., Jiang, R., Alberts, D.S., Greenberg, E.R., Gunter, E.W., Karagas, M.R., Lanza, E., Ratnasinghe, L., Reid, M.E., Schatzkin, A., Smith-Warner, S.A., Wallace, K., and Martinez, M.E., Selenium and colorectal adenoma: results of a pooled analysis, *J. Natl. Cancer Inst.,* 96:1669–1675, 2004.

Patrick, L., Selenium biochemistry and cancer: a review of the literature, *Altern. Med. Rev.,* 9:239–258, 2004.

Popova, N.V., Perinatal selenium exposure decreases spontaneous liver tumorogenesis in CBA mice, *Cancer Lett.,* 179:39–42, 2002.

Zagrodzki, P., Nicol, F., Arthur, J.R., and Slowiaczek, M., Selenoproteins in human thyroid tissues, *Biofactors,* 14:223–227, 2001.

Senega (*Polygara senega*) This perennial herb grows in central and western North America. The name of the genus, *Polygala*, means "much milk," alluding to its own profuse secretions and their effects. "Senega" is derived from the Seneca tribe of North American Indians, among

S

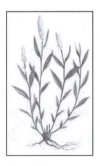

whom the roots were used as a remedy for snake bites. The root contains polygalic acid, virgineic acid, pectic and tannic acids, yellow, bitter, coloring matter, cerin-fixed oil, resin, traces of volatile oil (a mixture of valeric ether and methyl salicylate), 7 percent sugar, from 2 percent to 5 percent senegin (Saitoh et al., 1994), malatesgum, woody fiber, salts, aluminum, silica, magnesium, and iron (Moes, 1966). Fresh senega root has a pleasant odor due to its content of approximately 0.1 percent methyl salicylate. The active ingredient, however, is a complex mixture in the root of triterpenoid saponins in a concentration ranging from 8 percent to 16 percent (Yoshikawa et al., 1996). The saponins act by local irritation on the lining of the stomach, causing nausea that in turn stimulates both bronchial secretion and the sweat glands.

During the early 19th century, senega root was used as an expectorant cough remedy. Today, senega root is used to treat bronchitis, tracheitis, emphysema, and inflammation of the respiratory tract (Kuribara and Tadokoro, 1989). The saponins suppress coughing, while their detergent activity breaks up phlegm (Kantee, 1973). Senega is also believed to stimulate bronchial mucous-gland secretion. Saponins in senega root may hold some potential for treatment of noninsulin-dependent diabetes (Kako et al., 1996). Senegose A, senegin II, senegin III, and senegasaponin b, hair-regrowth substances, were isolated from *Polygara senega* by Ishida et al. (1999).

Recently, senega saponins were reported to display immunopotentiation activity to protein and viral antigens, suggesting their potential role as vaccine adjuvants to increase specific immune responses (Estrada et al., 2000)

References

Estrada, A., Katselis, G.S., Laarveld, B., and Barl, B., Isolation and evaluation of immunological adjuvant activities of saponins from *Polygala senega* L., *Comp. Immunol. Microbiol. Infect. Dis.*, 23:27–43, 2000.

Ishida, H., Inaoka, Y., Okada, M., Fukushima, M., Fukazawa, H., and Tsuji, K., Studies of the active substances in herbs used for hair treatment. III. Isolation of hair-regrowth substances from *Polygara senega* var. latifolia TORR. et GRAY, *Biol. Pharm. Bull.*, 22:1249–1250, 1999.

Kako, M., Miura, T., Nishiyama, Y., Ichimaru, M., Moriyasu, M., and Kato, A., Hypoglycemic effect of the rhizomes of *Polygala senega* in normal and diabetic mice and its main component, the triterpenoid glycoside senegin-II, *Planta Med.*, 62:440–443, 1996.

Kantee, H., Althaea, ipecac, senega and thyme as cough medicines, *Sairaanhoitaja*, 49:32, 1973.

Kuribara, H. and Tadokoro, S., Behavioral study on an antitussive and *expectorant*, and of its constituents. I. Effects on ambulatory activity and discrete lever-press avoidance response in mice, *Arukoru Kenkyuto Yakubutsu Ison*, 24:417–429, 1989.

Moes, A., A parallel study of the chemical composition of Polygala senega and of *"Securidaca longepedunculata"* Fres. var. parvifolia, a Congolese polygalacea, *J. Pharm. Belg.*, 21:347–362, 1966.

Saitoh, H., Miyase, T., Ueno, A., Atarashi, K., and Saiki, Y., Senegoses J-O, oligosaccharide multiesters from the roots of *Polygala senega* L., *Chem. Pharm. Bull.*, 42:641–645, 1994.

Yoshikawa, M., Murakami, T., Matsuda, H., Ueno, T., Kadoya, M., Yamahara, J., and Murakami, N., Bioactive saponins and glycosides. II. Senegae Radix. (2): Chemical structures, hypoglycemic activity, and ethanol absorption-inhibitory effect of E-senegasaponin c, Z-senegasaponin c, and Z-senegins II, III, and IV, *Chem. Pharm. Bull.*, 44:1305–1313, 1996.

Senna   Senna, a traditional Chinese medicine, possesses multiple pharmacological activities. In particular, it can promote the motility and secretion of the gastrointestinal tract (Krumbiegel and Schulz, 1993; Valverde et al., 1999). However, its application is greatly restricted by its toxicity (Stickel et al., 2001; Adam et al., 2001). The body-weight gain (males only) of animals receiving 750 or 1500 mg/kg per day was reduced significantly and, due to the laxative properties of senna, water consumption increased, and notable changes in electrolytes in both serum and urine were observed (Mengs et al., 2004). Senna plants are small shrubs of *Leguminosae*, cultivated in Somalia, the Arabian peninsula, and near the Nile River. Tinnevelly senna is obtained from cultivated plants, mainly in South India and Pakistan. The senna pods (fruits) are collected during the same

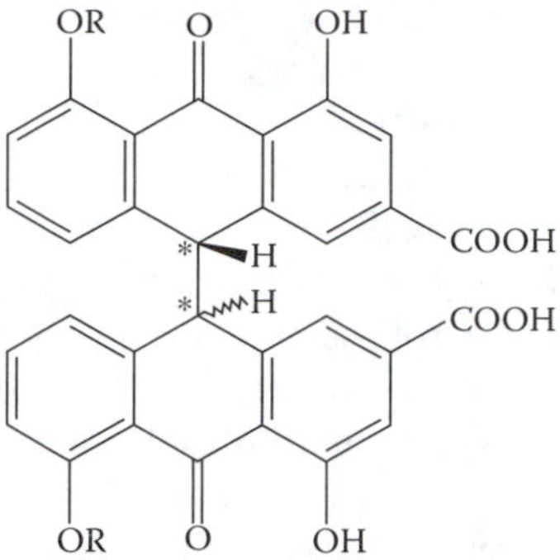

Compound	R
Sennidin A (10,10'-trans)	H
Sennidin B (10,10'-meso)	H
Sennoside A (10,10'-trans)	Glu
Sennoside B (10,10'-meso)	Glu

SCHEME S.56 Chemical structures of sennidins and sennosides. (From Hazra et al., *J. Chromatogr. B,* 812: 259–275, 2004. With permission.)

period as the leaves, then dried and separated into various qualities. The active principle of senna was first isolated and characterized by Stoll in 1941. The isolated glycosides were identified and attributed to the anthraquinone family (Scheme S.56). They were named sennosides A, B, C, and D. The active constituents in the pods and in the leaves are similar, but are present in larger quantities in the pods (Franz, 1993).

Much attention is being paid to senna effects on the regulation of gastrointestinal motility (Tian et al., 2000; Zhang et al., 2000). Wang et al. (2002) showed senna caused diarrhea and enhanced gastrointestinal motility through digestive-tract administration. Long-term gastric administration of senna induced inflammatory changes and cell damage in the whole gastrointestinal tract. The researchers suggested that the differential proteins screened from the colonic tissues of the model mice might mediate the enhancing effect of senna on gastrointestinal motility.

Quinquangulin and rubrofusarin are two known antimycobacterial natural products extracted from the stem and fruits of senna (Graham et al., 2004.). The piperidine alkaloid cassine is another antimicrobial compound isolated from the leaves of *Senna racemosa* (Sansores-Peraza et al., 2000).

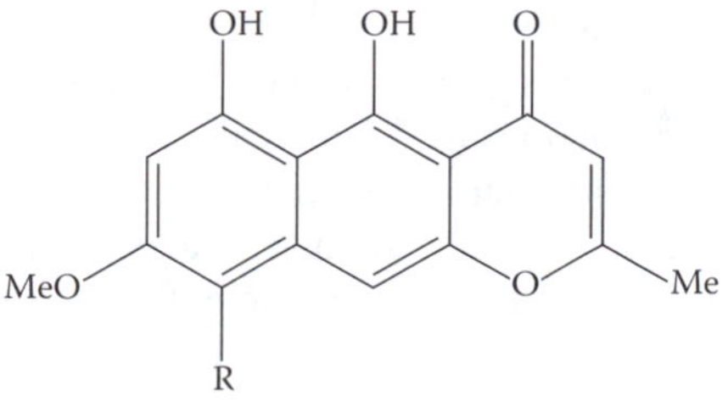

References

Adam, S.E., Al-Yahya, M.A., and Al-Farhan, A.H., Combined toxicity of *Cassia senna* and *Citrullus colocynthis* in rats, *Vet. Hum. Toxicol.,* 43:70–72, 2001.

Barbosa, F.G., da Conceicao, M., de Oliveira, F., Braz-Filho, R., and Silveira, E.R., Anthaquinones and naphthopyrones from *Senna rugosa, Biochem. System. Ecol.,* 32:363–365, 2004.

Franz, G., The senna drug and its chemistry, *Pharmacology,* 47:2–6, 1993.

Graham, J.G., Zhang, H., Pendland, S.L., Santarsiero, B.D., Mesecar, A.D., Cabieses, F., and Farnsworth, N.R., Antimycobacterial naphthopyrones from *Senna obliqua, J. Nat. Prod.,* 67:225–227, 2004.

Hazra, B., Das Sarma, M.D., and Sanyal, U., Separation methods of quinonoid constituents of plants used in Oriental traditional medicines, *J. Chromatogr. B,* 812:259–275, 2004.

Krumbiegel, G. and Schulz, H.U., Rhein and aloe-emodin kinetics from senna laxatives in man, *Pharmacology,* 47:120–124, 1993.

Mengs, U., Mitchell, J., McPherson, S., Gregson, R., and Tigner, J., A 13-week oral toxicity study of senna in the rat with an 8-week recovery period, *Arch. Toxicol.,* 78:269–275, 2004.

Sansores-Peraza, P., Rosado-Vallado, M., Brito-Loeza, W., Mena-Rejon, G.J., and Quijano, L., Cassine, an antimicrobial alkaloid from *Senna racemosa, Fitoterapia,* 71:690–692, 2000.

Quinquangulin (R = CH₃) and rubrofusarin (R = H). (From Barbosa et al., *Biochem. System. Ecol.,* 32: 363–365, 2004. With permission.)

Stickel, F., Seitz, H.K., Hahn, E.G., and Schuppan, D., Liver toxicity of drugs of plant origin, *Z. Gastroenterol.*, 39:225–232, 234–237, 2001.

Tian, X.L., Mourelle, M., Li, Y.L., Guarner, F., and Malagelada, J.R., The role of Chinese herbal medicines in a rat model of chronic colitis, *World J. Gastroenterol.*, 6:40, 2000.

Valverde, A., Hay, J-M., Fingerhut, A., Boudet, M-J., Petroni, R., Pouliquen, X., Msika, S., and Flamant, Y., Senna vs polyethylene glycol for mechanical preparation the evening before elective colonic or rectal resection: a multicenter controlled trial, *Arch. Surg.*, 134:514–519, 1999.

Wang, X., Zhong, Y.X., Lan, M., Zhang, Z.Y., Shi, Y.Q., Lu, J., Ding, J., Wu, K.C., Jin, J.P., Pan, B.R., and Fan, D.M., Screening and identification of proteins mediating senna induced gastrointestinal motility enhancement in mouse colon, *World J. Gastroenterol.*, 8:162–167, 2002.

Zhang, H.X., Ren, P., Huang, X., and Li, Y., Regulation of the traditional Chinese medicine on gastrointestinal hormone and motility, *Shijie Huaren Xiaohua Zazhi*, 8:10, 2000.

Sesame   Sesame (*Sesamum indicum* L.), an important oilseed crop in India, Sudan, China, and Burma, has been used as a healing oil for thousands of years. Sesame seeds have a higher oil and lower protein content than soybean, with the oil content ranging from 46.4–52.0 percent, and the protein content ranging from 19.8–24.2 percent. The fatty-acid composition of sesame seeds is oleic (40.4–44.9 percent), linoleic (37.7–43.4 percent), palmitic (9.1–9.8 percent), and stearic (4.8–6.1 percent).

The mechanism by which a diet containing 24 percent sesame oil reduces levels of serum and liver cholesterol, liver LDL cholesterol, and liver lipids is not known. However, the high degree of unsaturation (85 percent) of sesame oil and the presence of linoleic acid may be important factors (Satchithanandam et al., 1996). Linoleic acid is also known to have antineoplastic properties. When Salerno and Smith (1991) tested lipase-digested sesame oil and undigested sesame oil, they found that both inhibited the growth of three malignant colon-cell lines. Thus, sesame contains *in vitro* antineoplastic properties. Lignans and lignan glycosides, such

as sesamol dimer, sesamin, sesamolin, sesaminol triglucoside, and sesaminol diglucoside, isolated from sesame-methanolic extract, showed a high capacity for free-radical scavenging with the DPPH system (Suja et al., 2004). These lignans, in combination with α-tocopherol, showed a lag period in the time course of cumene hydroperoxide-mediated lipid peroxidation and a decreased rate of thiobarbituric acid reactive-product formation, suggesting recycling of α-tocopherol. Further work by Suja and coworkers (2005) showed the antioxidant activity of a crude methanol extract obtained from sesame cake was comparable to BHT at 200 ppm. In contrast, the corresponding

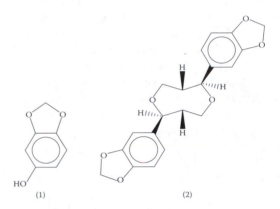

Sesamol (1) and sasamin (2). (From Chavali and Forse, *Prostaglandins Leukot. Essent. Fatty Acids*, 61:347–352, 1999. With permission.)

purified extract exhibited far superior antioxidant properties to BHT at 5, 10, 50, 100, and 200 ppm levels. A typical result is shown in Figure S.92 using the thiocyanate method linoleic-acid emulsion system. Prasad et al. (2005) reported that the antioxidant properties of sesamol provided potent phytoprotection to lymphocytes against UVB radiation.

An increase in reported sesame-induced allergic reactions led Wolff et al. (2004) to identify and characterize the linear B-cell epitopes, the major allergen of sesame seed, which might provide a better understanding of the functional role the allergens play and might have implications for immunodiagnosis and probably immunotherapy. A single dose of sesame oil reduced lipid peroxidation 6 h after endotoxin intoxication. Furthermore, sesame oil given 6 h after

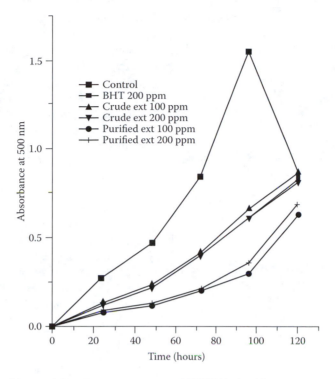

FIGURE S.92 Antioxidant activity of sesame extracts and BHT by the thiocyanate-cyanate method linoleic-acid system. (From Suja et al., *Food Chem.,* 91:213–219, 2005. With permission.)

cecal ligation and puncture significantly increased survival rate. These data suggest that sesame oil could be used as a potent antioxidant to reduce oxidative stress after the onset of sepsis in rats (Hsu and Liu, 2004).

Chen et al. (2005) recently suggested that the overall vascular fibrinolytic capacity may be enhanced by using sesamol, which regulates plasminogen activator gene expression. Sesamol is also known to reduce the synthesis of the coenzyme NADPH, which led Jacklin et al. (2003) to study the effect of oxidants on tumor and vascular endothelial cells. In preliminary studies on the effect of sesamol alone, it was clear that the compound demonstrated marked cytotoxicity.

References

Chavali, S.R. and Forse, R.A., Decreased production of interleukin-6 and prostaglandin E_2 associated with inhibition of Δ-5 desaturation of ω6 fatty acids in mice fed safflower oil diets supplemented with sasamol, *Prostaglandins Leukot. Essent. Fatty Acids,* 61:347–352, 1999.

Chen, P-R., Lee, C-C., Chang, H., and Tsai, C.E., Sesamol regulates plasminogen activator gene expression in cultured endothelial cells: a potential effect on the fibrinolytic system, *J. Nutr. Biochem.,* 16:59–64, 2005.

Hsu, D.Z. and Liu, M.Y., Effects of sesame oil on oxidative stress after the onset of sepsis in rats, *Shock,* 22:582–585, 2004.

Jacklin, A., Ratledge, C., Welham, K., Bilko, D., and Newton, C.J., The sesame seed oil constituent, sesamol, induces growth arrest and apoptosis of cancer and cardiovascular cells, *Ann. N.Y. Acad. Sci.,* 1010: 374–380, 2003.

Nakano, D., Itoh, C., Ishii, F., Kawanishi, H., Takaoka, M., Kiso, Y., Tsuruoka, N., Tanaka, T., and Matsumura, Y., Effects of sesamin on aortic oxidative stress and endothelial dysfunction in deoxycorticosterone acetate-salt hypertensive rats, *Biol. Pharm. Bull.,* 26:1701–1705, 2003.

Prasad, N.R., Mahesh, T., Menon, V.P., Jeevanram, R.K., and Pugalendi, K.V., Photoprotective effect of sesamol on UVB-radiation induced oxidative stress in human blood lymphocytes *in vitro, Environ. Toxicol. Pharmacol.,* 20:1–5, 2005.

S

Salerno, J.W. and Smith, D.E., The use of sesame oil and other vegetable oils in the inhibition of human colon cancer growth *in vitro*, *Anticancer Res.,* 11: 209–216, 1991.

Satchithanandam, S., Chanderbhan, R., Kharroubi, A.T., Calvert, R.J., Klurfeld, D., Tepper, S.A., and Kritchevsky, D., Effect of sesame oil on serum and liver lipid profiles in the rat, *Int. J. Vitam. Nutr. Res.,* 66:386–392, 1996.

Suja, K.P., Jayalekshmy, A., and Arumughan, C., Free radical scavenging behavior of antioxidant compounds of sesame (*Sesamum indicum* L.) in DPPH system, *J. Agric. Food Chem.,* 52:912–915, 2004.

Suja, K.P., Jayalekshmy, A., and Arumughan, C., Antioxidant activity of sesame cake extract, *Food Chem.,* 91:213–219, 2005.

Wolff, N., Yannai, S., Karin, N., Levy, Y., Reifen, R., Dalal, I., and Cogan, U., Identification and characterization of linear B-cell epitopes of β-globulin, a major allergen of sesame seeds, *J. Allergy Clin. Immunol.,* 114:1151–1158, 2004.

Sho-saiko-to Sho-saiko-to (SST), introduced into Japan as an oriental classical medicine from China approximately 1,500 years ago, is currently the most representative Kampo medicine (traditional Japanese medicine). SST is used to treat chronic hepatitis and cirrhosis. Many experimental and clinical studies have demonstrated the various pharmacological effects of SST (Kusunose et al., 2002; Tajiri et al., 1991; Geerts and Rogiers, 1999). SST is a mixture drug of medicinal herbs prepared from the hot-water extraction of seven raw materials. Fifteen major, low-molecular compounds (i.e., baicalin, wogonin-7-*O*-glucuronide, liquiritin, their three aglycons, liquiritin apioside, glycyrrhizin, saikosaponin b1, saikosaponin b2, ginsenoside Rg1, ginsenoside Rb1, (6)-gingerol, (6)-shogaol, and arginine) that have various pharmacological actions are assumed to be responsible, at least partly, for the pharmacological effects of SST (Scheme S.57) (Ohtake et al., 2004).

In prospective studies (Oka et al., 1995), SST was found to play a chemopreventive role in the development of hepatocellular carcinoma in cirrhotic patients. Recently, the mechanisms were studied, and SST was shown to function as a potent antifibrosuppressant via the inhibition of oxidative stress in hepatocytes and hepatic stellate cells. Its active components are baicalin and baicalein. SST also exhibited anticarcinogenic properties, as it inhibited chemical hepatocarcinogenesis in animals and suppressed the proliferation of hepatoma cells by inducing apoptosis and arresting the cell cycle (Shimizu, 2000).

SST may protect rats against lethality caused by endotoxin by its ability to regulate the heme metabolism in septic shock (Sakaguchi et al., 2005) or to inhibit TNF-α production in septic shock (Sakaguchi and Furusawa, 2004). It was also reported to reduce cholestasis in rats (Chen et al., 2004) and to suppress acute hepatic injury induced by CCl_4 and to bring about an early recovery in liver function (Taira et al., 2004).

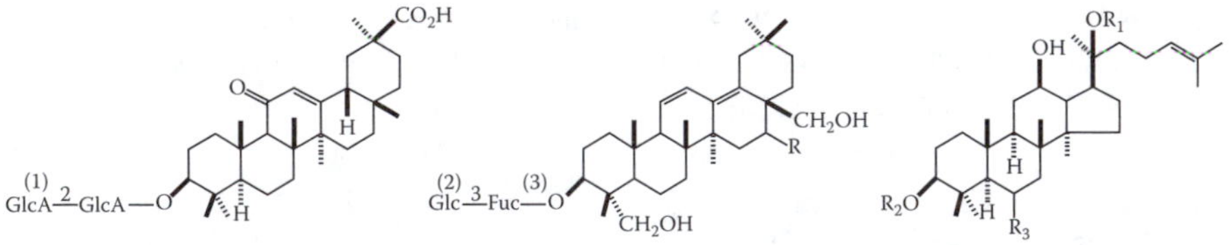

Glycyrrhizin

Saikosaponin b1 R= —OH
Saikosaponin b2 R= —OH

Ginsenoside Rbl
R_1=glc $\xrightarrow{6}$ glc
R_2=glc $\xrightarrow{2}$ glc
R_3=H

Ginsenoside Rgl
R_1=glc
R_2=H
R_3=----O-glc

SCHEME S.57 Structures of some detected compounds in Sho-saiko-to. (1) GlcA is D-glucuronic acid; (2) Glc is D-glucopyranese; (3) Fuc is fucose. (From Ohtake et al., *J. Chromatogr. B,* 812:135–148, 2004. With permission.)

References

Chen, M-H., Chen, J-C., Tsai, C-C., Wang, W-C., Chang, D-C., Lin, C-C., and Hsieh, H-Y., Sho-saiko-to prevents liver fibrosis induced by bile duct ligation in rats, *Am. J. Chin. Med.,* 32:195–207, 2004.

Geerts, A. and Rogiers, V., Sho-saiko-to: the right blend of traditional Oriental medicine and liver cell biology, *Hepatology,* 29:282–284, 1999.

Kusunose, M., Qiu, B., Cui, T., Hamada, A., Yoshioka, S., Ono, M., Miyamura, M., Kyotani, S., and Nishioka, Y., Effect of Sho-saiko-to extract on hepatic inflammation and fibrosis in dimethylnitrosamine induced liver injury rats, *Biol. Pharm. Bull.,* 25:1417–1421, 2002.

Ohtake, N., Nakai, Y., Yamamoto, M., Sakakibara, I., Takeda, S., Amagaya, S., and Aburada, M., Separation and isolation methods for analysis of the active principles of Sho-saiko-to (SST) oriental medicine, *J. Chromatogr. B,* 812:135–148, 2004.

Oka, H., Yamamoto, S., Kuroki, T., Harihara, S., Marumo, T., Kim, S.R., Monna, T., Kobayashi, K., and Tango, T., Prospective study of chemoprevention of hepatocellular carcinoma with Sho-saiko-to (TJ-9), *Cancer,* 76:743–749, 1995.

Sakaguchi, S. and Furusawa, S., Preventive effects of a traditional Chinese medicine (Sho-saiko-to) on endotoxin-induced cytotoxicity and tumor necrosis factor-alpha production in J774A.1 cells, *Biol. Pharm. Bull.,* 27:1468–1470, 2004.

Sakaguchi, S., Furusawa, S., and Iizuka, Y., Preventive effects of a traditional Chinese medicine (Sho-saiko-to) on septic shock symptoms; approached from Heme metabolic disorders in endotoxemia, *Biol. Pharm. Bull.,* 28:165–168, 2005.

Shimizu, I., Sho-saiko-to: Japanese herbal medicine for protection against hepatic fibrosis and carcinoma, *J. Gastroenterol. Hepatol.,* 15(Suppl. 1):D84–D90, 2000.

Taira, Z., Yabe, K., Hamaguchi, Y., Hirayama, K., Kishimoto, M., Ishida, S., and Ueda, Y., Effects of Sho-saiko-to extract and its components, baicalin, baicalein, glycyrrhizin and glycyrrhetic acid, on pharmacokinetic behavior of salicylamide in carbon tetrachloride intoxicated rats, *Food Chem. Toxicol.,* 42:803–807, 2004.

Tajiri, H., Kozaiwa, K., Ozaki, Y., Miki, K., Shimuzu, K., and Okada, S., Effect of Sho-saiko-to (Xiao-chai-hu-tang) on HBeAg clearance in children with chronic hepatitis B virus infection and with sustained liver disease, *Am. J. Chin Med.,* 19:121–129, 1991.

Silver birch (*Betula pendula*)   *Betula*, of the family Betulaceae, commonly known as silver

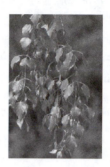

birch, grows mainly in the northern hemisphere from Eastern Europe to the northern parts of China and Japan. Different parts of *Betula* species have various medicinal applications, which in part is due to their essential oils. More than 50 compounds were identified in the essential oil from *Betula* species. The main components were α-copaene (12 percent and 10 percent), germacrene D (11 percent and 18 percent), and δ-cadinene (11 percent and 15 percent) (Betül et al., 2004). Some of the caryophyllene derivatives were evaluated for antimicrobial activity (Demirci et al., 2000a, b).

The medicinal parts are the bark, leaves, buds, sap, or juice or their processed products, which are used to treat diseases, such as urinary-tract disorders, skin diseases, severe infections, and inflammations. Furthermore, *B. pendula* flavors are used commercially as aroma and flavoring for alcoholic beverages. Other uses include applications in cosmetics.

Diverse phytochemical investigations of *Betula* species have shown they contain mainly phenolics, flavonoids, tannins, saponins, glycosides, sterols, and terpene derivatives (Demirci et al., 2000).

References

Demirci, B., Paper, D.H., Demirci, F., Baser, K.H.C., and Franz, G., Essential oil of *Betula pendula* Roth. Buds, *eCAM,* 1:301–303, 2004.

Demirci, B., Baser, K.H.C., Demirci, F., and Hamann, M.T., New caryophyllene derivatives from *Betula litwinowii, J. Nat. Prod.,* 63:902–904, 2000a.

Demirci, F., Demirci, F., Ozek, T., and Baser, K.H.C., Betulenols from *Betula* species, *Planta Med.,* 66: 490–493, 2000b.

S

Demirci, F., Demirci, B., Baser, K.H.C., and Güven, K., The Composition and antifungal bioassay of the essential oils of different *Betula* species growing in Turkey, *Khim Prir Soedin*, 2:126–130 (cited in *Chem. Nat. Comp.*, 36:159–165), 2000.

Sinigrin   Sinigrin, 2-propenyl glucosinolate, is a common glucosinolate in *Brassica* vegetables known to possess anticarcinogenic activity. Elfoul et al. (2001) showed that sinigrin can be

Singirin. (From Jen et al., *J. Chromatogr. A*, 912: 363–368, 2001. With permission.)

hydrolyzed by a *Bacteroides thetaiotaomicron* strain of human origin to yield allyl isothiocyanate (AITC) in the large bowel of rats inoculated with this bacterium. Three other strains of Bifidobacterium sp., *B. pseudocatenulatum*, *B. adolescentis*, and *B. longum*, from human intestinal tract were also able to digest sinigrin (Cheng et al., 2004). This local release of isothiocyanates may explain the protective effect of cruciferous vegetables on the colon epithelium.

Depending on target tissue and the type of compound, different mechanisms of action have been suggested to explain the anticarcinogenic actions of glucosinolates and their breakdown products, among which are the isothiocyanates (ITCs). The most frequently proposed cancer-preventive mechanisms are modulation of the activities of phase I (cytochrome P450s) and phase II (glutathione-*S*-transferase, UDP-glucuronosyl-transferase, and quinone reductase) biotransformation enzymes (Vang et al., 1999), redox regulation antiproliferation, and induction of cell-cycle arrest and by increasing the rate of apoptosis in cancer cells (Yu et al., 1998; Yang et al., 2002).

The production of allyl isothiocyanate from sinigrin was investigated in a dynamic, *in vitro* large-intestinal model, after inoculation with a complex microflora of human origin. Peak levels of allyl isothiocyanate were observed between 9 and 12 h after the addition of sinigrin. The conversion rate was remarkably higher if different individual human microflora were used. Between 10 percent and 30 percent (mean 19 percent) of the sinigrin was converted into allyl isothiocyanate (Krul et al., 2002)

References

Cheng, D.L., Hashimoto, K., and Uda, Y., *In vitro* digestion of sinigrin and glucotropaeolin by single strains of *Bifidobacterium* and identification of the digestive products, *Food Chem. Toxicol.*, 42:351–357, 2004.

Elfoul, L., Rabot, S., Khelifa, N., Quinsac, A., and Rimbault, A., Formation of allyl isothiocyanate from sinigrin by *Bacteroides thetaiotaomicron*, *FEMS Microbiol. Lett.*, 197:99–103, 2001.

Jen, J.-F., Lin, T.-H., Huang, J.-W., and Chung, W.-C., Direct determination of sinigrin in mustard seed without desulfatation by reversed-phase ion-pair liquid chromatography, *J. Chromatogr. A*, 912:363–368, 2001.

Krul, C., Humblot, C., Philippe, C., Vermeulen, M., van Nuenen, M., Havenaar, R. and Rabot, S., Metabolism of sinigrin (2-propenyl glucosinolate) by the human colonic microflora in a dynamic *in vitro* large-intestinal model, *Carcinogenesis*, 23:1009–1016, 2002.

Vang, O., Mehrota, K., Georgellis, A., and Andersen, O., Effects of dietary broccoli on rat intestinal xenobiotic metabolizing enzymes, *Eur. J. Drug. Metab. Pharmacokinet.*, 24:353–359, 1999.

Yang, Y.M., Conaway, C.C., Chiao, J.W., Wang, C.X., Amin, S., Whysner, J., Dai, W., Reinhardt, J., and Chung, F.L., Inhibition of benzo[a]pyrene-induced lung tumorigenesis in A/J mice by dietary *N*-acetylcysteine conjugates of benzyl and phenethyl isothiocyanates during the postinitiation phase is associated with activation of mitogen-activated protein kinases and p53 activity and induction of apoptosis, *Cancer Res.*, 62:2–7, 2002.

Yu, R., Mandlekar, S., Harvey, K.J., Ucker, D.S., and Kong, A.N., Chemopreventive isothiocyanates induce apoptosis and caspase-3-like protease activity, *Cancer Res.*, 58:402–408, 1998.

Sitostanol *see also* Phytosterols   Sitostanol, the saturated derivative of plant sterol β-sitosterol, is a natural dietary component with serum cholesterol-lowering properties (Perez-Jimenez et al., 1995; Terry et al., 1995; Jones et al., 1999). However, it is not found in significant amounts in plants but comprises up to 20 percent of the phytosterols extracted from tall oil (Ling and Joseph, 1995). The lowering of serum cholesterol by plant sterols is believed to be the

Sitostanol. (Adpated from Moreau et al., *Prog. Lipid Res.,* 41:457–500, 2002.)

result of an inhibition of cholesterol absorption in the small bowel (Normen et al., 2000), although increased bile-acid excretion has also been suggested (Becker et al., 1993). Recently, it has been reported that unesterified sitostanol is more effective in inhibiting cholesterol absorption and reducing LDL cholesterol than acetate or oleate esters (Sudhop et al., 2003).

References

Becker, M., Staab, D., and von Bergman, K., Treatment of severe familial hypercholesterolemia in childhood with sitosterol and sitostanol, *J. Pediatr.,* 122:292–296, 1993.

Jones, P.J.H., Ntanios, F.Y., Raeini-Sarjaz, M., and Vanstone, C.A., Cholesterol-lowering efficacy of a sitostanol-containing phytosterol mixture with a prudent diet in hyperlipidemic men, *Am. J. Clin. Nutr.,* 69:1144–1150, 1999.

Ling, W.H. and Jones, P.J.H., Enhanced efficacy of sitostanol-containing versus sitostanol-free phytosterol mixtures in altering lipoprotein cholesterol levels and synthesis in rats, *Atherosclerosis,* 118:319–331, 1995.

Moreau, R.A., Whitaker, B.D., and Hicks, K.B., Phytosterols, phytostanols, and their conjugates in food: structural diversity, quantitative analysis, and health-promoting properties, *Prog. Lipid Res.,* 41:457–500, 2002.

Normen, L., Dutta, P., Lia, A., and Andersson, H., Soy sterol esters and β-sitostanol ester as inhibitors of cholesterol absorption in human small bowel, *Am. J. Clin. Nutr.,* 71:908–913, 2000.

Perez-Jimenez, F., Espino, A., Lopez-Segura, F., Blanco, J, Ruiz-Gutierrez, V., Prada, J.L., Lopez-Miranda, J., Jimenez-Pereperez, J. and Ordovas, J.M., Lipoprotein concentration in normolipidemic males consuming oleic acid-rich diets from two different sources: olive oil and oleic acid-rich sunflower oil, *Am. J. Clin Nutr.,* 62:769–775, 2000.

Sudhop, T., Lutjohann, D., Agna, M., von Ameln, C., Prange, W., and von Bergmann, K., Comparison of the effects of sitostanol, sitostanol acetate, and sitostanol oleate on the inhibition of cholesterol absorption in normolipemic healthy male volunteers, a placebo controlled randomized cross-over study, *Arzneimittelforschung,* 53:708–713, 2003.

Terry, J.G., McGill, B.L., and Crouse, J.R., 3rd., Evaluation of the use of beta-sitostanol as a nonabsorbable marker for quantifying cholesterol absorption, *J. Lipid Res.,* 36:2267–2271, 1995.

Sitosterol *see also* **Phytosterols and Sitostanol** Sitosterol, or β-sitosterol, belongs to dietary phytosterols. The various biological activities of phytosterols, anti-inflammatory, cholesterol-lowering, antimicrobial, antibacterial, and antifungal effects, are reviewed by Tapiero et al. (2003), Ostlund (2004), and Quilez et al. (2003). Recently, the antitumor and chemopreventive activity of sitosterols were studied by Valchakova et al. (2004). They demonstrated that sitosterol inhibited colon and breast-cancer development at various stages of tumor development, including inhibition of tumorigenesis, inhibition of tumor promotion, and induction of cell differentiation. It also effectively inhibited invasion of tumor cells and

β-Sitosterol. (Adapted from Moreau et al., *Prog. Lipid Res.,* 41:457–500, 2002.)

metastasis. Ju et al. (2004) also reported that dietary β-sitosterol protected against E(2)-stimulated MCF-7 tumor growth and lowered circulating E(2) levels.

Circulating levels of β-sitosterol can be affected by dietary modification. Thus, β-sitosterol can be used as a biomarker of exposure in observational studies or as a compliance indicator in dietary-intervention studies of cancer prevention (Muti et al., 2003).

References

Ju, Y.H., Clausen, L.M., Allred, K.F., Almada, A.L., and Helferich, W.G., β-sitosterol, β-sitosterol glucoside, and a mixture of β-sitosterol and beta-sitosterol glucoside modulate the growth of estrogen-responsive breast cancer cells *in vitro* and in ovariectomized athymic mice, *J. Nutr.,* 134:1145–1451, 2004.

Moreau, R.A., Whitaker, B.D., and Hicks, K.B., Phytosterols, phytostanols, and their conjugates in food: structural diversity, quantitative analysis, and health-promoting properties, *Prog. Lipid Res.,* 41:457–500, 2002.

Muti, P., Awad, A.B., Schunemann, H., Fink, C.S., Hovey, K., Freudenheim, J.L., Wu, Y-W., Bellati, C., Pala, V., and Berrino, F., A plant food-based diet modifies the serum β-sitosterol concentration in hyperandrogenic postmenopausal women, *J. Nutr.,* 133:4252–4255, 2003.

Ostlund, R.E., Jr., Phytosterols and cholesterol metabolism, *Curr. Opin. Lipidol.,* 15:37–41, 2004.

QuIlez, J., GarcIa-Lorda, P., and Salas-Salvado, J., Potential uses and benefits of phytosterols in diet: present situation and future directions, *Clin. Nutr.,* 22:343–351, 2003.

Tapiero, H., Townsend, D.M., and Tew, K.D., Phytosterols in the prevention of human pathologies, *Biomed. Pharmacother.,* 57:321–325, 2003.

Vachalkova, A., Ovesna, Z. and Horvathova, K., Taraxasterol and β-sitosterol: A new natural compounds with chemoprotective/chemopreventive effects, *Neoplasma,* 51:407–414, 2004.

Skullcap (*Scutellaria lateriflora* L.)

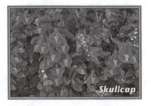

Skullcap

Skullcap is a perennial member of the mint family, with 300 *Scutellaria* species growing worldwide. It has been traditionally used as a sedative and to treat various nervous disorders, such as anxiety (Awad et al., 2003). Chinese skullcap is also used in Traditional Chinese Medicine to treat tumors. Early laboratory studies investigating this traditional use showed possible preventive involvement in bladder, liver, and other types of cancers (Udintsev et al., 1990). The main constituents found in the plant are scutellarin, a flavonoid glycoside, together with many other flavones, catalpol, other volatile oils, bitter iridoids, and tannins (Popova et al., 1972, Popova, 1974).

In vivo animal-behavior trials, performed to test anxiolytic effects in rats orally administered skullcap extracts, demonstrated that the flavonoid baicalin, its aglycone baicalein, and the amino acids GABA and glutamine may play a role in anxiolytic activity. This is not unexpected, as baicalin and baicalein are known to bind to the benzodiazepine site of the GABA receptor and GABA is the main inhibitory neurotransmitter (Awad et al., 2003).

Recently, Baikal-skullcap extract was reported to potentiate the anti-metastatic effect of cyclophosphamide in mice with Lewis lung carcinoma. It modulated cytotoxic activity of natural-killer cells and peritoneal macrophages during tumor growth (Kaplya et al., 2004).

References

Awad, R., Arnason, J.T., Trudeau, V., Bergeron, C., Budzinski, J.W., Foster, B.C., and Merali, Z., Phytochemical and biological analysis of skullcap (*Scutellaria lateriflora* L.): a medicinal plant with anxiolytic properties, *Phytomedicine,* 10:640–649, 2003.

Kaplya, O.A., Sherstoboev, E.Y., Zueva, E.P., Razina, T.G., Amosova, E.N., and Krylova, S.G., Effect of baikal skullcap extract administered alone or in combination with cyclophosphamide on natural cytotoxicity system in mice with Lewis lung carcinoma, *Bull. Exp. Biol. Med.,* 137:471–474, 2004.

Popova, T.P., Litvinenko, V.I., Gella, E.V., and Ammosov, O.S., Chemical composition and medicinal properties of common skullcap, *Farm Zh.,* 27: 58–61, 1972.

S

Popova, T.P., Flavone glycosides in the roots of the Baikal skullcap, *Farm Zh.*, 29:91–92, 1974.

Udintsev, S.N., Razina, T.G., and Iaremenko, K.V., The antitumor effect of Baikal skullcap, *Vopr Onkol.*, 36:602–607, 1990.

Sorghum (sorghum vulgare)   Sorghum is the major food crop in the semiarid regions of Africa and Asia. It provides a component to the diets of many people in the form of unleavened

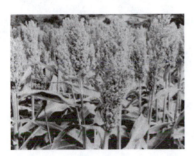

breads, boiled porridge or gruel, malted beverages, and specialty foods, such as popped grain and beer (Anglani, 1998). A syrup is produced from sweet sorghum. The crop is also used for building material, fencing, fodder for animals, and for brooms. In the United States, sorghum grain is used primarily for livestock feed, and the stems and foliage for green chop, hay, silage, and pasture.

A comparison of the nutritional and chemical parameters of 10 varieties of sorghum showed components to range from lipids (2.70–3.75 percent), raw fiber (60.0–64.7 percent), protein (9.01–11.43 percent), no nitrogen extract (77.65–83.07 percent), starch (60.5–64.20 percent), tannin (2.50–10.16 mg/g), and total calories (380–4000 kcal). Ash content, with values of 1.17–1.91 percent, protein digestibility (23.8–38.8 percent), and *in situ* starch (54.4–66.6 percent) were not statistically different (Torres Cepeda et al., 1996)

Sorghum is a rich source of various phytochemicals, including tannins, phenolic acids, anthocyanins, phytosterols, and policosanols (Awika and Rooney, 2004). These phytochemicals are known to impact human health. Sorghum fractions possess high antioxidant activity *in vitro*, relative to other cereals or fruits. Epidemiological studies suggest that, in comparison to other cereals, sorghum consumption reduces the risk of certain types of cancer in humans. Kamath et al. (2004), using the DPPH model system for assessing antiradical properties, recently identified various extracts from sorghum flour that exhibited significant, greater antioxidant activity than BHT (Figure S.93).

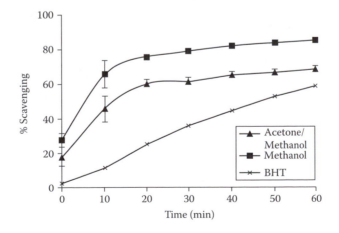

FIGURE S.93 Effect of subfractions of methanol extracts on quenching DPPH radicals-time related effect. 50 μL (0.2 mg) of either extract of sorghum was employed for quenching. An equal volume of respective solvents was used in control. 50 μL (10 mM) BHT was used. Each value represents mean ± standard error (n – 6). (From Kamath et al., *J. Cereal Sci.*, 40:283–288, 2004. With permission.)

Even though they were unable to correlate antioxidant activity and phenolic content, diets rich in sorghum could still be helpful in combating chronic diseases involving free radicals. This explains why sorghum phytochemicals promote cardiovascular health and are involved in cancer prevention (Awika and Rooney, 2004).

References

Anglani, C., Sorghum for human food — a review, *Plant Foods Hum. Nutr.,* 52:85–95, 1998.

Awika, J.M. and Rooney, L.W., Sorghum phytochemicals and their potential impact on human health, *Phytochemistry,* 65:1199–1221, 2004.

Kamath, V.G., Chandrashekar, A., and Ranjini, P.S., Antiradical properties of sorghum (*Sorghum bicolor* L. Moench) flour extracts, *J. Cereal Sci.,* 40:283–288, 2004.

Torres Cepeda, T.E., Alanis Guzman, M.G., and Maiti, R., Relationship between nutritional composition and anatomical parameters in sorghum (*Sorghum bicolor* L. Moench), *Arch. Latinoam. Nutr.,* 46: 253–259, 1996.

Southernwood (*Artemisia abrotanum*) There are two different cultivated strains of southernwood. The traditional type has a vague, lemon-like smell, while the more recently bred type has an even more intense and dominant smell. Despite their significant bitterness, the leaves of both types are well-suited for culinary usage. Various sources reported different compositions for the essential oil (0.2 percent), with some claiming absinthol as the main component, while others report the heterocyclic sesquiterpenes davanol and davanone plus carlinene and 1,8-cineol. Among the nonvolatile

constituents reported are the alkaloid abrotin and coumarins. Although southernwood contains significant amounts of bitter sesquiterpene lactones (absinthin) and the glycoside rutin, it is still less bitter than its close relative, wormwood.

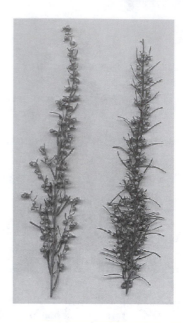

A nasal-spray formulation containing an extract of *Artemisia abrotanum* L. was developed for therapeutic use in patients with allergic rhinitis and other upper-airway disorders. The extract used contains a mixture of essential oils (4 mg/mL) and flavonols (2.5 microg/mL), of which some components have been shown to possess anti-inflammatory, expectorant, and spasmolytic, as well as antiseptic and antimicrobial, activities. The most important constituents in the essential-oil fraction are 1,8-cineole, linalool, and davanone, while the flavonol fraction contains centauredin, casticin, and quercetin dimethyl-ethers (Remberg, 2004).

Structures of 1,8-cineole (a) and davanone (b) (Adapted from Tisevec et al., *Biochem. Systems Ecol.,* 32:525–527, 2004; Silvester et al. *Ind. Crops Prod.,* 12: 53-56, 2000)

Lactones and sesquiterpenes, isolated from the methanol extract of the aerial parts of *Artemisia sylvatica,* displayed inhibitory activity on the LPS-induced NF-κB activation, NO production, and TNF-α production (Jin et al., 2004). *Artemisia iwayomogi* extract also inhibited mast-cell-derived, immediate-type allergic reactions and involvement of intracellular Ca(2+), proinflammatory cytokines, p38 MAPK, and NF-κB (Kim et al., 2005). These results support the pharmacological use of *Artemisia sylvatica* and *Artemisia iwayomogi*, which have been employed as herbal medicines for inflammation treatment.

References

Jin, H.Z., Lee, J.H., Lee, D., Hong, Y.S., Kim, Y.H., and Lee, J.J., Inhibitors of the LPS-induced NF-κB activation from *Artemisia sylvatica*, *Phytochemistry,* 65:2247–2253, 2004.

Kim, S.H., Choi, C.H., Kim, S.Y., Eun, J.S., and Shin, T.Y., Anti-allergic effects of *Artemisia iwayomogi* on mast cell-mediated allergy model, *Exp. Biol. Med.,* 230:82–88, 2005.

Remberg, P., Bjork, L., Hedner, T., and Sterner, O., Characteristics, clinical effect profile and tolerability of a nasal spray preparation of *Artemisia abrotanum* L. for allergic rhinitis, *Phytomedicine,* 11:36–42, 2004.

Silvestre, A.J.D., Valega, M. and Cavaliero, J.A.S., Chemical transformation of 1,8-cineole: Synthesis of seudenone, an insect pheromone, *Ind Crops Prod.,* 12:53–56, 2000.

Tisevec, V., Milosavljevie, S., Vajs, V., Janackovic, P., Jovic, D.L.J., Tetrahydroguran-type sesquiterpenes from *Artemisia lobelii* All Var. biasolettiana (Vis.) K. Malay., *Biochem. Systems Ecol.,* 32:527–532, 2004.

Soybeans *see also* Daidzein and Genistein

A large number of components contribute to the diverse biological activities of soybeans: hormonal, immunological, bacteriological, and digestive effects. These components include isoflavones (genistein, daidzein, biochanin), saponins, Kunitz inhibitor, Bowman–Birk inhibitor, soyacystatin, phytoestrogens, Maillard products, soybean hydrophobic protein, soy allergens, lecithins, allergens, raffinose, stachyose, and 2-pentyl pyridine (Csaky and Fekete, 2004).

Soy isoflavones (genistein, daidzein, biochanin) are known to protect against different cancers (Sarkar and Li, 2003), cardiovascular disease (Hasler, 2002), and bone loss (Harkness, 2004). Many studies have demonstrated the effect of soy isoflavones on specific target molecules and signaling pathways, cell proliferation and differentiation, cell-cycle regulation, apoptosis, angiogenesis, cell adhesion and migration, metastasis, and activity of different enzymes. Isoflavones are also classified as phytoestrogens with weak estrogenic properties (Valachovicova et al., 2004). Interleukin-6 is a pleiotropic cytokine that plays a crucial role in immune physiology and is tightly controlled by hormonal-feedback mechanisms. Isoflavones modulate IL-6 gene-expression levels and may have therapeutical benefit in preventing cancer progression, aging discomforts, and restoring immune homeostasis (Dijsselbloem et al., 2004).

A systematic review of randomized clinical trials performed to evaluate the benefit of soy for the treatment of perimenopausal symptoms provides some evidence for the efficacy of soy preparations for perimenopausal symptoms, but the heterogeneity of the studies performed makes it difficult to achieve a definitive statement (Huntley and Ernst, 2004).

The ability of soybean extracts to inhibit mouse mammary adenocarcinoma tumor growth was not only due to the presence of genistein but to other constituents present (Hewitt and Singletary, 2003). Recent studies demonstrated a direct effect of soy saponins on cancer cells, which further leads to elucidating the nature of soy constituents involved in cancer protection (Kerwin, 2004).

The Bowman–Birk inhibitor, a serine protease inhibitor derived from soybeans, is presently being evaluated in clinical trials for its ability to serve as a cancer preventive or anti-inflammatory agent (Kennedy et al., 2002). Kunitz inhibitor was also found to inhibit cell invasiveness through suppression of urokinase-type plasminogen activator signaling cascade (Kobayashi et al., 2004).

Soy infant formulas are widely used, but only a few studies have evaluated their long-term safety or specific forms of toxicity, such as the effects of genistein and daidzein in soy

S

infant formula, on the endocrine or immune systems. In addition, there is inconsistency in the existing data, which point to the need for more clinical and epidemiological studies (Chen and Rogan, 2004).

Soybean oil is the world's most widely used, edible oil. In the United States, soybean oil accounts for nearly 80 percent of edible-oil consumption. It contains 61 percent polyunsaturated fat and 24 percent monounsaturated fat. It is one of the few vegetable oils to contain linolenic acid, an omega-3 fatty acid (7.2 percent C18:3n-3) known to prevent cardiovascular diseases. Soybean oil also contains 54 percent C18:2n-6 linoleic acid, which is required for normal immune response (Meydani et al., 1991).

References

Csaky, I. and Fekete, S., Soybean: feed quality and safety. Part 1. Biologically active components, a review, *Acta Vet. Hung.*, 52:299–313, 2004.

Chen, A. and Rogan, W.J., Isoflavones in soy infant formula: a review of evidence for endocrine and other activity in infants, *Annu. Rev. Nutr.*, 24:33–54, 2004.

Dijsselbloem, N., Vanden Berghe, W., De Naeyer, A., and Haegeman, G., Soy isoflavone phyto-pharmaceuticals in interleukin-6 affections, Multi-purpose nutraceuticals at the crossroad of hormone replacement, anti-cancer and anti-inflammatory therapy, *Biochem. Pharmacol.*, 68:1171–1185, 2004.

Harkness, L., Soy and bone, where do we stand? *Orthop. Nurs.*, 23:12–17, 2004.

Hasler, C.M., The cardiovascular effects of soy products, *J. Cardiovasc. Nurs.*, 16:50–63, 2002.

Hewitt, A.L. and Singletary, K.W., Soy extract inhibits mammary adenocarcinoma growth in a syngeneic mouse model, *Cancer Lett.*, 192:133–143, 2003.

Huntley, A.L. and Ernst, E., Soy for the treatment of perimenopausal symptoms — a systematic review, *Maturitas*, 47:1–9, 2004.

Kennedy, A.R., Billings, P.C., Wan, X.S., and Newberne, P.M., Effects of Bowman-Birk inhibitor on rat colon carcinogenesis, *Nutr. Cancer*, 43:174–186, 2002.

Kerwin, S.M., Soy saponins and the anticancer effects of soybeans and soy-based foods, *Curr. Med. Chem. Anti-Canc. Agents*, 4:263–272, 2004.

Kobayashi, H., Suzuki, M., Kanayama, N., and Terao, T., A soybean Kunitz trypsin inhibitor suppresses ovarian cancer cell invasion by blocking urokinase upregulation, *Clin. Exp. Metastasis*, 21:159–166, 2004.

Meydani, S.N., Lichtenstein, A.H., White, P.J., Goodnight, S.H., Elson, C.E., Woods, M., Gorbach, S.L., and Schaefer, E.J., Food use and health effects of soybean and sunflower oils, *J. Am. Coll. Nutr.*, 10:406–428, 1991.

Sarkar, F.H. and Li, Y., Soy isoflavones and cancer prevention, *Cancer Invest.*, 21:744–757, 2003.

Valachovicova, T., Slivova, V., and Sliva, D., Cellular and physiological effects of soy flavonoids, *Mini Rev. Med. Chem.*, 4:881–887, 2004.

Soy fibers   Due to its neutral taste and light color, soy fiber can be incorporated into a variety of high-fiber and reduced-calorie products, such as baked goods, cereal, and beverages. Clinical studies showed soy fiber provided all the benefits associated with both soluble and insoluble fiber. A soy-fiber-rich diet (6 percent) significantly lowered serum total cholesterol (TC), LDL-C, and atherosclerotic index, increased the ratio of HDL-L/TC, lowered serum fibrinogen (FB), platelet aggregation, and prolonged clotting time in rats (Wang et al., 1996). Lo et al. (1987) suggested a complementary role for soy fibers and soy protein in preventing atherosclerosis in rabbits. Bile acids were markedly lower in bran-soy treated females with cholelithiasis (Belonovskaia and Kliashtornaia, 1992).

References

Belonovskaia, L.K. and Kliashtornaia, O.S., The effect of soy bran on the bile acid spectrum of patients with cholelithiasis, *Vopr Pitan.*, (4):15–17, 1992.

Lo, G.S., Evans, R.H., Phillips, K.S., Dahlgren, R.R., and Steinke, F.H., Effect of soy fiber and soy protein on cholesterol metabolism and atherosclerosis in rabbits, *Atherosclerosis*, 64:47–54, 1987.

S

Wang, C., Zhao, L., and Chen, Y., Hypolipidemic action of soy fiber and its effects on platelet aggregation and coagulation time in rats, *Zhonghua Yu Fang Yi Xue Za Zhi,* 30:205–208, 1996.

Soy protein   The U.S. Food and Drug Administration approved (1999) the association of soy proteins with coronary prevention. This claim was based on studies demonstrating that soy-protein components were primarily responsible for reducing cholesterolemia (Greaves et al., 1999; Sirtori et al., 1998; Nestel, 2002). Proteins appear to elicit the hypocholesterolemic response, mainly by activating liver LDL receptors (Baum et al., 1998), a mechanism tentatively attributed to specific protein components, i.e., the 7S globulin and its α-α′ subunits (Lovati et al., 2000).

Plant-derived proteins, such as soy protein, were shown by Damasceno and coworkers (2000) to have a beneficial effect on atherosclerosis. Using a soy-protein isolate, they found a reduction in the level of oxidized LDL, as well as in the production of oxidized LDL antibodies, in rabbits.

Proteomic comparison of soy proteins used for clinical studies on hypercholesterolemia, particularly in Europe and the United States, indicate differences in the protein composition. These results may explain the variability found in experimental and clinical studies (Gianazza et al., 2003).

References

Baum, J.A., Teng, H., Erdman, J.W., Jr., Weigel, R.M., Klein, B.P., Persky, V.W., Freels, S., Surya, P., Bakhit, R.M., Ramos, E., Shay, N.F., and Potter, S.M., Long-term intake of soy protein improves blood lipid profiles and increases mononuclear cell low-density-lipoprotein receptor messenger RNA in hypercholesterolemic, postmenopausal women, *Am. J. Clin. Nutr.,* 68:545–551, 1998.

Damasceno, N.R.T., Goto, H., Rodrigues, F.M.D., Dias, C.T.S., Okawabata, F.S., Abdalla, D.S.P., and Gidlund, M., Soy protein isolate reduces the oxidizability of LDL and the generation of oxidized LDL autoantibodies in rabbits with diet-induced atherosclerosis, *J. Nutr.,* 130:2641–2647, 2000.

Food and Drug Administration, Food labeling health claims: soy protein and coronary heart disease, Final rule, *Fed. Regist.,* 64:57699–57733, 1999.

Gianazza, E., Eberini, I., Arnoldi, A., Wait, R., and Sirtori, C.R., A proteomic investigation of isolated soy proteins with variable effects in experimental and clinical studies, *J. Nutr.,* 133:9–14, 2003.

Greaves, K.A., Parks, J.S., Williams, J.K., and Wagner, J.D., Intact dietary soy protein, but not adding an isoflavone-rich soy extract to casein, improves plasma lipids in ovariectomized cynomolgus monkeys, *J. Nutr.,* 129:1585–1592, 1999.

Lovati, M.R., Manzoni, C., Gianazza, E., Arnoldi, A., Kurowska, E., Carroll, K.K., and Sirtori, C.R., Soy protein peptides regulate cholesterol homeostasis in Hep G2 cells, *J. Nutr.,* 130:2543–2549, 2000.

Nestel, P., Role of soy protein in cholesterol-lowering: how good is it? *Arterioscler. Thromb. Vasc. Biol.,* 22:1743–1744, 2002.

Sirtori, C.R., Lovati, M.R., Manzini, C., Gianazza, E., Bondioli, A., Staels, B., and Auwerx, J., Reduction of serum cholesterol by soy proteins: clinical experience and potential molecular mechanisms, *Nutr. Metab. Cardiovasc. Dis.,* 8:334–340, 1999.

Spearmint   Like peppermint, spearmint (*Mentha spicata*) is a popular food-flavoring agent and a valuable medicinal herb. The essential oil of spearmint was reported to have antibacterial (Imai et al., 2001) and antifungal (Soliman and Badeaa, 2002) activities, as well as anti-inflammatory activities, possibly through the suppression of neutrophil recruitment into the peritoneal cavity, as demonstrated in mice (Abe et al., 2004).

A water extract from spearmint inhibited the mutagenic activity of the parent compound, 2-amino-3-methyl-3H-imidazo[4,5-f]quinoline (IQ), in the presence of rat liver. These findings suggest that spearmint extract protects against IQ, and possibly other heterocyclic amines, through inhibition of carcinogen activation and via direct effects on the activated metabolite (Yu et al., 2004). Spearmint was also found as an effective chemopreventive agent that may suppress benzoyl peroxide-induced cutaneous oxidative stress, toxicity, and hyperproliferative effects in the skin of mice (Saleem et al., 2000).

S

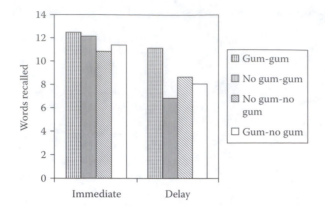

FIGURE S.94 Mean number of words recalled (maximum 15) after no retention interval ("Immediate") or after 24 h ("Delay"). Participants in two of the four groups chewed gum at initial learning (gum–gum, gum–no gum), and two of the groups chewed gum during both of the recall tests (gum–gum, no gum–gum). (From Baker et al., *Appetite*, 43:207–210, 2004. With permission.)

The constituents of anti-inflammatory and hemostatic active sites of *Mentha spicata* includes: ursane, 3-methoxy-4-methylbenzaldehyde, veratric acid, 5-hydroxy-3′,4′,6,7-tetramethoxyflavone, diosmetin, thymonin, and daucosterol (Zheng et al., 2002). Two monoterpenoid glycosides, spicatoside A and spicatoside B, were also isolated from whole herbs of *Mentha spicata* L. and found to have anti-inflammatory and hemostatic activities (Zheng et al., 2003). Recently, Akdogan et al. (2004) reported on lipid peroxidation and hepatic damage that occurs after *Mentha spicata* administration in rat liver and on nephrotoxic changes (Akdogan et al., 2003).

One of the major uses of spearmint is in chewing gum. A recent study by Baker et al. (2004) showed that chewing spearmint gum not only promoted initial learning but also led to context-dependent effects upon memory (Figure S.94). The same effects were also observed with sucking the gum.

References

Abe, S., Maruyama, N., Hayama, K., Intuye, S., Oshima, H., and Yamaguchi, H., Suppression of neutrophil recruitment in mice by geranium essential oil, *Mediators Inflamm.*, 13:21–24, 2004.

Akdogan, M., Ozguner, M., Aydin, G., and Gokalp, O., Investigation of biochemical and histopathological effects of *Mentha piperita* Labiatae and *Mentha spicata* Labiatae on liver tissue in rats, *Hum. Exp. Toxicol.*, 23:21–28, 2004.

Akdogan, M., Kilinc, I., Oncu, M., Karaoz, E., and Delibas, N., Investigation of biochemical and histopathological effects of *Mentha piperita* L. and *Mentha spicata* L. on kidney tissue in rats, *Hum. Exp. Toxicol.*, 22:213–219, 2003.

Baker, J.R., Bezance, J.B., Zellaby, E., and Aggleton, J.P., Chewing gum can produce context-dependent effects upon memory, *Appetite*, 43:207–210, 2004.

Imai, H., Osawa, K., Yasuda, H., Hamashima, H., Arai, T., and Sasatsu, M., Inhibition by the essential oils of peppermint and spearmint of the growth of pathogenic bacteria, *Microbios,*106:31–39, 2001.

Saleem, M., Alam, A., and Sultana, S., Attenuation of benzoyl peroxide-mediated cutaneous oxidative stress and hyperproliferative response by the prophylactic treatment of mice with spearmint (*Mentha spicata*), *Food Chem. Toxicol.*, 38:939–948, 2000.

Soliman, K.M. and Badeaa, R.I., Effect of oil extracted from some medicinal plants on different mycotoxigenic fungi, *Food Chem. Toxicol.*, 40:1669–1675, 2002.

Yu, T-W., Xu, M., and Dashwood, R.H., Antimutagenic activity of spearmint, *Environ. Mol. Mutagen.*, 44:387–393, 2004.

Zheng, J., Zhao, D.S., Wu, B., and Wu, L.J., A study on chemical constituents in the herb of *Mentha spicata*, *Zhongguo Zhong Yao Za Zhi*, 27:749–751, 2002.

Zheng, J., Wu, L.J., Zheng, L., Wu, B., and Song, A.H., Two new monoterpenoid glycosides from *Mentha spicata* L., *J. Asian Nat. Prod. Res.*, 5:69–73, 2003.

Spices *see also* **Individual spices**   Spices have been used for generations by humans as food and to treat ailments. Commonly used spices, such as garlic, black cumin, cloves, cinnamon, thyme, allspices, bay leaves, mustard, and rosemary, possess antimicrobial properties that, in some cases, can be used therapeutically. Other spices, such as saffron — a food colorant, turmeric — a yellow-colored spice, tea — either green or black — and flaxseed do contain potent phytochemicals, including carotenoids, curcumins, catechins, and lignan, respectively, which provide significant protection against cancer (Lai and Roy, 2004).

The improvement of food flavors was facilitated by the addition of different spices, such as garlic, red chili, and cloves. Subsequent research showed that it was the antioxidant activity of the spice extracts, due to the presence of high levels of antioxidants (Madsen and Bertelsen, 1995).

Spices have long been recognized for their digestive stimulant action. This action seems to be mediated by stimulating the liver to secrete bile rich in bile acids, components that are vital for fat digestion and absorption, and by stimulating enzymes that are responsible for digestion (reviewed by Platel and Srinivasan, 2004).

References

Madsen, H.L. and Bertelsen, G., Spices as antioxidants, *Trends Food Sci. Technol.,* 6:271–277, 1995.

Lai, P.K. and Roy, J., Antimicrobial and chemopreventive properties of herbs and spices, *Curr. Med. Chem.,* 11:1451–1460, 2004.

Platel, K. and Srinivasan, K., Digestive stimulant action of spices: a myth or reality? *Indian J. Med. Res.,* 119:167–179, 2004.

Spinach   Spinach leaves, another good source of flavonoids (Goldbohm et al., 1998), contain other active components that exhibit antioxidative (Kuti and Konuru, 2004), antiproliferative (Sani et al., 2004), and anti-inflammatory (Lomnitski et al., 2000) activities. Spinach extracts have numerous beneficial effects, including chemo and central nervous system protection and anticancer and antiaging functions (Galli et al., 2002; Lomnitski et al., 2003).

A water-soluble antioxidant mixture isolated from spinach leaves contained both flavonoids and p-coumaric-acid derivatives (Bergman et al., 2001). It was found to be nonmutagenic and to show promising anticarcinogenic effects in experimental models, such as skin and prostate cancer (Lomnitski et al., 2003). Spinach is relatively rich in nitrogenous substances, hydrocarbons, and iron sesqui-oxide, which account for 3.3 percent of the total ash.

References

Bergman, M., Varshavsky, L., Gottlieb, H.E., and Grossman, S., The antioxidant activity of aqueous spinach extract: chemical identification of active fractions, *Phytochemistry,* 58:143–152, 2001.

Galli, R.L., Shukitt-Hale, B., Youdim, K.A., and Joseph, J.A., Fruit polyphenolics and brain aging: nutritional interventions targeting age-related neuronal and behavioral deficits, *Ann. N.Y. Acad. Sci.,* 959:128–132, 2002.

Goldbohm, R.A., Hertog, M.G.L., Brants, H.A.M., van Poppel, G., and ven den Brandt, P.A., Intake of flavonoids and cancer risk: a prospective cohort study, in *Polyphenols in Foods, EUR18169-COST916-Bioactive Plant Cell Wall Components in Nutrition and Health,* Amado, R., Andersson, H., Bardocz, S., and Serra, F., Eds., European Commission, Luxembourg, 1998, pp. 159–166.

Kuti, J.O. and Konuru, H.B., Antioxidant capacity and phenolic content in leaf extracts of tree spinach (*Cnidoscolus* spp.), *J. Agric. Food Chem.,* 52:117–121, 2004.

Lomnitski, L., Bergman, M., Nyska, A., Ben-Shaul, V., and Grossman, S., Composition, efficacy, and safety of spinach extracts, *Nutr. Cancer,* 46:222–231, 2003.

Lomnitski, L., Carbonatto, M., Ben-Shaul, V., Peano, S., Conz, A., Corradin, L., Maronpot, R.R., Grossman, S., and Nyska, A., The prophylactic effects of natural water-soluble antioxidant from spinach and apocynin in a rabbit model of lipopolysaccharide-induced endotoxemia, *Toxicol. Pathol.,* 28:588–600, 2000.

Sani, H.A., Rahmat, A., Ismail, M., Rosli, R., and Endrini, S., Potential anticancer effect of red spinach (*Amaranthus gangeticus*) extract, *Asia Pac. J. Clin. Nutr.,* 13:396–400, 2004.

S

Squalene. (From Auwarter et al., *Forensic Sci. Int.,* 145:149–159, 2004. With permission.)

Squalene   Squalene, a unique hydrocarbon, was first discovered in shark-liver oil in 1906 and named after the Latin root "squalus" (shark). It is a very potent antioxidant because of its six double bonds. Desai and coworkers (1996) showed squalene and a squalene-containing compound, Roidex, both partially prevented the development of chemical-induced cancer and to cause the regression of some of the existing tumors in a mouse-skin model. Dietary squalene was also found to lower plasma cholesterol because of its ability to downregulate HMG-CoA reductase, a key enzyme in cholesterol synthesis. Chan et al. (1996) reported that squalene enhanced the effect of pravastatin (a cholesterol-lowering drug) in patients over 20 weeks. The anticancer properties of squalene, particularly its ability to scavenge free radicals and oxygen-reactive species, was also demonstrated in skin subjected to radiation (Morliere et al., 1995). A study by O'Sullivan and coworkers (2002) showed it was squalene, not ω-3 fatty acids eicosapentaenoic (EPA) and docosapentahexaenoic (DHA) acids, that protected Chinese hamster V79 fibroblast cells from H_2O_2-induced DNA damage.

The effectiveness of squalene as an adjuvant was recently demonstrated by Suli et al. (2004), who showed it increased the immunogenic activity of nonpotentiated rabies vaccine by approximately 1.8-fold.

References

Auwarter, V., Kiebling, B., and Pragst, F., Squalene in hair — a natural reference substance for the improved interpretation of fatty acid ethyl ester concentrations with respect to alcohol misuse, *Forensic Sci. Int.,* 145:149–159, 2004.

Chan, P., Tomlinson, B., Lee, C.B., and Lee, Y.S., Effectiveness and safety of low dose pravastin and squalene, alone and in combination, in elderly patients with hypercholesterolemia, *J. Clin. Pharmacol.,* 36:422–427, 1996.

Desai, K.N., Wei, H., and Lamartiniere, C.A., The preventative and therapeutic potential of the squalene-containing compound, Roidex, on tumor promotion and regression, *Cancer Lett.,* 101:93–96, 1996.

Morliere, P., Moysan, A., and Tirache, I., Action spectrum for UV-induced lipid peroxidation in cultured human skin fibroblast, *Free Rad. Biol. Med.,* 19:365–371, 1995.

O'Sullivan, L., Woods, J.A., and O'Brien, N.M., Squalene but not n-3 fatty acids protect against hydrogen peroxide-induced sister chromatid exchanges in Chinese hamster V79 cells, *Nutr. Res.,* 22:847–857, 2002.

Suli, J., Benisek, Z., Elias, D., Svrcek, S., Ondrejkova, A., Ondrejka, R., and Bajova, V., Experimental squalene adjuvant. I. Preparation and testing of its effectiveness, *Vaccine,* 22:3464–3469, 2004.

St. John's wort (*Hypericum perforatum*) *see also* Hyperforin and Hypericin   Hypericin is a naturally occurring substance found in the common St. John's wort that can also be synthesized from the anthraquinone derivative emodin. It has been used traditionally throughout the history of folk medicine. In the last three

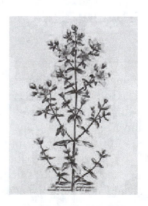

S

decades, St. John's wort has also become the subject of intensive biochemical research and is proving to be a multifunctional agent in drug and medicinal applications. Recent studies suggest it has antidepressive (Hirano et al., 2004; Zanoli, 2004; Muller et al., 2000), antineoplastic (Dona et al., 2004), antitumor (Gartner et al., 2004), and antiviral (human immunodeficiency and hepatitis C virus) properties (Jacobson et al., 2001; Kubin et al., 2005).

Hyperforins, a family of antimicrobial acylphloroglucinols, is thought to be a primary bioactive ingredient for antidepressive effects in the herb; and hypericins, a family of phototoxic anthraquinones, exhibits antimicrobial, antiviral, and antiherbivore properties *in vitro*, are two different classes of secondary metabolites produced by *Hypericum perforatum* L (Sirvent et al., 2003; Kirakosyan et al., 2004).

St. John's wort preparation has been used in large quantities in Germany for treating mild to moderate depression (Muller et al., 2000). Its efficacy has been demonstrated in several double-blind depression trials and some open-label studies with anxiety disorders. There is pharmacokinetic evidence for the serotonergic, domaminergic, and GABA minergic activity of hypericum, all of which are implicated in social anxiety disorder (Hirano et al., 2004; Zanoli, 2004).

References

Dona, M., Dell'Aica, I., Pezzato, E., Sartor, L., Calíbrese, F., Della Barbera, M., Donella-Deana, A., Appendino, G., Borsarini, A., Caniato, R., and Garbosa, S., Hyperforin inhibits cancer invasion and metastasis, *Cancer Res.*, 64:6225–6232, 2004.

Gartner, M., Muller, T., Simon, J.C., Giannis, A., and Sleeman, J.P., Aristoforin, a novel stable derivative of hyperforin, is a potent anticancer agent, *Chembiochem,* 6(1):171–177, 2004.

Hirano, K., Kato, Y., Uchida, S., Sugimoto, Y., Yamada, J., Umegaki, K., and Yamada, S., Effects of oral administration of extracts of *Hypericum perforatum* (St John's wort) on brain serotonin transporter, serotonin uptake and behaviour in mice, *J. Pharm. Pharmacol.*, 56:1589–1595, 2004.

Jacobson, J.M., Feinman, L., Liebes, L., Ostrow, N., Koslowski, V., Tobia, A., Cabana, B.E., Lee, D., Spritzler, J., and Prince, A.M., Pharmacokinetics, safety, and antiviral effects of hypericin, a derivative of St. John's wort plant, in patients with chronic hepatitis C virus infection, *Antimicrob. Agents Chemother.,* 45:517–524, 2001.

Kirakosyan, A., Sirvent, T.M., Gibson, D.M., and Kaufman, P.B., The production of hypericins and hyperforin by *in vitro* cultures of St. John's wort (*Hypericum perforatum*), *Biotechnol. Appl. Biochem.,* 39:71–81, 2004.

Kubin, A., Wierrani, F., Burner, U., Alth, G., and Grunberger, W., Hypericin — the facts about a controversial agent, *Curr. Pharm. Des.,* 11:233–253, 2005.

Muller, W.E., Singer, A., and Wonnemann, M., Mechanism of action of St. John's wort extract, *Schweiz Rundsch. Med. Prax.,* 89:2111–2121, 2000.

Sirvent, T.M., Krasnoff, S.B., and Gibson, D.M., Induction of hypericins and hyperforins in *Hypericum perforatum* in response to damage by herbivores, *J. Chem. Ecol.,* 29:2667–2681, 2003.

Zanoli, P., Role of hyperforin in the pharmacological activities of St. John's Wort, *CNS Drug Rev.,* 10:203–218, 2004.

Stilbenes *see also* **Resveratrol**   Stilbenes are nonflavonoid phenolics present primarily in grapes, berries, and wine products. Stilbenes are induced following stress, such as pathogenic attack and UV-C irradiation. One of the most extensively studied stilbenes is *trans*-resveratrol (3,5,4′-trihydroxystilbene), whose health benefits (Granados-Soto, 2003) include antioxidant (Caruso et al., 2004), antimutagenic (Orsini and Verotta, 1999), anti-inflammatory (Donnelly et al., 2004), antiestrogenic (Pozo-Guisado et al., 2004), antiarrhthymic, and cardioprotective (Dong and Ren, 2004), as well as anticancer agent (Aggarwal et al., 2004; Kundu and Surh, 2004) properties.

Resveratrol. (From Li et al., *Free Rad. Biol. Med.,* 38:243–257, 2005. With permission.)

Cantos and coworkers (2002) used UV-C irradiation pulses to enhance the production of stilbenes in four grape varieties. Using this procedure, the total resveratrol content increased from 3.4-fold in Flame to 2315-fold in Red Globe. Using this method, the UV-C-irradiated grapes were considered a new functional food because of its enrichment with stilbenes.

Recently, several active stilbenes (piceatannol, 3,5,4′-trimethylpiceatannol, resveratrol, trimethylresveratrol) were reported to exhibit antiallergic activities. They inhibited ionomycin-induced β-hexosaminidase release, suggesting that inhibition of Ca(2+) influx or degranulation mechanisms after Ca(2+) influx is important for their activities. Piceatannol, 3,5,4′-trimethylpiceatannol, resveratrol, and trimethylresveratrol also inhibited *in vitro* antigen-induced release of TNF-α and IL-4 significantly (Matsuda et al., 2004).

References

Aggarwal, B.B., Bhardwaj, A., Aggarwal, R.S., Seeram, N.P., Shishodia, S., and Takada, Y., Role of resveratrol in prevention and therapy of cancer: preclinical and clinical studies, *Anticancer Res.*, 24: 2783–2841, 2004.

Cantos, E., Epsin, J.C., and Tomas-Barberan, F.A., Postharvest stilbene-enrichment of red and white table grape varieties using UV-C irradiation pulses, *J. Agric. Food Chem.*, 50:6322–6329, 2002.

Caruso, F., Tanski, J., Villegas-Estrada, A., and Rossi, M., Structural basis for antioxidant activity of trans-resveratrol: *ab initio* calculations and crystal and molecular structure, *J. Agric. Food Chem.*, 52:7279–7285, 2004.

Dong, H.H. and Ren, H.L., New progression in the study of protective properties of resveratrol in anti-cardiovascular disease, *Bratisl Lek Listy.*, 105:225–229, 2004.

Donnelly, L.E., Newton, R., Kennedy, G.E., Fenwick, P.S., Leung, R.H.K., Ito, K., Russell, R.E.F., and Barnes, P.J., Anti-inflammatory effects of resveratrol in lung epithelial cells: molecular mechanisms, *Am. J. Physiol. Lung Cell Mol. Physiol.*, 287:L774–L783, 2004.

Granados-Soto, V., Pleiotropic effects of resveratrol, *Drug News Perspect.*, 16:299–307, 2003.

Kundu, J.K. and Surh, Y-J., Molecular basis of chemoprevention by resveratrol: NF-κB and AP-1 as potential targets, *Mutat. Res.*, 555:65–80, 2004.

Li, H.-L., Wang, A.-B., Huang, Y., Liu, D.-P., Wei, C., Williams, G.M., Zhang, C.-N., Liu, G., Liu, Y.-Q., Hao, D.-L., Hui, R.-T., Lin, M., and Liang, C.-C., Isorhapontigenin, a new resveratrol analog, attenuates cardiac hypertrophy via blocking signaling transduction pathways, *Free Rad. Biol. Med.*, 38: 243–257, 2005.

Matsuda, H., Tewtrakul, S., Morikawa, T., and Yoshikawa, M., Anti-allergic activity of stilbenes from Korean rhubarb (*Rheum undulatum* L.): structure requirements for inhibition of antigen-induced degranulation and their effects on the release of TNF-α and IL-4 in RBL-2H3 cells, *Bioorg. Med. Chem.*, 12:4871–4876, 2004.

Orsini, F. and Verotta, L., Stilbenes and bibenzyls with potential anticancer or chemopreventive activity, *Adv. Exp. Med. Biol.*, 472:169–186, 1999.

Pozo-Guisado, E., Lorenzo-Benayas, M.J., and Fernandez-Salguero, P.M., Resveratrol modulates the phosphoinositide 3-kinase pathway through an estrogen receptor α-dependent mechanism: Relevance in cell proliferation, *Int. J. Cancer*, 109:167–173, 2004.

Stinging nettle   The nettle tribe, *Urticaceae*, is spread throughout the world, with about 500 species, mainly tropical, though several, like the British species of stinging nettle, grows in temperate climates. The British species, belonging to the genus *Urtica* (the name derived from the Latin, *uro*, to burn), are known for their well-armed leaves with stinging hairs with the burning properties fluid.

Water extract of stinging nettle has powerful antioxidant activity, evaluated using different antioxidant tests, including reducing power, free-radical scavenging, superoxide-anion-radical scavenging, hydrogen-peroxide scavenging, and metal-chelating activities. It also showed antimicrobial activity against nine microorganisms, antiulcer activity against ethanol-induced ulcerogenesis, and analgesic effect on acetic acid-induced stretching (Gulcin et al., 2004).

The long-term use of the stinging nettle leaf extract, an adjuvant remedy in rheumatic diseases dependent on a cytokine suppressive effect, was found effective in the prevention of chronic murine colitis. This effect seems to be due to a decrease in the Th1 response and may be a new therapeutic option for prolonging remission in inflammatory-bowel disease (Konrad et al., 2005). The clinical efficacy of stinging-nettle-leaf extracts in treatment of rheumatoid arthritis is explained by the ability of 13-hydroxyoctadecatrienic acid, one of the more active anti-inflammatory substances in stinging-nettle-leaf extracts, to suppress the expression of matrix metalloproteinases, which are known to have a role in inflammatory joint diseases (Schulze-Tanzil et al., 2002).

The antiproliferative effect of a methanolic extract of stinging-nettle roots on human prostatic epithelial and stromal cells was observed both in *in vivo* and in *in vitro* systems (Konrad et al., 2000). In animal models, the induced growth of prostatic lobe could be reduced by the polysaccharide fraction of the methanolic extract of stinging-nettle roots by 33.8 percent (Lichius et al., 1999). In many European countries, phytopharmaceuticals are commonly used for managing benign prostatic hyperplasia and associated lower urinary-tract symptoms, with these products representing up to 80 percent of all drugs prescribed for this disorder. Extracts from the fruits of saw palmetto and the roots of stinging nettle are particularly popular.

Although extracts from the stinging nettle may provide therapeutic value for some inflammatory medical conditions, it can also cause a wide range of cutaneous reactions. Contact with the hairs or spines on the stems and leaves of the stinging nettle causes the release of several biologically active substances that cause itching, dermatitis, and urticaria within moments of contact (Anderson et al., 2003).

References

Anderson, B.E., Miller, C.J., and Adams, D.R., Stinging nettle dermatitis, *Am. J. Contact Dermat.*, 14:44–46, 2003.

Caliskaner, Z., Karaayvaz, M. and Ozturk, S., Misuse of a herb: stinging nettle (*Urtica urens*) induced severe tongue oedema, *Complementary Ther. Med.*, 12:57–58, 2004.

Gulcin, I., Kufrevioglu, O.I., Oktay, M., and Buyukokuroglu, M.E., Antioxidant, antimicrobial, antiulcer and analgesic activities of nettle (*Urtica dioica* L.), *J. Ethnopharmacol.*, 90(2–3):205–15, 2004.

Koch, E., Extracts from fruits of saw palmetto (*Sabal serrulata*) and roots of stinging nettle (*Urtica dioica*): viable alternatives in the medical treatment of benign prostatic hyperplasia and associated lower urinary tracts symptoms, *Planta Med.*, 67:489–500, 2001.

Konrad, A., Mahler, M., Arni, S., Flogerzi, B., Klingelhofer, S., and Seibold, F., Ameliorative effect of IDS 30, a stinging nettle leaf extract, on chronic colitis, *Int. J. Colorectal Dis.*, 20:9–17, 2005.

Konrad, L., Muller, H.H., Lenz, C., Laubinger, H., Aumuller, G., and Lichius, J.J., Antiproliferative effect on human prostate cancer cells by a stinging nettle root (*Urtica dioica*) extract, *Planta Med.*, 66: 44–47, 2000.

Lichius, J.J., Renneberg, H., Blaschek, W., Aumuller, G., and Muth, C., The inhibiting effects of components of stinging nettle roots on experimentally induced prostatic hyperplasia in mice, *Planta Med.*, 65:666–668, 1999.

Schulze-Tanzil, G., de, Souza P., Behnke, B., Klingelhoefer, S., Scheid, A., and Shakibaei M., Effects of the antirheumatic remedy Hox alpha — a new stinging nettle leaf extract — on matrix metalloproteinases in human chondrocytes *in vitro*, *Histol. Histopathol.*, 17:477–485, 2002.

Strawberries

Strawberries   Strawberries are rich in ascorbic acid and a wide range of phenolic compounds. The significant inhibition by strawberry juice of the endogenous formation of *N*-nitrosoamino acids in humans could not be solely attributed to ascorbic acid (Hesler et al., 1992). Subsequent research showed that strawberries were high in antioxidant activity and capable of enhancing antioxidant capacity in humans (Wang et al., 1996; Cao et al., 1998). Strawberry supplementation in the diet of *N*-nitroso-methyl-benzylamine-treated rats reduced the multiplicity of esophageal tumors (Stoner et al., 1997). Ellagic acid was subsequently identified as one of the chemopreventive components present in strawberries, responsible for inhibiting cancers. It appears to prevent the binding of the reactive-carcinogenic components with DNA, as well as stimulate detoxification enzymes (Teel, 1986; Ahn et al.,

S

1996). Treating Syrian hamster embryo (SHE) cells with the carcinogen benzo[*a*]pyrene for seven days, Xue and coworkers (2001) found that a methanolic extract from freeze-dried strawberries (*Fragara ananassa*) appeared to display chemopreventive activity by interfering with the uptake, activation, and detoxification of the carcinogen or by intervention of DNA binding and repair.

In strawberries, the most abundant bioactive compounds are ellagic acid and certain flavonoids: anthocyanin, catechin, quercetin, and kaempferol. These compounds in strawberries have potent antioxidant power, which helps to lower risk of cardiovascular events. Furthermore, strawberry extracts have been shown to inhibit COX enzymes *in vitro*, which would modulate the inflammatory process. Individual compounds in strawberries have demonstrated anticancer activity in several different experimental systems. Preliminary animal studies have indicated that diets rich in strawberries may also have the potential to provide benefits to the aging brain (Hannum, 2004).

References

Ahn, D., Putt, D., Kresty, L., Stoner, G.D., Fromm, D., and Hollenberg, P.F., The effects of dietary ellagic acid on rat hepatic and esophageal mucosal cytochromes P450 and phase II enzymes, *Carcinogenesis*, 17:821–828, 1996.

Cao, G., Russell, R.M., Lischner, N., and Prior, R.L., Serum antioxidant capacity is increased by consumption of strawberries, spinach, red wine or Vitamin C in elderly women, *J. Nutr.*, 128:2383–2390, 1998.

Hannum, S.M., Potential impact of strawberries on human health: a review of the science, *Crit. Rev. Food Sci. Nutr.*, 44:1–17, 2004.

Hesler, M.A., Hotchkiss, J.H., and Rose, D.A., Influence of fruit and vegetable juices on the endogenous formation of *N*-nitrosoproline and *N*-nitrosothiazolidine-4-carboxylic acid in humans on controlled diets, *Carcinogenesis*, 13:2277–2280, 1992.

Stoner, G.D., Kresty, L.A., Lu, J., Porter, C., Siglin, J.C., and Morse, M.A., Inhibitory effect of strawberries on esophageal tumorigenesis and O^6-methylguanine levels in the F344 rat, *Proc. Annu. Meet. Am. Assoc. Cancer Res.*, 38:A2462, 1997.

Teel, R.W., Dixit, R., and Stoner, G.D., The effect of ellagic acid on the uptake, persistence, metabolism

and DNA-binding of benzo[*a*]pyrene in cultured explants of strain A/J mouse lung, *Carcinogenesis*, 6:391–395, 1985.

Wang, H., Cao, G., and Prior, R.L., Total antioxidant capacity of fruits, *J. Agric. Food Chem.*, 44:701–705, 1996.

Xue, H., Aziz, R.M., Sun, N., Cassady, J.M., Kamendulis, L.M., Xu, Y., Stoner, G.D., and Klaunig, J.E., Inhibition of cellular transformation of berry extracts, *Carcinogenesis*, 22:351–356, 2001.

Sugar-beet fiber   Sugar-beet fiber, like wheat bran and flaxseed, is useful in the treatment of constipation, colon diverticulosis, and adiposity (Trepel, 2004). Rations containing sugar-beet pulp, given to broiler breeder females, were associated with higher water contents in the gastrointestinal tract, and it was proposed that this improved satiety and welfare (Hocking et al., 2004).

Mataumoto and coworkers (2001) showed that sugar-beet fiber reduced the ovariectomy-induced elevation in plasma cholesterol in 6-week-old ovariectomized female rats. Plasma total and non-HDL cholesterol were lowered significantly by 29 percent and 47 percent in rats fed sugar-beet fiber in comparison to the control diet.

References

Hocking, P.M., Zaczek, V., Jones, E.K., and Macleod, M.G., Different concentrations and sources of dietary fibre may improve the welfare of female broiler breeders, *Br. Poult. Sci.*, 45:9–19, 2004.

Mataumoto, J., Kishida, T., and Ebihara, K., Sugar beet fiber suppresses ovarian hormone deficiency-induced hypercholesterolemia in rats, *Nutr. Res.*, 21: 1519–1527, 2001.

Trepel, F., Dietary fibre: more than a matter of dietetics. II. Preventative and therapeutic uses, *Wien Klin. Wochenschr.*, 116:511–522, 2004.

Sulforaphane   Sulforaphane [1-isothiocyanato- (4R)-(methylsulfinyl) butane], an isothiocyanate present naturally in widely consumed vegetables, has a particularly high concentration in broccoli. It was isolated from

Sulforaphane. (Adapted from Wu et al., *Mutat. Res.,* 589:81–102, 2005.)

SAGA broccoli as the major phase II enzyme inducer, present in organic solvent extracts of this vegetable (Zhang et al., 1994). Sulforaphane was found to block chemical-initiated tumor formation in rats (Faulkner et al., 1998). The effectiveness of sulforaphane is based on induction of hepatic detoxifying enzymes. Sulforaphane is a very potent inducer of phase II enzymes, UDP-glucuronosyltransferase 1A1, and glutathione *S*-transferase A1 (Bacon et al., 2003). It was shown to inhibit cytochrome P-450 (CYP2E1) involved in the activation of a variety of carcinogens (Barcelo et al., 1996; Faulkner et al., 1998).

Recent studies report that induction of thioredoxin reductase by sulforaphane is mediated by putative antioxidant response elements found in the promoter similar to the upregulating mechanism of other antioxidant enzymes (Hintze et al., 2003). In highly proliferative HT29 cells, sulforaphane induces a cell-cycle arrest, followed by cell death caused by a proapoptotic protein bax-dependent pathway. These results suggest that in addition to the activation of detoxifying enzyme activities, specific mechanisms, such as apoptosis, are also involved in the sulforaphane-associated chemoprevention of cancer (Gamet-Payrastre et al., 2000; Misiewicz et al., 2004). Similar results were found in leukemic cells (Fimognari et al., 2002) and human melanoma cells (Misiewicz et al., 2003) with recent reports suggesting sulforaphane can halt human breast-cancer cells (Johnston, 2004). Animal studies demonstrated that sulforaphane significantly reduces the formation of total and multicrypt foci in azoxymethane-induced colonic aberrant crypt foci F344 rats, during both the initiation phase and the postinitiation treatment, indicative of its potential to prevent colon cancer (Chung et al., 2000). Recent studies demonstrated the potential of sulforaphane for treating pancreatic cancer (Pham et al., 2004). Jackson and Singletary (2004) reported sulforaphane was an effective inhibitor of human mcf-7 mammary-cancer cells.

A potent decrease in lipopolysaccharide-induced secretion of proinflammatory and procarcinogenic signaling factors (i.e., NO, prostaglandin E_2, and tumor-necrosis factor) in cultured Raw 264.7 macrophages after sulforaphane treatment suggested that anti-inflammatory mechanisms contribute to sulforaphane-mediated cancer chemoprevention (Heiss et al., 2001).

Sulforaphane was also shown to be a potent bactericidal agent against both extracellular and intracellular *H. pylori in vitro*. Haristoy et al. (2003) investigated the efficacy of sulforaphane *in vivo* against *H. pylori* by using a recently developed model, which uses human gastric xenografts in nude mice. They observed that *H. pylori* can be eradicated from human gastric xenografts after a short-term administration of sulforaphane at a dose that can be achieved in the human diet. Thus, sulforaphane delivered in the diet could be beneficial for the treatment of *H. pylori*-associated gastric diseases.

References

Bacon, J.R., Williamson, G., Garner, R.C., Lappin, G., Langouet, S., and Bao, Y., Sulforaphane and quercetin modulate PhIP-DNA adduct formation in human HepG2 cells and hepatocytes, *Carcinogenesis*, 24:1903–1911, 2003.

Barcelo, S., Gardiner, J.M., Gesher, A., and Chipman, J.K., CYP2E1-mediated mechanism of antigenotoxicity of the broccoli constituent sulforaphane, *Carcinogenesis*, 17:277–282, 1996.

Chung, F.-L., Conaway, C.C., Rao, C.V., and Reddy, B.S., Chemoprevention of colonic aberrant crypt foci in Fischer rats by sulforaphane and phenethyl isothiocyanate, *Carcinogenesis*, 21:2287–2291, 2000.

Faulkner, K., Mithen, R., and Williamson, G., Selective increase of the potential anticarcinogen 4-methylsulphinylbutyl glucosinolate in broccoli, *Carcinogenesis*, 19:605–609, 1998.

Fimognari, C., Nusse, M., Cesari, R., Iori, R., Cantelli-Forti, G., and Hrelia, P., Growth inhibition, cell-cycle arrest and apoptosis in human T-cell leukemia by the isothiocyanate sulforaphane, *Carcinogenesis*, 23:581–586, 2002.

Gamet-Payrastre, L., Li, P., Lumeau, S., Cassar, G., Dupont, M-A., Chevolleau, S., Gasc, N., Tulliez, J., and Terce, F., Sulforaphane, a naturally occurring isothiocyanate, induces cell cycle arrest and apoptosis in HT29 human colon cancer cells, *Cancer Res.,* 60:1426–1433, 2000.

Haristoy, X., Angioi-Duprez, K., Duprez, A., and Lozniewski, A., Efficacy of sulforaphane in eradicating *Helicobacter pylori* in human gastric xenografts implanted in nude mice, *Antimicrob. Agents Chemother.,* 47:3982–3984, 2003.

Heiss, E., Herhaus, C., Klimo, K., Bartsch, H., and Gerhauser, C., Nuclear factor κB is a molecular target for sulforaphane-mediated anti-inflammatory mechanisms, *J. Biol. Chem.,* 276:32008–32015, 2001.

Hintze, K.J., Wald, K.A., Zeng, H., Jeffery, E.H., and Finley, J.W., Thioredoxin reductase in human hepatoma cells is transcriptionally regulated by sulforaphane and other electrophiles via an antioxidant response element, *J. Nutr.,* 133:2721–2727, 2003.

Jackson, S.J.T. and Singletary, K.W., Sulforaphane inhibits human mcf-7 mammary cancer cell mitotic progression and tubulin polymerization, *J. Nutr.,* 134:2229–2236, 2004.

Johnston, N., Sulforaphane halts breast cancer cell growth, *Drug Discov. Today,* 9:908, 2004.

Misiewicz, I., Skupinska, K., and Kasprzycka-Guttman, T., Sulforaphane and 2-oxohexyl isothiocyanate induce cell growth arrest and apoptosis in L-1210 leukemia and ME-18 melanoma cells, *Oncol. Rep.,* 10:2045–2050, 2003.

Misiewicz, I., Skupinska, K., Kowalska, E., Lubinski, J., and Kasprzycka-Guttman, T., Sulforaphane-mediated induction of a phase 2 detoxifying enzyme NAD(P)H:quinone reductase and apoptosis in human lymphoblastoid cells, *Acta Biochem. Pol.,* 51: 711–721, 2004.

Pham, N.A., Jacobberger, J.W., Schimmer, A.D., Cao, P., Gronda, M., and Hedley, D.W., The dietary isothiocyanate sulforaphane targets pathways of apoptosis, cell cycle arrest, and oxidative stress in human pancreatic cancer cells and inhibits tumor growth in severe combined immunodeficient mice, *Mol. Cancer Ther.,* 3:1239–1248, 2004.

Wu, X., Kassie, F., and Mersch-Sundermann, V., Induction of apoptosis in tumor cells by naturally occurring sulfur-containing compounds, *Mutat. Res.,* 589:81–102, 2005.

Zhang, Y., Kensler, T.W., Cho, C.G., Posner, G.H., and Talalay, P., Anticarcinogenic activities of sulforaphane and structurally related synthetic norbornyl isothiocyanates, *Proc. Natl. Acad. Sci. U.S.A.,* 91:3147–3150, 1994.

Summer savory (*Satureja hortensis*) *Satureja hortensis* L. (Lamiaceae) is an annual herb, traditionally used in the Eastern Anatolia region of Turkey as folk medicine for treatment of different infectious diseases and disorders. In Iranian folk medicine, it was used as muscle- and bone-pain reliever.

Uslu and coworkers (2003) showed that the activity of nitric-oxide synthase enzyme, and concentration of nitric-oxide metabolites were both significantly reduced by topical administration of *S. hortensis* extract. Histological examination demonstrated reduced inflammation. Thus, their data suggest that *S. hortensis* extract may have the potential as an antiinflammation agent in the treatment of rhinosinusitis diseases. Antimicrobial test results showed that the essential oil of *S. hortensis* had great potential in antimicrobial activities against different bacteria, fungi, and yeast species. Thymol (29.0 percent), carvacrol (26.5 percent), γ-terpinene (22.6 percent), and p-cymene (9.3 percent) were the main components in essential oil of *S. hortensis* (Gulluce et al., 2003).

The essential oil of *S. hortensis* was also found as a relaxant of rat-isolated ileum. In addition to antispasmodic activity *in vitro*, it inhibited castor oil-induced diarrhea in mice. Thus, *S. hortensis* essential oil may have clinical benefits for treatment of some gastrointestinal disorders (Hajhashemi et al., 2000).

The polyphenolic fraction and the essential oil of *S. hortensis* L. were both shown to have antinociceptive and anti-inflammatory effects (Hajhashemi et al., 2002). The antioxidant capacities and total phenol content were demonstrated in the ethanol and acetone extracts of the dried material from a number of sources, including summer savory (Exarchou et al., 2002).

References

Exarchou, V., Nenadis, N., Tsimidou, M., Gerothanassis, I.P., Troganis, A., and Boskou, D., Antioxidant activities and phenolic composition of extracts from Greek oregano, Greek sage, and summer savory, *J. Agric. Food Chem.,* 50:5294–5299, 2002.

Gulluce, M., Sokmen, M., Daferera, D., Agar, G., Ozkan, H., Kartal, N., Polissiou, M., Sokmen, A., and Sahin, F., *In vitro* antibacterial, antifungal, and antioxidant activities of the essential oil and methanol extracts of herbal parts and callus cultures of *Satureja hortensis* L., *J. Agric. Food Chem.,* 51:3958–3965, 2003.

Hajhashemi, V., Ghannadi, A., and Pezeshkian, S.K., Antinociceptive and anti-inflammatory effects of *Satureja hortensis* L. extracts and essential oil, *J. Ethnopharmacol.,* 82:83–87, 2002.

Hajhashemi, V., Sadraei, H., Ghannadi, A.R., and Mohseni, M., Antispasmodic and anti-diarrhoeal effect of *Satureja hortensis* L. essential oil, *J. Ethnopharmacol.,* 71:187–192, 2000.

Uslu, C., Murat Karasen, R., Sahin, F., Taysi, S., and Akcay, F., Effects of aqueous extracts of *Satureja hortensis* L. on rhinosinusitis treatment in rabbit, *J. Ethnopharmacol.,* 88:225–228, 2003.

Sunflower *see* **Sunflower oil and Sunflower seed protein**

Sunflower oil   Alpaslan and Gunduz (2000) showed that growing conditions significantly affected the fatty-acid compositions of sunflower varieties. In the 1991 and 1992 crop years, they ranged for oil content 44.2–51.2 percent (on dry weight basis) and 43.0–51.5 percent (on dry weight basis); oleic acid 14.8–18.5 percent and 32.9–40.1 percent; linoleic acid 69.5–74.5 percent and 49.7–55.7 percent; and tocopherol content (as α-tocopherol) 648–860 mg/kg and 524–880 mg/kg, respectively.

A significantly higher LDL susceptibility to oxidation was observed after sunflower-oil intake in comparison with virgin olive oil, in spite of an increase in LDL α-tocopherol concentration in the sunflower-oil group. These results provide further evidence that sunflower-oil-enriched diets do not protect LDL against oxidation, as virgin olive oil does, in patients with peripheral vascular disease (Aguilera et al., 2004).

In comparison to other commercially available antimicrobial agents, ozonized sunflower oil demonstrated significant antimicrobial activity and anti-inflammatory and wound-healing properties (Rodrigues et al., 2004). Treatment of preterm infants < 34 weeks in Egypt with sunflower-seed oil resulted in a significant improvement in skin condition and a highly significant reduction in the incidence of nosocomial infections compared with infants not receiving topical prophylaxis. This study suggests the potential of topical therapy to reduce infections and save newborn lives in developing countries (Darmstadt et al., 2004).

Sesame oil and sunflower oil offered 20 percent and 40 percent protection, respectively, in mouse-skin tumor model. The antioxidant capabilities of these compounds could not solely explain the observed anticancer characteristics. Thus, the observed chemopreventive effects warrant more attention, since they already exist in the population with no known adverse effects (Kapadia et al., 2002).

References

Aguilera, C.M., Mesa, M.D., Ramirez-Tortosa, M.C., Nestares, M.T., Ros, E., and Gil, A., Sunflower oil does not protect against LDL oxidation as virgin olive oil does in patients with peripheral vascular disease, *Clin. Nutr.,* 23:673–681, 2004.

Alpaslan, M. and Gunduz, H., The effects of growing conditions on oil content, fatty acid composition and tocopherol content of some sunflower varieties produced in Turkey, *Nahrung,* 44:434–437, 2000.

Darmstadt, G.L., Badrawi, N., Law, P.A., Ahmed, S., Bashir, M., Iskander, I., Al Said, D., El Kholy, A., Husein, M.H., Alam, A., Winch, P.J., Gipson, R., and Santosham, M., Topically applied sunflower seed oil prevents invasive bacterial infections in preterm infants in Egypt: a randomized, controlled clinical trial, *Pediatr. Infect. Dis. J.,* 23:719–725, 2004.

Kapadia, G.J., Azuine, M.A., Tokuda, H., Takasaki, M., Mukainaka, T., Konoshima, T., and Nishino, H., Chemopreventive effect of resveratrol, sesamol, sesame oil and sunflower oil in the Epstein–Barr virus early antigen activation assay and the mouse skin two-stage carcinogenesis, *Pharmacol. Res.,* 45:499–505, 2002.

S

TABLE S.62
Lipid Concentrations (10^{-2}kgm^{-3}) in Plasma of Rats Fed Casein and Sunflower-Seed Protein Fraction (PF).

	Total Cholesterol	Triglyceride	MDL Cholesterol	VLDL Cholesterol	LDL Cholesterol	LDL Cholesterol/ HDL Cholesterol	Total Cholesterol/ HDL Cholesterol
Casein	53.9 ± 5.4	73.8 ± 3.5	9.3 ± 1.6	14.8 ± 2.2	29.9 ± 4.8	3.1 ± 0.4	5.8 ± 0.5
PF	37.2 ± 3.2*	60.0 ± 3.7**	5.5 ± 1.4***	12.0 ± 0.8	19.7 ± 3.4	3.6 ± 1.5	6.8 ± 0.6

Values are mean ±SEM, n =8, HDL, high-density lipoprotein, LDL-low-density lipoprotein, VLDL-very-low-density lipoprotein. *$p < 0.05$, **$p < 0.01$, ***$p < 0.001$.

Source: From Sen and Bhattacharyya, *J. Sci. Food Agric.,* 81:347–352, 2000. With permission.

Rodrigues, K.L., Cardoso, C.C., Caputo, L.R., Carvalho, J.C.T., Fiorini, J.E., and Schneedorf, J.M., Cicatrizing and antimicrobial properties of an ozonised oil from sunflower seeds, *Inflammopharmacology,* 12:261–270, 2004.

Sunflower-seed protein In addition to oil, sunflower also produces a protein. Over the past few decades, evidence has accrued that ingestion of plant proteins lowers plasma cholesterol in animals (Carroll, 1995). One mechanism suggests that plant proteins suppress the intestinal absorption or reabsorption of neutral lipids, reducing the cholesterol pool within the body (Van Deer Meer and Beynen, 1987). Sen and Bhattacharyya (2000) enzymatically extracted dehulled sunflower seeds with pectinase to produce a protein-rich fraction low in fiber and chlorogenic acid. The protein-rich fraction significantly reduced plasma cholesterol ($p < 0.02$) and triglyceride ($p < 0.02$) in rats fed the sunflower-seed protein fraction compared to casein (Table S.62). While the HDL-cholesterol levels were significantly reduced by the sunflower-seed protein fraction, the total cholesterol/HDL cholesterol and LDL cholesterol/HDL cholesterol ratios were not significantly different. Thus, the sunflower-seed protein fraction exhibited similar hypolipidemic effects to casein.

References

Carrol, K.K. and Kurowska, E.M., Soy consumption and cholesterol reduction, review of animal and human studies, *J. Nutr.,* 125:594S–597S, 1995.

Sen, M. and Bhattacharyya, D.K., Hypolipidemic effect of enzymatically extracted sunflower seed protein fraction, *J. Sci. Food Agric.,* 81:347–352, 2000.

Vandermeer, R. and Beynen, A.C., Species dependent responsiveness of serum cholesterol to dietary proteins, *J. Am. Oil Chem. Soc.,* 64:1172–1177, 1987.

Sweet basil Basil or sweet basil (*Ocimum basilicum*) is cultivated throughout India. It is rich in essential oils that have been the subject of numerous chemical studies (Grayer et al., 1996). Sweet basil was grown by local people as a medicinal plant, culinary herb, and antimicrobial agent. Some 30 monoterpenoids, sesquiterpenoids, and phenylpropanoids identified in basil oil as the major components (more than 20 percent of the total essential-oil composition) were linalool, methyl chavicol, eugenol, methyl eugenol, and geraniol (Grayer et al., 1996).

Basil essential oils and their principal constituents were found to exhibit antimicrobial activity against a wide range of Gram-negative and Gram-positive bacteria, yeast, and mold (Suppakul et al., 2003). Linalool alone showed a moderate antifungal activity, while eugenol showed no activity at all. Mixing the two components in a ratio similar to their concentrations

S

in the original oil was found to enhance the antifungal properties of basil oil, indicating a synergistic effect (Edris and Farrag, 2003).

The major antioxidant compound in the methanolic extract of sweet basil was confirmed as rosmarinic acid. The results showed that one rosmarinic acid can capture 1.52 radicals, and, furthermore, the existence of a synergistic effect between α-tocopherol and rosmarinic acid was revealed (Jayasinghe et al., 2003).

The effects of an alcoholic extract of the fresh leaves of sweet basil on Swiss albino mice were increasing the activity of xenobiotic metabolizing phase I and phase II enzymes, elevating antioxidant-enzyme response by increasing significantly the hepatic glutathione reductase, superoxide dismutase, and catalase activities, increasing glutathione content, and decreasing lipid peroxidation and lactate dehydrogenase activity in the liver after eight to nine weeks. Furthermore, chemopreventive response was evident from the reduced tumor, as well as from the reduced percentage of tumor-bearing animals (Dasgupta et al., 2004).

Recently Fang and coworkers (2004) reported that essential oil from sweet basil can act as skin-permeation enhancers to promote the percutaneous absorption of drugs. This might be mainly due to improvement in the partitioning of the drugs to the stratum corneum.

References

Dasgupta, T., Rao, A.R., and Yadava, P.K., Chemomodulatory efficacy of basil leaf (*Ocimum basilicum*) on drug metabolizing and antioxidant enzymes, and on carcinogen-induced skin and forestomach papillomagenesis, *Phytomedicine*, 11:139–151, 2004.

Edris, A.E. and Farrag, E.S., Antifungal activity of peppermint and sweet basil essential oils and their major aroma constituents on some plant pathogenic fungi from the vapor phase, *Nahrung*, 47:117–121, 2003.

Fang, J.Y., Leu, Y.L., Hwang, T.L., and Cheng, H.C., Essential oils from sweet basil (*Ocimum basilicum*) as novel enhancers to accelerate transdermal drug delivery, *Biol. Pharm. Bull.*, 27:1819–1825, 2004.

Grayer, R.J., Kite, G.C., Goldstone, F.J., Bryan, S.E., Paton, A., and Putievsky, E., Infraspecific taxonomy and essential oil chemotypes in sweet basil, *Ocimum basilicum*, *Phytochemistry*, 43:1033–1039, 1996.

Jayasinghe, C., Gotoh, N., Aoki, T., and Wada, S., Phenolics composition and antioxidant activity of sweet basil (*Ocimum basilicum* L.), *J. Agric. Food Chem.*, 51(15):4442–9, 2003.

Suppakul, P., Miltz, J., Sonneveld, K., and Bigger, S.W., Antimicrobial properties of basil and its possible application in food packaging, *J. Agric. Food Chem.*, 51:3197–3207, 2003.

Sweet flag (*Acorus calamus*)

Sweet flag (*Acorus calamus* L.) is a perennial shrub that grows in damp, marshy places in India, North America, and Europe. The rhizomes of *Acorus calamus* are empirically used for treating a wide variety of human diseases. It is recognized as an Indian drug with antibacterial, anticonvulsant, antiveratrinic, and antiarrhythmic action (Madan et al., 1960), as well as a tranquilizing agent (Menon and Dandiya, 1967).

The ethanol extract of *Acorus calamus* rhizomes exhibited a large number of actions on the CNS similar to α-asarone (an active principle of *A. calamus*) but differed from the latter in several other respects. These differences could be due to the effects of other chemicals in the plant extract (Vohora et al., 1990). The alcoholic extract also antagonized spontaneous motor activity and also amphetamine-induced hyperactivity in mice. It was less potent than chlorpromazine, but still exerted sedative and tranquilizing action (Panchal et al., 1989).

Neurobehavioral changes produced by acrylamide could be prevented following treatment with *Acorus calamus* rhizomes (Shukla et al., 2002). Administration of a 50 percent ethanolic extract (100 and 200 mg/kg), as well as saponins (10 mg/kg) isolated from the extract showed significant hypolipidemic activity (Parab and Mengi, 2002). Recently, Mehrotra and coworkers (2003) demonstrated the antiproliferative and immunosuppressive potential of an ethanolic extract from *Acorus calamus in vitro*.

References

Madan, B.R., Arora, B.B., and Kapila, K., Anticonvulsant, antiveratrinic and antiarrhythmic actions of *Acorus calamus* Linn. — an Indian indigenous drug, *Arch. Int. Pharmacodyn. Ther.*, 124:201–211, 1960.

S

Menon, M.K. and Dandiya, P.C., The mechanism of the tranquilizing action of asarone from *Acorus calamus* Linn., *J. Pharm. Pharmacol.,* 19:170–175, 1967.

Mehrotra, S., Mishra, K.P., Maurya, R., Srimal, R.C., Yadav, V.S., Pandey, R., and Singh, V.K., Anticellular and immunosuppressive properties of ethanolic extract of *Acorus calamus* rhizome, *Int. Immunopharmacol.,* 3:53–561, 2003.

Panchal, G.M., Venkatakrishna-Bhatt, H., Doctor, R.B., and Vajpayee, S., Pharmacology of *Acorus calamus* L., *Indian J. Exp. Biol.,* 27:561–567, 1989.

Parab, R.S. and Mengi, S.A., Hypolipidemic activity of *Acorus calamus* L. in rats, *Fitoterapia,* 73:451–455, 2002.

Shukla, P.K., Khanna, V.K., Ali, M.M., Maurya, R.R., Handa, S.S., and Srimal, R.C., Protective effect of *Acorus calamus* against acrylamide induced neurotoxicity, *Phytother. Res.,* 16:256–260, 2002.

Vohora, S.B., Shah, S.A., and Dandiya, P.C., Central nervous system studies on an ethanol extract of *Acorus calamus* rhizomes, *J. Ethnopharmacol.,* 28:53–62, 1990.

Sweet potatoes   Sweet potatoes, a crop native to South America, are easy to grow and have become a staple food in many African countries. The orange-fleshed sweet-potato variety is rich in β-carotene, which offers hope to the population who are currently beyond the reach of a vitamin A supplement. The effect of 60 days of daily supplementation with 750 mg retinol equivalents (RE) of pureed sweet potatoes were tested by Haskell et al. (2004). The overall geometric mean of initial vitamin A stores was 0.108 +/- 0.067 mmol. Relative to the low vitamin A control group, the estimated mean changes in vitamin A stores were 0.029 mmol. Vitamin A equivalency factors (β-carotene:retinol, wt:wt) were estimated as approximately 13:1 for sweet potato. Thus, daily consumption of pureed sweet potatoes has a positive effect on vitamin A stores in populations at risk of vitamin A deficiency (Haskell et al., 2004).

The major phenolic components contained in the 70 percent methanol extract of sweet potatoes with strong antioxidative activity were identified as chlorogenic acid and isochlorogenic acid-1, -2, and -3. The other minor free phenolics were identified as caffeic acid and 4-*O*-caffeoylquinic acid. Chlorogenic acid and isochlorogenic acids, however, had only a slight antioxidative activity. Thus, the effective antioxidant activity of the sweet-potato extract was proposed to be mainly based on the synergistic effect of phenolic compounds with amino acids (Hayase and Kato, 1984). The dietary fiber content of sweet potatoes was found to range from 9–12 percent for cured roots. Soluble and insoluble dietary fiber averaged 5·30 percent and 5·43 percent, respectively (Mullin et al., 1994).

Anthocyanins are the chemical components that give the intense color to sweet potatoes, as in many other fruits and vegetables. Epidemiological investigations have indicated that moderate consumption of anthocyanin products is associated with a lower risk of cardiovascular disease and improvement of visual functions (Hou, 2003). Recently, the leaves of sweet potatoes were found to be rich in nutritive and functional components. They were found to contain a large amount of protein, showing high amino-acid score, soluble dietary fibers and minerals, particularly iron, and vitamins, such as carotene, vitamin B_2, vitamin C, and vitamin E. Furthermore, polyphenol content in the leaves was comparatively high. These results suggest that the whole parts of sweet potatoes should be utilized as valuable foodstuffs (Ishida et al., 2000).

References

Haskell, M.J., Jamil, K.M., Hassan, F., Peerson, J.M., Hossain, M.I., Fuchs, G.J., and Brown, K.H., Daily consumption of Indian spinach (*Basella alba*) or sweet potatoes has a positive effect on total-body vitamin A stores in Bangladeshi men, *Am. J. Clin. Nutr.,* 80:705–714, 2004.

Hayase, F. and Kato, H., Antioxidative components of sweet potatoes, *J. Nutr. Sci. Vitaminol.,* 30:37–46, 1984.

Hou, D.X., Potential mechanisms of cancer. Dietary fibre in sweet potatoes, *Food Res. Int.,* 27:563–565, 1994.

Ishida, H., Suzuno, H., Sugiyama, N., Innami, S., Tadokoro, T. and Maekawa, A., Nutritive evaluation of chemical components of leaves, stalks and stems of sweet potatoes (*Ipomoea batatas poir*), *Food Chem.,* 68:359–367, 2000.

Mullin, J., Rosa, N. and Reynolds, L.B., Dietary fibre in sweet potatoes, *Food Res. Int.,* 27:563–565, 1994.

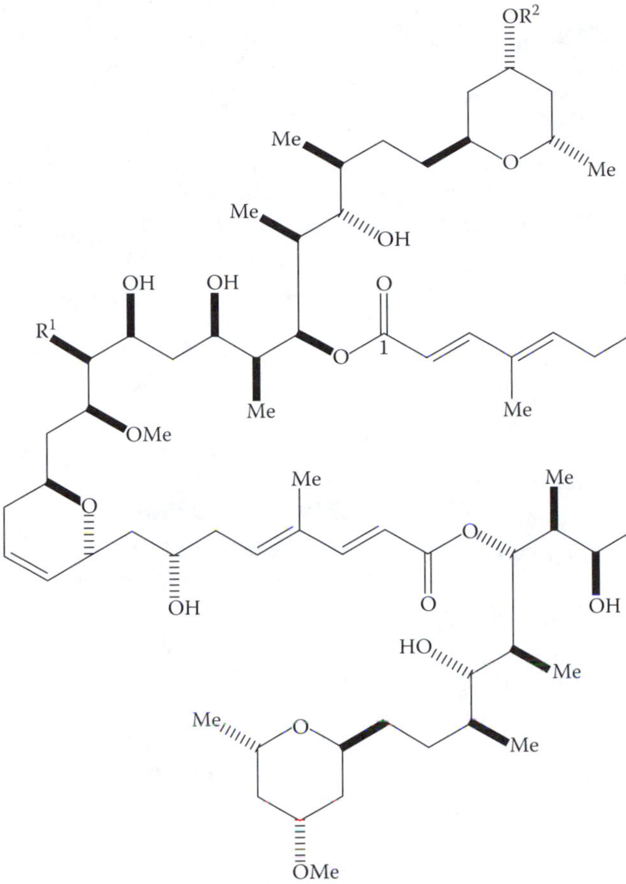

Swinholide A (1): n = 1, R¹=R²=Me
Swinholide B (2): n = 1, R¹=H, R²=Me
Swinholide C (3): n = 1, R¹=Me, R²=H

Swinholides A, B, and C. (From Hayakawa and Miyashita, *Tetrahedron Lett.*, 41:707–711, 2000. With permission.)

Swinholide The marine natural products swinholides A (**1**), B (**2**), and C (**3**), 44-membered dimeric macrolides isolated from the Okinawan marine sponge *Theonella swinhoei* (Carmely and Cashman, 1985), have been shown to exhibit potent cytotoxicity against a variety of human carcinoma-cell lines, as well as a broad spectrum of antifungal activity (Tanaka et al., 1990; Doi et al., 1991). Their structures are characterized by the C_2-symmetrical dimeric macrolides in which two polypropionate-derived chains take axial orientation on a tetrahydropyran ring. Their unique structures and potent anticancer activities have elicited much attention from synthetic organic chemists toward the synthesis of polypropionate-derived bioactive compounds (Paterson et al., 1994; Hiroyuki and Masaaki, 2000).

References

Carmely, S. and Kashman, Y., Structure of swinholide-a, a new macrolide from the marine sponge *Theonella swinhoei*, *Tetrahedron Lett.*, 26:511–514, 1985.

Doi, M., Ishida, T., Koybayashi, M. and Kitagawa, I. Molecular conformation of swinholide A, a potent cytotoxic dimeric macrolide from the Okinwan marine sponge *Theonella swinhoei*: X-ray crystal structure of its diketone, *J. Org. Chem.*, 56:3629–3643, 1991.

Hayakawa, H. and Miyashita, M., An efficient and stereoselective construction of the C(9)–C(17) dihydropyran segment of swinholides A–C via a novel reductive cleavage of an epoxy aldehyde, *Tetrahedron Lett.*, 41:707–711, 2000.

S

Tanaka, J., Higa, T., Kobayashi, M., and Kitagawa, I., Marine natural products. XXIV. The absolute stereo-structure of misakinolide A, a potent cytotoxic dimeric macrolide from an Okinawan marine sponge *Theonella* sp., *Chem. Pharm. Bull.*, 38:967–2970, 1990.

Paterson, I., Yeung, K.-S., Ward, R.A., Cumming, J.G., and Smith, J.D., Total synthesis of swinholide A and hemiswinholide A, *J. Am. Chem. Soc.*, 116: 9391–9392, 1994.

Synbiotic *see also* Prebiotics and Probiotics

Prebiotics, usually polysaccharides, exhibit strong bioactivity, and the ingestion of prebiotics has been shown to reduce the rate of infection and restore health in sick and postoperative patients. Probiotics are bacteria that reduce or eliminate potentially pathogenic microorganisms, as well as various toxins, mutagens, and carcinogens. They modulate the innate and adaptive immune defense mechanisms, promote apoptosis, and release many nutrients, antioxidants, growth, coagulation, and other factors necessary for recovery. A combination of prebiotics and probiotics is referred to as "synbiotics" if it has a stronger effect on intestinal diseases than probiotics or prebiotics alone (Holmes, 2003; Tuohy et al., 2003).

Synbiotics treatment was also found to contribute in the treatment of severe acute pancreatitis, chronic hepatitis, and liver transplantation (Bengmark, 2003). It was also reported as an alternative to lactulose for the management of minimal hepatic encephalopathy in patients with cirrhosis (Liu et al., 2004).

Roller and coworkers (2004) demonstrated that synbiotic supplementation in carcinogen-treated rats primarily modulated immune functions in the Peyer's patches, with a reduction in the number of colon tumors. Other evidence for the cancer-preventing properties of probiotics and prebiotics is derived from studies on fecal-enzyme activities in animals and humans, inhibition of genotoxicity of known carcinogens *in vitro* and *in vivo*, suppression of carcinogen-induced preneoplastic lesions and tumors in laboratory animals. Some of these studies indicate that combinations of probiotics and prebiotics are more effective than either one of these treatments (Burns and Rowland, 2000).

Synbiotic treatment to short-bowel patients with refractory enterocolitis was very promising. It improved the intestinal bacterial flora, increased short-chain fatty acids in the feces, and accelerated their body-weight gain (Kanamori et al., 2004). Oral supplements with synbiotic also increased energy intake and promoted weight gain in acutely ill children receiving antibiotics (Schrezenmeir et al., 2004).

References

Bengmark, S., Use of some pre-, pro- and synbiotics in critically ill patients, *Best Pract. Res. Clin. Gastroenterol.*, 17:833–848, 2003.

Burns, A.J. and Rowland. I.R., Anti-carcinogenicity of probiotics and prebiotics, *Curr. Issues Intest. Microbiol.*, 1:13–24, 2000.

Holmes, S., Are probiotics and other functional foods the medicines of the future? *Prof. Nurse*, 18:627–630, 2003.

Kanamori, Y., Sugiyama, M., Hashizume, K., Yuki, N., Morotomi, M., and Tanaka, R., Experience of long-term synbiotic therapy in seven short bowel patients with refractory enterocolitis, *J. Pediatr. Surg.*, 39:1686–1692, 2004.

Kanamori, Y., Hashizume, K., Sugiyama, M., Mortomi, M., Yuki, N., and Tanaka, R., A novel synbiotic therapy dramatically improved the intestinal function of a pediatric patient with laryngotracheo-esophageal cleft (LTEC) in the intensive care unit, *Clin. Nutr.*, 21:527–530, 2002.

Liu, Q., Duan, Z.P., Ha da, K., Bengmark, S., Kurtovic, J., and Riordan, S.M., Synbiotic modulation of gut flora: effect on minimal hepatic encephalopathy in patients with cirrhosis, *Hepatology*, 39:1441–1449, 2004.

Roller, M., Pietro Femia, A., Caderni, G., Rechkemmer, G., and Watzl, B., Intestinal immunity of rats with colon cancer is modulated by oligofructose-enriched inulin combined with *Lactobacillus rhamnosus* and *Bifidobacterium lactis*, *Br. J. Nutr.*, 92: 931–938, 2004.

Schrezenmeir, J., Heller, K., McCue, M., Llamas, C., Lam, W., Burow, H., Kindling-Rohracker, M., Fischer, W., Sengespeik, H.C., Comer, G.M., and Alarcon, P., Benefits of oral supplementation with and without synbiotics in young children with acute bacterial infections, *Clin. Pediatr.*, 43:239–249, 2004.

Tuohy, K.M., Probert, H.M., Smejkal, C.W., and Gibson, G.R., Using probiotics and prebiotics to improve gut health, *Drug Discov. Today*, 8:692–700, 2003.

S

T

Tangeretin Tangeretin is a flavone derivative (5,6,7,8,4′-pentamethoxyflavone) present in citrus-fruit peel. Pan and coworkers (2002) showed that it induces cell-cycle G_1 arrest in colorectal carcinoma COLO 205 cells. Exposure of cells to tangeretin resulted in inhibition

Tangeretin

(From Nielsen et al., *Food Chem. Toxicol.*, 38:739–746, 2000. With permission.)

of cyclin-dependent kinases 2 and 4 in a dose-dependent manner. Tangeretin also increased the level of Cdk inhibitor p21 and p27 protein. These studies showed that the growth inhibition was mediated by inhibiting the activities of cyclin-dependent kinases 2 and 4.

The modulation of apoB-containing lipoprotein metabolism by tangeretin was studied by Kurowska and coworkers (2004). A 24-h exposure of human hepatoma-cell line HepG2 to tangeretin decreased intracellular synthesis of cholesteryl esters, free cholesterol, and TAG, which were associated with decreased activities of DAG acyltransferase and microsomal triglyceride transfer protein. Tangeretin was also found to activate the peroxisome proliferator-activated receptor, a transcription factor with a positive regulatory impact on fatty acid oxidation and TAG availability. Tangeretin was also reported to upregulate the function of the E-cadherin/catenin complex in human breast carcinoma cells. This leads to firm cell–cell adhesion and inhibition of invasion *in vitro*.

The neuroprotective effects of tangeretin, found to cross the blood–brain barrier, were elucidated in the 6-hydroxydopamine lesion rat model of Parkinson's disease (Datla et al., 2001).

References

Datla, K.P., Christidou, M., Widmer, W.W., Rooprai, H.K., and Dexter, D.T., Tissue distribution and neuroprotective effects of citrus flavonoid tangeretin in a rat model of Parkinson's disease, *Neuroreport*, 12: 3871–3875, 2001.

Kurowska, E.M., Manthey, J.A., Casaschi, A., and Theriault, A.G., Modulation of HepG2 cell net apolipoprotein B secretion by the citrus polymethoxyflavone, tangeretin, *Lipids*, 39:143–151, 2004.

Nielsen, S.E., Breinholt, V., Cornett, C., and Dragsted, L.O., Biotransformation of the citrus flavone tangeretin in rats: Identification of metabolites with intact flavane nucleus, *Food Chem. Toxicol.*, 38:739–746, 2000.

Pan, M.-H., Chen, W.-J., Lin-Shiau, S.-Y.L., Ho, C.-T., and Lin, J.-K., Tangeretin induces cell-cycle G_1 arrest through inhibiting cyclin-dependent kinases 2 and 4 activities as well as elevating Cdk inhibitors p21 and p27 in human colorectal carcinoma cells, *Carcinogenesis*, 23:1677–1684, 2002.

Tangerine *see also* **Tangeretin** Tangerine is a member of the citrus family. In addition to vitamin C, it contains polymethoxylated flavones, such as tangeretin and nobiletin, found mainly in the peels of tangerines and oranges and in smaller amounts in the juices of these fruits. These flavones were shown to have cholesterol- and triacylglycerol-lowering potential (Kurowska and Manthey, 2004). Tangerines are also a rich source for β-carotene, folate, and potassium. Like other citrus fruits, tangerines contain *d*-limonene, another flavonoid.

Citrus nobiletin, a polymethoxylated flavone found in tangerine peels, was found to exhibit

Nobiletin. (From Iwase et al., *Cancer Lett.,* 163:7–9, 2001. With permission.)

chemopreventive ability against azoxymethane-induced rat colon carcinogenesis (Suzuki et al., 2004). β-Cryptoxanthin, a major source of vitamin A, is often second only to β-carotene in tangerines. Increasing amounts of free β-cryptoxanthin were detected in chylomicrons and serum of subjects following ingestion of tangerine juice (Wingerath et al., 1995). Subjects that frequently (> or = 3/d) consumed tropical fruits with at least 50 mg/100 g β-cryptoxanthin, such as papaya and tangerine, had twofold the plasma β-cryptoxanthin concentrations of those with intakes of < 4/wk (Irwig et al., 2002).

Jian and coworkers (2005) showed that an intake of citrus fruits was inversely associated with prostate-cancer risk. This risk declined with increasing consumption of α-carotene, β-carotene, β-cryptoxanthin, lutein, and zeaxanthin, all found in the tangerine. Previous work by Guo et al. (2000) isolated and identified hesperidin, neohesperidin, nobiletin, and tangeritin in tangerine peel.

References

Guo, X.L., Wang, T.J., Guo, M.J., and Chen, Y., Studies on chemical constituents of processed green tangerine peel, *Zhongguo Zhong Yao Za Zhi,* 25:146–148, 2000.

Irwig, M.S., El-Sohemy, A., Baylin, A., Rifai, N., and Campos, H., Frequent intake of tropical fruits that are rich in β-cryptoxanthin is associated with higher plasma β-cryptoxanthin concentrations in Costa Rican adolescents, *J. Nutr.,* 132:3161–3167, 2002.

Iwase, Y., Takemura, Y., Ju-ichi, M., Yano, M., Ito, C., Furukawa, H., Mukainaka, T., Kuchide, M., Tokuda, H., and Nishino, H., Cancer chemopreventive activity of 3,5,6,7,8,3′,4′-heptamethoxyflavone

from the peel of citrus plants, *Cancer Lett.,* 163:7–9, 2001.

Jian, L., Du, C-J., Lee, A.H., and Binns, C.W., Do dietary lycopene and other carotenoids protect against prostate cancer? *Int. J. Cancer,* 113:1010–1014, 2005.

Kurowska, E.M. and Manthey, J.A., Hypolipidemic effects and absorption of citrus polymethoxylated flavones in hamsters with diet-induced hypercholesterolemia, *J. Agric. Food Chem.,* 52:2879–2886, 2004.

Suzuki, R., Kohno, H., Murakami, A., Koshimizu, K., Ohigashi, H., Yano, M., Tokuda, H., Nishino, H., and Tanaka, T., Citrus nobiletin inhibits azoxymethane-induced large bowel carcinogenesis in rats, *Biofactors,* 21:111–114, 2004.

Wingerath, T., Stahl, W., and Sies, H., β-Cryptoxanthin selectively increases in human chylomicrons upon ingestion of tangerine concentrate rich in β-cryptoxanthin esters, *Arch. Biochem. Biophys.,* 324:385–390, 1995.

Taraxacum platycarpum *Taraxacum platycarpum* is a Chinese herb used in traditional Oriental medicine. The extracts from this herb have anti-inflammatory properties used for treating ulcers and colitis. Yun and coworkers (2002) isolated and characterized an anticoagulant from *T. platycarpum*. It appeared to be a protein monomer with a molecular weight of 31–33 kDa. The anticoagulant properties included delaying thrombin time and prothrombin time and activating partial-thromboplastin time. In addition, it activated murine macrophages to produce cyclooxygenase-2 and nitric-oxide synthase, as well as the secretion of tumor necrosis factor.

A polysaccharide fraction from *T. platycarpum* showed potent immunopotentiating activities, with antitumor activities. It inhibited the growth of solid tumor and increased peritoneal exudate cells and immunoorgan weights in normal mice, as well as increased hypersensitivities in tumor-bearing mice (Jeong et al., 1991).

Desacetylmatricarin was identified as the active principle responsible for the antiallergic property of *T. platycarpum* (Cheong et al., 1998).

References

Cheong, H., Choi, E.J., Yoo, G.S., Kim, K.M., and Ryu, S.Y., Desacetylmatricarin, an anti-allergic component from *Taraxacum platycarpum*, *Planta Med.,* 64(6):577–578, 1998.

Jeong, J.Y., Chung, Y.B., Lee, C.C., Park, S.W., and Lee, C.K., Studies on immunopotentiating activities of antitumor polysaccharide from aerial parts of *Taraxacum platycarpum*, *Arch. Pharm. Res.,* 14:68–72, 1991.

Yun, S.I., Cho, H.R., and Choi, H.S., Anticoagulant from *Taraxcum platycarpum*, *Biosci. Biotechnol. Biochem.,* 66:1859–1864, 2002.

Taurine   Taurine is a conditionally essential amino acid that has been shown to be involved in certain aspects of mammalian development (Sturman, 1993). The molecule contains a sulfonic-acid group, rather than the carboxylic

$$CH_2 — CH_2 — SO_3^-$$
$$|$$
$$+NH_3$$

acid moiety, that is not incorporated into proteins and is one of the most abundant free amino acids in many tissues, including skeletal and cardiac muscle and the brain (Huxtable, 1992). *In vitro* and animal studies demonstrated that low levels of taurine are associated with various pathological lesions, including cardiovascular disorders (Satoh and Sperelakis, 1998; Oudit et al., 2004), retinal degeneration (Sheik et al., 1981), and growth retardation (Geggel et al., 1985). Taurine is also involved in such metabolic activities as bile-acid conjugation (Smith et al., 1991; Carrasco et al., 1990), detoxification (Waterfield et al., 1993; Timbrell and Waterfield, 1996) membrane stabilization (Qi et al., 1995), osmoregulation (Olivero and Stutzin, 2004), and modulation of cellular calcium levels (Satoh and Sperelakis, 1998). Clinically, taurine has been used in the treatment of cardiovascular diseases (Azuma et al., 1992; Modi and Suleiman, 2004), ischemia-reperfusion injury (Kingston et al., 2004), hypercholesterolemia (Matsushima et al., 2003), epilepsy and other seizure disorders (Airaksinen et al., 1980), macular degeneration (Sturman, 1986), Alzheimer's disease (Csernansky et al., 1996), hepatic disorders (Matsuyama et al., 1983), alcoholism, and cystic fibrosis (Smith et al., 1991; Carrasco et al., 1990).

Taurine was recently shown by Takatani and coworkers (2004) to inhibit ischemic-induced apoptosis in cultured neonatal rat cardiomyocytes by increasing the activities of Akt kinase and inactivating caspase-9. Figure T.95A shows simulated ischemia induced a 4.5-fold and 11-fold increase in caspase-9 and caspase-3 compared to the control. In the presence of taurine caspase-9 and caspase-3, activities were significantly reduced. Thus, taurine treatment could be beneficial for treating heart failure.

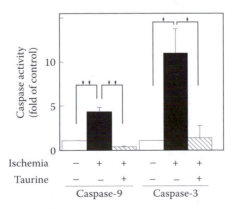

FIGURE T.95 Taurine prevents ischemia-induced caspase-9 and caspase-3 processing in cultured cardiomycetes. Cardiomyocytes were exposed to ischemia for 30 h in the absence (–) or in the presence (+) of 20 mM taurine. (From Takatani et al., *Biochem. Biophys. Res. Commun.,* 316:484–489, 2004. With permission.)

Recent *in vivo* and *in vitro* evidence found that taurine, through its ability to control sarcolemmal excitability and muscle contractibility, could have beneficial effects in many muscle dysfunctions (Conte Camerino et al., 2004).

References

Airaksinen, E.M., Oja, S.S., Marnela, K.M. et al., Effects of taurine treatment on epileptic patients, *Prog. Clin. Biol. Res.*, 39:157–166, 1980.

Azuma, J., Sawamura, A., and Awata, K., Usefulness of taurine in chronic congestive heart failure and its prospective application, *Jpn. Circ. J.*, 56:95–99, 1992.

Carrasco, S., Codoceo, R., Prieto, G. et al., Effect of taurine supplements on growth, fat absorption and bile acid on cystic fibrosis, *Acta Univ. Carol.*, 36: 152–156, 1990.

Conte Camerino, D., Tricarico, D., Pierno, S., Desaphy, J.F., Liantonio, A., Pusch, M., Burdi, R., Camerino, C., Fraysse, B., and De Luca, A., Taurine and skeletal muscle disorders, *Neurochem. Res.*, 29:135–142, 2004.

Csernansky, J.G., Bardgett, M.E., Sheline, Y.I. et al., CSF excitatory amino acids and severity of illness in Alzheimer's disease, *Neurology*, 46:1715–1720, 1996.

Geggel, H.S., Ament, M.E., and Heckenlively, J.R., Nutritional requirement for taurine in patients receiving long-term parenteral nutrition, *N. Engl. J. Med.*, 312:142–146, 1985.

Huxtable, R.J., Physiological actions of taurine, *Physiol. Rev.*, 72:101–163, 1992.

Kingston, R., Kelly, C.J., and Murray, P., The therapeutic role of taurine in ischaemia-reperfusion injury, *Curr. Pharm. Des.*, 10:2401–2410, 2004.

Matsushima, Y., Sekine, T., Kondo, Y., Sakurai, T., Kameo, K., Tachibana, M., and Murakami, S., Effects of taurine on serum cholesterol levels and development of atherosclerosis in spontaneously hyperlipidaemic mice, *Clin. Exp. Pharmacol. Physiol.*, 30:295–299, 2003.

Matsuyama, Y., Morita, T., Higuchi, M., and Tsujii, T., The effect of taurine administration on patients with acute hepatitis, *Prog. Clin. Biol. Res.*, 125:461–468, 1983.

Modi, P. and Suleiman, M-S., Myocardial taurine, development and vulnerability to ischemia, *Amino Acids*, 26:65–70, 2004.

Olivero, P. and Stutzin, A., Calcium modulates osmosensitive taurine efflux in HeLa cells, *Neurochem. Res.*, 29:169–176, 2004.

Oudit, G.Y., Trivieri, M.G., Khaper, N., Husain, T., Wilson, G.J., Liu, P., Sole, M.J., and Backx, P.H., Taurine supplementation reduces oxidative stress and improves cardiovascular function in an iron-overload murine model, *Circulation*, 109:1877–1885, 2004.

Qi, B., Yamagami, T., Naruse, Y., Sokejima, S. and Kogamimori, S., Effects of taurine on depletion of erythrocyte membrane Na-K ATPase activity due to ozone exposure or cholesterol enrichment, *J. Nutr. Sci. Vitaminol.*, 41:627–634, 1995.

Satoh, H. and Sperelakis, N., Review of some actions of taurine on ion channels of cardiac muscle cells and others, *Gen. Pharmacol.*, 30:451–463, 1998.

Sheik, K., Toskes, P., and Dawson, W., Taurine deficiency and retinal defects associated with small intestinal bacterial overgrowth, *Gastroenterology*, 80:1363, 1981.

Smith, U., Lacaille, F., and Lepage, G., Taurine decreases fecal fatty acid and sterol excretion in cystic fibrosis, a randomized double-blind study, *Am. J. Dis. Child*, 145:1401–1404, 1991.

Sturman, J.A., Taurine in development, *Physiol. Rev.*, 73:119–147, 1993.

Sturman, J.A., Nutritional taurine and central nervous system development, *Ann. N.Y. Acad. Sci.*, 477: 196–213, 1986.

Takatani, T., Takahasi, K., Uozumi, Y., Matsuda, T., Ito, T., Schaffer, S.W., Fujio, Y., and Azuma, J., Taurine prevents the ischemia-induced apoptosis in cultured neonatal rat cardiomycetes through Akt/caspase-9 pathway, *Biochem. Biophys. Res. Commun.*, 316:484–489, 2004.

Timbrell, J.A. and Waterfield, C.J., Changes in taurine as an indicator of hepatic dysfunction and biochemical perturbations, studies *in vivo* and *in vitro*, *Adv. Exp. Med. Biol.*, 403:125–134, 1996.

Waterfield, C.J., Turton, J.A., Scales, M.D., and Timbrell, J.A., Reduction of liver taurine in rats by beta-alanine treatment increases carbon tetrachloride toxicity, *Toxicology*, 77:7–20, 1993.

T

Tea *see also* **Black, Green, Oolong, and Rooibus tea**   Tea is the most-consumed drink in the world after water. Green, black, and oolong teas are the three major commercial types of teas and differ in how they are produced and in their chemical composition. Green tea is prepared by pan-frying or steaming fresh leaves to heat-inactivate oxidative enzymes and then the leaves are dried. By contrast, black tea is produced by crushing fresh tea leaves and allowing enzyme-mediated oxidation to occur. Green tea is chemically characterized by the presence of large amounts of polyphenolic compounds, known as catechins (Balentine et al., 1997). These include epicatechin, epigallocatechin, epicatechin-3-gallate, epigallocatechin-3-gallate (EGCG), caffeine, and theanine (Scheme T.58).

An accumulated number of population studies suggest that consumption of green- and black-tea beverages may have positive health benefits (Peters et al., 2001; Blumberg, 2003). Tea is an important source of flavonoids in the diet, with levels approaching 200 mg/cup for a typical brew of black tea (Lakenbrink et al., 2001). Tea flavonoids are potent antioxidants that are absorbed from the gut, leading to a significant increase in the antioxidant capacity of the blood. Beneficial effects of increased antioxidant capacity in the body include the reduction of oxidative damage to important biomolecules. The scientific support is strongest for the protection of DNA from oxidative damage after black- or green-tea consumption (Rietveld and Wiseman, 2003). The beneficial effect of tea on the cardiovascular system has been clearly established (Kris-Etherton et al., 2002). One mechanism is that it improves the vascular endothelium, which is known to play a central role in the regulation of vascular homeostasis, and that endothelial dysfunction contributes to the pathogenesis and clinical expression of cardiovascular disease (Vita, 2003).

As a source rich with antioxidants, tea is also involved in protection against the development of cancer (Kris-Etherton et al., 2002) and neurodegenerative diseases (Kakuda, 2002). Tea polyphenols seem able to modulate cell growth by arresting the cell cycle or inducing apoptosis. In addition, administration of green tea reduced the levels of 8-OHdG in the lung DNA. Other studies have also shown green tea inhibited the activity of phase I enzymes and induced phase II enzymes. Together, these mechanisms may be responsible for the protective effects of tea against carcinogenesis (Chung et al., 2003; Lambert and Yang, 2003).

Studies with human cancer-cell lines have demonstrated that epigallocatechin-3-gallate (EGCG), one of the major tea polyphenols, may be involved in its protective activities. It inhibits mitogen-activated protein kinases, cyclin-dependent kinases, growth factor-related cell signaling, activation of activator protein 1 (AP-1),

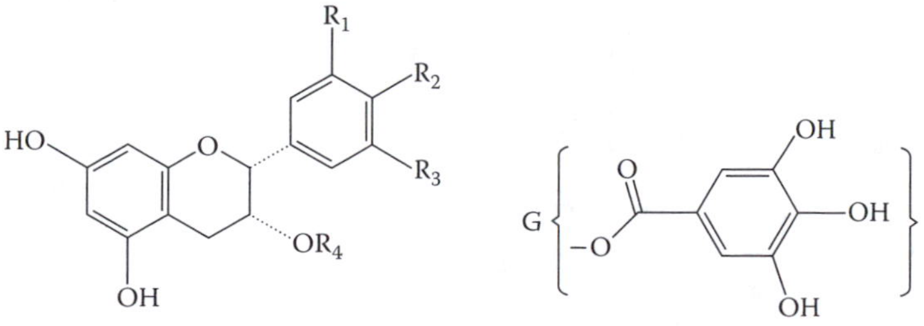

	R_1	R_2	R_3	R_4
EGCG: Epigallocatechin gallate	OH	OH	OH	G
ECG: Epicatechin gallate	OH	OH	H	G
EC: Epicatechin	OH	OH	H	OH
ECG: Epigallocatechin	OH	OH	OH	OH

SCHEME T.58 Structures of major polyphenols in green tea. (From Ghosh et al., *Biochem. Biophys. Res. Commun.*, 325:807–811, 2004. With permission.)

and nuclear factor κB (NF-κB), topoisomerase I, and matrix metalloproteinases, as well as other potential targets (Lambert and Yang, 2003).

References

Balentine, D.A., Wiseman, S.A., and Bouwens, L.C., The chemistry of tea flavonoids, *Crit. Rev. Food Sci. Nutr.,* 37:693–704, 1997.

Blumberg, J., Introduction to the proceedings of the Third International Scientific Symposium on Tea and Human Health: Role of Flavonoids in the Diet, *J. Nutr.,* 133:3244S–3246S, 2003.

Chung, F.L., Schwartz, J., Herzog, C.R., and Yang, Y.M., Tea and cancer prevention: studies in animals and humans, *J. Nutr.,* 133:3268S–3274S, 2003.

Ghosh, K.S., Maiti, T.K., and Dasgupta, S., Green tea polyphenols as inhibitors of ribonuclease A, *Biochem. Biophys. Res. Commun.*, 325:807–811, 2004.

Kakuda, T., Neuroprotective effects of the green tea components theanine and catechins, *Biol. Pharm. Bull.,* 25:1513–1518, 2002.

Kris-Etherton, P.M. and Keen, C.L., Evidence that the antioxidant flavonoids in tea and cocoa are beneficial for cardiovascular health, *Curr. Opin. Lipidol.,* 13:41–49, 2002.

Kris-Etherton, P.M., Hecker, K.D., Bonanome, A., Coval, S.M., Binkoski, A.E., Hilpert, K.F., Griel, A.E., and Etherton, T.D., Bioactive compounds in foods: their role in the prevention of cardiovascular disease and cancer, *Am. J. Med.,* 113(Suppl. 2):71S–88S, 2002.

Lakenbrink, C., Lapczynski, S., Maiwald, B., and Engelhardt, U.H., Flavonoids and other polyphenols in consumer brews of tea and other caffeinated beverages, *J. Agric. Food Chem.,* 48:2848–2852, 2000.

Lambert, J.D. and Yang, C.S., Mechanisms of cancer prevention by tea constituents, *J. Nutr.,* 133:3262S–3267S, 2003.

Peters, U., Poole, C., and Arab, L., Does tea affect cardiovascular disease? A meta-analysis, *Am. J. Epidemiol.,* 154:495–503, 2001.

Rietveld, A. and Wiseman, S., Antioxidant effects of tea: evidence from human clinical trials, *J. Nutr.,* 133: 3285S–3292S, 2003.

Vita, J.A., Tea consumption and cardiovascular disease: effects on endothelial function, *J. Nutr.,* 133: 3293S–3297S, 2003.

Tea tree (*Melaleuca alternifolia*) *Melaleuca alternifolia* is a tea tree native to Australia. The oil obtained by steam distillation of its leaves was reported to have antibacterial, antifungal, antiviral, anti-inflammatory, and analgesic properties (Carson et al. 1998; Messager et al., 2005). Currently, tea-tree oil is used in cosmetics, health-care products, and as an effective antiseptic (Williams et al., 1997). The concentrations of tea-tree oil found in commercially available products range from 2 percent to 5 percent. Terpinen-4-ol is the main antimicrobial component but other components, such as α-terpineol, also have antimicrobial activities similar to those of terpinen-4-ol (Carson and Riley, 1995). Studies on the antifungal mechanism of tea-tree oil and its components against *Candida albicans*, *Candida glabrata,* and *Saccharomyces cerevisiae* was due to the alteration in membrane properties and compromising membrane-associated functions (Hammer et al., 2004). The main antioxidants identified in tea-tree oil are α-terpinene, α-terpinolene, and γ-terpinene (Kim et al., 2004).

Recently, tea-tree oil was found to be effective as an adjunctive therapy in treating osteomyelitis and infected chronic wounds in case studies and small clinical trials (Halcon and Milkus, 2004).

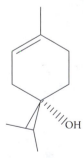

Terpinen-4-ol. (From Biju et al., *J. Pharmaceut. Biomed. Anal.,* 38:41–44, 2005. With permission.)

References

Biju, S.S., Ahuja, A., Rafullah, M.R.M., and Khar, R.K., A validated HPLTC method for determination of tea tree oil from cosmeceutical formulations, *J. Pharmaceut. Biomed. Anal.,* 38:41–44, 2005.

Carson, C.F., Riley, T.V., and Cookson, B.D., Efficacy and safety of tea tree oil as a topical antimicrobial agent, *J. Hosp. Infect.,* 40:175–178, 1998.

Carson, C.F. and Riley, T.V., Antimicrobial activity of the major components of the essential oil of *Melaleuca alternifolia*, *J. Appl. Bacteriol.,* 78:264–269, 1995.

Halcon, L. and Milkus, K., *Staphylococcus aureus* and wounds: a review of tea tree oil as a promising antimicrobial, *Am. J. Infect. Control,* 32:402–408, 2004.

Hammer, K.A., Carson, C.F., and Riley, T.V., Antifungal effects of *Melaleuca alternifolia* (tea tree) oil and its components on *Candida albicans, Candida glabrata* and *Saccharomyces cerevisiae, J. Antimicrob. Chemother.,* 53:1081–1085, 2004.

Kim, H-J., Chen, F., Wu, C., Wang, X., Chung, H.Y., and Jin, Z., Evaluation of antioxidant activity of Australian tea tree (*Melaleuca alternifolia*) oil and its components, *J. Agric. Food Chem.,* 52:2849–2854, 2004.

Messager, S., Hammer, K.A., Carson, C.F., and Riley, T.V., Assessment of the antibacterial activity of tea tree oil using the European EN 1276 and EN 12054 standard suspension tests, *J. Hosp. Infect.,* 59: 113–125, 2005.

Williams, L.R., Stockley, J.K., Home, V.N., and Yan, W., Therapeutic use for tea tree oil, *Aust. J. Pharm.,* 78:285–287, 1997.

Tedanolide   Tedanolide is a novel macrolide, isolated from the abundant Caribbean sponge, *Tedania ignis* (fire sponge). It was first reported by Schmitz and coworkers in 1984 to be a potent marine antitumor agent (Schmitz et al., 1983). A closely related compound, 13-deoxytedanolide, was reported by Fusetani et al. (1991) in the Japanese sponge, *Mycale adhaerens. In*

vitro studies revealed that tedanolide possessed an ED_{50} of 0.25 ng/mL and 1.6 pg/mL in KB and PS cells, respectively, causing cell accumulation in the S phase of the cell cycle at concentrations as low as 0.01 µg/mL (Schmitz et al., 1984). Similarly, 13-deoxytedanolide expressed an IC_{50} of 94 pg/mL against P388 murine leukemia cells (Fusetani et al., 1991).

Tedanolide increased the life span of mice implanted with lymphocytic leukemia by 23 percent when given 1.5 µg/kg of body weight (Schmitz et al., 1988). No information, however, is available on the biochemical mechanism of action of the tedanolides. A synthetic strategy for constructing potent marine antitumor agents, tedanolide and 13-deoxytedanolide, was recently described (Smith et al., 2004; Roush and Newcom, 2002).

References

Fusetani, N., Sugawara, T., Matsunaga, S., and Hirota, H., Bioactive marine metabolites, 35, Cytotoxic metabolites of the marine sponge Mycale-adhaerens Lambe, *J. Org. Chem.,* 56:4971–4974, 1991.

Roush, W.R. and Newcom, J.S., Studies on the synthesis of tedanolide. 2. Stereoselective synthesis of a protected C(1)-C(12) fragment, *Org. Lett.,* 4:4739–4742, 2002.

Schmitz, F.J., Vanderah, D.J., Hollenbeak, K.H., Enwall, C.E.L., Gopichand, Y., SenGupta, P.K., Hossain, M.B., and Van der Helm, D., Metabolites from the marine sponge Tedaniaignis — a new atisanediol and several known diketopiperazines, *J. Org. Chem.,* 48:3941–3945, 1983.

Schmitz, F.J., Gunasekera, S.P., Yalamanchili, G., Hossain, M.B., and Van der Helm, D., Tedanolide — a potent cytotoxic macrolide from the Caribbean sponge Tedaniaignis, *J. Am. Chem. Soc.,* 106:7251–7252, 1984.

Tedanolide and 13-deoxytedanolide. (From Taylor et al., *Tetrahedron Lett.,* 39:9361–9364, 1998. With permission.)

Schmitz, F.J., Gunasekera, S.P., Hossain, M.B., Van der Helm, D., and Yalamanchili, G., Tedanolide U.S. patent application 87–7347, 1988.

Smith, A.B., III, Adams, C.M., Barbosa, S.A., and Degnan, A.P., A unified approach to the tedanolides: total synthesis of (+)-13-deoxytedanolide, *Proc. Natl. Acad. Sci. U.S.A.*, 101:12042–12047, 2004.

Taylor, R.E., Ciavarri, J.P., and Hearn, B.R., A divergent approach to the myriaporones and tedanolide: enantioselective preparation of the common intermediate, *Tetrahedron Lett.*, 39:9361–9364, 1998.

Terpenes *see also* **Monoterpenes**   Terpenes are organic solvents, usually derived from natural sources, such as pine trees or citrus fruit, mainly as constituents of essential oils. Generally, they have strong, characteristic odors. Many terpenes are hydrocarbons, but oxygen-containing compounds, such as alcohols, aldehydes, or ketones (*terpenoids*) are also found. Their building block is the hydrocarbon isoprene, CH_2=C(CH_3)-CH=CH_2. Terpene hydrocarbons have a molecular formula of $(C_5H_8)_n$. They are volatile, organic compounds that are flammable or combustible.

In vitro and *in vivo* studies demonstrated terpenes had antibacterial (Alma et al., 2004), antifungal (Inoue et al., 2004), and anticancer activities. Specific terpenes used in cleaning are pinene, *d*-limonene, and turpentine. Menthol, a monoterpene (10 carbons) isolated from various mints, is a topical pain reliever and antipuretic (Wasner et al., 2004). Borneol, a monoterpene derived from pine oil, is used as a disinfectant and deodorant. Camphor is another monoterpene used as a counterirritant (Taniguchi et al., 1994), anesthetic (Kuroda et al., 2004), expectorant, and antipruritic (Shunying et al., 2005). Recently, serious pediatric toxicity resulting from exposure to small amounts of camphor-containing products were reported (Love et al., 2004).

One of the most well-known, medicinally valuable terpenes is the diterpene, taxol. It was first isolated from the bark of the Pacific yew, *Taxus brevifolia*, in the early 1960s, but its value as an anticancer drug was not determined until the late 1980s (Beijnen et al., 1994).

Taxol. (Adapted from Huang et al., *Bioorg. Med. Chem.*, 9:2237–2242, 2001.)

Taxol is thought to induce apoptosis through the release of cytochrome C and activation of caspases. However, the effect of taxol on dendritic cells was shown by Joo et al. (2003) to induce immunosuppression in patients with cancer by inhibition of dendritic cells-activated T cell proliferation. The effect of taxol on dendritic cells includes induction of immunosuppression in patients with cancer by inhibition of dendritic cells–activated T-cell proliferation (Joo et al., 2003).

Other examples of monoterpenes are nerol and citral, while sesquiterpenes include nerolidol and farnesol. An example of a diterpene is phytol, while squalene and carotene are examples of a triterpene and a tetraterpene, respectively.

References

Alma, M.H., Nitz, S., Kollmannsberger, H., Digrak, M., Efe, F.T., and Yilmaz, N., Chemical composition and antimicrobial activity of the essential oils from the gum of Turkish pistachio (*Pistacia vera* L.), *J. Agric. Food Chem.*, 52:3911–3914, 2004.

Beijnen, J.H., Huizing, M.T., Ten Bokkel Huinink, W.W., Veehof, C.H.N., Vermorken, J.B., Giaccone, G., and Pinedo, H.M., Bioanalysis, pharmacokinetics, and pharmacodynamics of the novel anticancer drug paclitaxel (Taxol), *Semin. Oncol.*, 21:53–62, 1994.

Huang, Q., Roesnner, C.A., Croteau, R., and Scott, A.I., Engineering *Escherichia coli* for the synthesis of taxadiene a key intermediate in the biosynthesis of taxol, *Bioorg. Med. Chem.*, 9:2237–2242, 2001.

Inoue, Y., Shiraishi, A., Hada, T., Hirose, K., Hamashima, H., and Shimada, J., The antibacterial effects of terpene alcohols on *Staphylococcus aureus* and their mode of action, *FEMS Microbiol. Lett.*, 237:325–331, 2004.

Joo, H-G., Altered maturation of dendritic cells by taxol, an anticancer drug, *J. Vet. Sci.*, 4:229–234, 2003.

Kuroda, M., Yoshikawa, D., Nishikawa, K., Saito, S., and Goto, F., Volatile anesthetics inhibit calcitonin gene-related peptide receptor-mediated responses in pithed rats and human neuroblastoma cells, *J. Pharmacol. Exp. Ther.*, 311:1016–1022, 2004.

Love, J.N., Sammon, M., and Smereck, J., Are one or two dangerous? Camphor exposure in toddlers, *J. Emerg. Med.*, 27:49–54, 2004.

Shunying, Z., Yang, Y., Huaidong, Y., Yue, Y., and Guolin, Z., Chemical composition and antimicrobial activity of the essential oils of *Chrysanthemum indicum*, *J. Ethnopharmacol.*, 96:151–158, 2005.

Taniguchi, Y., Deguchi, Y., Saita, M., and Noda, K., Antinociceptive effects of counterirritants, *Nippon Yakurigaku Zasshi*, 104:433–446, 1994.

Wasner, G., Schattschneider, J., Binder, A., and Baron, R., Topical menthol — a human model for cold pain by activation and sensitization of C nociceptors, *Brain*, 127:1159–1171, 2004.

Theaflavins Theaflavins (TFs) are specific, higher-molecular-weight polyphenol compounds arising from enzymatic oxidation (Scheme T.59). All phenolic compounds are highly unstable and are rapidly transformed into various reaction products when the plant cells are damaged (for instance, during food processing).

TFs are pigments found in both black and oolong teas. They are formed from polymerization of catechins at the fermentation or semifermentation stage during the manufacture of black or oolong tea (Subramanian et al., 1999). TFs contribute to the characteristic bright orange-red color of black tea. The major TF in black and oolong teas are theaflavin (TF$_1$), theaflavin-3-gallate (TF$_2$A), theaflavin-3′-gallate (TF$_2$B), and theaflavin-3,3′-digallate (TF$_3$). TFs have recently received much attention as protective agents against cardiovascular disease and cancer (Buschman, 1998; Yang, 1999; Boone et al., 2000). They are also believed to have a wide range of other pharmaceutical benefits, including antihypertensive (Henry and Stephens-Larson, 1984; Hara et al., 1987), antioxidative (Halder and Bhaduri, 1998; Leung et al., 2001), and hypolipidemic (Chan et al., 1999) activities.

Leung and coworkers (2001) demonstrated that TFs present in black tea possess at least the same antioxidant potency as catechins present in green tea, and that the conversion of catechins to TFs during fermentation in making black tea does not alter their free-radical-scavenging activity significantly. Way and coworkers (2004) showed that TF$_1$, TF$_2$, and TF$_3$ significantly inhibited human aromatase activities, the proliferation induced by dehydroepiandrosterone in MCF-7 cells (Figure T.96). In addition, they also had an inhibitory effect on breast-cancer cells with hormonal resistance. These findings suggest that black tea TFs may be beneficial in the chemoprevention of hormone-dependent breast tumors and represent a possible remedy to overcome hormonal resistance of hormone-independent breast tumors.

TF$_2$ and TF$_3$ were found to be slightly more potent in inducing apoptosis in murine myeloid leukemia cells and in reducing both the *in vitro* clonogenicity and *in vivo* tumorigenicity of these cells, representing potential candidates for the treatment of some forms of leukemia (Lung et al., 2004).

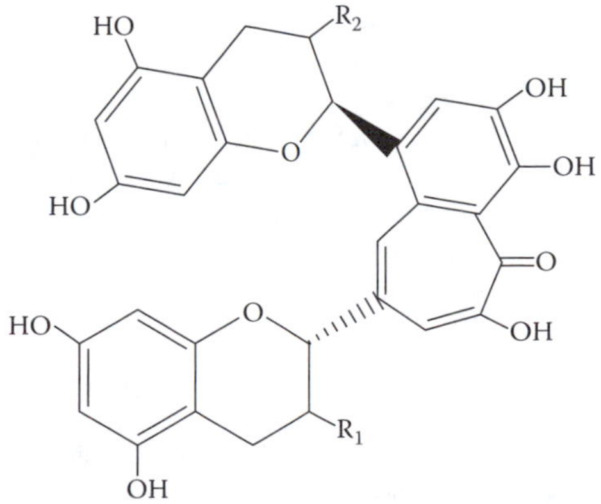

Theaflavin (TF$_1$): R$_1$ = R$_2$ = OH
Theaflavin-3-gallate (TF$_2$A): R$_1$ = Galloyl; R$_2$ = OH
Theaflavin-3′-gallate (TF$_2$B): R$_1$ = OH; R$_2$ = Galloyl
Theaflavin-3,3′-digallate (TF$_3$): R$_1$ = R$_2$ = Galloyl

SCHEME T.59 Structure of theaflavins. (From Lambert and Yang, *Mutat. Res.*, 523–524:201–208, 2003. With permission.)

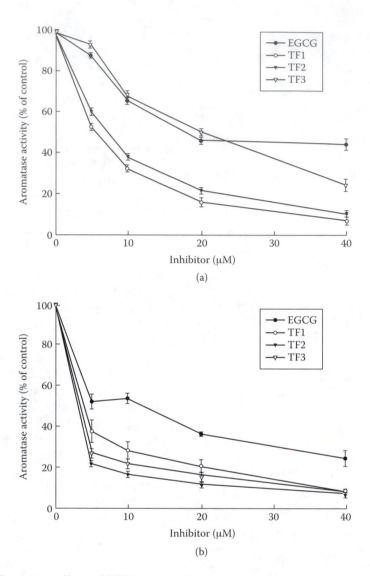

FIGURE T.96 The *in vitro* effects of EGCG and the flavins on aromatase activity from rat ovarian (a) and human placental (b) microsomes. Microsomal-tissue preparations were incubated with 0.05 μM [1b-3H] androstenedione and 1 mM nicotinamide adenine dinucleotide phosphate (NADPH) in the presence of EGCG (●), TF-1 (○), TF-2 (▼), or TF-3 (▽) at concentrations ranging from 5 to 40 μM. All measurements were performed in triplicate and represent ± standard error of the mean (SEM). (From Way et al., *Eur. J. Cancer*, 40: 2165–2174, 2004. With permission.)

References

Boone, C.W., Stoner, G.D., Bacus, J.V., Kagan, V., Morse, M.A., Kelloff, G.J., and Bacus, J.W., Chemoprevention with theaflavins of rat esophageal intraepithelial neoplasia quantitatively monitored by image tile analysis, *Cancer Epidemiol. Biomarkers Prev.*, 9:1149–1154, 2000.

Buschman, J.L., Green tea and cancer in humans: a review of the literature, *Nutr. Cancer*, 31:51–57, 1998.

Chan, P.T., Fong, W.P., Cheung, Y.L., Huang, Y., Ho W.K.K., and Chen, Z-Y., Jasmine green tea epicatechins are hypolipidemic in hamsters fed a high-fat diet, *J. Nutr.*, 129:1094–1101, 1999.

Halder, J. and Bhaduri, A.N., Protective role of black tea against oxidative damage of human red blood cells, *Biochem. Biophys. Res. Commun.*, 244:903–907, 1998.

Hara, Y., Matsuzaki, T., and Suzuki, T., Angiotensin I converting enzyme inhibiting activity of tea components, *J. Agric. Chem. Soc. Jpn.*, 61:803–808, 1987.

Henry, J.P. and Stephens-Larson, P., Reduction of chronic psychosocial hypertension in mice by decaffeinated tea, *Hypertension,* 6:437–444, 1984.

Lambert, J.D. and Yang, C.S., Cancer chemopreventive activity and bioavailability of tea and tea polyphenols, *Mutat. Res.,* 523–524:201–208, 2003.

Leung, L.K., Su, Y., Chen, R., Zhang, Z., Huang, Y., and Chen, Z.Y., Theaflavins in black tea and catechins in green tea are equally effective antioxidants, *J. Nutr.,* 131:2248–2251, 2001.

Lung, H.L., Ip, W.K., Chen, Z.Y., Mak, N.K., and Leung, K.N., Comparative study of the growth-inhibitory and apoptosis-inducing activities of black tea theaflavins and green tea catechin on murine myeloid leukemia cells, *Int. J. Mol. Med.,* 13:465–471, 2004.

Subramanian, N., Venkatesh, P., Ganguli, S., and Sinkar, V.P., Role of polyphenol oxidase and peroxidase in the generation of black tea theaflavins, *J. Agric. Food Chem.,* 47:2571–2578, 1999.

Way, T-D., Lee, H-H., Kao, M-C., and Lin, J-K., Black tea polyphenol theaflavins inhibit aromatase activity and attenuate tamoxifen resistance in HER2/neu-transfected human breast cancer cells through tyrosine kinase suppression, *Eur. J. Cancer,* 40:2165–2174, 2004.

Yang, C.S., Tea and health, *Nutrition,* 15:946–949, 1999.

Theopederin   Tsukamoto and coworkers (1999) isolated five new bioactive metabolites from the marine sponge *Theonella swinhoei,* theopederins F–J. Of these, theopederin F exhibited antifungal properties against *Saccharomyces cerevisie* and proved cytotoxic against P388 murine leukemia cells. Later work by Paul

1 R$_1$ = Me R$_2$ = H
2 R$_1$ = H   R$_2$ = H

Theopederins K (1) and L (2). (From Paul et al., *J. Nat. Prod.,* 65:59–61, 2002. With permission.)

et al. (2002) isolated theopederins K and L from the marine sponge *Discodermia* sp., collected from Honduras, with both showing *in vitro* cytotoxicity against P-388 and A-549 cell lines.

The amido trioxadecalin ring system is a common structural motif found in mycalamide, theopederin, and in onnamide families of natural products exhibiting pharmacological activities, including the insect chemical-defense agent pederin and the anticancer and immunosuppressive agents of the mycalamide, theopederin, and onnamide families of natural products (Vuong et al., 2001; Simpson et al., 2000; Rech and Floreancig, 2003).

References

Paul, G.K., Gunasekera, S.P., Longley, R.E., and Pomponi, S.A., Theopederins K and L, highly potent cytotoxic metabolites from a marine sponge *Discodermia* species, *J. Nat. Prod.,* 65:59–61, 2002.

Rech, J.C. and Floreancig, P.E., An oxidative entry into the amido trioxadecalin ring system, *Org. Lett.,* 5:1495–1498, 2003.

Simpson, J.S., Garson, M.J., Blunt, J.W., Munro, M.H., and Hooper, J.N., Mycalamides C and D, cytotoxic compounds from the marine sponge *Stylinos* n. species, *J. Nat. Prod.,* 63:704–706, 2000.

Tsukamoto, S., Matsunaga, S., Fusetani, N., and Tohe, A., Theopederins F–J: five new antifungal and cytotoxic metabolites from the marine sponge, *Theonella swinhoei, Tetrahedron,* 55:13697–13702, 1999.

Vuong, D., Capon, R.J., Lacey, E., Gill, J.H., Heiland, K., and Friedel, T., Onnamide F: a new nematocide from a southern Australian marine sponge, *Trachycladus laevispirulifer, J. Nat. Prod.,* 64:640–642, 2001.

Thyrsiferyl 23-acetate   Thyrsiferyl 23-acetate (TF23A) is a cytotoxic compound found in marine red alga that specifically inhibits serine/threonine protein phosphatase 2A (Matsuzawa et al., 1994). It induced rapid cell death in various leukemic T- and B-cell lines, which followed a typical apoptotic process (Matsuzawa et al., 1999).

References

Matsuzawa, S., Suzuki, T., Suzuki, M., Matsuda, A., Kawamura, T., Mizuno, Y., and Kikuchi, K., Thyr-

T

Thyrsiferyl 23-acetate

(From Matsuzawa et al., *FEBS Lett.,* 356:272–274, 1994. With permission.)

siferyl 23-acetate is a novel specific inhibitor of protein phosphatase PP2A, *FEBS Lett.,* 356:272–274, 1994.

Matsuzawa, S., Kawamura, T., Mitsuhashi, S., Suzuki, T., Matsuo, Y., Suzuki, M., Mizuno, Y., and Kikuchi, K., Thyrsiferyl 23-acetate and its derivatives induce apoptosis in various T- and B-leukemia cells, *Bioorg. Med. Chem.,* 7:381–387, 1999.

Thyme   Thyme (*Thymus vulgaris*; Labitae) is cultivated in central and southern Europe as a tea, spice, and herbal medicine. The leaf has been used as a stomachic, carminative, diuretic, urinary disinfectant, and vermifuge. Tea made from thyme leaf was reported to promote rest and relaxation (Van Den Broucke and Lemli, 1983; Wichtl, 1994). The essential oil in the leaf contains mainly isomeric monoterpenoid thymol (30–70 percent), carvacrol (3–15 percent), together with other monoterpenoids, such as γ-terpinene and *p-cymene* (Reddy et al., 1998; Rustaiyan et al., 2000; Hudaib et al., 2002) and exhibits strong antimicrobial and antifungal properties (Kalemba and Kunicka, 2003). Kitajima and coworkers (2004) isolated a number of monoterpenes and their glycosides from the polar portion of the methanolic extract of thyme leaf. Based on sprectral data, a novel glycoside,

thymuside, was identified as *p*-meth-4(5)-ene-1,2-diol and 2-hydroxyhexose, joined by two ether linkages.

Thymuside. (Adapted from Kitajima et al., *Phytochemistry,* 65:3279–3287, 2004.)

Rats maintained on thyme oil or a thyme supplement were found by Youdin and Deans (2002) to have significantly higher antioxidant-enzyme activities and total antioxidant status. The proportion of 22:6n-3 in brain phospholipids, which declined with age in control rats, was significantly higher in rats given either supplement. This latter finding is particularly important, as optimum levels of 22:6n-3 are needed for normal brain function.

Thyme has also been used in traditional medicine to treat bronchitis, asthma, and related respiratory diseases. It is well known that nitric

Structures of carvacrol (1) and thymol (2) γ-terpinene (3) and *p*-cymene (4). (Adapted from Burt, *Int. J. Food Microbiol.,* 94:223–253, 2004.)

oxide plays an important role in the pathogenesis of inflammatory diseases. Vigo and coworkers (2004) demonstrated that inhibition of net nitric-oxide production by thyme extract was probably due to its nitric-oxide scavenging activity and its inhibitory effects on inducible nitric-oxide synthase gene expression. Thymol, isolated from the leaves of thyme, was found to inhibit platelet aggregation induced by collagen, ADP, arachidonic acid, and thrombin (Okazaki et al., 2002).

Thyme oil was reported to inhibit the growth and aflatoxin production by *Aspergillus parasiticus* (Rasooli and Abyaneh, 2004), as well as the growth of *Shigella sonnei* and *Shigella flexneri* (Bagamboula et al., 2004). Aydin and coworkers (2005) recently showed that low concentrations (< 0.1 mM) of thyme volatiles, thymols and γ-terpinene, significantly reduced DNA damage in human lymphocytes induced by the heterocyclic amine, 2-amino-3-methylimidazo[4,5-f]-quinoline (IQ) and mitomycin (MMC). Carvacrol, an isomer of thymol, also protected lymphocytes from the genotoxic effects of IQ and MMC, but only at concentrations below 0.05 mM.

An acidic polysaccharide purified from the hot-water extract of thyme leaves was suggested to be a complement activator, which plays an important role in primary-host defense mechanisms (Chun et al., 2001).

References

Aydin, S., Basaran, A.A., and Basaran, N., The effects of thyme volatiles on the induction of DNA damage by the heterocyclic amine IQ and mitomycin C, *Mutat. Res./Gen. Toxicol. Environ. Mutagen.*, 581: 43–53, 2005.

Bagamboula, C.F., Uyttendaele, M., and Debevere, J., Inhibitory effect of thyme and basil oils, carvacrol, thymol, estragol, linalool and p-cymene towards *Shigella sonnei* and *S. flexneri*, *Food Micobiol.*, 21:33–42, 2004.

Burt, S., Essential oils: their antibacterial properties and potential applications in foods — a review, *Int. J. Food Microbiol.*, 94:223–253, 2004.

Chun, H., Shin, D.H., Hong, B.S., Cho, H.Y., and Yang, H.C., Purification and biological activity of acidic polysaccharide from leaves of *Thymus vulgaris* L., *Biol. Pharm. Bull.*, 24:941–946, 2001.

Hudaib, M., Speroni, E., Di Pietra, A.M., and Cavrini V., GC/MS evaluation of thyme (*Thymus vulgaris* L.) oil composition and variations during the vegetative cycle, *J. Pharm. Biomed. Anal.*, 29:691–700, 2002.

Kalemba, D. and Kunicka, A., Antibacterial and antifungal properties of essential oils, *Curr. Med. Chem.*, 10:813–829, 2003.

Kitajima, J., Ishikawa, T., Urabe, A., and Satoh, M., Monoterpenoids and glycosides from the leaf of thyme, *Phytochemistry*, 65:3279–3287, 2004.

Okazaki, K., Kawazoe, K., and Takaishi, Y., Human platelet aggregation inhibitors from thyme (*Thymus vulgaris* L.), *Phytother. Res.*, 16:398–399, 2002.

Rasooli, I. and Abyaneh, M.R., Inhibitory effects of thyme oils on growth and aflatoxin production by *Aspergillus parasiticus*, *Food Cont.*, 15:479–483, 2004.

Reddy, M.V.B., Angers, P., Gosselin, A., and Arul, J., Characterization and use of essential from *Thymus vulgaris* against *Botyris cinerea* and *Rhizopus stolonifer* in strawberry fruits, *Phytochemistry*, 47: 1515–1520, 1998.

Rustaiyan, A., Masoudi, S., Monfared, A., Kamalinejad, M., Lajevardi, T., Sedaghat, S., and Yari, M., Volatile constituents of three *Thymus* species grown wild in Iran, *Planta Med.*, 66:197–198, 2000.

Van Den Broucke, C.O. and Lemli, J.A., Spasmolytic activity of the flavonoids from *Thymus vulgaris*, *Pharm. Weekbl. Sci.*, 5:9–14, 1983.

Vigo, E., Cepeda, A., Gualillo, O., and Perez-Fernandez, R., *In-vitro* anti-inflammatory effect of *Eucalyptus globulus* and *Thymus vulgaris*: nitric oxide inhibition in J774A.1 murine macrophages, *J. Pharm. Pharmacol.*, 56:257–263, 2004.

Wichtl, M., Ed., *Herbal Drugs and Phytopharmaceuticals*, CRC Press, Stutgart, pp. 493–495, 1994.

Youdim, K.A. and Deans, S.G., Effect of thyme oil and thymol dietary supplementation on the antioxidant status and fatty acid composition of the ageing rat brain, *Br. J. Nutr.*, 83:87–93, 2000.

Tocopherols *see also* **Vitamin E**   In nature, vitamin E occurs in eight different forms (α-, β-, γ-, and Δ-tocopherols and α-, β-, γ-, and Δ-tocotrienols) with varying biological activities (Scheme T.60). All forms of vitamin E are present in the diet, e.g., γ-tocopherol in corn and

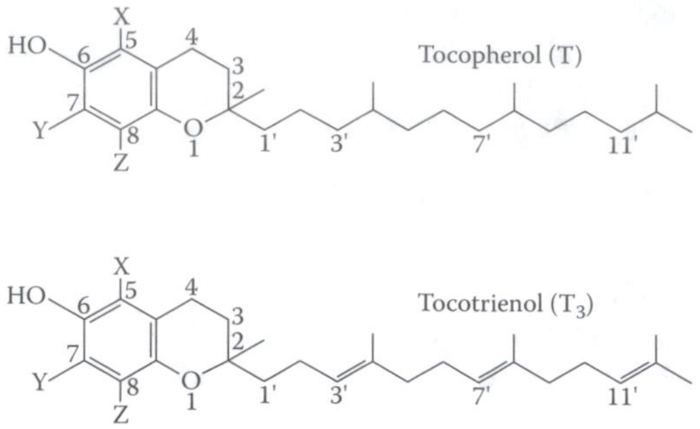

(A) α, X = CH$_3$, Y = CH$_3$, Z = CH$_3$

(B) β, X = CH$_3$, Y = H, Z = CH$_3$

(C) γ, X = H, Y = CH$_3$, Z = CH$_3$

(D) δ, X = H, Y = H, Z = CH$_3$

(E) ζ$_2$, X = CH$_3$, Y = CH$_3$, Z = H

(F) ε, X = H, Y = H, Z = H

SCHEME T.60 Structural formulae of tocopherols and tocotrienols. (From Abidi and Rewnnick, *J. Chromatogr. A*, 913:379–386, 2001. With permission.)

soybean oils, tocotrienols in cereal grains, bran, some nuts, and palm oil.

Epidemiological studies showed an inverse correlation between acute coronary events and high dietary intake of vitamin E (Rimm et al., 1993; Stampfer et al., 1993). Although α-tocopherol is the main vitamin E derivative in the diet, γ-tocopherol in particular has been shown to have potent antioxidant effects (Wolf, 1997) and was reduced in patients with coronary heart disease (Ohrvall et al., 1996). A preparation of mixed tocopherols rich in γ-tocopherol was found more potent than α-tocopherol alone in decreasing platelet aggregation and intraarterial thrombus formation in rats (Saldeen and Mehta, 1999), processes that play an important role in thrombosis and cardiovascular events.

Halliwell and coworkers (2005) recently argued that tocopherols and tocotrienols may exert direct, beneficial effects in the gastrointestinal tract and that their return to the gastrointestinal tract by the liver through the bile may be physiologically advantageous. These effects are suggested to include binding of prooxidant iron, scavenging of reactive nitrogen, chlorine, and oxygen species, and perhaps inhibition of cyclooxygenases and lipoxygenases.

References

Burlakova, E.B., Krashakov, S.A., and Khrapova, N.G., The role of tocopherols in biomembrane lipid peroxidation, *Membr. Cell. Biol.*, 12:173–211, 1998.

Halliwell, B., Rafter, J., and Jenner, A., Health promotion by flavonoids, tocopherols, tocotrienols, and other phenols: direct or indirect effects? Antioxidant or not? *Am. J Clin. Nutr.*, 81:268S–276S, 2005.

Ohrvall, M., Sundlof, G., and Vessby, B., Gamma, but not alpha, tocopherol levels in serum are reduced in coronary heart disease patients, *J. Intern. Med.*, 239:111–117, 1996.

Rimm, E.B., Stampfer, M.J., Ascherio, A., Giovannucci, E., Colditz, G.A., and Willett, W.C., Vitamin E consumption and the risk of coronary heart disease in men, *N. Engl. J. Med.*, 328:1450–1456, 1993.

Saldeen, T., Li, D., and Mehta, J.L., Differential effects of α- and γ-tocopherol on low-density lipoprotein oxidation, superoxide activity, platelet aggregation and arterial thrombogenesis, *J. Am. Coll. Cardiol.*, 34:1208–1215, 1999.

Stampfer, M.J., Hennekens, C.H., Manson, J.E., Colditz, G.A., Rosner, B., and Willett, W.C., Vitamin E consumption and the risk of coronary disease in women, *N. Engl. J. Med.*, 328:1444–1449, 1993.

Wolf, G., γ-Tocopherol: an efficient protector of lipids against nitric oxide-initiated peroxidative damage, *Nutr. Rev.*, 55:376–378, 1997.

Tomato *see also* **Lycopene** Epidemiology studies suggested that a higher intake of tomatoes and tomato products may protect against cardiovascular disease (Arab and Steck, 2000) and reduce the risk of several types of cancer, particularly prostate, lung, and digestive tract (Giovannucci et al., 1999). One of the mechanisms proposed is that tomato extracts inhibit platelet aggregation (Lazarus and Garg, 2004).

The most abundant carotenoid in tomatoes is lycopene (Agarwal and Rao, 2000). It appears to be responsible, in large part, for the potential health benefits of tomato products (Clinton, 1998). Tomatoes showed high antioxidant activities. For example, at the level of 1 g fresh sample, low-density lipoprotein peroxidation was inhibited by at least 90 percent by tomato meat. The total phenolic content was significantly correlated with antioxidant activities measured (Huang et al., 2004).

Lycopene. (From Duvoix et al., *Cancer Lett.*, 223:181–190, 2005.)

The consumption of tomato products is associated with reduced risk of prostate cancer. Lycopene, the primary red carotenoid in tomatoes, may be the principal phytochemical responsible for this reduction in risk. Lycopene can act as antioxidant, enhance cell-to-cell communication via increasing gap junctions between cells, and modulate cell-cycle progression. Tomatoes also contain folate, vitamin C, significant quantities of potassium, vitamin A, vitamin E, and various other carotenoids and phytochemicals, such as polyphenols, which may also be associated with lower cancer risk (Campbell et al., 2004).

It was recently demonstrated that tomato juice is a suitable raw material for the production of probiotic juice by four lactic-acid bacteria (*Latobacillus acidophilus* LA39, *Lactobacillus plantarum* C3, *Lactobacillus casei* A4, and *Lactobacillus delbrueckii* D7). This juice could serve as a health beverage for vegetarians or consumers who are allergic to dairy products (Yoon et al., 2004).

References

Agarwal, S. and Rao, A.V., Tomato lycopene and its role in human health and chronic diseases, *Can. Med. Assoc. J.,* 163:739–744, 2000.

Arab, L. and Steck, S., Lycopene and cardiovascular disease, *Am. J. Clin. Nutr.,* 71:1691S–1695S, discussion 1696S–1697S, 2000.

Campbell, J.K., Canene-Adams, K., Lindshield, B.L., Boileau, T.W.M., Clinton, S.K., and Erdman, J.W., Jr., Tomato phytochemicals and prostate cancer risk, *J. Nutr.,* 134:3486S–3492S, 2004.

Clinton, S.K., Lycopene: chemistry, biology, and implications for human health and disease, *Nutr. Rev.,* 56:35–51, 1998.

Duvoix, A., Blasius, R., Delhalle, S., Schneckenburger, M., Morceau, F., Henry, E., Dicato, M., and Diederich, M., Chemopreventive and therapeutic effects of curcumin, *Cancer Lett.,* 223:181–190, 2005.

Giovannucci, E., Tomatoes, tomato-based products, lycopene, and cancer: review of the epidemiologic literature, *J. Natl. Cancer Inst.,* 91:317–331, 1999.

Huang, H.Y., Chang, C.K., Tso, T.K., Huang, J.J., Chang, W.W., and Tsai, Y.C., Antioxidant activities of various fruits and vegetables produced in Taiwan, *Int. J. Food Sci. Nutr.,* 55(5):423–429, 2004.

Lazarus, S.A. and Garg, M.L., Tomato extract inhibits human platelet aggregation *in vitro* without increasing basal cAMP levels, *Int. J. Food Sci. Nutr.,* 55(3):249–256, 2004.

Yoon, K.Y., Woodams, E.E., and Hang, Y.D., Probiotication of tomato juice by lactic acid bacteria, *J. Microbiol.,* 42(4):315–318, 2004.

Triterpene saponins   Triterpene refers to a particular type of molecular structure that has a four- or five-ring, planar-base molecule containing 30 carbon atoms. Triterpene saponins are glycosides, with various sugar molecules attached to the triterpene unit. They have an acidic quality, an acrid–bitter taste, and their function in plants remains unknown. The triterpenes are subdivided into about 20 groups, depending on their particular structures. The base structure is the oleanane triterpene, which may be represented by four forms, oleanolic acid, ursolic acid, and α- and β-amyrin. Platycodin belongs to the very large class of oleanane triterpenes.

Triterpenoid saponins, which are present in plants and some marine animals, exert important pharmacological effects, including cytotoxicity (Haddad et al., 2004), antitumor activity (Setzer and Setzer 2003), antitumor-promoting activity (Yu et al., 2001), anti-inflammatory effects (Smolinski and Pestka 2003), antiallergy and immunomodulatory action (Yesilada et al., 2005), antiviral activity (Chiang et al., 2003), hepatoprotective effects (Kinjo et al., 2003), cardiac activities (Scott et al., 2001), antithrombotic activity (Xu et al., 1997), hypolipemic activity (Lee et al., 2000), central nervous system activity (Liao et al., 2002), and endocrine activity (Chan et al., 2002).

Yesilada and coworkers (2005) found triterpene saponins (Scheme T.61) isolated from

T

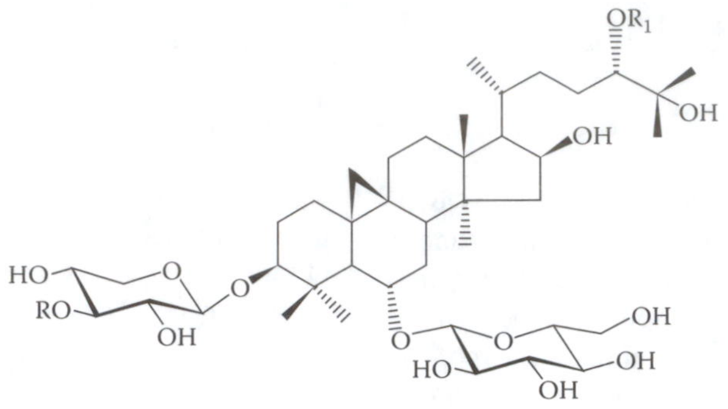

	R	R_1
1: Brachyoside A	β-D-xylocyr	H
2: Brachyoside C	H	β-D-glucopyr
3: Cyclocanthoside E	H	H

SCHEME T.61 Some triterpene saponins isolated from *Astragalus* species. (From Yesilada et al., *J. Ethnopharmacol.*, 96:71–77, 2005. With permission.)

Turkish *Astragalus* species exhibited prominent IL-2-inducing activity, ranging from 35.9–139.6 percent. This may be the mechanism responsible for its immunomodulatory and anticancer effects.

Triterpene saponins obtained from *Albizia adianthifolia* were found to exhibit a cytotoxic effect on human leukemia T cells by induction of apoptosis (Haddad et al., 2004).

Hypoglycemic actions have been reported for the triterpenes of platycodon, bupleurum, polygala, and ginseng (Suttisri et al., 1995). The methanolic extract of the leaves of the Vietnamese plant *Maesa balansae* Mez. (*Myrsinaceae*) was found to possess strong antileishmanial potential, and pentacyclic triterpene saponins were identified as the active constituents (Maes et al., 2004).

References

Chan, R.Y.K., Chen, W-F., Dong, A., Guo, D., and Wong, M-S., Estrogen-like activity of ginsenoside Rg1 derived from *Panax notoginseng, J. Clin. Endocrinol. Metab.*, 87:3691–3695, 2002.

Chiang, L.C., Ng, L.T., Liu, L.T., Shieh, D.E., and Lin, C.C., Cytotoxicity and anti-hepatitis B virus activities of saikosaponins from Bupleurum species, *Planta Med.*, 69:705–709, 2003.

Haddad, M., Laurens, V., and Lacaille-Dubois, N-A., Induction of apoptosis in a leukemia cell line by triterpene saponins from *Albizia adianthifolia, Bioorg. Med. Chem.*, 12:4725–4734, 2004.

Kinjo, J., Hirakawa, T., Tsuchihashi, R., Nagao, T., Okawa, M., Nohara, T., and Okabe, H., Hepatoprotective constituents in plants. 14. Effects of soyasapogenol B, sophoradiol, and their glucuronides on the cytotoxicity of tert-butyl hydroperoxide to HepG2 cells, *Biol. Pharm. Bull.*, 26:1357–1360, 2003.

Lee, K.T., Sohn, I.C., Kim, D.H., Choi, J.W., Kwon, S.H., and Park, H.J., Hypoglycemic and hypolipidemic effects of tectorigenin and kaikasaponin III in the streptozotocin-induced diabetic rat and their antioxidant activity *in vitro, Arch. Pharm. Res.*, 23:461–466, 2000.

Liao, B., Newmark, H., and Zhou, R., Neuroprotective effects of ginseng total saponin and ginsenosides Rb1 and Rg1 on spinal cord neurons *in vitro, Exp. Neurol.*, 173:224–234, 2002.

Maes, L., Vanden Berghe, D., Germonprez, N., Quirijnen, L., Cos, P., De Kimpe, N., and Van Puyvelde, L., *In vitro* and *in vivo* activities of a triterpenoid saponin extract (PX-6518) from the plant *Maesa balansae* against visceral *Leishmania* species, *Antimicrob. Agents Chemother.*, 48:130–136, 2004.

Scott, G.I., Colligan, P.B., Ren, B.H., and Ren, J., Ginsenosides Rb1 and Re decrease cardiac contraction in adult rat ventricular myocytes: role of nitric oxide, *Br. J. Pharmacol.*,134:1159–1165, 2001.

T

Setzer, W.N. and Setzer, M.C., Plant-derived triter-penoids as potential antineoplastic agents, *Mini. Rev. Med. Chem.*, 3:540–56, 2003.

Smolinski, A.T. and Pestka, J.J., Modulation of lipopolysaccharide-induced proinflammatory cytokine production *in vitro* and *in vivo* by the herbal constituents apigenin (chamomile), ginsenoside Rb_1 (ginseng) and parthenolide (feverfew), *Food Chem. Toxicol.*, 41:1381–1390, 2003.

Suttisri, R., Lee, I.S., and Kinghorn, A.D., Plant-derived triterpenoid sweetness inhibitors, *J. Ethnopharmacol.*, 47:9–26, 1995.

Xu, H.L., Liu, W.B., and Rao, M.R., Effect of sanchinoside Rg1 on experimental thrombosis and its mechanisms, *Yao Xue Xue Bao*, 32:502–505, 1997.

Yesilada, E., Bedir, E., Calis, I., Takaishi, Y., and Ohmoto, Y., Effects of triterpene saponins from *Astragalus* species on *in vitro* cytokine release, *J. Ethnopharmacol.*, 96:71–77, 2005.

Yu, T.X., Ma, R.D., and Yu, L.J., Structure-activity relationship of tubeimosides in anti-inflammatory, antitumor, and antitumor-promoting effects, *Acta Pharmacol. Sin.*, 22:463–468, 2001.

consume approximately three servings per day of whole-grain foods are also less likely to develop T2DM than low consumers (< 3 servings per week) with a risk reduction in the order of 20–30 percent (Venn and Mann 2004).

References

Adam, A., Levrat-Verny, M.A., Lopez, H.W., Leuillet, M., Demigne, C., and Remesy, C., Whole wheat and triticale flours with different viscosities stimulate cecal fermentations and lower plasma and hepatic lipid in rats, *J. Nutr.*, 131:1770–1776, 2001.

Jacobs, D.R., Jr., Meyer, H.E., and Solvoll, K., Consumption of whole grain foods and chronic disease, *Tidsskr. Nor. Laegeforen.*, 124:1399–1401, 2004.

Jensen, M.K., Koh-Banerjee, P., Hu, F.B., Franz, M., Sampson, L., Gronbaek, M., and Rimm, E.B., Intakes of whole grains, bran, and germ and the risk of coronary heart disease in men, *Am. J. Clin. Nutr.*, 80:1492–1499, 2004.

Venn, B.J. and Mann, J.I., Cereal grains, legumes and diabetes, *Eur. J. Clin. Nutr.*, 58:1443–1461, 2004.

Triticale   Triticale is a hybrid grain that takes its name from the botanical names for wheat *(triticum)* and rye *(secale)*. It is known for its higher protein content and it is now grown throughout the United States, primarily in the Midwest. Triticale is found in cereals and in baked goods. It is also available in flake form or as a whole grain or flour. It is a good source of thiamine (0.416 mg), magnesium (130 mg), and folate (73 mg) (in 100 grams).

Recent epidemiological investigations found that whole-grain intake is associated with a reduced risk of chronic diseases, especially cardiovascular disease and diabetes (Jacobs et al., 2004). Three servings of whole-grain foods daily is associated with a reduced risk of coronary heart disease (Jensen et al., 2004). In addition, triticale flours were found to be effective plasma cholesterol-lowering agents (Adam et al., 2001).

Epidemiological studies strongly support the suggestion that high intakes of whole-grain foods protect against the development of type 2 diabetes mellitus (T2DM). People who

Trypsin inhibitor *see also* **Bowman–Birk protease inhibitor**   The pancreatic Kunitz inhibitor, also known as aprotinin, bovine basic pancreatic trypsin inhibitor, and trypsin-kallikrein inhibitor, is one of the most extensively studied globular proteins. Trypsin activity in the pancreas is mainly controlled by the pancreatic secretory trypsin inhibitor, which acts as a potent natural inhibitor of trypsin in order to prevent the occurrence of pancreatitis. When trypsinogen is activated into trypsin in the pancreas, trypsin inhibitor immediately binds to trypsin to prevent further activation of pancreatic enzymes. The inhibitor also blocks the further activation of pancreatic cells via the trypsin receptor (Hirota et al., 2003).

Pancreatic trypsin inhibitor has a relatively broad specificity, inhibiting trypsin-like, as well as chymotrypsin-like and elastase-like, serine (pro)enzymes endowed with very different primary specificity. It reacts rapidly with serine proteases to form stable complexes. This inhibitor, the Bowman–Birk trypsin inhibitor (BPTI) inhibits the nitric-oxide synthase type I and type II action and impairs K+ transport by Ca2+-

T

activated K+ channels. Clinically, the use of BPTI in selected surgical interventions, such as cardiopulmonary surgery and orthotopic liver transplantation, is advised, as it significantly reduces hemorrhagic complications and thus blood-transfusion requirements (Ascenzi et al., 2003).

Tumor-associated trypsin inhibitor was initially isolated from the urine of a patient with ovarian cancer. It is a peptide produced at high concentrations by several tumors. It is identical to pancreatic secretory trypsin inhibitor. It is a prognostic marker for ovarian, bladder, and kidney cancer, which may be associated with the participation of trypsin in protease cascades contributing to tumor invasiveness (Stenman, 2002.)

Trypsin inhibitors are widely distributed in plant seeds; the most examined plant inhibitors are found in the species of the families *Leguminosae*, *Graminae*, and *Solanaceae*. Feeding experiments on diets containing isolated soybean trypsin caused insignificant growth depression in rats and chicks, but induced enlargement of the pancreas in rats, chicks, and mice but not in pigs, dogs, calves, monkeys, and presumably humans (Birk, 1996). Findings on the involvement of trypsin inhibitor (Kunitz) and of the Bowman–Birk trypsin inhibitor (BBTI), which possesses two independent sites of inhibition, one against trypsin and the other against chymotrypsin (Birk, 1985), in prevention of tumorigenesis suggest a possible positive contribution of the inhibitors. BBTI is also an effective inhibitor of nephrotoxicity induced by the antibiotic gentamicin. It does not cause side effects and does affect the antimicrobial activity (Birk, 1996). Recently, it has been reported that a trypsin inhibitor from Peltophorum dubium seeds caused apoptosis of concanavalin A-stimulated mouse lymphocytes, whereas it had no effect on normal mouse splenocytes or lymphocytes (Fernanda et al., 2003). The *in vitro* effects of these inhibitors on animals should be interpreted with caution when related to humans. Trypsin inhibitor from the seeds of *Clausena lansium* reduced the activity of HIV-1 reverse transcriptase and exerted antifungal activity toward *Physalospora piricola* (Ng et al., 2003).

References

Ascenzi, P., Bocedi, A., Bolognesi, M., Spallarossa, A., Coletta, M., De Cristofaro, R., and Menegatti, E., The bovine basic pancreatic trypsin inhibitor (Kunitz inhibitor): a milestone protein, *Curr. Protein Pept. Sci.,* 4:231–251, 2003.

Birk, Y., The Bowman-Birk inhibitor, trypsin- and chymotrypsin-inhibitor from soybeans, *Int. J. Pept. Protein Res.,* 25(2):113–131, 1985.

Birk, Y., Protein proteinase inhibitors in legume seeds — overview, *Arch. Latinoam. Nutr.,* 44(4 Suppl. 1):26S–30S, 1996.

Fernanda Troncoso, M., Zolezzi, G.P., Hellman, U., and Wolfenstein-Todel, C., A novel trypsin inhibitor from *Peltophorum dubium* seeds, with lectin-like properties, triggers rat lymphoma cell apoptosis, *Arch. Biochem. Biophys.,* 411:93–104, 2003.

Hirota, M., Kuwata, K., Ohmuraya, M., and Ogawa, M., From acute to chronic pancreatitis: the role of mutations in the pancreatic secretory trypsin inhibitor gene, *JOP,* 4:83–88, 2003.

Ng, T.B., Lam, S.K., and Fong, W.P., A homodimeric sporamin-type trypsin inhibitor with antiproliferative, HIV reverse transcriptase-inhibitory and antifungal activities from wampee (*Clausena lansium*) seeds, *Biol. Chem.,* 384:289–293, 2003.

Stenman, U.H., Tumor-associated trypsin inhibitor, *Clin. Chem.,* 48:1206–1209, 2002.

Turmeric *see also* **Curcumin** Turmeric is a spice that comes from the root *Curcuma longa*, a member of the ginger family, *Zingaberaceae*. In Indian traditional medicine, turmeric has been used for its medicinal properties for treating various ailments, such as biliary disorders, anorexia, coryza, cough, diabetic wounds, hepatic disorder, rheumatism, and sinusitis (Ammon et al., 1992) and through different routes of administration, including topically, orally, and by inhalation.

Clinical studies demonstrated that administration of turmeric powder to different patients with respiratory diseases relieves symptoms like dyspnea, cough, and sputum or physical signs. Treatment of patients with rheumatoid arthritis also showed a real improvement (Ammon and Wahl, 1991). Turmeric can lower lipid peroxidation by maintaining the activities of antioxidant enzymes like superoxide dismutase, catalase, and glutathione peroxidase at higher levels (Pulla Reddy & Lokesh, 1992).

Curcuminoids are major components of turmeric, which include mainly curcumin (diferuloyl methane), demethoxycurcumin, and bisdemethoxycurcumin. A large number of studies on the antioxidant (Unnikrishnan and Rao 1999), anti-inflammatory (Chainani-Wu, 2003), antiviral (Mazumder et al., 1995), anticancer (Aggarwal et al., 2003), and antifungal properties of curcuminoids were identified. Curcumin has been shown to be safe in six human trials and has demonstrated anti-inflammatory activity by inhibition of a number of different molecules, such as phospholipase, lipooxygenase, cyclooxygenase 2, leukotrienes, thromboxane, prostaglandins, nitric oxide, collagenase, elastase, hyaluronidase, monocyte chemoattractant protein-1, interferon-inducible protein, tumor necrosis factor, and interleukin-12, that play a role in inflammation (Chainani-Wu, 2003). In addition, the wound-healing and detoxifying properties of curcumin have also received considerable attention (Joe et al., 2004).

Recently, curcumin was shown to have radio-sensitizing effects on squamous carcinoma cells by arresting at the S/G2M phases of the cell cycle (Khafif et al., 2005). Treatment with curcumin prior to radiation significantly decreased the ability of cancerous cells to colonize compared to the control (without added curcumin). These results were consistent with earlier studies in which curcumin induced apoptosis and cell death in colon carcinoma cells and human cancer-cell lines (Jiang et al., 1996; Chen et al., 1999).

References

Aggarwal, B.B., Kumar, A., and Bharti, A.C., Anticancer potential of curcumin: preclinical and clinical studies, *Anticancer Res.,* 23(1A):363–398, 2003.

Ammon, H.P.T. and Wahl, M.A., Pharmacology of *Curcuma longa, Planta Med.,* 57:1–7, 1991.

Ammon, H.P.T., Anazodo, M.I., Safayhi, H., Dhawan, B.N., and Srimal, R.C., Curcumin: a potent inhibitor of leukotriene B_4 formation in rat peritoneal polymorphonuclear neutrophils (PMNL), *Planta Med.,* 58:26, 1992.

Chainani-Wu, N., Safety and anti-inflammatory activity of curcumin: a component of turmeric (*Curcuma longa*), *J. Altern. Complement. Med.,* 9:161–168, 2003.

Chen, H., Zhng, Z.S., and Zhang, Y.L., Curcumin inhibits cell proliferation by interfering with the cell cycle and inducing apoptosis in colon carcinoma cells, *Anitcancer Res.,* 19:3675–3680, 1999.

Jiang, M.C., Yang-Yen, H.F., and Yen, J.J., Curcumin induces apoptosis in immortalized NIH 3T3 and malignant cancer cell lines, *Nutr. Cancer,* 26:111–120, 1996.

Joe, B., Vijaykumar, M., and Lokesh, B.R., Biological properties of curcumin-cellular and molecular mechanisms of action, *Crit. Rev. Food Sci. Nutr.,* 44(2):97–111, 2004.

Khafif, A., Hurst, R., Kyker, K., Fliss, D.M., Gil, Z., and Medina, J.E., Curcumin: a new radio-sensitizer of squamous cell carcinoma cells, *Otolaryngol. Head Neck Surg.,* 132:317–21, 2005.

Manikandan, P., Sumitra, M., Aishwarya, S., Manohar, B.M., Lokanadam, B., and Puvanakrishnan, R., Curcumin modulates free radical quenching in myocardial ischaemia in rats, *Int. J. Biochem. Cell Biol.,* 36:1967–1980, 2004.

Mazumder, A., Raghavan, K., Weinstein, J., Kohn, K.W., and Pommer, Y., Inhibition of human immunodeficiency virus type-1 integrase by curcumin, *Biochem. Pharmacol.,* 49:1165–1170, 1995.

Turmeric curcumin [1,7,-bis(4-hydroxy-3-methoxyphenyl)-1,6-heptadiene-3,5-dione]. (From May et al., *Anal. Biochem.,* 337:62–69, 2005. With permission.)

May, L.A., Tourkina, E., Hoffman, S.R., and Dix, T.A., Detection and quantitation of curcumin in mouse lung cell cultures by matrix-assisted laser desorption ionization time of flight mass spectrometry, *Anal. Biochem.,* 337:62–69, 2005.

Pulla, R.A. and Lokesh, B.R., Studies on spice principles as antioxidants in the inhibition of lipid peroxidation of rat liver microsomes, *Mol. Cell. Biochem.,* 111:117–124, 1992.

Unnikrishnan, M.K. and Rao, M.N.A., Inhibition of nitrite induced oxidation of hemoglobin by curcuminoids, *Pharmazie,* 50:490–492, 1995.

Tyrosinase inhibitor   Tyrosinase is known to be a key enzyme in melanin biosynthesis, involved in determining the color of mammalian skin and hair. Various dermatological disorders, such as melasma, age spots, and sites of actinic damage, arise from the accumulation of an excessive level of epidermal pigmentation. Tyrosinase inhibitors have become increasingly important in medication and in cosmetics to prevent hyperpigmentation by inhibiting enzymatic oxidation.

A number of naturally occurring tyrosinase inhibitors have been described (Curto et al., 1999; Matsuda et al., 1996; Kubo and Kinst-Hori, 1999: Kim et al., 2005). Many are polyphenol derivatives of flavonoids or of *trans*-stilbene (*t*-stilbene), such as resveratrol and its derivatives, which have been investigated intensively. They are usually constructed from one of two distinct substructures, which dictate their mechanism of tyrosinase inhibition: containing either a 4-substituted resorcinol moiety or catechol. The 4-substituted resorcinol group has been reported to be a potent tyrosinase inhibitor (Shimizu et al., 2000).

Another group of compounds, with a similar structure to *t*-stilbene, is the chalcones, which are widely distributed in higher plants and were recently demonstrated as potential inhibitors of tyrosinase (Nerya et al., 2003, 2004). Other potentially active agents, such as kojic acid (5-hydoxy-4-pyran-4-one-2-methyl), a fungal metabolic product, and arbutin (hydroquinone-beta-D-glucopyranoside), a glycosylated hydroquinone found at high concentrations in certain plants, have not yet been demonstrated as clinically efficient (Nakagawa and Kawai, 1995). Hydroquinone, a widely used skin-lightening agent, is a compound considered to be cytotoxic to melanocytes and, hence, potentially mitogenic (Frenk, 1995; Dooley, 1997; Hermanns et al., 2000). As a result of these and other side effects, there has been increasing impetus to find alternative herbal depigmenting agents.

Azelaic acid is a naturally occurring, saturated dicarboxylic-acid originally isolated from *Pityrosporum ovale* and is a rather weak competitive inhibitor of tyrosinase *in vitro*. In addition, azelaic acid has a cytotoxic effect on melanocytes (Schallreuter and Wood, 1990). Several other natural compounds (Seo et al., 1999; Shin et al., 1998), such as quercetin, myricetin, and glycoside of myricetin, have been reported to have various degrees of inhibitory activity toward tyrosinase (Matsuda et al., 1996), and flavonoids and stilbenes obtained from *Artocarpus incisus* and other plants also suggest that compounds having the 4-substituted resorcinol skeleton have potent tyrosinase inhibitory ability (Shimizu et al., 2000). However, the effective topical concentration of these compounds in disorders of hyperpigmentation is not yet known. Among the licorice constituents, glabridin exhibited superior activity compared to that of glabren, isoflavene, and ILC, a chalcone (Nerya et al., 2003).

References

Chakraborty, A.K., Funasaka, Y., Komoto, M., and Ichihashi, M., Effect of arbutin on melanogenic proteins in human melanocytes, *Pigment Cell Res.,* 11: 206–212, 1998.

Curto, E.V., Kwong, C., Hermersdorfer, H., Glatt, H., Santis, C., Virador, V., Hearing, V.J., Jr., and Dooley, T.P., Inhibitors of mammalian melanocyte tyrosinase: *in vitro* comparisons of alkyl esters of gentisic acid with other putative inhibitors, *Biochem. Pharmacol.,* 57:663–672, 1999.

Dooley, T.P., Topical skin depigmentation agents: current products and discovery of novel inhibitors of melanogenesis, *J. Dematol. Treat.,* 8:275–279, 1997.

Frenk, E., Treatment of melasma with depigmenting agents, in *Melasma: New Approaches to Treatment*, Martin Dunitz Ltd, London, 1995, pp. 9–15.

Hermanns, J.F., Petit, L., Martalo, O., Pierard-Franchimont, C., Cauwenbergh, G., and Pierard, G.E., Unraveling the patterns of subclinical pheomelanin-enriched facial hyperpigmentation: effect of depigmenting agents, *Dermatology,* 201:118–122, 2000.

Kim, Y.J., No, J.K., Lee, J.H., and Chung, H.Y., 4,4′-Dihydroxybiphenyl as a new potent tyrosinase inhibitor, *Biol. Pharm. Bull.,* 28(2):323–327, 2005.

Kubo, I. and Kinst-Hori, I., Tyrosinase inhibitory activity of the olive oil flavor compounds, *J. Agric. Food Chem.,* 47:4574–4578, 1999.

Kubo, I. and Kinst-Hori, I., 2-Hydroxy-4-methoxybenzaldehyde: a potent tyrosinase inhibitor from African medicinal plants, *Planta Med.,* 65:19–22, 1999.

Matsuda, H., Higashino, M., Nakai, Y., Iinuma, M., Kubo, M., and Lang, F.A., Studies of cuticle drugs from natural sources. IV. Inhibitory effects of some *Arctostaphylos* plants on melanin biosynthesis, *Biol. Pharm. Bull.,* 19:153–156, 1996.

Nakagawa, M. and Kawai, K., Contact allergy to kojic acid in skin care products, *Contact Dermatit.,* 32:9–13, 1995.

Nerya, O., Vaya, J., Musa, R., Izrael, S., Ben-Arie, R., and Tamir, S., Glabrene and isoliquiritigenin as tyrosinase inhibitors from licorice roots, *J. Agric. Food Chem.,* 51:1201–1207, 2003.

Nerya, O., Musa, R., Khatib, S., Tamir, S., and Vaya, J., Chalcones as potent tyrosinase inhibitors: the effect of hydroxyl positions and numbers, *Phytochemistry,* 65:1389–1395, 2004.

Schallreuter, K.U. and Wood, J.W., A possible mechanism of action for azelaic acid in the human epidermis, *Arch. Dermatol. Res.,* 282:168–171, 1990.

Seo, B., Yun, J., Lee, S., Kim, M., Hwang, K., Kim, J., Min, K.R., Kim, Y., and Moon, D., Barbarin as a new tyrosinase inhibitor from *Barbarea orthocerus, Planta Med.,* 65:683–686, 1999.

Shimizu, K., Kondo, R., and Sakai, K., Inhibition of tyrosinase by flavonoids, stilbenes and related 4-substituted resorcinols: structure-activity investigations, *Planta Med.,* 66:11–15, 2000.

Shin, N.H., Ryu, S.Y., Choi, E.J., Kang, S.H., Chang, I.M., Min, K.R., and Kim, Y., Oxyresveratrol as the potent inhibitor on dopa oxidase activity of mushroom tyrosinase, *Biochem. Biophys. Res. Commun.,* 243:801–803, 1998.

T

U

Uncaria tomentosa see also Cat's claw, Quinic acid Hot-water extracts from the vine *Uncaria tomentosa* were reported to affect immune function (Aquino et al., 1991; Lemaire et al., 1999). Such effects were later shown to include inhibition of TNFa (Sandoval et al., 2000) and activation of the central transcription nuclear factor κB (NF-κB) (Sandoval-Chacon et al., 2002; Akesson et al., 2003). A hot-water extract from the bark of *Uncaria tomentosa*, C-Med 100®, in which large molecules, such as tannins and flavonoids, had been removed, still enhanced DNA repair (Sheng et al., 2000) and protected against "spontaneous" apoptosis induction *in vitro* (Akesson et al., 2003). It also inhibited proliferation of tumor cells without inducing apoptosis or necrotic cell death. Subsequent work by Akesson et al. (2005) identified quinic acid as one of the components responsible for these effects.

References

Aquino, R., De Feo, V., De Simona, F., Pizza, C., and Cirino, G., Plant metabolites. New compounds and anti-inflammatory activity of *Uncaria tomentosa*, *J. Nat. Prod.,* 54:453–459, 1991.

Akesson, C., Lindgren, H., Pero, R.W., Leanderson, T., and Ivars, F., An extract from *Uncaria tomentosa* inhibiting cell division and NF-κB activity without inducing cell death, *Int. Immunopharmacol.,* 3: 1889–1900, 2003.

Akesson, C., Lindgren, H., Pero, R.W., Leanderson, T., and Ivars, F., Quinic acid is a biologically active component of the *Uncaria tomentosa* C-Med 100®, *Int. Immunopharmacol.,* 5:219–229, 2005.

Lemaire, I., Assinewe, V., Cano, P., Awang, D.V., and Arnason, J.T., Stimulation of interleukin-1 and -6 production in alveolar macrophages by the neotropical liana, *Uncaria tomentosa* (una de gato), *J. Ethnopharmacol.,* 64:109–115, 1999.

Sandoval-Chacon, M., Thompson, J.H., Zhang, X.J., Liu, X., Mannick, E.E., Sadowski-Krowicka, H., Charbonnet, R.M., Clark, D.A., and Miller, M.J.S., Anti-inflammatory actions of cat's claw: the role of NF-κB. *Aliment. Pharmacol. Ther.,* 12:1279–1289, 1998.

Sheng, Y., Bryngelsson, C., and Pero, R.W., Enhanced DNA repair, immune function and reduced toxicity of C-Med 100®, a novel aqueous extract from *Uncaria tomentosa*, *J. Ethnopharmacol.,* 69: 115–126, 2000.

Uva ursi see also Bearberry Uva ursi is a compound extracted from the bearberry plant (*Arctostaphylos uva ursi* L.). This herb is used for treating lower urinary-tract infections and is currently recommended for the treatment and prophylaxis of cystitis (Larsson et al., 1993; Yarnell, 2002). Uva ursi, however, causes depigmentation by inhibiting tyrosinase kinase and hence melanin synthesis (Matsuda et al., 1996). Wang and Del Priore (2004) recently reported a case of bilateral bull's eye maculopathy in a patient ingesting tea made from uva ursi over a three-year period to treat a recurrent urinary-tract infection. Based on these results, they cautioned against the use of uva ursi, which should be considered a retinal toxic drug.

References

Larsson, B., Jonasson, A., and Fianu, S., Prophylactic effect of UVA E in women with recurrent cystitis: A preliminary report, *Curr. Ther. Res. Clin. Exp.,* 53: 441–443, 1993.

Matsuda, H., Higashino, M., Nakai, Y., Iinuma, M., Kubo, M., and Lang, F.A., Studies of cuticle drugs from natural sources. IV. Inhibitory effects of some *Arctostaphylos* plants on melanin biosynthesis, *Biol. Pharm. Bull.,* 19:153–156, 1996.

Wang, L. and Del Priore, L.V., Bull's eye maculopathy secondary to herbal toxicity from uva ursi, *Am. J. Ophthamol.,* 137:1135–1137, 2004.

Yarnell, E., Botanical medicines for the urinary tract, *World J. Urol.,* 20:285–293, 2002.

U

V

Valerenic acid *see also* **Valerian**   Valerenic acid, a hydrophilic sesquiterpenoid, and its derivatives are the major active constituents in the herb valerian (*Valeriana officinalis*). Valerian, an herbal medicine, is used primarily for its sleep-enhancing and sedative effects (McCabe, 2002). Gao and Bjork (2000) found valerenic-acid derivatives varied from 11.65–0.15 mg/g in different varieties of Valeriana.

Valerenic acid

Adapted from Fernandez, S., et al., *Pharmacol. Biochem. Behav.*, 77:399–404, 2004.

Micropropagation proved to be a much more reliable and effective method for optimizing the bioactive constituents in *V. officinalis* compared to seed-propagated plants. Valerenic acid was shown by Reidel et al. (1982) to inhibit the enzyme system, causing GABA breakdown in the brain. The resulting increase in GABA is associated with sedation and decrease in CNS activity.

References

Gao, X.Q. and Bjork, L., Valerenic acid derivatives and valepotriates among individuals, varieties and species of Valeriana, *Fitoterapia*, 71:19–24, 2000.

McCabe, S., Complimentary herbal and alternative drugs in clinical practice, *Perspect. Psychiatr. Care,* 38:98–107, 2002.

Reidel, E., Hansel, R., and Erkhe, G., Hemmung des Aminobuttersaureabbaus durch Valerensaurederivate*, Planta Med.,* 46:219–220, 1982.

Valepotriates *see also* **Valerian**   Valepotriates, naturally occurring iridoids or cyclopentan-c-pyran monoterpenoids, are found in many plants, including the herb valerian. Together with valerenic-acid derivatives, they are considered to be the active constituents of valerian (Gao and Bjork, 2000). Unlike the hydrophilic valerenic-acid derivatives, valepotriates are hydrophobic and can be divided into four main groups based on their chemical structure. These include diene, monoene, valtrate-hydrine, and desoxy monoene types. The diene types are shown in Scheme V.62 (Bos et al., 2002). Valepotriates, mainly present in the roots, are thought to dampen the central-nervous system by exhibiting activity between sedation and tranquilization and are referred to aequilans (Von Eickstedt and Rahman, 1969). Bos et al. (2002) reviewed the properties of valepotriates, as well as the qualitative and quantitative methods used for their analysis.

References

Bos, R., Woerdenbag, H.J., and Pras, N., Determination of valepotriates, *J. Chromatogr.,* A., 967:131–146, 2002.

Fernandez, S., Wasowski, C., Paladini, A.C., and Marder, M., Sedative and sleep-enhancing properties of linarin, a flavonoic-isolated from *Valeriana officinalis. Pharm. Biochem. Behav.,* 77:399–404, 2004.

Gao, X.Q. and Bjork, L., Valerenic acid derivatives and valepotriates among individuals, varieties and species of Valeriana, *Fitoterapia*, 71:19–24, 2000.

Von Eickstedt, K.W. and Rahman, S., Psychopharmacologic effects of valepotriates, *Arzneim Forsch.,* 19:316–319, 1969.

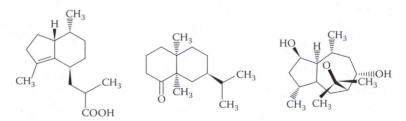

	R_1	R_2	R_3	
1	Iv	Iv	Ac	Valtrate
2	Iv	Ac	Iv	Isovaltrate
3	Aiv	Iv	Ac	Acevaltrate
4	Iv	Ac	Ac	Diavaltrate
5	Iv	Aiv	Ac	Homoacevaltrate
6	Miv	Iv	Ac	1-Homovaltrate
7	Iv	Ac	Miv	7-Homovaltrate
8	Iv	Ac	Aiv	11-Acevaltrate
9	Iv	Hiv	Ac	Hydroxyvaltrate
10	Cr	Iv	Ac	1-Seneciovaltrate (isohomoacevaltrate)
11	Iv	H	Iv	Deacetylisovaltrate

SCHEME V.62   Valepotriates (diene type). (From Bos et al., *J. Chromatogr.,* A 967:131–146, 2002. With permission.)

Valerian *see also* **Valerenic acid and Valepotriates**   Valerian (*Valeriana officinalis*), an herbal medicine, is used primarily as a tranquilizer and sleep inducer (Reynolds, 1996). The effects of valerian are attributed to a number of different compounds present as volatile-oil components. These include monoterpenes, although it is the biological activity of the sesquiterpene components that have received the most attention. The latter includes valerenic acid, valeranone, and kessyl glycol.

Valerenic acid and kessyl-ring systems are unique to valerian. Valerenic acid appears to inhibit the enzymatic degradation of GABA in the brain (Reidel et al., 1982). This results in increased GABA levels that are associated with sedation and CNS activity (Houghton, 1999). In contrast, valeranone acts primarily on the muscle rather than on the CNS (Hazelhoff et al., 1982).

A novel group of irioid-like monoterpenes, the valepotriates, were also identified in *Valeriana* (Mannerstatter et al., 1966; Thies, 1966). These were esters with moderate polarity, requiring extraction with alcoholic solvents. The tranquilizing effects of valepotriates, as measured by a decrease in spontaneous motility in mice, was clearly shown by Von Eikstedt (1969) and Von Eikstedt and Rahman (1969). The major degradation product of valepotriates by the intestinal bacteria flora was homobaldrinal and related products. Homobaldrinal was found by Wagner et al. (1980) to have a greater effect on spontaneous motility in mice compared to the parent valepotriates, suggesting valepotriates may act as prodrugs.

Valerenic acid, Valeranone, Kessyl glycol

Adapted from Fernandez et al., *Pharmacol. Biochem. Behav.,* 77:399–404, 2004, and Tori et al., *Phytochemistry,* 41:977–979, 1996.

Homobaldrinal. (From Hui-lian et al., *Toxicol. Appl. Pharmacol.*, 188:36–41, 2003. With permission.

There is considerable controversy, however, over the efficacy of valerian in the treatment of insomnia. A systematic review of the effect of valerian on insomnia in nine randomized clinical trials by Stevinson and Ernst (2000) showed great discrepancies among trials. Some studies showed promising but inconclusive results, while others found valerian had no acute and cumulative effects on sleep. Using a series of randomized trials, Coxeter and coworkers (2003) found no improvement of valerian over the placebo in reducing chronic insomnia symptoms in patients. A recent study on healthy volunteers by Gutierrez et al. (2004) found acute administration of valerian had no mood-altering or psychomotor/cognitive effects. Poyares and coworkers (2002), however, reported valerian had a beneficial effect on improving the sleep of insomniacs after benzodiazepine withdrawal. Problems associated with the long-term use of this drug are dependency, tolerance, long-term memory, and altered sleep structure. Low doses of dichloromethane extracts of valerian were not found by Hui-lian et al. (2003) to have any significant cytoxicity or genotoxicity on human endothelial ECV304 cells, but did cause moderate DNA damage at higher doses as a result of oxidative stress. Both vitamins E and C attenuated the effect of high doses of the valerian extract, suggesting definite guidelines are needed for clinical therapy with valerian.

References

Bos, R., Woerdenberg, H.J., and Pras, N., Determination of valepotriates, *J. Chromatogr.*, A., 967:131–146, 2002.

Coxeter, P.D., Schluter, P.J., Eastwood, H.L., Nickles, C.J., and Glasziou, P.P., Valerian does not appear to reduce symptoms for patients with chronic insomnia in general practice using a series of randomized n-of-1 trials, *Complement. Ther. Med.*, 11:215–222, 2003.

Fernandez, S., Wasowski, C., Paladini, A.C., and Marder, M., Sedative and sleep-enhancing properties of linarin, a flavonoid-isolated from *Valeriana officinalis. Pharm. Biochem. Behav.*, 77:399–404, 2004.

Gutierrez, S., Ang-Lee, M.K., Walker, D.J., and Zacny, J.P., Assessing subjective and psychomotor effects of the herbal medication valerian in healthy volunteers, *Pharmacol. Biochem. Behav.*, 78:57–64, 2004.

Hazelhoff, B., Malingre, T.M., and Meijer, D.F.K., Antispasmodic effects of valerian compounds: an *in-vivo* and *in-vitro* study on the guinea-pig ileum, *Arch. Int. Pharmacodyn.*, 257:274–287, 1982.

Houghton, P.J., The scientific basis for the reputed activity of valerian, *J. Pharm. Pharmacol.*, 51:505–512, 1999.

Hui-lian, W., Dong-fang, Z., Zhao-feng, L., Yang, L., Quai-rong, L., and Yu-zhen, W., *In vitro* study on the genotoxicity of dichloromethane extracts of valerian (DEV) in human endothelial ECV304 cells and the effect of vitamins E and C in attenuating the DEV-induced DNA damages, *Toxicol. Appl. Pharmacol.*, 188:36–41, 2003.

Mannenstatter, E., Gerlach, H., and Poethke, W., Phytochemical studies on *Centranthus ruber, Pharmazie*, 21:321–327, 1996.

Poyares, D.R., Guilleminault, C., Ohayon, M.M., and Tufik, S., Can valerian improve the sleep of insomniacs after benzodiazepine withdrawal, *Prog. Neuro-Psychopharmacol. Biol. Psychiatry*, 26:539–545, 2002.

Reidel, E., Hansel, R., and Ehrke, G., Hemmung desAminobuttersaureabbaus durch Valerensaurederivate, *Planta Med.*, 46:219–220, 1982.

Reynolds, J.E.F., *Martindale: The Extra Pharmacipiae*, 31st ed., Pharmaceutical Press, London, 1996.

Stevinson, C. and Ernst, E., Valerian for insomnia: a systematic review of randomized clinical trials, *Sleep Med.*, 1:91–99, 2000.

Thies, P.W., Uber die wirkstoffe des baldrians 2: Mitteilung zur konstitution der isovaleriansaureester valepotriaten, acetoxyvalepotriat und dihydrovalepotriat, *Tetrahedron Lett.*, 11:1163–1170, 1966.

Tori, M., Yoshida, M., Yokoyama, M., and Asakawa, Y., A guaiane-type sequiterpene valeracetate from *Valeriana officinalis. Phytochemistry.* 41:977–979, 1996.

Von Eickstedt, K.W., Die Beeinflussung der Alkohol-Wirkung durch Valepotriate, *Arzneim. Forsch.*, 19:316–319, 1969.

Von Eickstedt, K.W. and Rahman, S., Psychopharmacological effects of valepotriates, *Arzneim. Forsch.*, 19:316–319, 1969.

V

Wagner, H., Jurcic, K., and Schaette, R., Vergleichende Untersuchungen uber die sedierende Wirkung von Baldrianextrakten, Valepotriaten und ihren Abbauprodukten, *Planta Med.,* 38:358–365, 1980.

Vegetable oils   *see* Canola, Corn, Flax, Soybean, and Sunflower oils

---

Vegetables   *see also* Individual vegetables
The presence of bioactive phytochemicals, in addition to vitamins and provitamins, in vegetables and fruits is associated with a decreased risk of cancer (Block et al., 1992; Steinmetz and Potter, 1991) and cardiovascular disease (Grey et al., 1993; Gramenzi et al., 1990; Hertog et al., 1993). Broekmans and coworkers (2000) showed that the consumption of fruits and vegetables by 47 male and female volunteers significantly increased plasma carotenoids and vitamins, while decreasing homocysteine. The latter has become a useful biomarker, as epidemiological studies have shown an inverse relationship between plasma homocysteine and cardiovascular disease. Chu and coworkers (2002) examined 10 common vegetables based on their consumption per capita data in the United States. Broccoli contained the highest levels of total phenols (101.6 mg/g), followed by spinach, yellow onion, red pepper, carrot, cabbage, potato, lettuce, celery, and cucumber. Using the Total Oxygen Scavenging (TOSC) assay, red pepper had the highest antioxidant activity (46.95 mmol of vitamin C equiv/g of sample), followed by broccoli, carrot, spinach, cabbage, yellow onion, celery, potato, lettuce, and cucumber. These researchers also proposed a phenolic-antioxidant index (PAI) for evaluating the quantity/quality of phenolics in these vegetables by eliminating vitamin C's antioxidant contributions. Using HepG$_2$ liver-cancer cells, spinach was found to have the highest antiproliferative activity, followed by cabbage, red pepper, onion, and broccoli. Based on these results, a bioactivity index (BI) for cancer prevention was proposed to help consumers select vegetables on the basis of their health benefits. For example, because red pepper and spinach had the highest antioxidant and antiproliferative

activities, they were used as controls to calculate BI.

A recent study by Ismail et al. (2004) was unable to find any relationship between antioxidant activity and total phenolics for commonly selected vegetables in Malaysia. Spinach was very high in total phenols, followed by swamp cabbage, kale, shallots, and cabbage. A 1-min thermal treatment, involving boiling 300 g of each vegetable in 500 mL water, significantly ($p < 0.05$) decreased the total phenolic content in all the vegetables examined.

Rijken et al. (1999), using aberrant crypt multiplicity as the marker for colorectal cancer, found that vegetable consumption (freeze-dried peas, spinach, sprouts, and broccoli) had a beneficial effect on colorectal cancer by inhibiting early postinitiation events, but were more pronounced in the advanced lesions. These researchers, however, found that α- and β-carotenoids made only a marginal contribution to the observed beneficial effects.

References
Block, G., Patterson, B., and Subar, A., Fruits, vegetables, and cancer prevention: a review of epidemiological evidence, *Nutr. Cancer*, 18:1–29, 1992.

Broekmans, W.M.R., Klopping-Ketelaars, I.A.A., Schuurman, C.R.W.C., Verhagen, H., van den Berg, H., Kok, F.J., and van Poppel, G., Fruits and vegetables increase plasma carotenoids and vitamins and decrease homocysteine in humans, *J. Nutr.,* 130:1578–1583, 2000.

Chu, Y-F., Sun, J., Wu, X., and Liu, R.H., Antioxidant and antiproliferative activities of common vegetables, *J. Agric. Food Chem.*, 50:6910–6916, 2002.

Gramenzi, A., Gentile, A., Fasoli, M., Negri, E., Parazzini, F., and La Vecchia, C., Association between certain foods and risk of acute myocardial infarction in women, *Br. Med. J.,* 300:771–773, 1990.

Gey, K.F., Moser, U.K., Stahelin, H.B., Eicholzer, M., and Ludin, E., Increased risk of cardiovascular disease at suboptimal plasma concentrations of essential antioxidants: an epidemiological update with special attention to carotene and vitamin C, *Am. J. Clin. Nutr.,* 57:787S–797S, 1993.

Hertog, M.G.L., Feskens, E.J.M., Kromhout, D., Hollman, P.C.H., and Katan, M.B., Dietary antioxidant flavonoids and risk of cardiovascular disease, The Zutphen Elderly Study, *Lancet,* 342:1007–1011, 1993.

Ismail, A., Marjan, Z.M., and Foong, C.W., Total antioxidant activity and phenolic content in selected vegetables, *Food Chem.,* 2004 (in press).

Rijken, P.J., Timmer, W.G., van de Kooij, A.J., van Benschop, I.M., Wiseman, S.A., Meijers, M., and Tijburg, B.M., Effect of vegetable and carotenoid consumption on aberrant crypt multiplicity, a surrogate end-point marker for colorectal cancer in azoxymethane-induced rats, *Carcinogenesis,* 20: 2267–2272, 1999.

Vinegar *see also* **Kurosu**   As an acidic seasoning, vinegar is reported to have medicinal properties due to its physiological functions, such as digestive, appetite-stimulating, and exhaustion-recovering effects. One of the most common traditional Japanese vinegars obtained from unpolished rice is kurosu. In addition to preventing hypertension by improving blood fluidity, Nishidai et al. (2000) showed an ethylacetate extract of kurosu exhibited antitumor properties arising, in part, from its suppression of lipid peroxidation.

Vinegar is also a by-product of Sherry wines by a dynamic aging process known as "*solaras and criaderas.*" Recent work by Alonso et al. (2004) demonstrated the antioxidant power of vinegar, which was highly influenced by its polyphenolic content (Figure V.97). Correlation analysis was obtained for compounds identified in more than two samples. Gallic acid was particularly important in vinegar without aging, while *cis-p*-coumaric acid, 1-ferulic and syringic acids, together with vanillin and *p*-hydroxy-benzaldehyde, exhibited high correlations for vinegars aged in wood.

References

Alonso, A.M., Castro, R., Rodriguez, M.C., Guillen, D.A., and Barroso, C.G., Study of the antioxidant power of brandies and vinegars derived from Sherry wines and correlation with their content in polyphenols, *Food Res. Inter.,* 37:715–722, 2004.

Nishidai, S., Nakamura, Y., Torikai, K., Yamamoto, N., Ishihara, N., Mori, H., and Ohigashi, H., Kurosu, a traditional vinegar produced from unpolished rice suppresses lipid peroxidation *in vitro* and in mouse skin, *Biosci. Biotechnol. Biochem.,* 64:1909–1914, 2000.

Vitamins *see also* **Individual vitamins, as well as Niacin and Folate**   Oxidative stress is the major contributor to many degenerative or chronic diseases, such as coronary heart disease, cancers, and neurodegenerative diseases. These result from the biological damage to lipids, proteins, and nucleic acids brought about by the production of reactive-oxygen species. To protect the body from the deleterious effects of reactive-oxygen species, endogenous antioxidants are present, including antioxidant vitamins. A review by McCall and Frei (1999), however, pointed out that studies on smokers and non-smokers revealed that only vitamin A, and possibly vitamin C, could reduce lipid-oxidative damage. Kriharides and Stocker (2002), in reviewing the data from a number of major, randomized studies, were unable to find any evidence for recommending α-tocopherol or β-carotene supplements in treating coronary heart disease.

A review of a number of randomized trials by Mitchell et al. (2003) found that supplementation with vitamins and minerals enhanced immune function of the elderly. The primary

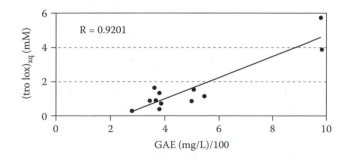

FIGURE V.97 Correlation line between total polyphenolic index (GAE) and antioxidant power ([Trolox]$_{eq}$) of vinegars. (From Alonso et al., *Food Res. Int.,* 37:715–722, 2004. With permission.)

vitamins involved were vitamins E, C, A, and β-carotene. In a double-blind, placebo-controlled trial with 1078 Tanzanian women infected with HIV, Fawzi et al. (2004) showed that a daily multivitamin supplement of vitamins (vitamins A [preformed and β-carotene], B, C, and E), slowed down the progression of HIV. The supplement significantly reduced fatigue, rash, and upper-respiratory infections and provided a low-cost strategy for delaying implementation of antiretroviral therapy.

The evidence for the protective nature of vitamin supplements in humans is mixed and still requires further studies.

References

Fawzi, W.W., Msamanga, G.I., Spiegelman, D., Wei, R., Kapiga, S., Villamor, E., Mwakagile, D., Mugusi, F., Hertzmark, E., Essex, M., and Hunter, D.J., A randomized trial of multivitamin supplemented and HIV disease progression and mortality, *N. Engl. J. Med.*, 351:23–32, 2004.

Kritharides, L. and Stocker, R., The use of antioxidant supplements in coronary heart disease, *Atherosclerosis*, 164:211–219, 2002.

McCall, M.R. and Frei, B., Can antioxidant vitamins materially reduce oxidative damage in humans? *Free Rad. Biol. Med.*, 26:1034–1053, 1999.

Mitchell, B.L., Ulrich, C.M., and McTiernan, A., Supplementation with vitamins or minerals and immune function: can the elderly benefit? *Nutr. Res.*, 23:1117–1139, 2003.

Vitamin A *see also* **β-Carotene, Retinoic acid, and Retinol**   Vitamin A was one of the first vitamins discovered, but many of its functions are still poorly defined. The physiological active forms of vitamin A are retinol, retinal, and retinoic acid (Scheme V.63). The hydrophobic polyene chain in vitamin A is responsible for its ability to quench singlet oxygen, neutralize thiyl radicals, and combine and stabilize peroxyl radicals (Palace et al., 1999). These researchers reported that while epidemiological and experimental studies support the possible benefits of vitamin A in reducing heart disease, several large, intervention studies did not. Further confusion was provided by the fact that β-carotene supplementation can actually increase cardiovascular and cancer-related mortality.

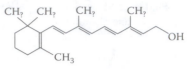

All-*trans* retinol

All-*trans* retinal

All-*trans* retinoic acid

SCHEME V.63 Structure of all-*trans*-retinol, all-*trans*-retinal, and all-*trans*-retinoic acid. (From Ono et al., *Exp. Neurol.*, 189:380–392, 2004. With permission.)

Talas et al. (2003), however, demonstrated the benefits of vitamin A therapy in healing tracheal anastomoses in adult Wistar rats by reversing the deleterious effects of the corticosteroid dexamethasone. A recent study by Ono et al. (2004) speculated that vitamin A and β-carotene could prevent the development of Alzheimer's disease. This disease is characterized by the deposition of amyloid β-peptide (Ab) as amyloid plaques and vascular amyloid and neurofibillary tangles (Selkoe, 2001). *In vitro* studies by Ono et al. (2004) showed that vitamin A and β-carotene inhibited the formation of β-amyloid fibrils (fAb) from fresh amyloid β-peptide (Ab), as well as their extension. In addition, vitamin A and β-carotene destabilized preformed fAb in a dose-dependent manner. The relative potency of their antiamyloidogenic and fibril-destabilizing effects ranged from highest for retinol and retinal, followed by β-carotene, and then retinoic acid. These results pointed to the application of these molecules in the prevention and therapy of Alzheimer's disease.

References

Ono, K., Yoshiike, Y., Takashima, A., Hasegawa, K., Naiki, H., and Yamada, M., Vitamin A exhibits potent antiamyloidogenic and fibril-destabilizing effects *in vitro*, *Exp. Neurol.*, 189:380–392, 2004.

Palace, V.P., Khaper, N., Qin, Q., and Singal, P.K., Antioxidant potentials of vitamin A and carotenoids and their relevance to heart disease, *Free Rad. Biol. Med.*, 26:746–761, 1999.

Selkoe, D.J., Alzheimer's disease: genes, protein, and therapy, *Physiol. Rev.*, 81:741–766, 2001.

Talas, D.U., Nayci, A., Atis, S., Comelekoglu, U., Polat, A., Bagdatoglu, C., and Renda, N., The effects of corticosteroids and vitamin A on the healing of tracheal anastomoses, *Int. J. Pediatr. Otohinolaryngol.*, 67:109–116, 2003.

Vitamin B$_3$ *see* Niacin

Vitamin B$_6$

The different natural forms of vitamin B$_6$, pyridoxine, pyridoxal, and pyridoxamine, are all converted *in vivo* to the active coenzyme form, pyridoxal-5'-phosphate (Scheme V.64). Pyridoxal-5'-phosphate is involved in a wide range of synthetic and catabolic processes, as well as the interconversion of amino acids, biosynthesis of carbohydrates, proteins, lipids, and nucleic acids (Brody, 1999). In addition, pyridoxal-5'-phosphate-dependent enzymes are also involved in the synthesis of such neurotransmitters as GABA, norepinephrine, dopamine, serotonin, and polyamines. The possible role of B$_6$ in normal neuronal development became evident when vitamin B$_6$ was deficient (Kirskey et al., 1990). Geng and coworkers (1997) reported pyridoxal phosphate protected cultured hippocampal neurons from glucose deprivation-induced damage. Wang et al. (2002) found vitamin B$_6$ protected monkey retinal neurons from ischemic damage, with the potential as a novel pharmacotherapy.

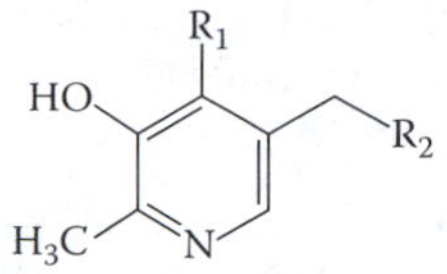

Previous studies on the suppression of animal and human cancer cells *in vitro* by high levels of vitamin B$_6$ pointed to its ability to act as a chemopreventive agent (DiSorbo and Litwack, 1983; Di Sorbo et al., 1985; DiSorbo and Nathanson, 1983; Molina et al., 1997). The anticancer properties of vitamin B$_6$ against colon cancer were first reported in case-control studies in the United States by Slattery et al. (1997). They found an inverse association

Compound	R$_1$	R$_2$
1:	–CHO	–OH
2:	–CH$_2$OH	–OH
3:	–CH$_2$NH$_2$	–OH
4:	–CHO	$-O-\overset{\overset{O}{\|\|}}{\underset{\|}{P}}-OH$ OH

SCHEME V.64 Chemical structures of vitamin B$_6$ compounds. Compound 1, pyridoxal (PL); compound 2, pyridoxine (PN); compound 3, pyridoxamine (PM); and compound 4, pyridoxal 5'-phosphate (PLP). (Mizushina et al., *Biochem. Biophys. Res. Commun.*, 312:1025–1032, 2003. With permission.)

between the risk for colon cancer and vitamin B$_6$ intake. Confirmation of the protective role of vitamin B$_6$ against colorectal cancer was provided by Jansen et al. (1999) based on case-control studies conducted in seven European countries. An inverse relationship was also reported between vitamin B$_6$ and the risk for prostate and lung cancers (Hartman et al., 2001; Key et al., 1997). Moderate doses of vitamin B$_6$ were also reported by Komatsu et al. (2001) to significantly suppress the development of colonic tumors in azoxymethane (AOM)-treated mice. The anticancer effect of vitamin B$_6$ was shown by Matsubara et al. (2001) to be due, in part, to inhibition of angiogenesis. Further elucidation of the antiangiogenesis and anticancer mechanisms of vitamin B$_6$ by Mizushina et al. (2003) showed pyridoxal-5'-phosphate-inhibited, replicative DNA polymerases and human cancer-cell proliferation.

References

Brody, T., *Nutritional Biochemistry*, 2nd ed., Academic Press, San Diego, 1999, pp. 541–554.

DiSorbo, D.M. and Litwack, G., Vitamin B$_6$ kills hepatoma cells in culture, *Nutr. Cancer*, 5:10–15, 1983.

DiSorbo, D.M. and Nathanson, L., High-dose pyridoxal supplemented cultured medium inhibits the growth of human malignant melanoma cell line, *Nutr. Cancer*, 5:10–15, 1983.

DiSorbo, D.M., Wagner, R., Jr., and Nathanson, L., *In vivo* and *in vitro* inhibition of B16 melanoma growth by vitamin B$_6$, *Nutr. Cancer*, 7:43–52, 1985.

Geng, M.Y., Saito, H., and Nishiyama, N., Protective effects of pyridoxal phosphate against glucose deprivation-induced damage in cultured brain neurons, *J. Neurochem.*, 68:2500–2506, 1997.

Hartman, T.J., Woodson, K., Stolzenberg-Solomon, R., Virtamo, J., Selhub, J., Barrett, M.J., and Albanes, D., Association of the B-vitamins pyridoxal 5′-phosphate (B(6)), B(12) and folate with lung cancer risk in older men, *Am. J. Epidemiol.*, 153:688–694, 2001.

Jansen, M.C.J.F., Bueno-de-Mesquita, H.B., Buzina, R., Fidanza, F., Menotti, A., Blackburn, H., Nissinen, A.M., Kok, F.J., and Kromhout, D., Dietary fiber and plant foods in relation to colorectal mortality: the seven countries study, *Int. J. Cancer*, 81:174–179, 1999.

Key, T.J., Silcocks, P.B., Davey, G.K., Appleby, P.N., and Bishop, D.T., A case-control study of diet and prostate cancer, *Br. J. Cancer*, 76:678–687, 1997.

Kirskey, A., Morre, D.M., and Wasynczuk, A.Z., Neuronal development in vitamin B$_6$ deficiency, *Ann. N.Y. Acad. Sci.*, 585:202–218, 1990.

Matsubara, K., Mori, M., Matsuura, Y., and Kato, N., Pyridoxal 5′-phosphate and pyridoxal inhibit angiogenesis in the serum-free rat aortic ring assay, *Int. J. Mol. Med.*, 8:505–508, 2001.

Mizushina, Y., Xu, X., Matsubara, K., Murakami, C., Kuriyama, I., Oshige, M., Takemura, M., Kato, N., Yoshida, H., and Sakaguchi, K., Pyridoxal 5′-phosphate is a selective inhibitor *in vivo* of DNA polymerases, *Biochem. Biophys. Res. Commun.*, 312: 1025–1032, 2003.

Molina, A., Ako, T., Munoz, S.M., Chikamori-Aoyama, M., Kuwahata, M., and Natori, Y., Vitamin B$_6$ suppresses growth and expression of albumin gene in a human hepatoma cell line HepG2, *Nutr. Cancer*, 28:206–211, 1997.

Slattery, M.L., Potter, J.D., Coates, A., Ma, K.N., Berry, T.D., Duncan, D.M., and Caan, B.J., Plant foods and colon cancer: an assessment of specific foods and their related nutrients (United States), *Cancer Causes Cont.*, 8:575–592, 1997.

Wang, X.-D., Kashii, S., Zhao, L., Tonchev, A.B., Katsuki, H., Akaike, A., Honda, Y., Yamashita, J., and Yamashima, T., Vitamin B$_6$ protects primate retinal neurons from ischemic injury, *Brain Res.*, 940: 36–43, 2002.

Vitamin B$_{12}$ Vitamin B$_{12}$, or cobalamin, is a complex molecule containing a cobalt-centered, corrin nucleus. It functions as a coenzyme by resynthesizing methionine from homocysteine with 5-methyl tetrahydrofolic acid as the methyl-group donor (Marsh, 1999). In addition, it provides tetrahydrofolic acid for other folate-dependent reactions (Selub, 2002). Animal organ meats, such as liver and kidney, are particularly rich sources of cobalamin, although it is synthesized exclusively by bacteria (Herbert, 1996; Raux et al., 2000). Because the synthesis of cobalamin by intestinal bacteria is insufficient, dietary sources of vitamin B$_{12}$ must be provided in the diet (Herbert, 1988).

Traditionally, vitamin B$_{12}$ deficiency has been associated with pernicious anemia, a condition characterized by poorly formed, large red blood cells and demyelinization of sheaths of nerve cells (Gropper, 2000). Current research associates deficiency of vitamin B$_{12}$ with increased risk for atherosclerosis (Nygard et al., 1999; Brattstrom and Wilcken, and Jackson, 2000; Mangoni et al., 2002) and neurodegenerative diseases (Selhub et al., 2000; Rosenberg et al., 2001). Wolters et al. (2004) pointed out that vitamin B$_{12}$ deficiency is particularly prevalent among the elderly population and recommends supplementation of > 50 mg/day.

A review of Alzheimer' disease by Luchsinger and Mayeux (2004) reported that some studies suggest that a high intake of vitamins, including B$_{12}$, lowered the risk for this disease. However, based on a number of different studies, no definite conclusions or recommendations could be made. This was borne out in a recent study by Mizrachi et al. (2004), who found no significant association between plasma total homocysteine, B$_{12}$, and folate levels in either healthy or Alzheimer's patients in Israel.

An abnormal vitamin B$_{12}$ status was reported in depressed patients by Bell et al. (1991), while epidemiological data from a Women's Health and Aging Study suggested a twofold risk of severe depression was associated with a deficiency of this vitamin (Pennix et al., 2000). However, a recent three-month, randomized, placebo-controlled study of 140 individuals deficient in vitamin B$_{12}$, assessed by an increase in plasma methyl-malonic acid, found no improvement in cognitive function or symptoms of depression following supplementation with the vitamin.

Even though few studies evaluated visual-evoked potential (VEP) changes after vitamin B_{12} supplementation, Pandy and coworkers (2004) showed that visual pathways were vulnerable to vitamin B_{12} deficiency. The prolonged VEP associated with patients suffering from vitamin B_{12} deficiency was found to return to normal following vitamin B_{12} supplementation.

References

Bell, I.R., Erdman, J.S., Morrow, F.D., Marby, D.W., Mirages, S., Kayne, L.H., and Cole, J.O., Perrone, G., B complex vitamin patterns in geriatric and young adult inpatients with major depression, *J. Am. Geriatr. Soc.,* 39:252–257, 1991.

Brattstrom, L. and Wilcken, D.E., Homocysteine and cardiovascular disease: cause or effect? *Am. J. Clin. Nutr.,* 72:315–323, 2000.

Gropper, S.S., *The Biochemistry of Human Nutrition,* Wadsworth Thomas Learning, 2000, pp. 250–252.

Herbert, V., Vitamin B_{12}: plant sources, requirements, and assay, *Am. J. Clin. Nutr.,* 48:852–858, 1988.

Herbert, V., B_{12}, in *Present Knowledge on Nutrition,* Ziegler, E.E. and Filer, I.F., Eds., International Life Science Institute Press, Washington, D.C., 1996. pp. 191–205.

Hvas, A.-M., Juul, S., Lauritzen, L., Nexo, E., and Ellegaard, J., No effect of vitamin B-12 treatment on cognitive function or depression: a randomized placebo controlled study, *J. Affect. Disord.,* 81:269–273, 2004.

Luchsinger, J.A. and Mayeux, R., Factors and Alzheimer's disease, *Lancet Neurol.,* 3:579–587, 2004.

Mangoni, A.A. and Jackson, S.H.D., Homocysteine and cardiovascular disease: current evidence and future prospects, *Am. J. Med.,* 112:556–655, 2002.

Mizrachi, E.H., Bowirrat, A., Jacobsen, D.W., Korczyn, A.D., Traore, F., Petot, G.J., Lerner, A.J., Debanne, S.M., Adunsky, A., DiBello, P.M., and Friedland, R.P., Plasma homocysteine, vitamin B12 and folate in Alzheimer's patients and healthy arabs in Israel, *J. Neurol. Sci.,* 227:109–113, 2004.

Marsh, E.N., Coenzyme B12 (cobalamin)-dependent enzymes, *Essays Biochem.,* 34:139–154, 1999.

Pandy, S., Kalita, J., and Misra, U.K., A sequential study of visual evoked potential in patients with vitamin B12 deficiency neurological syndrome, *Clin. Neurophysiol.,* 115:914–818, 2004.

Penninx, B.W., Guralnik, J.M., Ferrucci, L., Fried, L.P., Allen, R.H., and Stabler, S.P., Vitamin B(12) deficiency and depression in physically disabled older women: epidemiologic evidence from the Women's Health and Aging Study, *Am. J. Psychiatry,* 157:715–721, 2000.

Raux, E., Schubert, H.L., and Warren, M.J., Biosynthesis of cobalamin (vitamin B_{12}): a bacterial conundrum, *Cell Mol. Life Sci.,* 57:1880–1893, 2000.

Rosenberg, I.H., B vitamins, homocysteine, and neurocognitive function, *Nutr. Rev.,* 9:S69–S73, 2001.

Selhub, J., Folate, vitamin B_{12} and vitamin B_6 and one carbon metabolism, *J. Nutr. Health & Aging,* 6: 39–42, 2002.

Selhub, J., Bagley, L.C., Miller, J., and Rosenberg, I.H., B vitamins, homocysteine, and neurocognitve function in the elderly, *Am. J. Clin. Nutr.,* 71:614S–620S, 2000.

Wolters, M., Strohle, A., and Hahn, A., Cobalamin: a critical vitamin in the elderly, *Prev. Med.,* 39:1256–1266, 2004.

Vitamin C *see also* **Ascorbic acid**   Vitamin C, or L-ascorbic acid, is a water-soluble antioxidant widely distributed in fruits and vegetables. Alul et al. (2003) showed vitamin C protected LDL from homocysteine-mediated oxidation via dehydroascorbic acid. Homocysteine, an atherogenic amino acid, appears to promote iron-dependent oxidation of LDL. Thus, vitamin C may have a role in the prevention of cardiovascular disease. Guaiquil et al. (2003) confirmed the prominent cardioprotective effect of vitamin C in ischemic myocardium. Rat cardiomyocytes accumulated vitamin C by transporting only dehydroascorbic acid (DHA), the oxidized form of vitamin C. Thus, treatment with DHA inhibited hypoxia-induced damage and decreased apoptosis by preventing expression of Bax, caspase-3 activation, and cytochrome C translocation into the cytoplasm. These results pointed to the potential therapeutic value of DHA. A recent study by Wu et al. (2004) showed that the microvascular benefits

V

of vitamin C in septic patients may be due to its inhibition of inducible nitric-oxide synthetase (iNOS).

Epidemiological studies pointed to the protective role of antioxidants in fruits and vegetables against cancer (Michels et al., 2000; Vecchia et al., 2001). Of the major antioxidants in fruits and vegetables, vitamin C was reported to prevent oxidative-stress-mediated chronic diseases, including cancer, cardiovascular disease, hypertension, stroke, and neurodegenerative diseases. The U.S. Department of Agriculture and National Cancer Institute recommend a minimum consumption of five servings of fruits and vegetables per day to prevent cancer. Based on this recommendation, 200–280 mg of vitamin C would be consumed. However, conflicting results have been obtained regarding the beneficial effects of vitamin C in cancer prevention. *In vitro* studies by Lee et al. (2001) showed vitamin C-induced decomposition of

lipid hydroperoxides to endogenous genotoxins capable of causing DNA damage. These results suggested that the amount needed in the diet was equivalent to a daily consumption of 200 mg of vitamin C. However, the amount of lipid peroxides used in the study was 400 mmol/L, which far exceeded the levels normally found in human blood, which ranged from 10–500 nmol/L (Zamburlini et al., 1995). In addition, endogenous antioxidants, such as glutathione peroxidase and catalase, are also present. Nevertheless, questions have been raised regarding the effectiveness of vitamin C in cancer prevention. Lee et al. (2003) reappraised the role of vitamin C in cancer prevention, suggesting that it is the flavonoid components in fruits and vegetables that are primarily responsible for the observed chemopreventive effects.

Wenzel and coworkers (2004) showed that as an antioxidant, ascorbic acid interfered with drug-induced (camptothecin or flavonoid flavone) apoptosis of HT-29 human colon-carcinoma cells. By dramatically reducing the production of reactive-oxygen species in the mitochondria, ascorbic acid blocked apoptosis of the cancer cells by inhibiting disintegration of the plasma membrane (Figure V.98). In addition,

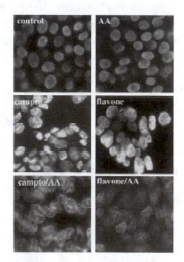
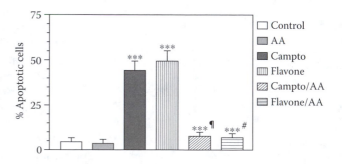

FIGURE V.98 Camptothecin-mediated and flavone-mediated plasma-membrane disintegration is reduced by ascorbic acid. Membrane disintegration in cell treated with medium alone (control), or with 1 mM ascorbic acid, or with 50 mM camptothecin (campto), or 150 mM flavone in the absence or presence of 1 mM ascorbic acid (AA) was assessed by uptake of Hoechst 33342 after 24 h. The percentage of apoptotic cells at 24 h is given in the lower panel. $^{***}p < 0.001$ versus control cells or versus cells treated with and camptothecin or # flavone. (From Wenzel et al., *Carcinogenesis*, 25:703–712, 2004. With permission.)

ascorbic acid prevented caspase-3 stimulation, downregulation of the mitochondrial antiapoptic protein bcl-X_L, and NF-κB mRNA levels. Thus, there may be a need to reduce ascorbic-acid intake in patients undergoing a course of chemotherapy for tumors.

Verrax and coworkers (2003) reported that a combination of vitamins C and K_3 effectively killed cancer cells by a new type of cancer-cell death known as autoschizis. This process was caspase-3-independent and characterized by oxidative stress, DNA fragmentation, and cell-membrane damage, with progressive loss of organelle-free cytoplasm. These researchers proposed vitamins C and K_3 be considered coadjuvants for cancer therapy. Park and coworkers (2004) reported that L-ascorbic acid induced apoptosis in acute myeloid-leukemia cells. The daily administration of up to 100 g of L-ascorbic acid proved beneficial to patients with acute myeloid leukemia. The mechanism appeared to involve the production of H_2O_2 from the oxidation of reduced glutathione by L-ascorbic acid.

References

Alul, R.H., Wood, M., Longo, J., Marcotte, A.L., Campione, A.L., Moore, M.K., and Lynch, S.M., Vitamin C protects low-density lipoprotein from homocysteine-mediated oxidation, *Free Rad. Biol. Med.,* 34:881–891, 2003.

Guaiquil, V.H., Golde, D.W., Beckles, D.L., Mascareno, E.J., and Siddiqui, M.A.Q., Vitamin C inhibits hypoxia-induced damage and apoptic signaling pathways in cardiomyocytes and ischemic hearts, *Free Rad. Biol. Med.,* 37:1419–1429, 2004.

Lee, K.W., Lee, H.-J., Surh, Y.-J., and Lee, C.Y., Vitamin C and cancer chemoprevention: reappraisal, *Am. J. Clin. Nutr.,* 78:1074–1078, 2003.

Lee, S.H., Oe, T., and Blair, I.A., Vitamin C-induced decomposition of lipid hydroperoxides to endogenous genotoxins, *Science,* 292:2083–2086, 2001.

Michels, K.B., Givanucci, E., Joshipura, J.K., Rosner, B.A., Stamfor, M.J., Fuchs, C.S., Colditz, G.A., Speizer, F.E., and Willett, W.C., Prospective study of fruit and vegetable consumption and incidence of colon and rectal cancers, *J. Natl. Cancer Inst.,* 92:1740–1752, 2000.

Park, S., Han, S.-S., Park, C.H., Hahm, E.-R., Lee, S.J., Park, H.K., Lee, S.-H., Kim, W.S., Jung, C.W.,

Park, K., Riordan, H.D., Kimler, B.F., Kim, K., and Lee, J.-H., L-Ascorbic acid induces apoptosis in acute myeloid leukemia cells via hydrogen peroxide-mediated mechanisms, *Int. J. Biochem. Cell Biol.,* 26:2180–2195, 2004.

Ruiz, E., Siow, R.C.M., Bartlett, S.R., Jenner, A.M., Sato, H., Bannai, S., and Mann, G.E., Vitamin C inhibits diethylmaleate-induced L-cysteine transport in human vascular smooth muscle cells, *Free Rad. Biol. Med.,* 34:103–110, 2002.

Vecchia, C.L., Alitieri, A., and Tavani, A., Vegetables, fruit, antioxidants and cancer: a review of Italian studies, *Eur. J. Nutr.,* 40:261–267, 2001.

Verrax, J., Cadrobbi, J., Delvaux, M., Jamison, J.M., Gilloteaux, J., Summers, J.L., Taper, H.S., and Calderon, P.B., The association of vitamins C and K3 kills cancer cells mainly by autoschizis, a novel form of cell death, basis for their potential use as coadjuvants in anticancer therapy, *Eur. J. Med. Chem.,* 38:451–457, 2003.

Wenzel, U., Nickel, A., Kuntz, S., and Daniel, H., Ascorbic acid suppresses drug-induced apoptosis in human colon cancer cells by scavenging mitochondrial superoxide anions, *Carcinogenesis,* 25:703–712, 2004.

Wu, F., Wilson, J.X., and Tyml, K., Ascorbate protects against impaired constriction in sepsis by inhibiting inducible nitric oxide synthase expression, *Free Rad. Biol. Med.,* 37:1282–1289, 2004.

Zamburlini, A., Maiorino, M., Barbera, P., Roveri, A., and Ursini, F., Direct measurement of single photon counting of lipid hydroperoxides in human plasma and lipoproteins, *Anal. Biochem.,* 232:107–113, 1995.

Vitamin D   Vitamin D consists of a family of 9,10 secosteroids differing in their side-chain structure (Mehta and Mehta, 2002). The main one, vitamin D_3, in its biological form, is inactive but metabolizes into the active form, 1-alpha-25-dihydroxy D_3, which plays a crucial role in calcium and bone homeostasis. The active form has been shown to prevent the growth of many neoplastic cells in prostate cancer (Lokeshwar et al., 1999), breast cancer (Pirianov and Colston, 2001), osteosarcoma (Hansen et al., 2001), and colon carcinoma (Diaz et al., 2000), but its use in cancer prevention is limited by its calcemic activity. The levels needed to suppress the growth of neoplasmic cells would cause hypercalcemia and death

(Mehta et al., 1997). To overcome this problem, a number of vitamin D_3 analogues were developed to reduce calcemic activity without compromising its antiproliferative activity. The vitamin D structure consists of four parts, including A, B, C, and D rings, plus the side chain. Most of the analogs involved modification in the A and B rings, such as calcipotiol, 2,2-oxacalcitrol, KH 1060, 1-alpha-25 $(OH)_2D_3$, and EB 1089, as shown in Scheme V.65.

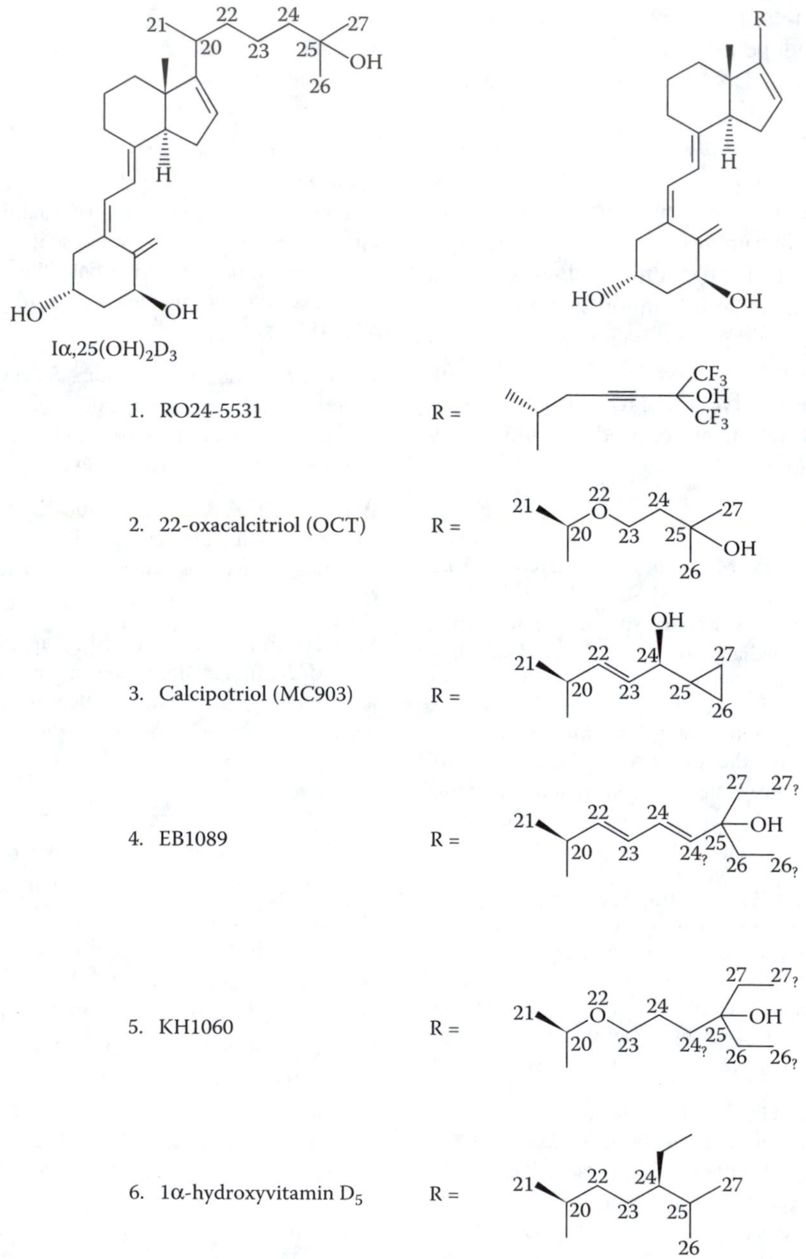

1. RO24-5531   R =
2. 22-oxacalcitriol (OCT)   R =
3. Calcipotriol (MC903)   R =
4. EB1089   R =
5. KH1060   R =
6. 1α-hydroxyvitamin D_5 R =

SCHEME V.65 Chemical structure of some active analogs of vitamin D. (From Mehta and Mehta, *J. Nutr. Biochem.*, 13:252–264, 2002. With permission.)

References

Diaz, G.D., Paraskeva, C., Thomas, M.G., Binderup, L., and Hague, A., Apoptosis is induced by the active metabolite of vitamin D-3 and its analogue EB1089 in colorectal adenoma and carcinoma cells: possible implications for prevention and therapy, *Cancer Res.*, 60:2304–2312, 2000.

Hansen, C.M., Hansen, D., Holm, P.K., and Binderup, L., Vitamin D compounds exert anti-apoptotic effects in human osteosarcoma cells *in vitro*, *J. Steroid Biochem. Mol. Biol.*, 77:1–11, 2001.

Lokeshwar, B.L., Schwartz, G.G., Selzer, M.G., Burnstein, K.L., Zhuang, S.H., Block, N.L., and Binderup, L., Inhibition of prostate cancer metastasis *in vivo*: a comparison of 1,25-dihydroxyvitamin D (calcitriol) and EN 1089, *Cancer Epidemiol. Biomark. Prevent.*, 8:241–248, 1999.

Mehta, R.G. and Mehta, R.R., Vitamin D and cancer, *J. Nutr. Biochem.*, 13:252–264, 2002.

Mehta, R.G., Mariarty, M.R., Mehta, R.R., Penmastys, R., Lazzaro, G., Constantinou, A., and Gou, L., Prevention of preneoplasmic mammary lesion development by a novel vitamin D analogue, 1-alpha-hydroxyvitamin D$_5$, *J. Nat. Cancer Inst.*, 89:212–218, 1997.

Pirianov, G. and Colston, K.W., Interaction of vitamin D analogs with signaling pathways leading to active cell death in breast cancer cells, *Steroids*, 66:309–318, 2001.

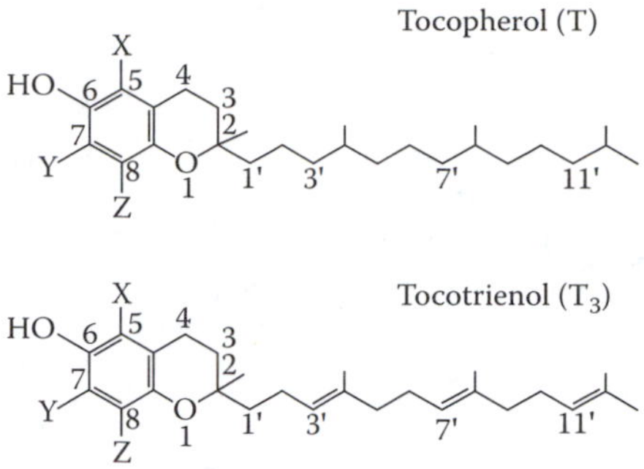

Vitamin E *see also* **Tocopherols** Vitamin E is a mixture of fat-soluble vitamins classified as tocopherols or tocotrienols. Tocopherols have a 16-carbon isoprenoid side chain, while tocotrienols have three, unsaturated double bonds in the 16-carbon isoprenoid side chain. Four different isomers are recognized, based on the number and position of the methyl groups in the ring structure, and are designated α, β, γ, and δ (Scheme V.66). While tocopherols are widely distributed in foods, tocotrienols are found in only a limited number of foods, such as palm oil. The major tocopherol in mammalian foods is α-tocopherol, followed by γ-tocopherol. They both act as chain-breaking antioxidants by the phenoxylic group, interacting with scavenging free radicals. There is strong epidemiological evidence between elevated tocopherol levels in the blood and protection against

Tocopherol (T)

Tocotrienol (T$_3$)

(A) α,X = CH$_3$, Y = CH$_3$, Z = CH$_3$
(B) β,X = CH$_3$, Y = H, Z = CH$_3$
(C) γ,X = H, Y = CH$_3$, Z = CH$_3$
(D) δ,X = H, Y = H, Z = CH$_3$

SCHEME V.66 Structural formulae of tocopherol and tocotrienol isomers. (From Abidi and Rennick, *J. Chromatogr. A*, 913:379–386, 2001. With permission.)

the development of cardiovascular disease, cancer, and dementia. Most of the attention on vitamin E has been focused on α-tocopherol; however, recent studies have pointed to the anti-inflammatory, antineoplastic, and natriuretic functions associated with γ-tocopherol (Hensley et al., 2004). Clermont et al. (2001) showed the use of vitamin E-coated dialyzer reduced oxidative stress in hemodialysis patients. Further work by Chao and coworkers (2002) found that supplementation of vitamins C and E dramatically improved the oxidation status in hemodialysis patients by decreasing the formation of lipid peroxides. The neuroprotective effect of vitamin E was demonstrated by Roghani and Behzadi (2001) by its ability to rapidly protect nigrostriatal dopaminergic neurons in an early model of Parkinson's disease in rat. Fariss and Zhang (2003) proposed that a chronic, high dose of vitamin E supplementation administered parenterally could provide an effective strategy for preventing or treating Parkinson's disease.

In addition to its role as an antioxidant, a number of nonantioxidant roles were highlighted for vitamin E by Azzi and Stocker (2000), including inhibition of protein kinase C and cell proliferation. Of the different vitamin E isomers, Osakada et al. (2004) recently found α-tocotrienol exhibited the most potent antiapoptotic neuroprotective effect on CNS neurons. These effects were attributed to its nonantioxidant

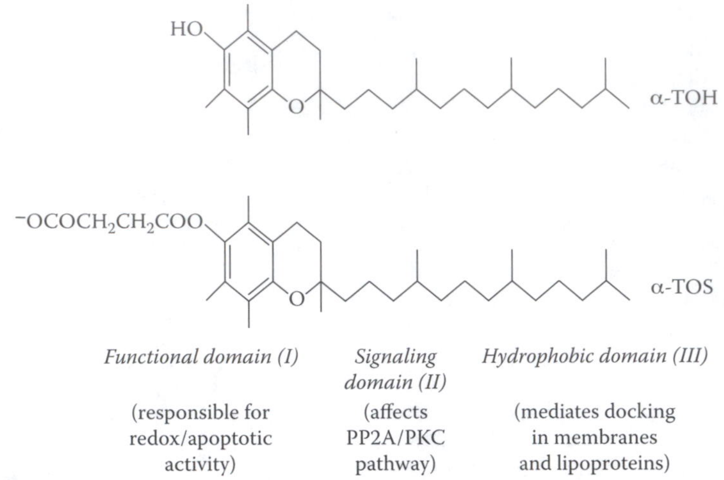

SCHEME V.67 in vitamin E (α-TOH) and vitamin E analog (α-TOS).

α-TOH

α-TOS

Functional domain (I)	Signaling domain (II)	Hydrophobic domain (III)
(responsible for redox/apoptotic activity)	(affects PP2A/PKC pathway)	(mediates docking in membranes and lipoproteins)

SCHEME V.67 Functional domains in vitamin E (α-TOH) and vitamin E analog (α-TOS). (From Birringer et al., *Br. J. Cancer,* 88:1948–1955, 2003. With permission.)

function and could also explain the beneficial effects of vitamin E, such as α-tocopherol, in treating Alzheimer's disease (Sano et al., 1997; Morris et al., 1998). Since neurodegenerative disorders involve both oxidative stress and apoptosis of neurons, these vitamin E isomers may play an important role in treating these diseases.

Epidemiological and intervention studies examining the possible role of vitamin E in cancer prevention found little or no association between disease incidence and vitamin E intake (Albanes et al., 1996, 2000; Heart Protection Study Collaborative Group, 2002). While vitamin E supplementation can be manipulated, it is limited by the hepatic system, which maintains the circulating/tissue levels within a narrow range by preventing both hypervitaminosis and hypovitaminosis. In addition, Neuzil et al. (1999) suggested that the lack of anticancer properties in vitamin E were due to its biological activity as a redox-active substance, which does not cause apoptosis of malignant cells. However, a new class of vitamin E analogs, such as α-tocopheryl succinate (α-TOS), was identified as effective antineoplastic agents with high selectivity for malignant cells and low toxicity (Birringer et al., 2003; Neuzil et al., 2001a, b, 2004; Jha et al., 1999). α-Tocopheryl succinate also efficiently killed cancer cells deficient in tumor-suppressor genes p53 and p21 [Wafl/Cipl] (Weber et al., 2002). As shown in Scheme V.67, vitamin E can be divided into three distinct

functional domains (Neuzil et al., 2002). Domain I, which involves the hydroxyl group in position C6 of the chromanol ring, is required for redox activity. However, α-TOH does not induce apoptosis even when acetylated at C6 (Neuzil et al., 2001a).

Succinylation at the C6 position, however, makes it (α-TOS) a strong apoptogen (Neuzil et al., 2001b). Further modifications, such as replacing the succinyl group with a maleyl group, enhanced apoptotic activity, while methylation of the succinyl group removed this property (Birringer et al., 2003). Extensive studies have since established the efficacy of these vitamin E analogs as anticancer agents, including their recent, novel treatment of fatal human malignant mesothelioma and breast cancer (Tomasetti et al., 2004; Wang et al., 2005).

References

Abidi, S.L. and Rennick, K.A., Capillary electro-chromatographic evaluation of vitamin E-active oil constituents: tocopherols and tocotrienols, *J. Chromatogr. A,* 913:379–386, 2001.

Albanes, D., Heinonen, O.P., Taylor, P.R., Virtamo, J., Edwards, B.K., Rautalahti, M., Hartman, A.M., Palmgren, J., Freedman, L.S., Haapakoski, J., Barret, M.J., Pietinen, P., Malila, N., Tala, E., Erozan, Y., Greenwald, P., and Huttunen, J.K., Tocopherol and β-carotene cancer prevention study: effects of baseline characteristics and study compliance, *J. Natl. Cancer Inst.,* 88:1560–1570, 1996.

Albanes, D., Malila, N., Taylor, P.R., Huttunen, J.K., Virtamo, J., Edwards, B.K., Rautalahti, M., Hartman, A.M., Barret, M.J., Pietinen, P., Hartman, T.J., Sipponen, P., Lewin, K., Teerenhovi, L., Hietanen, P., Tangrea, J.A., Virtanen, M., and Heinonen, O.P., Effects of supplemental α-tocopherol and β-carotene on colorectal cancer: results from a controlled trial, *Cancer Causes Cont.,* 11:197–205, 2000.

Azzi, A. and Stocker, A., Vitamin E: non-antioxidant roles, *Prog. Lipid Res.,* 39:231–255, 2000.

Birringer, M., Ey Tina, J.H., Salvatore, B.A., and Neuzil, J., Vitamin E analogs as inducers of apoptosis: structure-function relation, *Br. J. Cancer,* 88: 1948–1955, 2003.

Chao, J.C.-J., Yuan, M.-D., Chen, P.-Y., and Chien, S.-W., Vitamin C and E supplements improve the impaired antioxidant status and decrease plasma lipid peroxides in hemodialysis patients, *J. Nutr. Biochem.,* 13:653–663, 2002.

Clermont, G., Lecour, S., Cabanne, J.-F., Motte, G., Guilland, J.-C., Chevet, D., and Rochette, L., Vitamin E-coated dialyzer reduces oxidative stress in hemodialysis patients, *Free Rad. Biol. Med.,* 31:233–241, 2001.

Fariss, M.W. and Zhang, J.-G., Vitamin E therapy in Parkinson's disease, *Toxicology,* 189:129–146, 2003.

Heart Protection Study Collaborative Group, MRC/BHF Heart Protection study of antioxidant vitamin supplementation in 20,536 high risk individuals: a randomized placebo-controlled trial, *Lancet,* 360:23–33, 2002.

Hensley, K., Benakas, E.J., Bolli, R., Comp, P., Grammas, P., Hamdhekdari, L., Mou, S., Pye, Q.N., Stoddard, M.F., Wallis, G., Williamson, K.S., West, M., Wechter, W.J., and Floyd, R.A., New perspectives on vitamin E: γ-tocopherol and carboxyethylchroman metabolites in biology and medicine, *Free Rad. Bol. Med.,* 36:1–15, 2004.

Jha, M.N., Bedford, J.S., Cole, W.C., Edward-Prasad, J., and Prasad, K.N., Vitamin (d-α-tocopheryl succinate) decreases mitotic accumulation in g-irradiated human tumor, but not in normal cells, *Nutr. Cancer,* 35:189–194, 1999.

Morris, M.C., Beckeet, L.A., Scherr, P.A., Herbert, L.E., Bennett, D.A., Field, T.S., and Evans, D.A., Vitamin E and vitamin C supplement use and risk of incident of Alzheimer's disease, *Dis. Assoc. Disord.,* 12:121–126, 1998.

Neuzil, J., Kagedal, K., Andera, L., Weber, C., and Brunk, U.T., Vitamin E analogs: A new class of multiple action agents: anti-neoplastic and anti-atherogenic activity, *Apoptosis,* 7:177–185, 2002a.

Neuzil, J., Weber, T., Gellent, N., and Weber, C., Selective cancer cell killing by α-tocopheryl succinate, *Br. J. Cancer,* 84:87–89, 2001b.

Neuzil, J., Schroeder, A., von Hundelshausen, P., Zerrecke, A., Weber, T., Gellent, N., and Weber, C., Inhibition of inflammatory endothelial responses by a pathway involving caspase activation and p65 cleavage, *Biochem.,* 40:4686–4692, 2001a.

Neuzil, J., Weber, T., Schroeder, A., Lu, M., Ostermann, G., Gellent, N., Mayne, G.C., Olejnicka, B., Negre-Salvayre, A., Sticha, M., Coffrey, R.J., and Weber, C., Induction of apoptosis in cancer cells by α-tocopheryl succinate: molecular pathways and structural requirement, *FASEB,* 15:403–415, 2001c.

Neuzil, J., Svensson, J., Weber, T., Weber, C., and Brunk, U.T., α-Tocopheryl succinate-induced apoptosis of Jurkat T cells involves caspase-3 activation, and both lysosomal and mitochondrial destabilization, *FEBS Lett.,* 445:295–300, 1999.

Osakada, F., Hashino, A., Kume, T., Katsuki, H., Kaneko, S., and Akaike, A., α-Tocotrienol provides the most potent neuroprotection among vitamin E analogs on cultured striatal neurons, *Neuropharmacology,* 47:904–915, 2004.

Roghani, M. and Behzadi, G., Neuroprotective effect of vitamin E on the early model of Parkinson's disease in rat: behavioral and histochemical evidence, *Brain Res.,* 892:211–217, 2001.

Sano, M., Ernesto, C., Thomas, R.G., Klauber, M.R., Schafer, K., Grundman, M., Woodbury, P., Growdon, J., Cotman, C.W., Pfeiffer, E., Schneider, L.S., and Thal, L.J., A controlled trial of selegiline, alpha-tocopherol, or both as treatment for Alzheimer's disease, *N. Eng. J. Med.,* 336:1216–1222, 1997.

Tomasetti, M., Rippo, M.R., Alleva, R., Moretti, S., Andera, L., Neuzil, J., and Procopio, A., α-Tocopheryl succinate and TRAIL selectivity synergise in induction of apoptosis in human malignant meothelioma cells, *Br. J. Cancer,* 90:1644–1653, 2004.

Wang, X.-F., Witting, P.K., Salvatore, B.A., and Neuzil, J., Vitamin E analogs trigger apoptosis in HER2/erbB2-overexpressing breast cancer cells by signaling via the mitochondrial pathway, *Biochem. Biophys. Res. Commun.,* 326:282–289, 2005.

Weber, T., Lu, M., Andera, L., Lahm, H., Gellert, N., Farris, M.W., Korinek, V., Sattler, W., Ucker, D.S., Terman, A., Schroder, A., Erl, W., Brunk, U.T., Coffrey, R.J., Weber, C., and Neuzil, J., Vitamin E succinate is a potent novel anti-neoplastic agent with high tumor selectivity and cooperativity with tumor necrosis factor-related apoptosis-inducing ligand (Apo 2 ligand) *in vivo*, *Clin. Cancer Res.*, 8:863–869, 2002.

Vitamin K *see also* **Menadione**   Vitamin K is a family of fat-soluble vitamins with a number of important biological functions, including the formation of prothrombin and other blood-clotting factors. It is not a single compound but a group of quinones based on their source of origin. For example, phylloquinones (vitamin K_1) are found in plants, menaquinones (vitamin K_2) are synthesized by bacteria, while synthetic forms of vitamin K include menadione (K_3) (Scheme V.68). Leafy, green vegetables are good sources of vitamin K, which is also synthesized by bacteria in the small intestine. The presence of glutamic-acid residues in prothrombin (factor II) and other blood-clotting factors VII,

IX, and X requires vitamin K for their carboxylation. This converts glutamic acid to γ-carboxyglutamic, enabling it to bind calcium, an essential step in the blood-clotting process (Furie and Furie, 1988, 1990).

In addition to their important physiological role, vitamins K_1 and K_2 were also found to inhibit the growth of a hepatoma cell line Hep 3B (Wang et al., 1995). The low potency of the natural vitamins, however, led Wang et al. (1995) to synthesize 2-(2-mercapto-ethanol)-3-methyl-1,4-napthoquinone, a vitamin K analog with 20 times the potency against Hep 3B cells. Inhibition of the induction of extracellular signal-regulated kinase (ERK) phosphorylation by this analog appeared to be one of the mechanisms involved in the apoptosis of rat hepatocytes (Wang et al., 2002). Ge et al. (2004) recently showed that mediation of c-Myc phosphorylation by this vitamin K analog resulted in enhancement of c-Myc protein degradation and reduced c-Myc protein levels, which may contribute to inhibition of the cell growth of human Hep 3B hepatoma lines.

Vitamin K_3 or menadione (2-methyl-1,4-napthaquinone) has been used together with

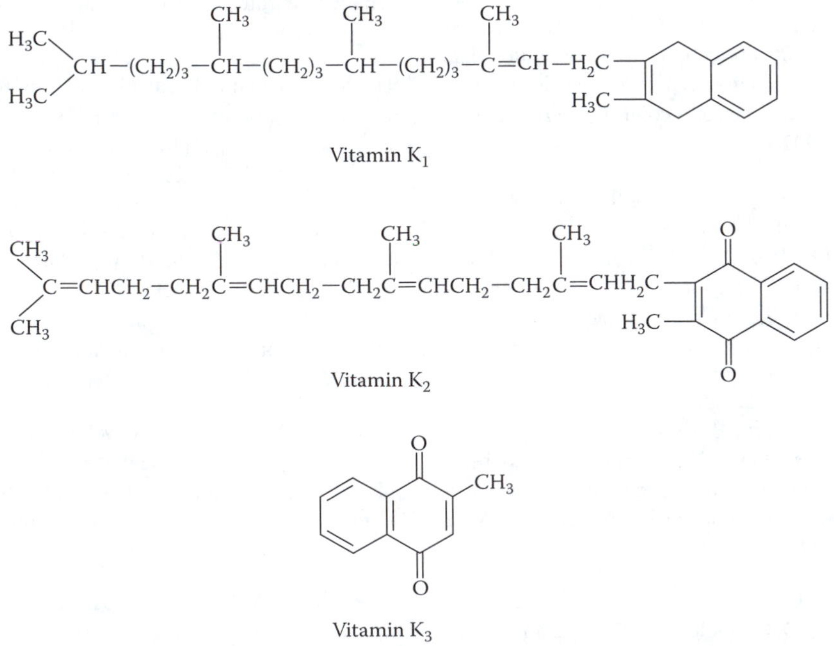

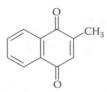

Vitamin K_1

Vitamin K_2

Vitamin K_3

SCHEME V.68 Structures of vitamins K_1 and K_2. (From Serfis and Katzenberger, Colloids and Surfaces, A., *Physicochem. Eng. Aspects*, 138:91–95, 1998. With permission.)

chemotherapeutic agents to treat cancers (Tetef et al., 1995). More recent studies by McAmis et al. (2003) showed menadione caused oxidative stress and endothelial-cell cytotoxicity by altering intracellular thiols rather than increasing the amount of reactive-oxygen species (ROS). When vitamin C and vitamin K_3 were administered in a ratio of 100:1, synergistic antitumor activity was observed, in which the tumor cells were killed by a novel type of necrosis, autoschizis (Jamison et al., 2002). The latter is characterized by membrane damage and progressive loss of organelle-free cytoplasm.

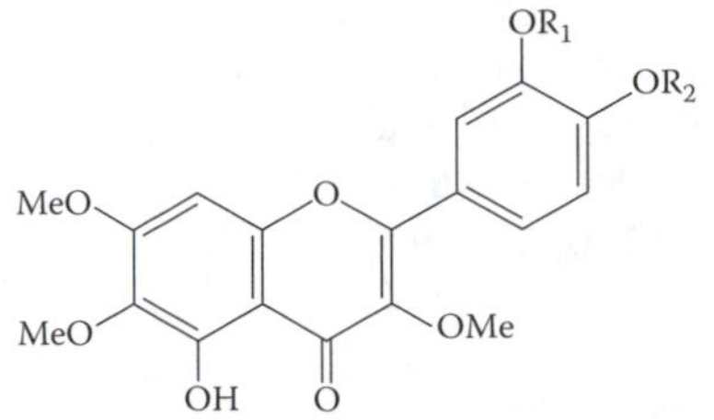

Compounds	R_1	R_2
2',3',5'-trihydroxy-3,6,7-trimethoxyflavone (Vx-1)	OH	OH
Vitexicarpin (Vx-5)	OH	OMe
Arternetin (Vx-6)	OMe	OMe

SCHEME V.69 Structural formulae of the polymethoxy-flavonoids isolated from *V. rotundifolia*. (From Ko et al., *Food Chem. Toxicol.*, 38:861–865, 2000. With permission.)

Vitex rotundifolia *Vitex rotundifolia* or Beach vitex, is a plant native to the Pacific region with silvery-green, rounded leaves and purple flowers over the summer. During the winter, however, the plant remains dormant, producing berries. It has been traditionally used in Asia to treat colds, headaches, migraine, sore eyes, and myalgia (But et al., 1996). A polymethoxyflavonoid, vitocarpin, was isolated from *V. rotundifolia* by You et al. (1998), which inhibited the proliferation of lymphocyte and the growth of some cancer cells.

Further work by Ko et al. (2000) isolated three polymethoxyflavonoids from the fruit of *V. rotundifolia*, which were characterized as 2',3',5'-trihydroxy-3,6,7 trimethoxy-flavone (Vx-1), vitexicarpin (Vx-5), and artemetin (Vx-6) (Scheme V.69). These compounds all inhibited proliferation of human myeloid leukemia (HL-60) cells by inducing apoptosis.

References

Furie, B. and Furie, C. M., Molecular basis of vitamin-K-dependent γ-carboxylation, *Blood*, 75:1753–1762, 1990.

Furie, B. and Furie, C., Vitamin K-dependent biosynthesis of g-carboxyglutamatic acid, *Blood*, 75: 1753–1762, 1990.

Ge, L., Wang, Z., Wang, M., Kar, S., and Carr, B.I., Involvement of c-Myc in growth inhibition of Hep 3B human hepatoma cells from a vitamin K analog, *J. Hepatol.*, 41:823–829, 2004.

Jamison, J.M., Gilloteaux, J., Taper, H.S., Calderon, P.B., and Summers, J.L., Autoschizis: a novel cell death, *Biochem. Pharmacol.*, 63:1773–1783, 2003.

McAmis, W.C., Schaeffer, R.C., Jr., Baynes, J.W., and Wolf, M.B., Menadione causes endothelial barrier failure by direct effect on intracellular thiols, independent of reactive oxidant production, *Biochem. Biophys. Acta*, 164:43–53, 2003.

Serfis, A.B. and Katzenberger, R., A comparison of the behavior of vitamin K_1 and K_2 monolayers at the air-water interface. Colloids and surfaces A, *Physicochem, Aspects*, 138:91–95, 1998.

Tetef, M., Margolin, K., Ahn, C., Ackman, S., Chow, W., Coluzzi, P., Hamasaki, V., Leon, L., Morgan, R.J. Jr., Rascho, J., Shibata, S., Somlo, G., Yen, Y., and Doroshow, J.H., Mitomycin C and menadione for the treatment of Jung cancer. A phase II trial, *Invest. New Drugs*, 13:157–162, 1995.

Wang, Z., Wang, M., Finn, F., and Carr, B.I., The growth inhibitory effects of vitamins K and their actions on gene expression, *Hepatol.*, 22:876–881, 1995.

Wang, Z., Nishikawa, Y., Wang, M., and Carr, B.I., Induction of apoptosis via mitogen-activated protein kinase pathway by a K vitamin analog in rat hepatocytes, *J. Hepatol.*, 36:85–92, 2002.

References

But, P.P.H., Guo, J.X., and Sung, C.K., *International Collation of Traditional and Folk Medicine*, World Scientific Publishing, Singapore, 1998, p. 141.

Ko, W.G., Kang, T.H., Lee, S.J., Kim, N.Y., Kim, Y.C., Sohn, D.H., and Lee, B.H., Polymethoxyflavonoids from *Vitex rotundifolia* inhibit proliferation by inducing apoptosis in human myeloid leukemia cells, *Food Chem. Toxicol.*, 38:861–865, 2000.

V

You, K.M., Son, K.H., Chang, H.W., Kang, S.S., and Kim, H.P., Vitexicarpin, a flavonoid from the fruits of *Vitex rotundifolia*, inhibits mouse lymphocyte proliferation and growth of cell lines *in vitro*, *Planta Med.*, 64:546–550, 1998.

Vulgin   Ye and Ng (2001) identified an antifungal polypeptide from pinto beans with a molecular weight of 5 kDa and a sequence homology to cowpea. This polypeptide, subsequently referred to as vulgin, had an N-terminal sequence with some similarities to chitinases (Ye and Ng, 2003) These researchers also found vulgin inhibited HIV-1 reverse transcriptase activity, with an IC_{50} of 58 mM.

References

Ye, X.Y. and Ng, T.B., Peptides from pinto bean and red bean with sequence of homology to cowpea 10 kDa protein precursor exhibit antifungal, mitogenic and HIV-1 reverse transcriptase-inhibitory activities, *Biochem. Biophys. Res. Commun.*, 285:424–429, 2001.

Ye, X.Y. and Ng, T.B., Isolation of vulgin, a new antifungal polypeptide with mitogenic activity from P into bean, *J. Peptide Sci.*, 9:114–119, 2003.

V

W

Walnuts Walnuts, the seeds of *Juglans regia* L., have been used as a folk medicine in Europe and Asia for treating coughs and stomach ache (Perry, 1980) and cancer (Duke, 1989). Hu et al. (1998) showed that frequent consumption of nuts may offer some protection from coronary heart disease. Nuts, such as walnuts, are relatively high in polyunsaturated fatty acids, particularly omega-3 fatty acids. Iwamoto and coworkers (2000) examined the effect of walnuts on the serum cholesterol of Japanese men and women. A moderate intake of walnuts of 43–57 g/d, equivalent to 12.5 percent of energy, significantly reduced LDL cholesterol levels in both Japanese men and women by 0.18 mmol/L and 0.22 mmol/L, respectively. The ratio of LDL to HDL cholesterol was also significantly lowered, as was the apolipoprotein B concentration. A subsequent study by Almario et al. (2001) confirmed the ability of walnuts to beneficially reduce LDL cholesterol in patients with combined hyperlipidemia. Another study by Iwamoto et al. (2002) confirmed that a diet containing 44–58 g/day of walnuts fed to normal Japanese men and women lowered serum cholesterol, as well as had a beneficial effect on lipoproteins. In addition to lowering cholesterol, Ros and coworkers (2004) found that substituting walnuts for monounsaturated fat in a Mediterranean diet also improved endothelium vasodilation in hypercholesterolemic subjects. This suggested that the benefits of nuts went beyond just lowering cholesterol.

In addition to the oil, a polyphenolic-rich walnut extract containing ellagic acid, gallic acid, and flavonoids was shown by Anderson et al. (2001) to be a potent antioxidant by inhibiting oxidation of human plasma and LDL *in vitro*. The presence of ellagic acid suggested to Fukuda et al. (2003) the possible presence of tannins, such as ellagitannins. These researchers isolated a number of tannins from the butanol extract of walnut, including three hydrolyzable tannins, glansrins A–C, together with 13 known tannins. Glansrins A–C proved to be ellagitannins, with a tergalloyl or related poly-phenolic acyl group. Fukuda et al. (2003) demonstrated the antioxidant properties of these polyphenols by their SOD-like and radical-scavenging activities. A recent study by Kearny et al. (2004) showed that a diet enriched with 64 g/day of walnuts fed to hypercholesterolemic patients over six weeks significantly reduced total cholesterol (–5 percent) and LDL cholesterol (–9 percent). An additional trend observed was a 20 percent reduction in the large VLDL particle subclass. This study further demonstrated the cardiovascular health benefits of a daily diet enriched with walnuts.

References

Almario, R.U., Vonghavaravat, V., Wong, R., and Kasim-Karakas, S.E., Effect of walnut consumption on plasma fatty acids and lipoproteins in combined hyperlipidemia, *Am. J. Clin. Nutr.,* 74:72–79, 2001.

Anderson, K.J., Teuber, S.S., Gobielle, A., Cremin, P., Waterhouse, A.L., and Steinberg, F.M., Walnut polyphenolics inhibit *in vitro* human plasma and LDL oxidation, *J. Nutr.,* 131:2837–2842, 2001.

Feldman, E.B., The scientific evidence for a beneficial health relationship between walnuts and coronary heart disease, *J. Nutr.,* 132:1062–1101, 2002.

Fukuda, T., Ito, H., and Yoshida, T., Antioxidative polyphenols from walnuts (*Juglans regia* L.), *Phytochemistry,* 63:795–801, 2003.

Hu, F.B., Sampfer, M.J., Manson, J.E., Colditz, G.A., Rimm, E.B., Rosner, B.A., Speizer, F.E., Hennekens, C.H., and Willett, W.C., Frequent nut consumption and risk of coronary heart disease in women: prospective cohort study, *Br. J. Med. J.,* 317:1341–1345, 1998.

Iwamoto, M., Imaizumi, K., Hirooka, Y., Sakai, K., Takeshit, A., and Kono, M., Serum lipid profiles in Japanese women and men during consumption of walnuts, *Eur. J. Clin. Nutr.,* 56:629–637, 2002.

W

Iwamoto, M., Sato, M., Kono, M., Hirooka, Y., Sakai, K., Takeshita, A., and Imaizumi, K., Walnuts lower serum cholesterol in Japanese men and women, *J. Nutr.,* 130:171–176, 2000.

Kearny, D., Dulaney, K., Carey, C., Capuzzi, and Morgan, J., Effects of walnut consumption as part of a heart healthy diet on atherogenic lipoprotein subclasses, *J. Am. Dietet. Assoc.,* 104(Suppl. 2):20, 2004.

Ros, E., Nunez, I., Perez-Heras, A., Serra, M., Gilabert, R., Casals, E., and Deulofeu, R., A walnut diet improves endothelial function in hypercholesterolemic subjects: A randomized crossover trial. *Circulation,* 109:1609–1614, 2004.

Wasabi (*Wasabia japonica*)   Wasabi, a member of the Japanese horseradish family with a number of important, health-related compounds, is usually served as a condiment with Japanese cuisine. Sinigrin was shown by Yu et al. (2001) to be the main, sulfur-containing species in wasabi initially hydrolyzed by myrosinase, followed by a nonenymatic step, the Lossen rearrangement, to form isothiocyanates (Scheme W.70). Yano et al. (2000) showed isothiocyanate, 6-methylthiohexyl isothiocyanate (6MHITC), isolated from wasabi inhibited 4-(methylnitrosamino)-1-(3-pyridyl)-1-butanone (NNK)-induced lung tumorigenesis in mice, suppressing the initiation phase, that is

the formation of O^6-methylguanine (O^6MG) (Figure W.99). O^6MG is a promutagen adduct formed from activation of NNK via a-hydroxylation. 6MHIT significantly reduced the level of O^6MG by 55 percent, very similar to the control containing phenylethyl isothiocyanate.

Morimitsu and coworkers (2000) isolated 6-methylsulfinylhexyl isothiocyanate from wasabi and showed it possessed antiplatelet and anticancer properties. Subsequent work by Watanabe et al. (2003) identified the active component in an ethanol extract capable of inducing apoptosis as 6-methylsulfinylhexyl isothiocyanate by its ability to inhibit the cell growth of human monoblastic leukemia U937 cells.

Shin et al. (2004) recently observed the bactericidal properties of wasabi against *Helicobacter pylori*. In addition to allyl isothiocyante, several other components were also responsible for the effectiveness of wasabi.

References

Morimitsu, Y., Hayashi, K., Nakagawa, Y., Fujii, H., Horio, F., Uchida, K., and Osawa, T., Antiplatelet and anticancer isothiocyanates in Japanese domestic horseradish, Wasabi, *Mech. Aging Develop.,* 116: 125–134, 2000.

Shin, I.S., Masuda, H., and Naohide, K., Bacteriocidal activity of wasabi (*Wasabia japonica*) against *Helicobacter pylori, Inter. J. Food Microbiol.,* 94: 255–261, 2004.

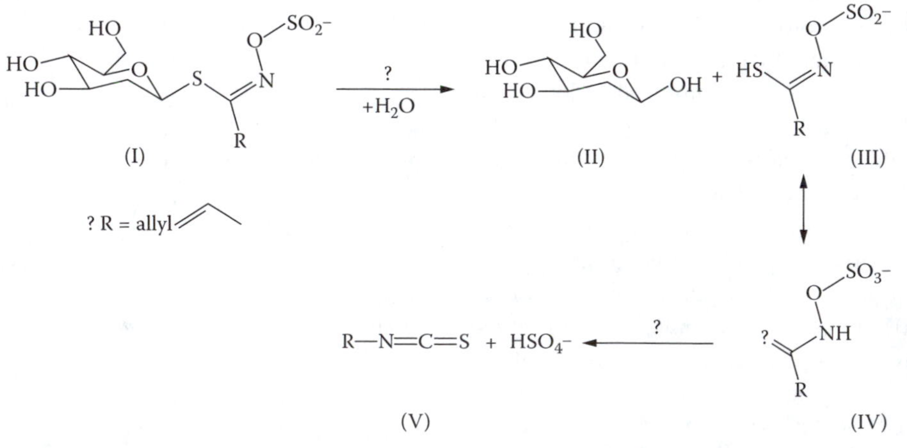

SCHEME W.70 Degradation of β-D-*S*-glucosides (I) by myrosinase (β-thioglucoside glucohydrolase) and related biochemistry. The initial hydrolysis of (I) yields glucose (II) and (III), which will be in equilibrium with (IV), is then thought to undergo a Lossen rearrangement to produce the isothiocyanate (V) and sulfate. (From Yu et al., *Biochim. Biophys. Acta,* 1527:156–160, 2001.)

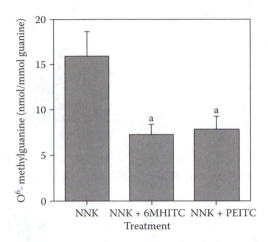

FIGURE W.99 The effect of 6MHITC treatment on pulmonary O^6-methyl guanine level in mice treated with NNK. Values are expressed as the mean ± SE from five mice. (a) Significantly different from the NNK-treated group ($p < 0.05$). (From Yano et al., *Cancer Lett.,* 155:115–120, 2000. With permission.)

Watanabe, M., Ohata, M., Hayakawa, S., Isemura, M., Kumazawa, S., Nayakama, T., Furugori, M., and Kinae, N., Identification of 6-methtylsulfinylhexyl isothiocyanate as an apoptosis-inducing component in wasabi, *Phytochemistry,* 62:733–739, 2003.

Yano, T., Yajima, S., Virgona, N., Yano, Y., Otani, S., Kumagai, H., Sakurai, M., and Ichikawa, T., The effect of 6-methylthiohexyl isothiocyanate isolated from *Wasabia japonica* (wasabi) on 4-(methylnitrosamino)-1-(3-pyridyl)-1-(butanone-induced lung tumorigenesis in mice, *Cancer Lett.,* 155:115–120, 2000.

Yu, E.Y., Pickering, I.J., George, G.N., and Prince, R.C., *In situ* observation of the generation of isothiocyanates from sinigrin in horseradish and wasabi, *Biochem. Biophys. Acta,* 1527:156–160, 2001.

Wheat bran Wheat bran was shown to decrease the mucosal formation of aberrant crypt foci, an important marker for determining the efficacy of colon cancer preventative agents (Earnest et al., 1999). In fact, wheat bran was found to be the most effective fiber for protecting against colon cancer. Whether this was related to fermentation of the fiber and the release of short-chain fatty acids, particularly butyric acid, a known inhibitor of tumor growth, remains unclear. Zile and coworkers (1998) also showed that inclusion of wheat bran suppressed mammary-gland tumorigenesis in experimental animals. Wheat dietary fiber comprises less than

wheat bran, so that other nutrients besides dietary fiber may also protect against cancer. Such components were thought to be phenolic acids, lignans, and flavonoids (Ferguson and Harris, 1999). The effectiveness of different dietary components, wheat bran (WB), curcumin (CUR), rutin (RUT), and benzyl isothiocyanate (BIT), on the formation aberrant crypt foci (ACF), colorectal tumors, and selected gene expression in azoxymethane-treated F344 rats were compared by Wijnands et al. (2004). Of the different dietary components, only WB and CUR protected against colorectal cancer compared to RUT and BIT.

Wheat bran has also been associated with considerable antioxidant activity due to the concentration of phenolics in the bran portion of the grain (Zhou and Yu, 2004). Bran extracts of hard wheat varieties, Akron and Trego, grown at three different locations in Colorado, were shown by Yu et al. (2004) to significantly reduce lipid peroxidation in human LDL *in vitro*. They also found that the bran absorbed oxygen radicals, with the potential of preventing them from attacking biological molecules. Yuan et al. (2004) showed that the water-soluble feruloyl oligosaccharides in the insoluble dietary fiber of wheat bran scavenged 2,2-diphenyl-1-picrylhydrazine (DPPH) free radicals, as well as inhibited oxidative hemolysis of rat erythrocytes induced by 2,2-azobis-2-amidinopropane dihydrochloride (AAPH) by 91.7 percent.

Thus, incorporation of wheat-bran products may provide functional foods capable of preventing atherosclerosis and related diseases, as well as a new source of natural antioxidants.

References

Earnest, D.L., Einspahr, J.G., and Alberts, D.S., Protective role of wheat bran fiber: data from marker trials, *Am. J. Med.*, 106:32S–37S, 1999.

Ferguson, L. and Harris, P.J., Protection against cancer by wheat bran: role of dietary fiber and phytochemicals, *Eur. J. Cancer Prev.*, 8(Suppl. 1):17–25, 1999.

Wijnands, M.V.W., van Erk, M.J., Doorbos, R.P., Krul, C.A.M., and Woutersen, R.A., Do aberrant crypt foci have predictive value for the occurrence of colorectal tumors? Potential of gene expression profiling tumors, *Food Chem. Toxicol.*, 42:1629–1639, 2004.

Yu, L., Zhou, K., and Parry, J.W., Inhibitory effects of wheat bran extracts on human LDL oxidation and free radicals, *Lebensm.-Wiss. U.-Technol.*, 38:463–470, 2005.

Yuan, X., Wang, J., Yao, H., and Chen, F., Free radical-scavenging capacity and inhibitory activity on rat erythrocyte hemolysis of feruloyl oligosaccharides from wheat bran insoluble dietary fiber, *Lebensm.-Wiss U.-Technol.*, 38:877–883, 2005.

Zhou, K. and Yu, L., Effects of extraction solvent on wheat bran antioxidant activity estimation. *Lebensm.-Wiss U.-Technol.*, 37:717–721m, 2004.

Zile, M.H., Welsch, C.W., and Welsch, M.A., Effect of wheat bran on the development of mammary tumors in female mice intact and ovariectomized treated with 7,12-dimethylbenz(a)anthracene and in mice with spontaneously developing mammary tumors, *Int. J. Cancer*, 75:439–443, 1998.

Wheat flour   Whole-wheat flour was reported by Adam and coworkers (2001) to lower plasma and hepatic lipids in rats. Since whole-wheat flour is normally consumed in a processed product, such as bread, Adams et al. (2003) showed breadmaking (fermentation, starch gelatinization, heating) had a hypolipidemic effect compared to native whole-wheat flour. Rats fed a semipurified diet containing 70 percent whole-wheat flour (WWF) or 70 percent desiccated whole-wheat bread (WWB) had significantly ($p < 0.05$) lower plasma and liver

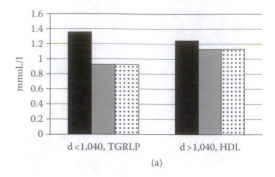

(a)

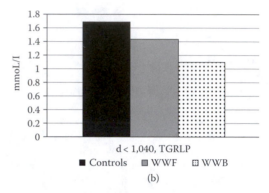

(b)

FIGURE W.100 Differences in the repartition of cholesterol (panel a) in plasma lipoprotein fractions of rats fed the control, WWF, and WWB diets. Each value is a mean of triplicate analyses of a pool of plasma. The fractions with a density of less than 1.040 kg/L corresponded to triacylglycerol-rich lipoproteins with a lower contribution of LDL. The fractions with a density higher than 1.040 kg/L corresponded essentially to HDL. (From Adam et al., *Food Chem.*, 80:337–344, 2003. With permission.)

cholesterol levels compared to a control fiber-free starch diet. A closer examination of the plasma lipoproteins showed the triacylglycerol fraction (TGRLP, d < 1.040 kg/L) was 33 percent lower in animals fed WWF or WWB diets compared to the control, accounting for decreases of 14 percent and 24 percent, respectively. No differences were evident in the HDL fraction (Figure W.100). Total steroid excretion was significantly ($p < 0.01$) higher in the cereal diets, but was higher with the WWB diet. This corresponded to a reduction in cholesterol absorption of 26 percent for WWB compared to 38 percent and 52 percent for the WWF and control diets.

References

Adam, A., Levrat-Verny, M-A., Lopez, H.W., Leuillet, M., Demigne, C., and Remesy, C., Whole wheat and triticale flours with different viscosities stimulate cecal fermentations and lower plasma and hepatic lipid in rats, *J. Nutr.,* 131:1770–1776, 2001.

Adam, A., Lopez, H.W., Leuillet, M., Demigne, C., and Remesy, C., Whole wheat flour exerts cholesterol-lowering in rats in its native form and after use in bread-making, *Food Chem.,* 80:337–344, 2003.

Whey *see also* α-Lactalbumin and Lactoferrin

The whey fraction of bovine milk is rich source of immunomodulators, including the β-lactoglobulin, α-lactalbumin, lactoferrin, lactoperoxidase, and such tissue growth factors as TGF-β (Buonous et al., 1981; Stoeck et al., 1986; Dababbi et al., 1998; Wong et al., 1997, 1998). The unique immunomodulatory properties of a whey-protein concentrate (WPC) obtained from rennet casein whey was shown by Low et al. (2001) to markedly increase the intestinal-tract antibody responses in BALB/c mice over a 12-week period. Further research by Low and coworkers (2003) showed WPC increased humoral immune response in BALB/c mice immunized with such antigens as influenza virus, diphtheria, tetanus toxoids, poliomyelitis vaccine, ovalbumin, and cholera toxin subunit. The ability of dietary WPC to boost immune response in mice may be applicable for boosting postvaccination in humans, especially in children and the elderly with suboptimal immunity.

Tong et al. (2000) examined the antioxidant activity of a high-molecular-weight (HMW) fraction from whey. Using a salmon-oil emulsion, the antioxidant activity of the HMW fraction appeared dependent on the availability of sulfhydryl groups. However, even when the sulfhydryl groups were blocked, whey proteins still exhibited significant antioxidant activity. This was attributed to the scavenging activity of other amino acids in whey proteins by the HMW fraction's ability to scavenge peroxyl radicals generated by β-PE decay. An additional antioxidant mechanism of whey proteins was reported to be metal chelation.

References

Bounous, G., Stevenson, M.M., and Kongshavn, P.A.L., Influence of dietary α-lactalbumin hydrolysate on the immune system of mice and resistance to salmonellosis, *J. Infect. Dis.,* 144:281, 1981.

Debabbi, H., Dubarry, M., Rautureau, M., and Tome, D., Bovine lactoferrin induces both mucosal and systemic immune responses in mice, *J. Dairy Res.,* 65: 283–293, 1998.

Low, P.P.L., Rutherfurd, K.J., Gill, H.S., and Gross, M.L., Effect of dietary whey protein concentrate on primary and secondary antibody responses in immunized BALB/c mice, *Int. Immunopharmacol.,* 3:393–401, 2003.

Low, P.P.L., Rutherfurd, K.J., Gross, M.L., and Gill, H.S., Enhancement of mucosal antibody responses by dietary whey protein concentrate, *Food Agric. Immunol.,* 13:255–264, 2001.

Stoeck, M., Ruegg, V., Miescher, S., Carrel, S., Cox, D., van Fliedner, V., and Alkanis, Comparison of the immunosuppressive properties of milk growth factor and transforming growth factors β1 and β2, *J. Immunol.,* 143:3258–3265, 1989.

Tong, L.M., Sasaki, S., McClements, D.J., and Decker, E.A., Mechanisms of the antioxidant activity of a high molecular weight fraction of whey, *J. Agric. Food Chem.,* 48:1473–1478, 2000.

Wong, C.W., Seow, H.F., Husband, A.J., Regester, G.O., and Watson, D.L., Effects of purified bovine whey factors on cellular immune functions in ruminants, *Vet. Immunol. Immunopathol.,* 56:85–96, 1997.

Wong, K.F., Middleton, N., Montgomery, M., Dey, M., and Carr, R.I., Immunostimulation of murine spleen cells by materials associated with bovine milk protein fractions, *J. Dairy Sci.,* 81:1825–1835, 1998.

Wheat germ

A commercial wheat germ was enzymically hydrolyzed by Arrigoni et al. (2002) and then subjected to fermentation with fresh human feces under anaerobic conditions. The short-chain fatty acids produced were high in proprionates, suggesting wheat germ behaved as a prebiotic by its support of bifidobacteria.

References

Arrigoni, E., Jorger, F., Kolloffel, B., Roulet, I., Herenspeger, M., Meile, L., and Amado, R., *In vitro* fermentability of a commercial wheat germ preparation and its impact on the growth of bifidobacteria, *Food Res. Intern.,* 35:475–481, 2002.

Whole grains *see also* **Wheat, Barley, Maize or Corn, Millet, Oats, Sorghum, and Triticale**

Epidemiological evidence supports an inverse relationship between consumption of cereal fiber or whole grains and type 2 diabetes (Meyer et al., 2000; Liu et al., 2000; Salmeron et al., 1997a, b), cardiovascular disease (Jacobs et al., 1998, 1999), and total mortality (Jacobs et al., 1998, 1999). Whole grains from cereals (wheat, rice, maize, oats, barley, triticale, sorghum, and millet) are rich in phytochemicals, such as dietary fiber, resistant starch, oligosaccharides, and phytoestrogens, some exhibiting anticarcinogenic activity (Slavin et al., 1999). Table W.63 summarizes the range of components and their health-related properties.

Phytoestrogens appear to play a role in reducing the risk of cardiovascular disease, diabetes, and some cancers. The regular consumption of whole grains significantly reduces the risk of coronary heart disease (Rimm et al., 1996; Jacobs et al., 1998; Liu et al., 1999). Jacobs and coworkers (2002) reported that whole-grain elevated serum enterolactone in hyperinsulinemic women. Previous studies showed that the risk of incidence of heart disease was reduced in Finnish men when serum enterolactone was in the upper quartile (Vanharanta et al., 1999). McKeown et al. (2002) reported that increased intake of whole grains had a favorable effect on the metabolic risk factors associated with cardiovascular disease and type 2 diabetes. Pereira and coworkers (2002) confirmed the improvement of insulin insensitivity in hyperinsulinemic and obese adults following the consumption of whole grains. A prospective study in men by Fung et al. (2002) also found that diets high in whole grains reduced the risk of type 2 diabetes and should replace refined grains.

TABLE W.63
Selected Components in Whole Grains and Their Postulated Mechanisms

Components	Antioxidant	Tumor Growth Suppressor	Enzyme Modulator	Binding ???????	Chemical	Cholesterol-lowering	Gut Modifier	Hormonal Effects
Dietary fiber			✔			✔	✔	✔
Oligosaccharides			✔	✔		✔	✔	
Flavonoids	✔	✔	✔					
Inositols	✔							
Lignin	✔							
n-3 Fatty acids		✔				✔		
Phenolics	✔	✔	✔					
Phytates	✔							
Phytoestrogens	✔	✔						✔
Protease inhibitor		✔						
Saponins		✔						
Selenium	✔	✔						
Tocopherol	✔		✔					
Zinc	✔				✔			

[1] Source: Adapted from Slavin et al. (1997) and Kohlmeier et al. (1995).
[2] Source: Taken from Slavin et al., *Am. J. Clin Nutr.* 70:459S–463S, 1999. With permission.

References

Fung, T.T., Hu, F.B., Pereira, M.A., Liu, S., Stampfer, M.J., Colditz, G.A., and Willett, W.C., Whole-grain intake and the risk of type 2 diabetes: a prospective study in men, *Am. J. Clin. Nutr.,* 76:535–540, 2002.

Jacobs, D.R., Jr., Meyer, K.A., Kushi, L.H., and Folsom, A.R., Whole-grain intake may reduce risk of ischemic heart disease death in postmenopausal women: Iowa Women's Health Study, *Am. J. Clin. Nutr.,* 68:248–257, 1998.

Jacobs, D.R., Pereira, M.A., Stumpf, K., Pins, J.J., and Adlecreutz, H., Whole grain food intake elevates serum enterolactone, *Br. J. Nutr.,* 88:111–116, 2002.

Kohlmeier, L., Simonsen, N., and Mohus, K., Dietary modifiers of carcinogenesis, *Environ. Health Perspect.,* 103(Suppl):177–184, 1995.

Liu, S., Stampfer, M.J., Hu, F.B., Giovannucci, E., Rimm, E., Manson, J.E., Hennekens, C.H., and Willett, W.C., Whole-grain consumption and risk of coronary heart disease: results from Nurses' Health Study, *Am. J. Clin. Nutr.,* 70:412–419, 1999.

Liu, S., Stampfer, M.J., and Hu, F.B., A prospective study of whole grain intake and risk of type 2 diabetes in women, *Am. J. Pub. Hlth.,* 90:1409–1415, 2000.

McKeown, N.M., Meigs, J.B., Liu, S., Wilson, P.W.F., and Jacques, P.F., Whole-grain intake is favorably associated with metabolic risk factors for type 2 diabetes and cardiovascular disease in the Framingham offspring study, *Am. J. Clin. Nutr.,* 76:390–398, 2002.

Meyer, K.A., Kushi, L.H., Jacobs, Jr., D.R., Slavin, J.S., Sellers, T.A., and Folsom, A.R., Carbohydrates, dietary fiber and incident of 2 diabetes in older women, *Am. J. Clin. Nutr.,* 71:921–930, 2000.

Pereira, M.A., Jacobs, D.A., Pins, J.J., Raatz, S.K., Gross, M.D., Slavin, J.L., and Seaquist, E.R., Effect of whole grains on insulin sensitivity in overweight, hyperinsulinemic adults, *Am. J. Clin. Nutr.,* 75:848–855, 2002.

Rimm, E.B., Ascherio, A., Giovannucci, E., Spiegelman, D., Stampfer, M.J., and Willett, W.C., Vegetable, fruit, and cereal intake and risk of coronary heart disease among men, *JAMA,* 275:447–451, 1996.

Salmeron, J., Ascherio, A., Rimm, E.B., Colditz, G.A., Spiegelman, D., Jenkins, D.J., Stampfer, M.J., Wing, A.L., and Willett, W.C., Dietary fiber, glycemic load, and risk of NIDDM in men, *Diabet. Care,* 20:545–550, 1997.

Salmeron, J., Manson, J.E., Stampfer, M.J., Colditz, G.A., Wing, A.L., and Willett, W.C., Dietary fiber, glycemic load and risk of non-insulin-dependent diabetes mellitus in women, *JAMA,* 277:472–477, 1997.

Slavin, J.L., Jacobs, D., and Marquart, L., Whole-grain consumption and chronic disease: protective mechanisms, *Nutr. Cancer,* 27:14–21, 1997.

Slavin, J.L., Martini, M.C., Jacobs, D.R., Jr., and Marquart, L., Plausible mechanisms for the protectiveness of whole grains, *Am. J. Clin. Nutr.,* 70:459S–463S, 1999.

Vanharanta, M., Voutilainen, S., Lakka, T.A., van der Lee, M., Adlecruetz, H., and Salonen, J.T., Risk of acute coronary events according to serum concentrations of enterolactone: a prospective population-based case-control study, *Lancet,* 354:2112–2115, 1999.

Wine *see also* **Red wines and Resveratrol**
The relationship between wine and cardiovascular disease arose from the fact that in certain parts of France, where people consumed greater amounts of animal fats, the incidence of cardiovascular disease was remarkably low compared to North America. This phenomenon, referred to as the "French Paradox," was subsequently attributed to the greater consumption of red wine. Frankel and coworkers (1993) showed it was the phenolics in wine that inhibited oxidation of human LDL cholesterol and, hence, the progression of atherosclerosis. This observation was confirmed by other researchers, including Tedesco et al. (2000), who demonstrated the beneficial effects of the nonalcoholic wine components, mainly polyphenols, in protecting red blood cells against oxidative stress. Fernandez-Pachon et al. (2004) assessed the antioxidant activity of different wine samples and found it was higher in red wine compared to either white or sherry wines. Auger et al. (2001) showed a phenolic extract from red wine reduced atherosclerosis in hypercholesterolemic Golden Syrian hamsters. One of the major polyphenols found in red wine is resveratrol (3,5,4′-trihydroxystilbene) present as *trans* and *cis* isomers, depending on the type of wine (Scheme W.71). Most studies, however, have focused on the *trans* isomer and its antioxidant and antiproliferative activities *in vitro* (Briviba et al., 2002;

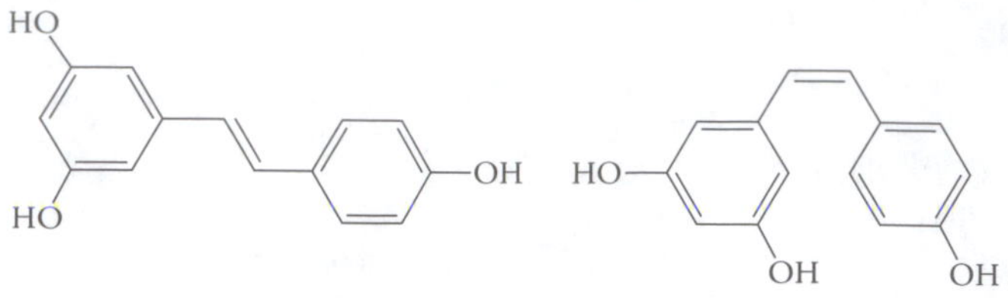

SCHEME W.71 Structure of the *trans-* (a) and *cis-* (b) isomers of resveratrol. (From Kolouchova-Hanzlikova et al., *Food Chem.,* 87:151–158, 2004. With permission.)

Olas and Wachowicz, 2002; Zoberi et al., 2002). Resveratrol also inhibits angiogenesis, the process of new blood-cell growth associated with tumor growth and metastasis (Cao et al., 2002).

Among the proposed mechanisms for the protective action of red wine is its effect on HDL metabolism (Gaziano et al., 1993; Lavy et al., 1994). HDL not only reverses cholesterol transport but also inhibits accumulation of lipid peroxides on LDL (Aviram et al., 1998a). Paraoxonase (PON), an enzyme on HDL particles, is responsible for the antioxidant properties of HDL by inhibiting or preventing oxidation of LDL and HDL. In addition, PON was thought to stimulate cholesterol efflux, the first step in reversing cholesterol transport (Aviram et al., 1998a, b; Mackness et al., 1993). Sarandol et al. (2004) examined the effect of wine consumption on the serum paraoxonase/arylesterase activities of PON, as well as lipoprotein oxidizability in 14 healthy males between the ages of 25 and 38 years. While there was no change in paraoxonase activity, there was a 22 percent decrease in arylesterase activity following wine consumption. However, the ability of red wine to protect lipoproteins from oxidation was clearly evident by the significant (29 percent) decrease in oxidation of apolipoprotein B-containing lipoproteins. Gomez-Cordoves et al. (2001) also showed wine phenolics could decrease melanogenic activity, suggesting their potential as therapeutic agents in the treatment of human melanoma.

References

Auger, C., Caporiccio, B., Landrault, N., Teissedre, P.L., Laurent, C., Cros, G., Besancon, P., and Rouanet, J.-M., Red wine phenolic compounds reduce plasma lipids and apolipoprotein B and prevent early aortic atherosclerosis in hypercholesterolemic Golden Syrian hamsters (*Mesocricetus auratus*), *J. Nutr.,* 132:1207–1213, 2002.

Aviram, M., Billecke, S., Sorenson, R., Bisgaier, C., Newton, R., Rosenblat, M., Erogul, J., Hsu, C., Dunlop, C., and La Du, B., Paraoxonase active site required for the protection against LDL oxidation involves its free sulfhydryl group and is different from that required for its arylesterase/paraoxonase activities: selective action of human paraoxonase allozymes Q and R, *Arterioscler. Thromb. Vasc. Biol.,* 18:1617–1624, 1998a.

Aviram, M., Rosenblat, M., Bisgaier, C.L., Newton, R.S., Primo-Parmo, S.L., and La Du, B.N., Paraoxonase inhibits high density lipoprotein oxidation and preserves its functions. A possible peroxidative role for paraoxonase, *J. Clin. Invest.,* 101:1581–1590, 1998b.

Briviba, K., Pan, L., and Rechkemmer, G., Red wine polyphenols inhibit the growth of colon carcinoma cells and modulate the activation pattern of mitogen activated protein kinases, *J. Nutr.,* 132:2814–2828, 2002.

Cao, Y., Cao, R., and Brakenhielm, E., Antiangiogenic mechanisms of diet-derived polyphenols, *J. Nutr. Biochem.,* 13:380–390, 2002.

Fernandez-Pachon, M.S., Villano, D., Garcia-Parrilla, M.C., and Troncoso, A.M., Antioxidant activity of wines and relation with their polyphenolic composition, *Anal. Chim. Acta,* 513:113–118, 2004.

Frankel, E.N., Kinsella, J.E., German, J.B., Parks, E., and Kinsella, J.E., Inhibition of oxidation of human low density lipoprotein by phenolic substances in red wine, *Lancet,* 341:454–457, 1993.

Gaziano, J.M., Buring, J.E., Breslow, J.L., Goldhaber, S.Z., Rosner, B., VanDenburgh, M., Willett, W., and Hennekens, C.H., Moderate alcohol consumption intake, increased levels of high-density lipoprotein and its subfractions and decreased risk of myocardial infarction, *N. Engl. J. Med.,* 329:1829–1834, 1993.

Gomez-Cordoves, C., Bartolome, B., Vieira, W., and Virador, V.M., Effects of wine phenolics and sorghum tannins on tyrosinase activity and growth of melanoma cells, *J. Agric. Food Chem.*, 49:1620–1624, 2001.

Kolouchova-Hanzlikova, I., Melzoch, K., Filip, V., and Smidrkal, J., Rapid method for resveratrol by HPLC with electrochemical and UV detections in wines, *Food Chem.*, 87:151–158, 2004.

Lavy, A., Fuhrman, N.B., Markel, A., Danker, G., Ben-Amotz, A., Presser, D., and Aviram, M., Effect of dietary supplementation of red or white wine on human blood chemistry, hematology and coagulation: favorable effect of red wine on plasma high-density lipoprotein, *Ann. Nutr. Metab.*, 38:287–294, 1994.

Mackness, M.I., Arrol, S., Abbott, X., and Durrington, P.N., Protection of low-density lipoprotein against oxidative modification by high-density lipoprotein associated paraoxonase, *Atherscler.*, 104:129–135, 1993.

Olas, B. and Wachowicz, B., Resveratrol and vitamin C as antioxidants in blood platelets, *Thromb. Res.*, 106:143–148, 2002.

Sarandol, E., Serdar, Z., Dirican, M., and Safak, O., Effects of red wine consumption on serum paraoxonase/arylesterase activities and lipoprotein oxidizability in healthy-men, *J. Nutr. Biochem.*, 14:507–512, 2003.

Tedesco, I., Russo, M., Russo, P., Iacomino, G., Russo, G.L., Carraturo, A., Faruolo, C., Moio, L., and Palumbo, R., Antioxidant effect of red wine polyphenols on red blood cells, *J. Nutr. Biochem.*, 11:114–119, 2000.

Zoberi, I., Bradbury, C.M., Curry, H.A., Bisht, K.S., Goswami, P.C., Roti, J.L., and Gius, D., Radiosensitizing and antiproliferative effects of resveratrol in two human cervical tumor lines, *Cancer Lett.*, 175:165–173, 2002.

Winter savory   Winter savory (*Satureja montana* L.), an aromatic and medicinal herb used as a folk remedy for many diseases, grows along the Adriatic coast and parts of Croatia. It contains a number of biologically active components including triterpenes, flavonoids, and rosmarinic acid (Escudero et al., 1985; Thomas-Barberan et al., 1987; Reschke, 1983). Madsen et al. (1996) found extracts from a number of plants, including winter savory, were high in antioxidants. The broad-spectrum antimicrobial activity of the essential oil and ethanol extracts from winter savory was demonstrated in several studies, including its ability to control potential pathogenic and spoilage yeasts (Pepeljnak et al., 1999; Ciani et al., 2000).

The value of savory oil was attributed by Lawrence (1979) to its high carvacrol content and fresh, spicy phenolic notes reminiscent of oregano and thyme. Carvacrol was approved as a flavoring agent by the FDA and the Council of Europe at a level of 2 ppm in beverages, 5 ppm in fold, and 25 ppm in candy (De Vincent et al., 2004). These researchers pointed out the need for long-term toxicological studies to establish its safety. Mastelic and Kerkovic

Carvacrol. (From De Vicenzi et al., *Fitoterapia*, 75:801–804, 2004. With permission.)

(2003) found a moderate correlation between the chemical composition of savory oil and its volatile aglycones. The compounds identified were thymol, *p*-cymene-9-ol, geraniol, 1-octen-3-ol, carvacrol, and nerol.

References

Ciani, M., Menghini, L., Mariani, F., Pagiotti, R., Menghini, A., and Fatichenti, F., Antimicrobial properties of essential of *Satureja montana* L. on pathogenic and spoilage yeasts, *Biotechnol. Lett.*, 22:1007–1010, 2000.

De Vincenzi, M., Stammati, A., De Vencenzi, A., and Silano, M., Constituents of aromatic plants carvacol, *Fitoterapia*, 75:801–804, 2004.

Escudero, J., Lopez, J.C., Rabanal, R.M., and Valverde, S., Secondary metabolites from *Satureja* species. New triterpenoid from Satureja-Acionos, *J. Nat. Prod.*, 48:128–132, 1985.

Lawrence, B.M., *Essential Oils*, Allured Publishing, Wheaton, IL, 1979.

Madsen, H.L., Nielsen, B.R., Bertelsen, G., and Skibsted, L.H., Screening of antioxidative activity of spices. A comparison between assays based on ESR spin trapping and electrochemical measurement of oxygen consumption, *Food Chem.*, 57:331–337, 1996.

Mastelic, J. and Jerkovic, I., Gas chromatography-mass spectrometry analysis of free and glycoconjugated aroma compounds of seasonally collected *Satureja montana* L., *Food Chem.*, 80:135–140, 2003.

Pepeljnjak, S., Stanic, G., and Potocki, P., Antimicrobial activity of the ethanol extract of *Satureja montana* sp. montana, *Acta Pharm.*, 49:65–69, 1999.

Reschke, A., Capillary gas chromatographic determination of rosmarinic acid in leafy spices, *Z. Lebensm. Unters Forsch.*, 176:116–119, 1983.

Thomas-Barberan, F.A., Husain, S.Z., and Gil, M.J., The distribution of methylated flavones in the *Lamiaceae*, *Biochem. Sys. Ecol.*, 16:43–46, 1987.

Witch hazel   Witch hazel (*Hamamelis virginiana* L.), a deciduous shrub native to Eastern North America and Canada, has been used in skin-care products and for treating sunburn, irritated skin, and atopic eczema (Korting et al., 1995). One of the main components in the bark extract from witch hazel is hamamelitannin, a compound composed of two gallate moieties and the sugar hamamelose (Hartisch and Kolodzie, 1996). Hamamelitannin was reported to protect cells from ultraviolet B radiation and to scavenge superoxide and hydroxyl radicals

Structure of hamamelitannin (2,5′-di-*O*-galloyl hamamelose). (Adapted from Dauer et al., *Phytochemistry*, 63:199–207, 2003.)

(Masaki et al., 1995a, b). *In vitro* studies by Habtermariam (2002) found hamamelitannin inhibited the activity of the tumor necrosis factor (α-TNF), preventing its cytotoxic induction of endothelial cell death. An important prerequisite of endothelial cell death is DNA fragmentation. Hamamelitannin prevented DNA fragmentation by α-TNF in a concentration-dependent manner, as shown in Figure W.101. However, it had no effect on TNF-induced upregulation of endothelial adhesiveness. In addition to tannins, Dauer et al. (2003) reported that catechin present in the bark of *Hamamelis virginiana* also protected human hepatoma cells (Hep G2) from benz(a)pyrene (BP) and (±)-*anti*-benz(a)pyrene-7,8-dihydrodiol-9,10-epoxide (BPDE)-induced DNA damage by inactivation of the mutagen. These compounds may prevent genetic damage caused by genotoxins present in the diet or environment.

References

Dauer, A., Hensel, A., Lhoste, E., Knasmuller, S., and Mersch-Sundermann, V., Genotoxic and antigenotoxic effects of catechin and tannins from the bark of *Hamamelis virginiana* L. in metabolically competent human hepatoma cells (Hep G2) using single cell electrophoresis, *Phytochemistry,* 63:199–207, 2003.

Habtemariam, S., Hamamelitannin from *Hamamelis virginiana* inhibits the tumor necrosis factor-α-TNF-induced endothelial cell death *in vitro*, *Toxicon.*, 40:83–88, 2002.

Hartisch, C. and Kolodziej, H., Galloylhamameloses and proanthocyanidins from *Hamamelis virginiana,* *Phytochemistry,* 42:191–198, 1996.

Korting, H.C., Schafer-Korting, M., Kloverlorn, W., Kloverlorn, G., Martin, C., and Laux, P., Comparative efficacy of hamamelis distillate and hydrocortisone cream in atopic eczema, *Eur. J. Clin. Pharmacol.*, 48:461–465, 1995.

Masaki, H., Atsumi, T., and Sakurai, H., Protective activity of hamamelitannin on cell damage of murine skin fibroblasts induced by UVB irradiation, *J. Dermatol. Sci.*, 10:25–34, 1995a.

Masaki, H., Atsumi, T., and Sakurai, H., Peroxyl radical scavenging activities in hamamelitannin in chemical and biological systems, *Free Rad. Res.*, 22:419–430, 1995b.

W

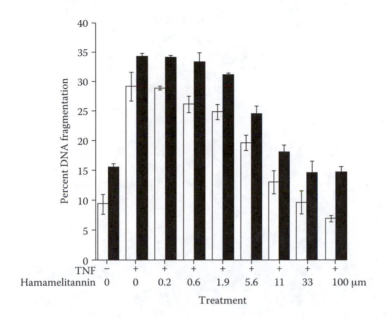

FIGURE W.101 Inhibition of TNF-mediated DNA fragmentation by hamamelitannin. Endothelial cells were treated with TNF and actinomycin D in the presence or absence of hamamelitannin. DNA leakage was assessed to the medium (open bars), and DNA fragmentation is quantified from cell lysates (solid bars). Results are mean values ± SEM from four separate experiments. (From Habtemariam, *Toxicon.*, 40:83–88, 2003. With permission.)

W

Xanthan gum Xanthan, an industrial microbial gum produced by aerobic fermentation of *Xanthomonas campestris,* consists of a β-(164)-D-glucopyranose glucan backbone with side chains composed of (163)-α-linked D-mannopyranose-(261)-β-D-glucuronic acid-(461)-β-D-mannopyranose on alternate residues (Scheme X.72). The rheological properties of xanthan makes it an ideal emulsifier and thickener in foods, as well as in cosmetics and pharmaceuticals (Garcia-Ochoa et al., 2000). As a complex polysaccharide, it would be expected to have a low glycemic index. Sun and Griffiths (2000) reported that immobilization of *Bifidobacteria* on a novel, acid-stable bead made from gellan gum and xanthan gum significantly enhanced their tolerance to high-acid environments compared to the free cells when added to pasteurized yogurt and stored for five weeks at refrigerated temperatures. This technology could be useful for delivering probiotic cultures to the gastrointestinal tract of humans and animals.

Xanthan gum also has drug release-retarding properties, which are enhanced in the presence of galactomannan gums, such as guar gum (Melia, 1991). This property is important, as it permits the delivery of drugs to a particular site, which not only reduces the side effects of the drug but increases its pharmacological response. Sinha et al. (2004) prepared tablets of 50 mg fluoracil compression coated with a mixture of xanthan and guar gums. 5-Fluoracil, an established pyrimidine drug for treating colon cancer, inhibits RNA function and the processing and synthesis of thymidylate. The compressed tablet, coated with a xanthan gum: guar gum combination of 10:20, permitted 5-fluoracil to move down the upper part of the gastrointestinal tract without exposing it to its toxic side effects, releasing it specifically in the colon.

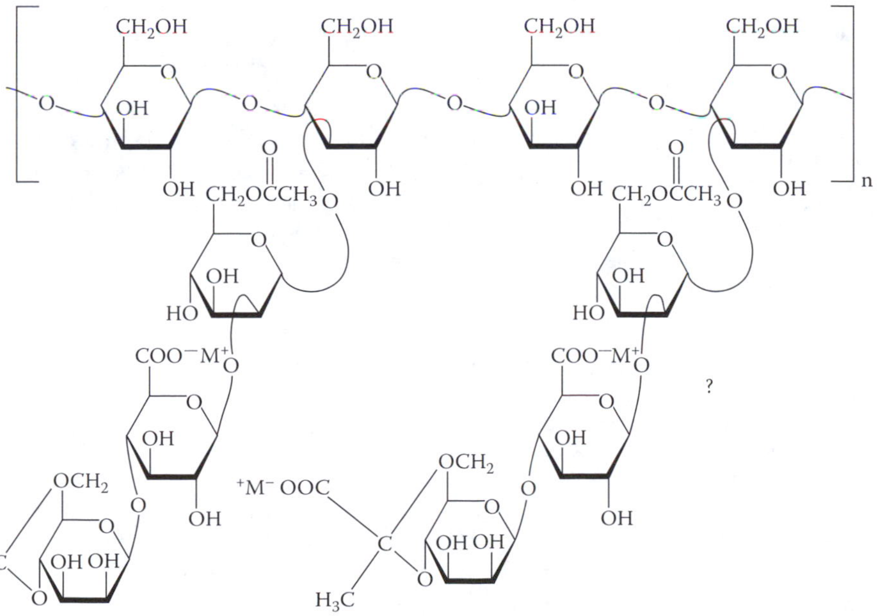

SCHEME X.72 Structure of xanthan gum. (From Garcia-Ochoa et al., *Biotechnol. Adv.,* 18:549–579, 2000. With permission.)

References

Garcia-Ochoa, F., Santos, V.E., Casas, J.A., and Gomez, E., Xanthan gum: production, recovery and properties, *Biotechnol. Adv.,* 18:549–579, 2000.

Melia, C.D., Hydrophilic matrix sustained release systems based on polysaccharide carriers, *Crit. Rev. Ther. Drug Carrier Syst.,* 8:391–421, 1991.

Sinha, V.R., Mittal, B.R., Bhutani, K.K., and Kumria, R., Colonic drug delivery of 5-fluoracil: an *in vitro* evaluation, *Int. J. Pharmacol. Sci.,* 269:101–108, 2004.

Sun, W. and Griffiths, M.W., Survival of bifidobacteria in yogurt and simulated gastric juice following immobilization in gellan-xanthan beads, *Int. J. Food Microbiol.,* 61:17–25, 2000.

Xanthophylls *see* **Carotenoids, Lutein, and Zeaxanthin**   Xanthophylls are oxygenated carotenoids found in plants. One of the richest sources is the marigold flower. Xanthophylls are important nutraceuticals, because they prevent cancer (Chew et al., 1996) and oxidation of cellular lipids (Zhang et al., 1991), as well as age-related macular degeneration (Fullmer and Shao, 2001). The two most important xanthophylls are lutein and zeaxanthin.

References

Chew, P.P., Wong, M.W., and Wong, T.S., Effect of lutein from marigold extract on immunity and growth of mammary tumors in mice, *Anticancer Res.,* 16: 3689–3694, 1996.

Fullmer, L.A. and Shao, A., The role of lutein in eye health and nutrition, *Cereal Chem.,* 46:408–413, 2001.

Zhang, L.X., Cooney, R.V., and Bertram, J.S., Carotenoids enhance gap functional communication and inhibit lipid peroxidation in C3H/10TY/2 cells: relationship to their cancer chemopreventive action, *Carcinogenesis,* 12:2109–2114, 1991.

Xanthorrhizol   Xanthorrhizol, a sesquiterpenoid compound, is one of the major constituents in the rhizome of *Curcuma* species. Hwang and coworkers (2000) found that xanthorrhizol had the highest antibacterial activity against *Streptococcus* species responsible for dental caries.

Structure of xanthorrhizol. (From Choi et al., *Biochem. Biophys. Res. Commun.,* 326:210–217, 2005. With permission.)

Xanthorrhizol has been used as a folk medicine for treating rheumatic and stomach ailments. Lee et al. (2002) showed xanthorrhizol suppressed COX-2 and iNOS activities in mouse-macrophage cells, while Kim et al. (2004) reported it attenuated induction of COX-2 and iNOS genes in cisplatin-induced hepatoxicity in mouse-macrophage cells. Cisplatin, a widely used cancer drug, suffers from serious side effects, such as nephrotoxicity. The prevention of hepatoxicity and nephrotoxicity induced by high doses of cisplatin could be alleviated by combining it with xanthorrhizol. This combination could enhance the safety of cisplatin in cancer therapy. Using an experimental mouse-lung metastasis model, Choi et al. (2004) reported xanthorrhizol exerted its antimatastic properties *in vivo* through the possible expression of COX-2 and the activity of MM-9.

Campos et al. (2000) observed that xanthorrhizol, isolated from the dried roots of *Iostephane heterophylla,* relaxed smooth-muscle cells in the rat aorta previously contracted with high-KCl, $CaCl_2$, or noradrenaline. This was the first report of a vasorelaxant bioactive compound from the Cachani complex of medicinal plants.

References

Campos, M.G., Oropeza, M.V., Villaneuva, T., Aguilar, M.I., Delgado, G., and Ponce, H.A., Xanthorrhizol induces endothelium-independent relaxation of rat thoracic aorta, Life Sci., 67:327–333, 2000.

Choi, M.-A., Kim, S.K., Chung, W.-Y., Hwang, J.-K., and Park, K.-K., Xanthorrhizol, a natural sesquiterpenoid from *Curcuma xanthorrhiza,* has an antimetastatic potential in experimental lung metastasis model, *Biochem. Biophys. Res. Commun.,* 326:210–217, 2004.

Hwang, J.K., Shim, J.S., and Pyun, Y.R., Antibacterial activity of xanthorrhizol from *Curcuma xanthorrhiza* against oral pathogens, *Fitoterapia,* 71:321–323, 2000.

Kim, S.H., Hong, K.O., Hwang, J.K., and Park, K.-K., Xanthorrhizol has a potential to attenuate the high dose of cisplatin-induced nephrotoxicity in mice, *Food Chem. Toxicol.*, 43:117–122, 2005.

Lee, S.K., Hong, C.H., Huh, S.K., Kim, S.S., Oh, O.J., Min, H.Y., Park, K.-K., Chung, W.Y., and Hwang, J.K., Suppressive effect of natural sesquiterpenoids on inducible cyclooxygenase (COX-2) and nitric oxide synthase (iNOS) activity in mouse macrophage cells, *J. Environ. Pathol. Toxicol. Oncol.*, 21:141–148, 2002.

Xestospongin Xestospongins, a group of macrocyclic *bis*-1-oxaquinolizidines isolated from the Australian sponge *Xestospongi* species, are potent blockers of inositol 1,4,5-triphosphate (IP$_3$)-induced Ca^{2+} mobilization in cerebellar and intact cells (Gafni et al., 1997). They proved valuable tools for studying the molecular pharmacology of the myo-inositol 1,4,5-triphosphate receptor in intact-cell preparations. The most potent antagonist of *myo*-inositol IP$_3$ proved to be xestospongin C. The vasodilatory properties of xestospongin were first recognized more than 20 years ago by Nakagawa et al. (1984). Subsequent research has rationalized these properties to xestospongins' IP$_3$ receptor-blocking activity within the vasculature. Xestospongin C was suggested by Dassen et al. (2003) as a possible new therapy for

treating Detrusor overactivity (DO). DO is a condition defined as the presence of involuntary detrusor (the main bladder muscle) contractions leading to urinary incontinence. Dassen et al. (2003) found that the ability of xestospongin C to inhibit IP$_3$ pathway reduced spontaneous detrusor contractions. Kajioka et al. (2005), however, reported there were two mechanisms, an IP$_3$-dependent and an IP$_3$-independent, responsible for the phasic and tonic contractions of the urinary bladder associated with DO.

Wilcox et al. (1998) suggested that the antihypertensive potential should lead to the synthesis and pharmacological assessment of analogs of xestospongins. Rao and coworkers (1998) examined a number of marine biomolecules on rat brain nitric-oxide synthase (NOS) activity. Nitric oxide mediates a variety of physiological functions and is considered a messenger molecule. Xestospongin D proved to be one of only two compounds that significantly inhibited NOS activity, which might explain its toxicity due to impairment in neurotransmission.

References

Dassen, E., van Koeveringe, G., and Kerrebroeck, P., Inhibition of intracellular IP3(inositol-tri-phosphate) pathway blocks oxidative stress induced overactivity but far less effect on the stimulated contractions in detrusor smooth muscle, ICS 2003, conference report, Abstr. 142, 2003.

Gafni, J., Munsch, J.A., Lam, T.H., Catlin, M.C., Costa, L.G., Molinski, T.F., and Pessah, I.N., Xestospongins: potent membrane permeable blockers of the inositol 1,4,5-triphosphate receptor, *Neuron*, 19: 723–733, 1997.

Kajioka, S., Nakayama, S., Asano, H., and Brading, A.F., Involvement of ryanoside receptors in muscarinic receptor-mediated membrane current oscillation in urinary bladder smooth muscle, *Am. J. Physiol.*, 288:C100–C108, 2005.

Nakagawa, Tanaka, N., Endo, M., Tanaka, N., and Gen-Pei, L., Structures of xestospongin A, B, C and D, novel vasodilative compounds from marine sponge, *Tetrahedron Lett.*, 25:3227–3230, 1984.

Rao, J.V., Desaiiah, D., Vig, P.J.S., and Venkateswarlu, Y., Marine biomolecules inhibit brain nitric oxide synthase activity, *Toxicology*, 129:103–112, 1998.

Xestospongin C. (From Wilcox et al., *TiPS*, 19:467–475, 1998. With permission.)

X

Wilcox, R.A., Primrose, W.U., Nahorski, S.R., and Challiss, R.A.J., New developments in the molecular pharmacology of the *myo*-inositol 1,4,5-trisphosphate receptor, *TiPS,* 19:467–475, 1998.

Xylooligosaccharides Xylooligosaccharides, sugar oligomers composed of xylose units, are found naturally in bamboo shoots, fruits, vegetables, milk, and honey. They are utilized in pharmaceuticals, feed formulations, for agricultural purposes, and in foods (Vazquez, 2001). Xylooligosaccharides are extremely stable over a wide pH range (2.5–8.0) compared to the nondigestible fructooligosaccharides.

The primary health properties of xylooligosaccharides are related to their effect on the gastrointestinal flora. Xylooligosaccharides enhance the growth of *Bifidobacterium* spp. in the gastrointestinal tract (Suwa et al., 1999), as well as increases the production of short-chain fatty acids in the rat caecum (Campbell et al., 1997; Imaizumi et al., 1991). As prebiotics, they stimulate *Bifidobacterium* in the gastrointestinal tract, which provides a number of important health benefits.

Ando et al. (2004) published the first report on the effect of bamboo xylooligosaccharides on the viability of leukemia cells. Several hot-compressed, water-fractionated bamboo products were separated, including Fraction A. This fraction, composed of xylose, xylooligosaccharides, and water-soluble lignin, markedly reduced the viability of leukemia-cell lines derived from acute lymphoblastic leukemia (ALL), Jurkat, and MOLT-4. Induction of apoptosis induced by Fraction A on ALL-derived cells was attributed to xylooligosaccharides. However, the cytoxicity of the hot-compressed, water-fractionated bamboo products were less than that observed for other natural products, such as lectins.

References

Ando, H., Ohba, H., Sakaki, T., Takamine, K., Kamino, Y., Moriwaki, S., Bakalova, R., Uemura, Y., and Hatate, Y., Hot-compressed decomposed products from bamboo manifest a selective cytotoxicity against acute lymphoblastic leukemia cells, *Toxicol. in Vitro,* 18:765–771, 2004.

Campbell, J.M., Fahey, G.C., Jr., and Wolf, B.W., Selected indigestible oligosaccharides affect large bowel mass, cecal and fecal short-chain fatty acids, pH and microflora in rats, *J. Nutr.,* 127:130–136, 1997.

Imaizumi, K., Nakatsu, Y., Sato, M., Sedamawati, Y., and Sugano, M., Effects of xylooligosaccharides on blood glucose, serum and liver lipids and cecum short-chain fatty acids in rats, *Agric. Biol. Chem.,* 55:199–205, 1991.

Suwa, Y., Koga, K., Fujikawa, S., Okazaki, M., Irie, T., and Nakada, T., *Bifidobacterium Bifidum* Proliferation, Promoting Composition Containing Xyloliogosaccharide, U.S.A. Patent US5939309, 1999.

Vazquez, M.J., Alonso, J.L., Dominguez, H., and Parajo, J.C., Xylooligosaccharides: manufacture and applications, *Trends Food Sci. Technol.,* 11:387–393, 2001.

X

Y

Yarrow Yarrow (*Achillea millefolium*) is a perennial plant native to Europe and Asia, with a number of species growing in temperate North America (Konemann, 1999). It has been used in folk medicine as an appetizer, wound healer, diuretic, carminative, or menstrual regulator (Botys, 1999). Yarrow contains flavonoids, alkaloids, triterpenes, coumarins, and tannins, as well as sesquiterpene lactones. Tozyo et al. (1994) identified three sequiterpenes in yarrow, achimillic acids A, B, and C, all of which acted as antitumor agents against mouse P-388 leukemia cells *in vivo*. An earlier study by Zitterl-Eglseer et al. (1992) reported the presence of rupicolin and 11, 13-dehydrodeacetyl-matricarin in yarrow, both of which had anti-inflammatory activity.

Candan et al. (2003) evaluated the antioxidant and antimicrobial properties in the essential oil and methanolic extract of *Achillea millefolium* sub. Millefollium (*Asteracea*). Of 36 compounds identified in the essential oil, eucalyptol, camphor, α-terpineol, β-pinene, and borneol accounted for 60.7 percent of the oil. The oil had moderate antimicrobial activity against of number of organisms, including *Staphyllococcus pneumonia*, *Clostridium perfringens*, and *Candida albicans*. The antimicrobial properties were attributed, in part, to the presence of eucalyptol (1,8-cineole), camphor, and borneol (Pattnaik et al., 1997; Tzakou et al., 2001; Tabanca et al., 2001).

Montanari and coworkers (1998) monitored the morphological changes in the germinal epithelium of Swiss mice treated with ethanolic and hydroalcoholic extracts of *A. millefolium* flowers. The antispermatogenic action of *A. millefolium* suggested it might be used as an antifertility agent. Dalsenter et al. (2004) pointed out the need for long-term animal reproductive and toxicological studies and that further studies were needed to determine the real risk to humans.

References

Baytop, T., Ed., *Turkiye de bitkiler le tedavi* (*Treatment with Plants in Turkey*), Istanbul University, Istanbul, Pub. No. 3255:40 1999, p. 176.

Candan, F., Unlu, M., Tepe, B., Daferera, D., Polissou, M., Sokmen, A., and Akpulat, H.A., Antioxidant and antimicrobial activity of the essential oil and methanol extracts of *Achillea millefolium* subsp. millefolium Afan (*Asteracea*), *J. Ethnopharmacol.*, 87:218–220, 2003.

Dalsenter, P.R., Cavalcanti, A.M., Andrade, A.J.M., Araujo, S.L., and Marques, M.C.A., Reproductive evaluation of aqueous crude extract of *Achillea millefolium* L. (*Asteraceae*) in Wistar rats, *Reprod. Toxicol.*, 18:819–823, 2004.

Konermann, *Botanica: The Illustrated A-Z of other 10,000 Garden Plants and How to Cultivate Them*, Gordon Cheers Pub., Hong Kong, 1999, pp. 51–53.

Montanari, T., de Cervalho, J.E., and Dolder, H., Antospermatogenic effect of *Achillea millefolium* in mice, *Contraception*, 58:309–313, 1998.

Pattnaik, S., Subramanyam, V.R., Bapaji, V.R., and Kole, C.R., Antibacterial and antifungal activity of aromatic constituents of essential oils, *Microbios.*, 89:39–46, 1997.

Tabanca, N., Kiriner, N., Demirci, B., Demirci, F., and Baser, K.H.C., Composition and antimicrobial activity of the essential oils of *Micromeria cristata* subsp. phyrgia and the enantiomeric distribution of borneol, *J. Agric. Food Chem.*, 49:4300–4303, 2001.

Tzakou, O., Pitarokili, D., Chinou, I.B., and Harvala, C., Composition and antimicrobial activity of the essential oil of *Salvia ringens*, *Planta Med.*, 67:81–83, 2001.

Tozyo, T., Yoshimura, Y., Sakurai, K., Uchida, N., Nakai, H., and Ishii, H., Novel antitumor sesquiterpenoids in *Achillea millefolium*, *Chem. Pharm. Bull.*, 42:1096–1100, 1994.

Zitterl-Eglseer, K., Jurenitsch, J., Korhammer, S., Haslinger, E., Sosa, S., Della Loggia, R., Kubelka, W., and Franz, C., Sesquiterpene lactones of *Achillea setacea* with antiphlogistic activity, *Planta Med.*, 57:444–446, 1991.

Yellow mustard (*Sinapis alba*) "White" or "yellow" mustard is grown extensively in western Canada for use as a condiment (Cui and Eskin, 1998). Of the two principal species grown, oriental and yellow mustard, yellow mustard contains less oil but is much richer in mucilage. A detailed examination of yellow-mustard gum identified a unique water-soluble 1,4 linked β-glucose with ethyl and propyl groups randomly distributed at the C2, 3, and 6 positions (Cui et al., 1993). Yellow-mustard gum is the only natural gum that resembles xanthan gum by exhibiting shear, thinning behavior at low concentrations, forming weak-gel structures and interacting synergistically with galactommans (Cui et al., 2005).

Since yellow-mustard gum is a dietary fiber, it would be expected to regularize colonic function, normalize serum lipids, and attenuate postprandial glucose response and possibly suppress appetite. Begin et al. (1988) showed yellow-mustard gum, guar gum, oat β-glucan, and carboxymethylcellulose all significantly decreased postprandial insulin levels by slowing glucose absorption. In addition, yellow-mustard gum decreased insulemia by delaying gastric emptying. Incorporating yellow-mustard fiber into white bread at levels not affecting palatability showed a modest by significant reduction in the glycemic index on the bread in normal and diabetic volunteers (Jenkins et al., 1987).

The anticancer potential of yellow mustard was recently demonstrated by Eskin and Bird (unpublished data) in male Sprague–Dawley rats injected with the specific colon carcinogen, azoxymethane (AOM). Animals were maintained on a diet with or without 5 percent yellow-mustard gum over a six-week period. A significant ($p < 0.05$) decrease in the number of advanced aberrant crypt foci (ACF > 7 crypts) was observed in the yellow-mustard-fed rats, which accounted for a reduction of more than 90 percent. Further work is under way to explore the anticancer properties of yellow-mustard gum.

References

Begin, F., Vachon, C., Jones, J., Wood, P.J., and Savoie, L., Effect of dietary fibers on glycemia and insulinemia and on gastrointestinal function in rats, *Can. J. Physiol. Pharmacol.*, 67:1265–1271, 1988.

Cui, W. and Eskin, N.A.M., Processing and properties of mustard products and components, in *Functional Foods: Biochemical & Processing Aspects*, Technomic Pub. Co. Inc., 1998, chap. 7.

Cui, W., Eskin, N.A.M., and Biliaderis, C.G., NMR characterization of a 1,4-linked b-D-glucan having ether groups from yellow mustard (*Sinapis alba* L.) mucilage, *Carbohydr. Polym.*, 27:117–122, 1993.

Cui, S.W., Ikeda, S., and Eskin, N.A.M., Seed polysaccharide gums, in *Food Carbohydrates*, Biliaderis, C.G. and Izydorczyk, M., Eds., CRC Press, Boca Raton, Florida, 2005.

Jenkins, A.L., Jenkins, D.J.A., Ferrari, F., Collier, G., Rao, A.V., Samuels, S., Jones, J.D., Wong, G.S., and Josse, R.G., Effect of mustard seed fiber on carbohydrate tolerance, *J. Clin. Nutr. Gastroenterol.*, 2:81–86, 1987.

Yucca *Yucca* species (*Agavaceae*) are found growing in arid areas. Of these, *Yucca periculosa*, F. Baker, known as palmitos or izote, is a tree found in semiarid regions of Mexico. Torres and coworkers (2003) isolated stilbenes from the bark of *Yucca periculosa*, such as in the Tehuacan-Cuicatlan Valley, with only a few being of medicinal interest. Of the various *Yucca* species, *Y. schidigera* had the highest saponin content (Oleszek et al., 2001a), with its condensed juice widely used as food, cosmetic, and pharmaceutical additives (Cheeke, 1998). *Y. schidigera*, a folk medicine by American Indians and early settlers, has GRAS (generally regarded as safe) status by the FDA for human use. A number of phenolic compounds have been identified in the methanolic extract from the bark of *Y. schidigera*, including yuccaol A-C, a C15 unit derived from a flavonoid skeleton and a stilbenic portion, closely related to resveratrol (Scheme Y.73) (Oleszek et al., 2001b).

Tsai et al. (1999) showed resveratrol strongly inhibited the production of nitric oxide (NO) in activated macrophages, as well as downregulated the cytosolic inducible isoform of nitric-oxide synthase (iNOS), a key mediator in inflammatory processes. Subsequent research by Olas and coworkers (2002) reported yuccaol A-C exhibited antiplatelet activity. Recent research by Marzocco et al. (2004) showed yuccaol C inhibited iNOS protein

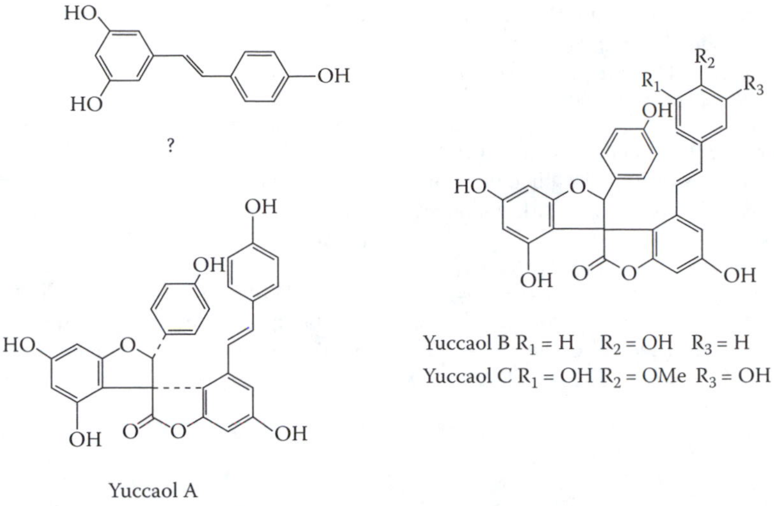

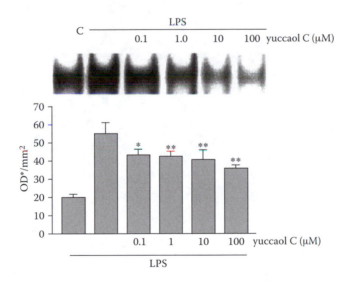

SCHEME Y.73 Chemical structures of *Yucca schidigera*-derived yucaol A–C and resveratrol. (From Marzocco et al., *Life Sci.*, 75:1491–1501, 2004. With permission.)

FIGURE Y.102 Effect of yuccaol C (0.1–100 mM) on NF-κB activation in LPS-stimulated J774.A1 macrophages. Values, mean ± S.E.M. are expressed as optical density/mm² of at least three independent experiments with three replicates each. Comparisons were performed using one-way ANOVA test. $^*p < 0.05$ and $^{**}p < 0.01$. (From Marzocco et al., *Life Sci.*, 75:1491–1501, 2004. With permission.)

expression, preventing activation of NF-κB (Figure Y.102). Induction of specific NF-κB binding activity by LPS was significantly reduced by yuccaol C (0.1 – 100 mM) added to cells 1 h prior to LPS challenge. Yuccaol A had no effect on NF-κB expression. The ability of yuccaol to prevent NF-κB activation sug-

gests that, together with resveratrol, it could be used to control the inflammatory process.

References

Cheeke, P.P., Saponins: surprising benefits of desert plants. The Linus Pauling Institute Newsletter, Oregon State University, Corvallis, Oregon, 1998, pp. 4–5.

Marzocco, S., Piacente, S., Pizza, C., Oleszek, W., Stochmal, A., Pinto, A., Sorrentino, R., and Autore, G., Inhibition of inducible nitric oxide synthase expression by yuccaol C from *Yucca Schidigera* roezl, *Life Sci.,* 75: 1491–1501, 2004.

Olas, B., Wachowicz, B., Stochmal, A, and Oleszek, W., Anti-platelet effects of different phenolic compounds from *Yucca schidigera* Roezl bark, *Platelets,* 13:167–173, 2002.

Oleszek, W., Sitek, M., Stochmal, A., Piacente, S., Pizza, C., and Cheeke, P., Steroidal saponins of *Yucca Schidigera* Roezl, *J. Agric. Food Chem.,* 49:4392–4397, 2001a.

Oleszek, W., Sitek, M., Stochmal, A., Piacente, S., Pizza, C., and Cheeke, P., Resveratrol and other phenolics from the bark of *Yucca schidigera* Roezl, *J. Agric. Food Chem.,* 49:747–752, 2001b.

Torres, P., Avila, J.G., de Vivar, A.R., Garcia, A.M., Marin, J.C., Aranda, E., and Cespedes, C.L., Antioxidant and insect growth regulatory activities of stilbenes and extracts from *Yucca periculosa*, *Phytochemistry,* 64:463–473, 2003.

Tsai, S.H., Lin-Shiau, S.Y., and Lin, J.K., Suppression of nitric oxide synthase and the down regulation of the activation of NFκB in macrophages by resveratrol, *Br. J. Pharmacol.,* 126:673–680, 1999.

Y

Z

Zeaxanthin Zeaxanthin, a hydroxylated carotenoid, is an important plant food xanthophyll. Together with lutein, they are found in the macula pigment of the central retina of the eye responsible for the yellow coloration (Snodderly et al., 1986). Since the source of the macular pigment is solely dietary-based, studies have examined the possible relationship between the pigment and dietary intake. The majority of dietary zeaxanthin and lutein (78 percent) are obtained from such vegetables as spinach and orange pepper, although they are also found in egg yolk (Summerburg et al., 1998; USDA, 1998). The importance of the macula pigment is its protection against age-related maculopathy, one of the major causes of blindness in Western countries (Klaver et al., 1998). Modified diets that are supplemented with zeaxanthin and lutein were shown to augment or enhance the macular pigment optical density (Hammond et al., 1997; Johnson et al., 2000). Both zeaxanthin and lutein are strong antioxidants, as age-related maculopathy is due to a combination of cumulative blue-light damage or oxidative stress (Beatty et al., 2000). Thus, oxidative stress appears to play a role in such neurodegenerative diseases as age-related macular degeneration (ARMD), the primary cause of blindness in seniors in developed countries (Leibowitz et al., 1980; Klein et al., 1992).

Wrona and coworkers (2004) examined the ability of zeaxanthin to protect the outer layer of the retina containing photoreceptor outer segments and retinal pigment epithelium (RPE), possible targets of oxidative damage. Using ARPE 19 cells from the globes of a 19-year-old male donor, they showed that zeaxanthin, in the presence of ascorbic acid and α-tocopherol, significantly enhanced resistance to photo-induced oxidative stress. Compared to cells without added antioxidants, these cells had enhanced cell viability and accumulated fewer lipid hydroperoxides. A synergism was evident between zeaxanthin and vitamin E or C, which could play a role in protecting the cell membranes from oxidative damage. The reduction in the decay of zeaxanthin in the presence of either vitamin C or E, following photo-sensitized oxidation of ARPE-19 cells, pointed to their protective effects. The synergism between these antioxidants was responsible for preventing the depletion of zeaxanthin by free-radical degradation and repair of the semioxidized zeaxanthin molecules. Chen et al. (2005) recently reported the successful use of high-speed, counter-current chromatography for isolating and purifying zeaxanthin from the microalga *Microcystis aeruginosa*. For a further review of the relationship between serum and dietary levels of zeaxanthin, lutein, and macular pigment optical density, the article by Beatty et al. (2004) is recommended.

Zeaxanthin. (From Chen et al., *J. Chromatogr. A*, 1064:183–186, 2005. With permission.)

References

Beatty, S., Koh, H., Phil, M., Henson, D., and Boulton, M., The role of oxidative stress in the pathogenesis of age-related macular degeneration, *Surv. Ophthalmol.*, 45:115–134, 2000.

Beatty, S., Nolan, J., Kavanagh, H., and O'Donovan, O., Macular pigment optical density and its relationship with serum and dietary levels of lutein and zeaxanthin, *Arch. Biochem. Biophys.*, 430:70–76, 2004.

Chen, F., Li, H.-B., Wong, R. N.-K., Ji, B., and Jiang, Y., Isolation and purification of the bioactive carotenoid zeaxanthin from the microalga *Microcystis aeruginosa* by high-speed counter-current chromatography, *J. Chromatogr. A*, 1064:183–186, 2005.

Hammond, B.R., Jr., Johnson, E.J., Russell, R.M., Krinsky, N.I., Yeurn, K.J., Edwards, R.B., and Snodderly, D.M., Dietary modification of human macular pigment density, *Invest. Ophthalmol. Vis. Sci.*, 38: 1795–1801, 1997.

Johnson, E.J., Hammond, B.R., Jr., Yeurn, K.J., Quin, J., Wang, X.D., Castaneda, C., Snodderly, D.M., and Russel, R.M., Relation among serum and tissue concentrations of lutein and zeaxanthin and macular pigment density, *Am. J. Clin. Nutr.*, 71:1555–1562, 2000.

Klaver, C.C.W., Wolfs, R.C.W., Vingerling, J.R., Hofman, A., and de Jong, P.T.V.M., Age-specific prevalence and causes of blindness and visual impairment in an older population: The Rotterdam Study, *Arch. Ophthalmol.*, 116:653–658, 1998.

Klein, R., Klein, B.E.K., and Linton, K.L.P., Prevalence of age-related maculopathy: the Beaver Dam Eye Study, *Ophthalmol.*, 99:933–943, 1992.

Leibowitz, H.M., Kreuger, D.E., and Maunder, L.R., Framingham Eye Study Monograph. VI. Macular degeneration, *Surv. Ophthalmol.*, 24:428–457, 1980.

Snodderly, D.M., Auran, J.D., and Delori, F.C., The macular pigment. II. Spatial distribution in primate retinas, *Invest. Ophthalmol. Vis. Sci.*, 25:674–685, 1984.

Sommerburg, O., Keunen, J.E., Bird, A.C., and van Kujik, F.J., Fruits and vegetables that are sources of lutein and zeaxanthin; the macular pigment in human eye, *Br. J. Ophthalmol.*, 82:907–910, 1998.

USDA Agriculture Research Service, Nutrient Data Laboratory Home Page, http://www.nal.usda.gov/fnic/foodcomp, 1998.

Wrona, M., Rozanowski, M., and Jarna, T., Zeaxanthin in combination with ascorbic acid and a-tocopherol protects ARPE-19 cells against photosensitized peroxidation of lipids, *Free Rad. Biol. Med.*, 36:1094–1101, 2004.

Zerumbone   Zerumbone is a sesquiterpene obtained from a Southeast Asian edible ginger plant, *Zingiber zerumbet* Smith. The rhizomes of this plant were used for antiinflammation (Farnsworth and Bunyapraphatasara, 1992) while the young shoots and inflorescence were used in condiments (Jacquat and Bertossa, 1990). Murakami et al. (1999) first reported that the rhizomes of *Zingiber zerumbet* suppressed the tumor promoter 12-*O*-tetradecanoylphorbol-13-acetate (TPA)-induced Epstein–Barr virus activation in Raji cells. Further work by Murakami et al. (2002) showed that zerumbone suppressed carcinogenesis in a number of different models, including TPA-induced superoxide anion generation from both NADPH oxidase in dimethylsulfoxide-differentiated HL-60

Zerumbone. (From Tanaka et al., *Life Sci.*, 69:1935–1945, 2001. With permission.)

human acute promyelocytic leukemia cells and xanthine oxidase in AS52 Chinese hamster ovary cells. Zerumbone also induced apoptosis in human colonic adenocarcinoma cell lines. A structural analog of zerumbone, α-humulene, which lacked the αβ-unsaturated carbonyl group in zerumbone, points to the importance of this group in the anti-inflammatory and chemopreventive properties of this nutraceutical.

Tanaka et al. (2001) showed dietary zerumbone reduced the development of colon cancer in male F344 rats injected with azoxymethane (AOM). Their results in Table Z.64 show a significant reduction in aberrant crypt foci (ACF) when fed 0.05 percent zerumbone. Of particular importance is the significant reduction in the number of large ACF from 11.1 in the control group to 2.3 and 0.7 in animals fed 0.01 and 0.05 percent zerumbone. Thus, zerumbone appeared to have strong chemopreventive properties,

TABLE Z.64

Incidence of Aberrant Crypt Foci (ACF) in Rats Treated with AOM and/or Zerumbone

Group no.	Treatment		Total no. of ACF/Colon	No. of Aberrant Crypts/Focus	No. of Large ACF (More than 4 Crypts/Focus)
	AOM	Zerumbone in diet (w/w)			
1	+	—	84 ± 13[a]	2.0 ± 0.2	11.1 ± 2.6
2	+	0.01%	72 ± 17	1.6 ± 0.2[b]	2.3 ± 1.4[c]
3	+	0.05%	45 ± 18[c]	1.5 ± 0.1	0.7 ± 0.5[c]

Note: Analysis of ACF was done in 8 rats each of groups 1–3 and 4 rats each of groups 4 and 5. There were no ACF in rats of groups 4 and 5.

[a] Mean ± SD.

[b,c] Significantly different vs. group 1 ([b]$p < 0.05$, and [c]$p < 0.001$).

Source: Tanaka et al., *Life Sci.,* 69:1935–1945, 2001. With permission.

resulting from the suppression of COX-2 expression and proliferation of colonic mucosa and induction of phase II detoxification enzymes.

Further work by Nakamura et al. (2004) on the potential of zerumbone as a promising chemopreventive agent against colon and skin cancer confirmed its ability to reduce oxidative stress by inducing endogenous antioxidants, such as phase II enzymes.

References

Farnsworth, N.R. and Bunyapraphatasara, N., *Thai Medicinal Plants*, Prachachon, Bangkok, Thailand, 1992.

Jacquat, C. and Bertossa, C., *Plants from the Markets of Thailand*, Dung Kamol, Bangkok, Thailand, 1990.

Murakami, A., Takahashi, M., Jiwajinda, S., Koshimizu, K., and Ohigashi, H., Identification of zerumbone in *Zingiber zerumbet* as a potent inhibitor of 12-*O*-tetradecanoylphorbol-13-acetate-induced Epstein–Barr virus activation, *Biosci. Biotechnol. Biochem.,* 63:1811–1812, 1999.

Murakami, A., Takahashi, D., Kinoshita, T., Koshimizu, K., Kim, H.W., Yoshihiro, A., Nakamura, Y., Jiwajinda, S., Terao, J., and Ohigashi, H., Zerumbone, a Southeast Asian sesquiterpene, markedly suppresses free radical generation, proinflammatory protein production, and cancer cell proliferation accompanied by apoptosis: the αβ-unsaturated carbonyl group is a prerequisite, *Carcinogenesis,* 23: 795–802, 2002.

Nakamura, Y., Yoshida, C., Murakami, A., Ohigashi, H., Osawa, T., and Uchida, K., Zerumbone, a tropical ginger sesquiterpene, activates phase II drug metabolizing enzymes, *FEBS Lett.,* 572:245–250, 2004.

Tanaka, T., Shimizu, M., Kohno, H., Yoshitani, S., Tsukio, Y., Murakami, A., Safitri, R., Takahashi, D., Yamamoto, K., Koshimizu, K., Ohigashi, H., and Mori, H., Chemoprevention of azoxymethane-induced rat aberrant crypt foci by dietary zerumbone isolated from *Zingiber zerumbet*, *Life Sci.,* 69:1935–1945, 2001.

Zingiber officinale *see* **Ginger**

Zucchini see Bryonolic acid

Z